535965

HSHS

AF441824

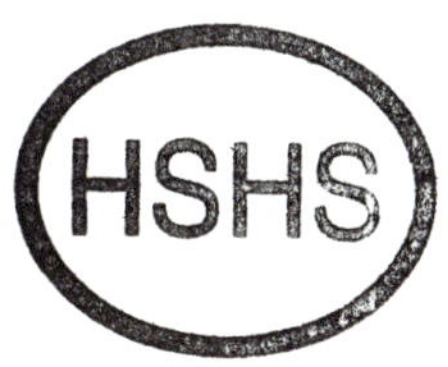

Homerton Health Library, Peterborough
Education Centre, PDH
Thorpe Road, Peterborough PE3 6DA
Telephone: 01733 874766

Dermatology Therapy
A–Z Essentials

Springer

*Berlin
Heidelberg
New York
Hong Kong
London
Milan
Paris
Tokyo*

Norman Levine · Carol C. Levine

Dermatology Therapy

A–Z Essentials

FOR
REFERENCE ONLY

With 96 Figures and 87 Tables

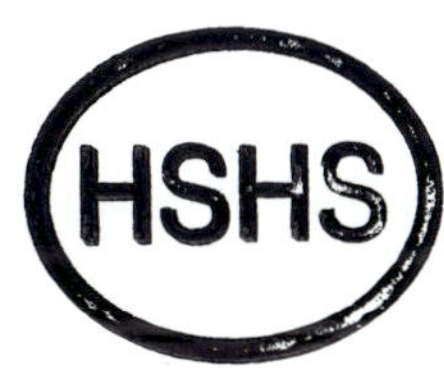

Homerton Health Library, Peterborough
Education Centre, PDH
Thorpe Road, Peterborough PE3 6DA
Telephone: 01733 874766

Acc.	535965	Site	HD
Date	17/9/04	Loc.	Reference
Order	2/6651	Cat.	Reference only Ref.
Inv.	57903	Shelf mark	WR 13
Price	£69-00		Lev
	/55-70		

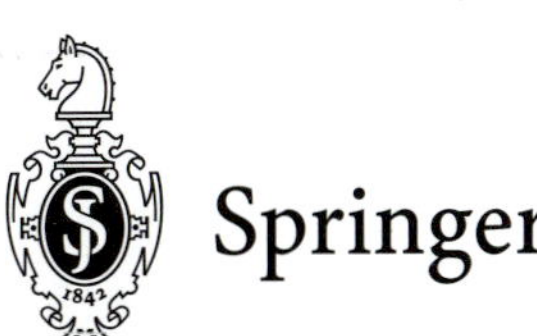

Springer

Prof. Dr. N. Levine
University of Arizona
Section of Dermatology
P.O. Box 5038
Tucson AZ, 85724
USA

C. C. Levine
University of Phoenix
5099 East Grant Road
85712 Tucson AZ
USA

ISBN   3-540-00864-0   Springer-Verlag Berlin Heidelberg New York

Library of Congress Cataloging-in-Publication Data

Dermatology therapy : a-z essentials / Norman Levine & Carol C. Levine.
p.cm.
Includes bibliographical references.
ISBN 3-540-00864-0 (alk. paper)
1. Dermatopharmacology. 2. Skin--Diseases--Chemotherapy. I. Levine, Norman, 1945 Mar. 18- II Levine, Carol C.

RL801.D475 2003-08-29 615'.778--dc22

2003059065

This work is subject to copyright. All rights are reserved, whether the whole or part of the material is concerned, specifically the rights of translation, reprinting, reuse of illustrations, recitation, broadcasting, reproduction on microfilms or in other ways, and storage in data banks. Duplication of this publication or parts thereof is only permitted under the provisions of the German Copyright Law of September 9, 1965, in its current version, and permission for use must always be obtained from Springer-Verlag. Violations are liable for prosecution under the German Copyright Law.

Springer-Verlag Berlin Heidelberg New York

springeronline.com

© Springer-Verlag Berlin Heidelberg 2004
Printed in Germany

The use of registered names, trademarks, etc. in this publication does not imply, even in the absence of a specific statement, that such names are exempt from the relevant protective laws and regulations and therefore free for general use.

Product liability: The publishers cannot guarantee the accuracy of any information about the application of operative techniques and medications contained in this book. In every individual case the user must check such information by consulting the relevant literature.

Production Editor and Typesetting: Frank Krabbes, Heidelberg
Cover design: design & production, Heidelberg
Gedruckt auf säurefreiem Papier   SPIN: 10886806   14/3109 - 5 4 3 2 1 0

Foreword

The concept of a therapeutic dictionary is somewhat novel for a dermatology text. In the past, a limited number of books defined the myriad terms used in dermatology, but they did not provide detail about each entity. Of course, there are many excellent volumes which discuss all aspects of given diseases, but in a format which might be daunting for a hurried practitioner. This book provides a concise view of more than 800 diseases; in just a few moments, one can understand the basics of these conditions and begin therapy.

This text stresses therapeutics when treatments are indicated and helpful. To this end, more than 80 drugs in common use in dermatology are presented in significant detail, in outline form, to provide a quick and handy reference. A table accompanies each of these agents, with detailed information about dosages. Side effects, precautions, contraindications, and drug interactions are also discussed. Many other drugs occasionally used in treating certain dermatologic conditions are noted in the discussion of the specific disease. Numerous therapies described in the literature are included. When there is a clear treatment of choice, it has been denoted by means of a blue asterisk. We have chosen not to list modalities of treatment that remain on lists of therapeutic options in spite of little or no evidence of beneficial effects.

Although thousands of sources were tapped for important data, only one or two references are cited at the end of each entry. These articles are primarily reviews of the diseases for those who wish to read a more detailed discussion. The Internet, an almost unlimited factual source on medical issues, has been utilized to ensure that all of the information given there is current.

No modern dermatologic text is complete without color images. We have chosen approximately 90 photographs that illustrate either dramatic examples of common conditions or diagnostic features of less common skin problems.

Finally, the many generic medication are listed along with common trade names in tabular form for ease of reference at the end of the book.

We are hopeful that the body of material presented here will be a tool that assists practitioners in providing the most complete and up-to-date care for patients with skin disease.

NORMAN LEVINE, MD
CAROL C. LEVINE

Tucson, Arizona

A

Abrikossof's tumor

▸ Granular cell tumor

Abscess

Definition
Accumulation of pus in tissue, usually caused by a bacterial infection

▸ Furuncle

References
Lowy, FD (1998) Staphylococcus aureus infections. New England Journal of Medicine 339:520–532

Academy rash

▸ Erythema infectiosum

Acanthamebiasis

Synonym(s)
None

Definition
Cutaneous and/or systemic infection caused by one of several species of acanthamoeba

Pathogenesis
Opportunistic infection, most often in an immunocompromised host, particularly with HIV disease

Clinical manifestation
Multiple pustules; infiltrated papules and plaques; subcutaneous nodules; non-healing cutaneous ulcers; distribution mainly on the extremities

Differential diagnosis
Furunculosis; disseminated varicella/zoster infection; deep fungal infection; bacillary angiomatosis; myctobacterial infection; pyoderma gangrenosum

Therapy
Multidrug regimen for systemic disease: pentamidine; flucytosine; fluconazole; sulfadiazine

References
Murakawa GJ, McCalmont T, Altman J, Telang GH, Hoffman MD, Kantor GR, Berger TG (1995) Disseminated acanthamebiasis in patients with AIDS. A report of five cases and a review of the literature. Archives of Dermatology 131(11):1291–1296

Acanthoma fissuratum

Synonym(s)
Granuloma fissuratum; spectacle frame granuloma; acanthoma fissuratum cutis

Definition
Keratotic papule or nodule which develops at the site of chronic irritation, such as under eye glasses or in the oral cavity

Pathogenesis
Chronic contact irritation; includes other factors such as local anatomic changes, seborrheic dermatitis, and hyperhidrosis

Clinical manifestation
Oral cavity: solitary smooth-surfaced papule at the juncture of the lip and gum
Face or post-auricular fold: pink papule with a longitudinal central fissure

Differential diagnosis
Oral cavity: squamous cell carcinoma.
Skin: basal cell carcinoma; foreign body granuloma; chondrodermatitis nodularis helicis

Therapy
Removal of stimulus by changing eye glasses, dentures, etc.; surgical excision in recalcitrant cases

References
Frey T, Bartak P (1992) Acanthoma supratrochantericum. Cutis 49(6):412–416

Acanthoma fissuratum cutis

▶ Acanthoma fissuratum

Acanthome à cellules claires

▶ Clear cell acanthoma

Acanthosis nigricans

Synonym(s)
None

Definition
Hyperpigmented, velvety thickening of the skin; most commonly on the neck, in the axillae, and in the groin

Pathogenesis
Caused by factors that stimulate epidermal keratinocyte and dermal fibroblast proliferation, such as insulin or an insulin-like growth factor

Clinical manifestation
Symmetrical, hyperpigmented, velvety plaques, which most commonly appear in the intertriginous areas; skin tags in the vicinity of the plaques

Differential diagnosis
Becker nevus; confluent and reticulated papillomatosis of Gougerot and Carteaud; Dowling-Degos disease; seborrheic keratosis; ichthyosis hystrix; linear epidermal nevus; parapsoriasis en plaque; pemphigus vegetans; hemochromatosis; Addison's disease; pellagra

Therapy
Correction of underlying disease process; weight reduction in obese patients; tretinoin 0.025% cream; adapalene 0.1% gel; calcipotriene; dietary fish oils; dermabrasion

References
Hud JA Jr, Cohen JB, Wagner JM, Cruz PD Jr (1992) Prevalence and significance of acanthosis nigricans in an adult obese population. Arch Dermatol 128: 941–944

Accessory nipples

▶ Supernumerary nipple

Accessory tragus

Synonym(s)
Supernumerary ear; supernumerary auricle; accessory external ear; rudimentary auricle; accessory auricle; auricular appendage; cervical auricle; preauricular appendage; cutaneous cervical tag; preauricular appendage; wattle

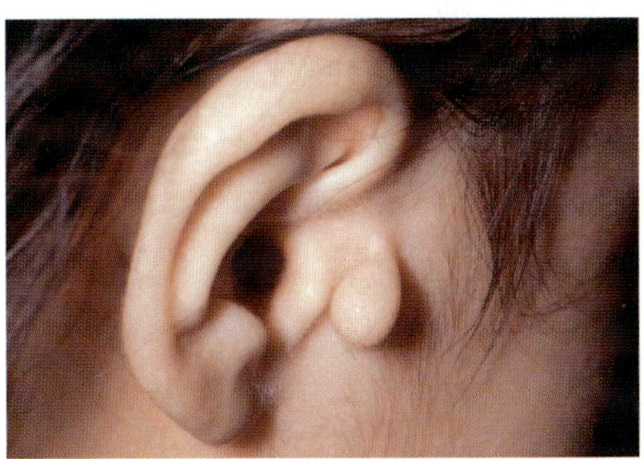

Accessory tragus. Solitary preauricular flesh-colored papule

Definition
Congenital anomaly of branchial arch development, producing a preauricular papule

Pathogenesis
Abnormal development of portions of one of the branchial arches

Clinical manifestation
Asymptomatic, solitary, flesh-colored papule, usually in the preauricular area; vellus hairs arise from the papule

Differential diagnosis
Preauricular cyst or sinus; thyroglossal duct cyst; branchial cyst or sinus; bronchogenic cyst; acrochordon; melanocytic nevus; epidermoid cyst; neurofibroma

Therapy
Surgical excision

References
Jansen T; Romiti R; Altmeyer P (2000) Accessory tragus: report of two cases and review of the literature. Pediatric Dermatology 17:391–394

Accutane

▶ Isotretinoin

Acetowhite test

Synonym(s)
None

Definition
Application of 3% acetic acid to lesions suspicious for human papillomavirus infection; positive test indicated by lesion turning white

References
Kitchener HC, Symonds P (1999) Detection of cervical intraepithelial neoplasia in developing countries. Lancet 353:869–873

Achromic nevus

▶ Nevus depigmentosus

Acinetobacter infection

Synonym(s)
None

Definition
Infection caused by Acinetobacter, a gram negative organism

Pathogenesis
Opportunistic infection from an organism which is often a part of the normal flora in the axilla and groin; increased sweating resulting in higher carriage levels; skin involvement usually colonization rather than infection

Clinical manifestation
No physical findings in colonized patients; skin pustules, cellulitis with clinical infection

Differential diagnosis
Other gram negative infections; ecthyma; staphyloccal cellulitis

Therapy
No therapy for colonization; treatment of active infection dependent on sensitivities of the organism in the individual patient

References
Cunha BA, Klein NC (1995) Pseudoinfections: a review. Infectious Disease Clinical Practice 4:95–103

Acitretin

Trade name(s)
Soriatane

Generic available
No

Drug class
Retinoid

Mechanism of action
Induction of cellular differentiation; anti-inflammatory; anti-proliferative

Dosage form
10 mg, 25 mg capsule

Dermatologic indications and dosage
See table

Common side effects
Cutaneous: cheilitis, sticky skin, alopecia, dry skin, pruritus, paronychia, desquamation of hands and feet
Laboratory: hyperlipidemia
Musculoskeletal: myalgias; arthralgias
Ocular: dry eyes

Serious side effects
Gastrointestinal: pancreatitis, hepatotoxicity
Miscellaneous: major birth defects
Musculoskeletal: spinal hyperostosis
Neurologic: pseudotumor cerebri

Drug interactions
Norethindrone; methotrexate

Other interactions
Alcohol

Contraindications/precautions
Hypersensitivity to drug class or component; pregnancy; renal or hepatic dysfunction; children may be more sensitive to the drug's effect on bones, which may prevent normal bone growth during puberty

References
Katz HI, Waalen J, Leach EE (1999) Acitretin in psoriasis: an overview of adverse effects. Journal of the American Academy of Dermatology 41(3 Pt 2):S7–S12

Ackerman tumor

▶ Verrucous carcinoma

Ackerman's tumor

▶ Verrucous carcinoma

Acitretin. Dermatologic indications and dosage

Disease	Adult dosage	Child dosage
Balanitis xerotica obliterans	25–50 mg PO daily as a single dose; after four weeks, 25–75 mg PO daily	10–25 mg PO daily
Berardinelli-Seip syndrome	75 mg PO daily	10–25 mg PO daily
Darier disease	25–50 mg PO daily as a single dose; after four weeks, 25–75 mg PO daily	10–25 mg PO daily
Epidermolytic hyperkeratosis	0.5–1 mg per kg PO daily indefinitely	0.5 mg per kg PO daily indefinitely
Erythrokeratodermia variabilis	25–50 mg PO daily indefinitely	10–25 mg PO daily
Graft-versus-host disease	1 mg per kg PO daily	10–25 mg PO daily
Hairy tongue	25–50 mg daily for up to 5 months	10–25 mg PO daily
Harlequin ichthyosis	1 mg per kg PO daily	1 mg per kg PO daily indefinitely
Hidradenitis suppurativa	1 mg per kg PO daily for 4–8 months	10–25 mg PO daily
Hyperkeratosis lenticularis perstans	25–50 mg PO daily indefinitely	10–25 mg PO daily
Kyrle's disease	1 mg per kg PO daily for 4–8 months	10–25 mg PO daily
Lamellar ichthyosis	1 mg per kg PO daily	10–25 mg PO daily
Lichen planus	25–50 mg PO daily as a single dose; after four weeks, 25–75 mg PO daily	10–25 mg PO daily
Lichen sclerosus	25–50 mg PO daily as a single dose; after four weeks, 25–75 mg PO daily	10–25 mg PO daily
Lipoid proteinosis	25–50 mg daily for up to 5 months	10–25 mg PO daily
Lupus erythematosus	25–50 mg PO daily as a single dose; after four weeks, 25–75 mg PO daily	10–25 mg PO daily
Mal de Meleda	25–50 mg PO daily as a single dose; after four weeks, 25–75 mg PO daily	10–25 mg PO daily
Nevus verrucosus	25–50 mg daily for up to 5 months	10–25 mg PO daily
Olmsted syndrome	1 mg per kg PO daily	10–25 mg PO daily
Pachonychia congenita	25–50 mg PO daily as a single dose; after four weeks, 25–75 mg PO daily	10–25 mg PO daily
Palmoplantar keratoderma	25–50 mg PO daily as a single dose; after four weeks, 25–75 mg PO daily	10–25 mg PO daily
Papillon-Lefévre syndrome	25–50 mg PO daily as a single dose; after four weeks, 25–75 mg PO daily	10–25 mg PO daily
Papular mucinosis	1 mg per kg PO daily	10–25 mg PO daily
Pityriasis rubra pilaris	25–50 mg PO daily as a single dose; after four weeks, 25–75 mg PO daily	10–25 mg PO daily
Progressive symmetric erythrokeratodermia	25–50 mg PO daily indefinitely	10–25 mg PO daily

Acitretin. Dermatologic indications and dosage (Continued)

Disease	Adult dosage	Child dosage
Psoriasis	25–50 mg PO daily as a single dose; after four weeks, 25–75 mg PO daily	10–25 mg PO daily
Reiter syndrome	25–50 mg PO daily as a single dose; after four weeks, 25–75 mg PO daily	10–25 mg PO daily
Striate keratoderma	0.5–1 mg per kg daily indefinitely	10–25 mg PO daily
Subcorneal pustular dermatosis	1 mg per kg PO daily	10–25 mg PO daily
Tyrosinemia II	0.5–1 mg per kg daily indefinitely	10–25 mg PO daily
Vohwinkel's syndrome	25–50 mg PO daily as a single dose; after four weeks, 25–75 mg PO daily	10–25 mg PO daily

Acne aestivalis

Synonym(s)
Mallorca acne

Definition
Monomorphous follicular papular eruption which occurs after sun exposure

Pathogenesis
Sun exposure appears to produce the lesions; may be a variant of polymorphous light eruption; hypersensitivity reaction to sunscreens or cosmetics possible contributing factor

Clinical manifestation
Monomorphous follicular papules over the shoulders, arms, chest, and neck; no comedones present

Differential diagnosis
Folliculitis; acne vulgaris; steroid acne; insect bite reaction; polymorphous light eruption

Therapy
Tretinoin 0.025% cream; benzoyl peroxide 5% gel; prophylaxis by increasing exposures to artificial ultraviolet radiation to "harden" the skin to the effects of sunlight

References
Plewig G, Jansen T (1998) Acneiform dermatoses. Dermatology 196:102–107

Acne atrophica

▶ Acne necrotica

Acne comedonica

Synonym(s)
Comedonal acne; blackheads; whiteheads

Definition
Open and closed comedones on the face, chest, and back

Pathogenesis
Accumulation of corneocytes in the follicular infundibulum, producing a spherical dermal papule (see acne vulgaris); cause unknown but may involve stimulation of the follicular lining and sebaceous duct by exogenous compounds, an endogenous hormonal stimulus, or a neurologic stimulus

A

Clinical manifestation

Open comedone: skin-colored or white, slightly elevated papule with a punctate central opening

Closed comedone: slightly raised papule with a central black keratotic plug

Differential diagnosis

Milium; epidermoid cyst; giant pore of Winer; nevus comedonicus; Favre-Racouchot disease; radiation acne; acne cosmetica; chloracne; trichostasis spinulosa; flat warts; appendageal tumors (syringoma, etc.); sebaceous gland hyperplasia

Therapy

Tretinoin cream 0.025%[*]; tazarotene 0.1%; adapalene 0.1% gel[*]; benzoyl peroxide 5% gel; azelaic acid 20% cream; salicylic acid 1–2% cream or gel; alpha hydroxy acid preparation; trichloroacetic acid 10–20% peel

References

Webster, GF (1999) Acne vulgaris. Archives of Dermatology 135:1101–1102

Acne conglobata

Synonym(s)

Conglobate acne

Definition

Inflammatory disease characterized by cysts, double-headed comedones, abscesses, sinus tracts, and severe scarring; occurs almost exclusively in adult men

Pathogenesis

Unknown

Clinical manifestation

Numerous large comedones with multiple openings; multiple inflammatory papules, pustules, nodules, and cysts; distribution of lesions over back, chest, buttocks, arms, abdomen, and thighs; heals with deep pitted scars and hypertrophic scars

Differential diagnosis

Acne inversa; acne fulminans; chloracne; tropical acne

Therapy

Isotretinoin[*]; prednisone for extreme acute flares; dapsone; incision and drainage of suppurative cysts and nodules; triamcinolone 3–5 mg per ml intralesional to inflamed cysts; liquid nitrogen cryotherapy for hemorrhagic nodules; surgical excision and skin grafting of chronically involved sites

References

Chicarilli ZN (1987) Follicular occlusion triad: hidradenitis suppurativa, acne conglobata, and dissecting cellulitis of the scalp. Annals of Plastic Surgery 18:230–237

Acne decalvans

▶ Folliculitis decalvans

Acne excoriée

Synonym(s)

Picker's acne; excoriated acne

Definition

Acne lesions which are excoriated

Pathogenesis

Self-induced lesions, often in patients whose acne becomes a source of extreme mental distress

Clinical manifestation

Irregular crusts at sites of acne which have been excoriated

Differential diagnosis

Atopic neurodermatitis; depression with self-mutilation; ecthyma; herpes simplex virus infection

Therapy

Treatment of underlying acne (see acne vulgaris); discussion of the cause of the excoriations; psychotherapy in selected patients

References

Arnold LM, Auchenbach MB, McElroy SL (2001) Psychogenic excoriation. Clinical features, proposed diagnostic criteria, epidemiology and approaches to treatment. CNS Drugs 15:351–359

Acne frontalis

▶ Acne necrotica

Acne inversa

▶ Hidradenitis suppurativa

Acne keloid

▶ Acne keloidalis

Acne keloidalis

Synonym(s)

Acne keloidalis nuchae; folliculitis keloidalis; folliculitis keloidalis nuchae; acne keloid

Definition

Chronic inflammatory process of the hair follicles leading to keloidal papules and plaques on the occipital scalp and posterior neck

Pathogenesis

Theories: injury produced by short haircuts; irritation from shirt collars; chronic low-grade bacterial infections; autoimmune process; primary scarring alopecia; weakened follicular wall with subsequent rupture and foreign body reaction

Clinical manifestation

Firm, dome-shaped, follicular papules, which develop on the nape of the neck and/or on the occipital scalp; papules coalesce into plaques; scarring alopecia and subcutaneous abscesses with draining sinuses occur later in the course

Differential diagnosis

Folliculitis; acne vulgaris; perifolliculitis capitis abscedens et suffodiens; nevus sebaceous of Jadassohn; keloid; pediculosis capitis; hidradenitis suppurativa; seborrheic dermatitis; squamous cell carcinoma; basal cell carcinoma

Therapy

Avoidance of trauma to the neck and posterior scalp area; triamcinolone (5–10 mg per ml) intralesional after softening the site with light liquid nitrogen cryotherapy; CO_2 laser vaporization followed by intralesional triamcinolone (5–10 mg per ml) or imiquimod 5% cream applied daily for 6–8 weeks; punch excision of individual papules; horizontal ellipical excision with or without primary closure

References

Gloster HM Jr (2000). The surgical management of extensive cases of acne keloidalis nuchae. Archives of Dermatology 136:1376–1379

Acne keloidalis nuchae

▶ Acne keloidalis

Acne medicamentosa

Synonym(s)
None

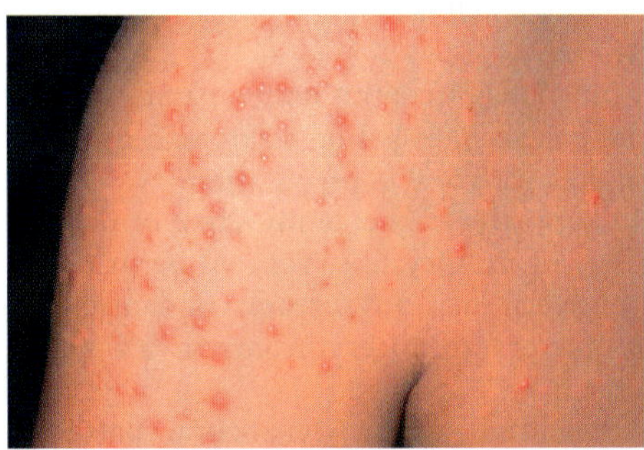

Acne Medicamentosa. Monomorphous red papules on the arm and lateral chest wall

Definition
Acneiform eruption related to ingestion of a medication

Pathogenesis
Unknown; not an allergic reaction to the medication; not a variant of acne vulgaris

Clinical manifestation
Acute onset of inflammatory papules in the the same stage of development with few or no comedones; occurs on the chest, back, and upper extremities; causative agents include systemic corticosteroids, anabolic steroids, B vitamins, anticonvulsants, lithium, isoniazid, quinidine, azathioprine, cyclosporine, etretinate, and halides

Differential diagnosis
Acne vulgaris; folliculitis; chloracne; tropical acne; acne aestavalis

Therapy
Discontinue offending medication, if possible; tetracycline; tretinoin 0.025% cream

References
Webster, GF (2002) Acne. British Medical Journal 325:475–479

Acne necrotica

Synonym(s)
Acne necrotica miliaris; acne variolaformis; acne frontalis; acne atrophica; necrotizing lymphocytic folliculitis; pustular perifolliculitis

Definition
Papulopustular follicular eruption which heals with depressed scars

Pathogenesis
Genetic factors possibly operative

Clinical manifestation
Recurrent grouped perifollicular papules and pustules which heal with variolaform scars; most often located in the temporal scalp, but also on the face, chest, and back

Differential diagnosis
Bacterial folliculitis; tinea capitis; vasculitis; papulonecrotic tuberculid; hydroa vacciniforme

Therapy
Tetracycline; isotretinoin 1 mg per kg PO combined with prednisone 1 mg per kg per day PO*; antibacterial washes with chlorhexadine or hexachlorophene 2–3 times daily; daily shampooing

References
Kossard S, Collins A, McCrossin I (1987) Necrotizing lymphocytic folliculitis: the early lesion of acne necrotica. Journal of the American Academy of Dermatology 16:1007–1014

Acne necrotica miliaris

▶ Acne necrotica

Acne rosacea

▶ Rosacea

Acne variolaformis

▶ Acne necrotica

Acne varus

▶ Acne vulgaris

Acne vulgaris

Synonym(s)
Acne varus

Definition
Common, self-limited eruption characterized by abnormal follicular keratinization, comedones, inflammatory papules, pustules, and nodular abscesses

Pathogenesis
Multiple contributing factors including inheritance, hormonal effects on follicles, increased sebum production, bacteria, abnormal follicular keratinization, and response to environmental stimuli such as oils and frictional trauma

Clinical manifestation
Closed comedones (whitehead); open comedones (blackhead); inflammatory papules and pustules; nodules; draining sinuses; postinflammatory scars; lesions in areas with abundant sebaceous follicles: face, back, upper chest wall

Differential diagnosis
Acne aestivalis; rosacea; perioral dermatitis; folliculitis; acne medicimentosa; occupational acne; tropical acne; acne cosmetica; syndrome of Favre-Racouchot; flat warts; trichostasis spinulosa

Therapy
Comedonal acne: tretinoin 0.025% cream or adapalene 0.1% gel or tazarotene 0.1% gel; alpha hydroxy acid preparation
Inflammaroty acne: tetracycline or doxycycline or minocycline; benzoyl peroxide 5% gel; azelaic acid 20% cream; clindamycin 1% lotion or cream; erythromycin 2% gel or cream
Recalcitrant acne in women: oral contraceptive containing norgestimate 0.25 mg and ethinyl estradiol 0.035 mg; spironolactone; prednisone
Acne where sweating is an aggravating factor: aluminium chloride solution
Severe nodulocystic acne unresponsive to other therapies: isotretinoin[*]
Acne surgery: comedone expression; incision and drainage of fluctuant cysts and abscesses; chemical peel; microdermabrasion; intralesional triamcinolone 2–4 mg/ml

References
Webster GF (2002) Acne vulgaris. British Medical Journal 325:475–479

Acoustic neuroma

▶ Granular cell tumor

Acquired digital fibrokeratoma

Synonym(s)
Garlic glove fibroma

Definition
Benign, acquired, hyperkeratotic projection, usually on one of the digits

Pathogenesis
Trauma possibly a contributing factor

Clinical manifestation
Solitary, smooth, asymptomatic, dome-shaped, skin-colored papule with a collarette of skin encircling the base of the growth, creating a moat-like effect; lesion usually arising on one of the digits of the hand, but also occurring on the palms and soles, dorsum of the hand, wrist, calf, toe, or pre-patellar area

Differential diagnosis
Wart; periungual fibroma (Koenen tumor); pyogenic granuloma; fibroma; supernumerary digit

Therapy
Simple excision*

References
Vinson RP, Angeloni VL (1995): acquired digital fibrokeratoma. American Family Physician 52:1365–1367

Acquired epidermolysis bullosa

▶ Epidermolysis bullosa acquisita

Acquired generalized anhidrosis

Synonym(s)
Tropical anhidrotic asthenia

Definition
Generalized loss of sweat function following prolonged sun exposure

Pathogenesis
Unknown

Clinical manifestation
Loss of sweat function after prolonged exposure to the sun

Differential diagnosis
None

Therapy
Avoidance of situations where core body temperature may rise (exercise, sun exposure, etc.)

References
Tsuji T, Yamamoto T (1976) Acquired generalized anhidrosis. Archives of Dermatology 112:1310–1314

Acquired hypertrichosis

Definition
Excess hair growth in androgen-independent sites; occurs in men and women

References
Manders SM (1995) Acquired hypertrichosis. In: demis DJ (ed) Clinical Dermatology. Lippincott Williams and Wilkins, Philadelphia, Section 2–27, pp 1–4

Acquired partial lipodystrophy

▶ Progressive lipodystrophy

Acquired perforating dermatitis

▶ Perforating folliculitis

Acquired perforating dermatosis

▶ **Perforating folliculitis**

Acquired perforating disease

▶ **Reactive perforating collagenosis**

Acquired progressive lipodystrophy

▶ **Progressive lipodystrophy**

Acquired reactive perforating dermatosis

▶ **Reactive perforating collagenosis**

Acquired tufted angioma

▶ **Tufted angioma**

Acral lentiginous melanoma

Synonym(s)
Acral melanoma

Definition
Melanoma affecting the palms, soles, subungual, and periungual skin or the mucous membranes

Pathogenesis
Unknown

Clinical manifestation
Subungual melanoma: diffuse nail discoloration or a longitudinal pigmented band within the nail plate, with bleeding of pigment onto the nail fold (Hutchinson's sign)
Palmer or plantar melanoma: irregularly pigmented plaque with variable nodularity and late erosion or ulceration
Mucosal melanoma: unevenly pigmented macule, patch, or plaque, with an asymmetric shape and irregular borders and surface

Differential diagnosis
Lentigo; subungual hematoma; chronic paronychia; nevus; melanonychia striata; benign mucosal melanosis; traumatic tattoo; Kaposi's sarcoma; pyogenic granuloma

Therapy
See melanoma

References
Rogers RS 3rd, Gibson LE (1997) Mucosal, genital, and unusual clinical variants of melanoma. Mayo Clinic Proceedings 72:362–366

Acral melanoma

▶ **Acral lentiginous melanoma**

Acral persistent papular mucinosis

Synonym(s)
None

Definition
Chronic localized papular mucinous eruption of the upper extremities

Pathogenesis
Unknown

A

Clinical manifestation
Multiple, discrete, flesh-colored or ivory-colored papules of the hands, wrists, and forearms; occurs in middle-aged women; not associated with systemic findings

Differential diagnosis
Cutaneous focal mucinosis; lupus erythematosus; mucocoele; digital mucous cyst; reticular erythematous mucinosis; cutaneous myxoma; urticarial follicular mucinosis

Therapy
None

References
Flowers SL, Cooper PH, Landes HB (1989) Acral persistent papular mucinosis. Journal of the American Academy of Dermatology 21:293–297

Acroangiodermatitis

Synonym(s)
Pseudo Kaposi's sarcoma; Mali's disease; acroangiodermatitis of Mali; angiodermité de Favre et Chaix; Favre-Chaix disease; Stewart-Bluefarb syndrome

Definition
Hyperplasia of preexisting vasculature in patients with chronic venous insufficiency

Pathogenesis
Severe chronic venous stasis and insufficiency of the calf muscle pump resulting in an elevated capillary pressure; insufficiency of both the muscular pump of the calf and the venous pump of the foot, producing relative tissue anoxia which may cause secondary vascular proliferation

Clinical manifestation
Blue or purple papules and nodules occurring in chronically edematous skin; may be associated with other signs of venous insufficiency, such as varicose veins, elephantiasis nostra, and leg ulcers

Differential diagnosis
Kaposi's sarcoma; pigmented purpuric dermatosis; lichen planus; hemangioma; vasculitis

Therapy
Treatment of underlying vascular insufficiency: support hose; sequential compression device; Unna boots; leg elevation; weight loss; exercise program
Surgical therapy: excision of individual lesions

References
Pires A, Depairon M, Ricci C (1999) Effect of compression therapy on a pseudo-Kaposi sarcoma. Dermatology 198:439–441

Acroangiodermatitis of Mali

▶ Acroangiodermatitis

Acrocephalosyndactyly

Synonym(s)
Apert's syndrome; Pfeiffer's syndrome; Saethre-Chotzen syndrome

Definition
Tower skull deformity; facial peculiarities; syndactyly of the hands and feet; increased incidence of mental retardation

Pathogenesis
Genetic defect (autosomal dominant); localized mutations of FGFR2 gene

Clinical manifestation
Apert's syndrome: high peaked or conical skull; flattened face; hypertelorism; poor vision; low set ears with poor hearing acuity; severe syndactyly; mitten hand deformity; severe acne vulgaris
Pfeiffer's syndrome: similar to Apert's syndrome, but less severe

Saethre-Chotzen syndrome: similar to Apert's syndrome, but less severe; dental defects; often normal intelligence

Differential diagnosis
Acrocephalopolysyndactyly syndromes; Rubinstein-Taybi syndrome; D1 trisomy; hereditary brachymegalodactyly; Léri's pleonostenosis

Therapy
Reconstructive skull surgery; isotretinoin for severe acne vulgaris*

References
Park WJ, Theda C, Maestri NE, Meyers GA, et al. (1995) Analysis of phenotypic features and FGFR2 mutations in Apert syndrome. American Journal of Human Genetics 57:321–328

Acrochordon

Synonym(s)
Skin tag; soft wart; fibroepithelial polyp

Definition
Tumor of loose fibrous tissue, occurring mostly on the neck and in flexural areas

Pathogenesis
Frequent irritation; obesity; epidermal growth factor (EGF) and α-tissue growth factor (TGF) possibly involved; hormone imbalances, such as that seen in pregnancy or acromegaly possibly facilitating growth

Clinical manifestation
Round, soft, pedunculated papules, which are either flesh-colored or hyperpigmented

Differential diagnosis
Wart; neurofibroma; seborrheic keratosis, particularly the dermatosis papulosa nigra variety; melanocytic nevus; melanoma; fibroepithelioma of Pinkus; pseudosarcomatous polyp

Therapy
Scissors excision; liquid nitrogen cryotherapy; destruction by electrodesiccation

References
Hood AF. Lumadue J (1992) Benign vulvar tumors. Dermatologic Clinics 10:371–385

Acrocyanosis

Synonym(s)
None

Definition
Persistent dusky discoloration and coolness of the hands and feet

Pathogenesis
Decreased basal flow through the acral cutaneous microcirculation; theories of causation: defective arteriolar physiology; blood viscosity abnormalities; elevated endothelin-1 levels and exaggerated responses of this molecule to cold stimulation

Clinical manifestation
Violaceous discoloration of the distal extremities; nose, lips, nipples, and ears possibly also involved; worsens with cold exposure; may be associated with cold agglutinin disease, cryoglobulinemia, certain medications, malignancies, and infections

Differential diagnosis
Chilblains; livedo reticularis; Raynaud phenomenon; erythromelalgia; lupus erythematosus; scleroderma

Therapy
Protection of acral areas of the body from the cold; minoxidil 5% solution; bromocriptine; nicotinic acid; biofeedback training

References
Nousari HC, Kimyai-Asadi A, Anhalt GJ (2002) Chronic idiopathic acrocyanosis. Journal of the

American Academy of Dermatology 45:S207–208

Acrodermatitis chronica atrophicans

Synonym(s)
Chronic atrophic acrodermatitis; Lyme borreliosis, late phase

Definition
Fibrosing skin process due to the effect of continuing active infection with Borrelia afzelii

Pathogenesis
Several nonspecific reactions with a specific immune response possibly contributing to its manifestations; progressive, restricted pattern of cytokine expression, including deficient interferon-γ, possibly contributing to its chronicity

Clinical manifestation
Insidious onset of reddish-brown plaques and nodules on the distal extremities; lesions expanding outward with resultant central atrophy

Differential diagnosis
Morphea; venous insufficiency; lichen sclerosus et atrophicus; eosinophilic fasciitis; pernio; endemic syphilis

Therapy
Absence of signs of systemic disease: doxycyline[*]; amoxicillin.
Signs and symptoms of systemic disease: ceftriaxone 2 g IV every 24 hours for 14–21 days; cefotaxime 1–2 g IV every 8 hours for 14–21 days; penicillin G 3–4 million units IV every 4 hours for 21 days

References
Melski JW (2000) Lyme borreliosis. Seminars in Cutaneous Medicine & Surgery 19:10–18

Acrodermatitis enteropathica

Synonym(s)
Acrodermatitis enteropathica; Danbolt-Closs syndrome; acrodermatitis enteropathica-like syndrome; transient symptomatic zinc deficiency; iatrogenic acrodermatitis enteropathica; zinc deficiency syndrome; zinc depletion syndrome; self-limiting acrodermatitis enteropathica

Definition
Autosomal recessive disorder with skin lesions, diarrhea, alopecia, photophobia, irritability, and failure to thrive

Pathogenesis
Deficient intestinal absorption of zinc from the small intestine

Clinical manifestation
Signs and symptoms appearing shortly after discontinuation of breast-feeding; red patches, scaly plaques, and eczematous skin that may evolve into crusted, vesiculobullous, erosive, and pustular plaques; distribution in a periorificial and acral pattern, on the face, scalp, hands, feet, and anogenital areas; alopecia of the scalp and eyebrows; secondary staphylococcal and candidal skin infections

Differential diagnosis
Biotin and multiple decarboxylase deficiencies; essential fatty acid deficiencies; Langerhans cell histiocytosis; cystic fibrosis; mucocutaneous candidiasis; glucagonoma syndrome; seborrheic dermatitis; atopic dermatitis

Therapy
Zinc dietary supplementation 1 mg per kg per day for life

References
Radja N, Charles-Holmes R (2002) Acrodermatitis enteropathica: lifelong follow-up and zinc

monitoring. Clinical & Experimental Dermatology 27:62–63

Acrodermatitis enteropathica-like syndrome

▶ Acrodermatitis enteropathica

Acrodermatitis of Dore

▶ Psoriasis

Acrodermatitis papulosa

▶ Gianotti-Crosti syndrome

Acrodermatitis papulosa eruptiva infantilis

▶ Gianotti-Crosti syndrome

Acrodermatitis papulosa infantum

▶ Gianotti-Crosti syndrome

Acrodynia

Synonym(s)
Pink disease

Definition
Multisystem disease related to mercury intoxication

Pathogenesis
Sympathovasomotor dysfunction secondary to mercury intoxication, perhaps on an idiosyncratic basis

Clinical manifestation
Pain in the hands and feet; hyperhidrosis; excess salivation; gingivitis; early tooth loss; pink discoloration of the nose and distal digits; peripheral neuronitis; hypotonia of the muscles; renal insufficiency

Differential diagnosis
Acrocyanosis; chilblains; acrodermatitis enteropathica; glucagonoma syndrome Kawasaki disease; polio; intoxication with thallium, copper, arsenic, or gold

Therapy
Removal of source of mercury from the environment; DMSA (meso 2,3-dimercaptosuccinic acid) used as a chelating agent; hemodialysis or peritoneal dialysis for renal insufficiency

References
Graeme KA, Pollack CV Jr (1998) Heavy metal toxicity, Part I: arsenic and mercury. Journal of Emergency Medicine 16(1):45–56

Acroerythrokeratoderma

▶ Mal de Meleda

Acrogeria

Synonym(s)
Gottron's syndrome

Definition
Premature aging of the skin, predominately affecting the distal extremities, without other features of premature aging

Pathogenesis
Autosomal recessive inheritiance; may be related to type IV Ehlers-Danlos syndrome

Clinical manifestation
Dry, thin, wrinkled skin; most prominent over the distal extremities; dystrophic nails; short stature; normal life expenctancy

Differential diagnosis
Werner's syndrome (pangeria); progeria

Therapy
None

References
Greally JM, Boone LY, Lenkey SG, Wenger SL, Steele MW (1992) Acrometageria: a spectrum of "premature aging" syndromes. American Journal of Medical Genetics 44(3):334–339

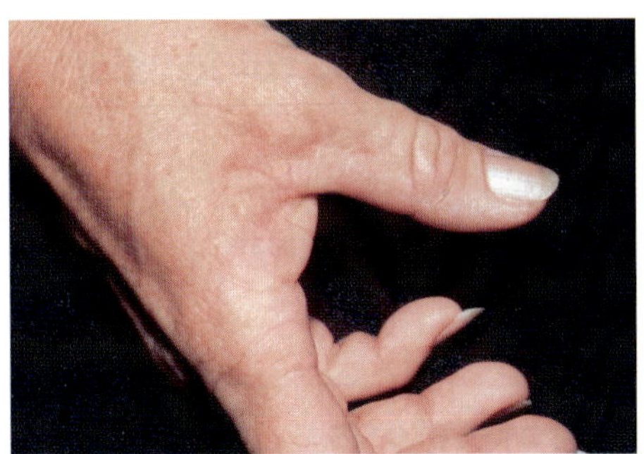

Acrokeratoelastoidosis. Confluent scaly plaques on the sides of the digits

Acrokeratoderma hereditarium punctatum

▸ Acrokeratoelastoidosis

Acrokeratoelastoidosis

Synonym(s)
Acrokeratoelastoidosis marginalis; acrokeratoelastoidosis of Costa; acrokeratoderma hereditarium punctatum; hereditary papulotranslucent acrokeratoderma

Definition
Papular eruption which occurs on the margins of the hands and feet

Pathogenesis
Autosomal dominant transmission in some cases

Clinical manifestation
Keratotic translucent papules which arise on the margins of the hands and feet; lesions often occur in a linear distribution

Differential diagnosis
Keratoelastoidosis marginalis; focal acral hyperkeratosis; flat warts; acrodynia; acrokeratosis verruciformis of Hopf

Therapy
Tretinoin 0.025% cream

References
Rongioletti F, Betti R, Crosti C, Rebora A (1994) Marginal papular acrokeratodermas: a unified nosography for focal acral hyperkeratosis, acrokeratoelastoidosis and related disorders. Dermatology 188(1):28–31

Acrokeratoelastoidosis marginalis

▸ Acrokeratoelastoidosis

Acrokeratoelastoidosis of Costa

▶ Acrokeratoelastoidosis

Acrokeratosis paraneoplastica

▶ Paraneoplastic acrokeratosis

Acrokeratosis paraneoplastica of Bazex

▶ Paraneoplastic acrokeratosis

Acrokeratosis verruciformis

Synonym(s)
Acrokeratosis verruciformis of Hopf

Definition
Autosomal dominant disease consisting of flat wart-like papules over the dorsal aspects of the hands and feet

Pathogenesis
Appears to be a variant of an epithelial nevus

Clinical manifestation
Multiple, asymptomatic, flesh-colored to reddish-brown, flat-topped polygonal papules over the dorsal aspects of the hands and feet; occasional whitish discoloration and thickening of the nail plates

Differential diagnosis
Flat warts; epidermodysplasia verruciformis; stucco keratosis; lichen planus; keratosis follicularis (Darier disease); arsenical keratosis; granuloma annulare; colloid milia

Therapy
Destruction with liquid nitrogen cryotherapy; CO_2 laser or Nd:YAG laser; tretinoin 0.025% cream; adapalene 0.1% gel

References
Chapman-Rolle L, DePadova-Elder SM, Ryan E, Kantor GR (1994) Persistent flat-topped papules on the extremities. Acrokeratosis verruciformis (AKV) of Hopf. Archives of Dermatology 130(4):508–509, 511–512

Acrokeratosis verruciformis of Hopf

▶ Acrokeratosis verruciformis

Acromegalic gigantism (prepubertal children)

▶ Acromegaly

Acromegaly

Synonym(s)
Hyperpituitarism; acromegalic gigantism (prepubertal children)

Definition
A metabolic disorder caused by excess growth hormone that results in gradual enlargement of body tissues, including the bones of the face, jaw, hands, feet, and skull

Pathogenesis
Growth-hormone-secreting pituitary tumors; rarely caused by ectopic growth hormone overproduction by lung or pancreas tumors

Clinical manifestation
Coarsening of facial features; darkening of the skin; large, spade-like hands and feet; excessive sweating; hypertrichosis; oily skin; enlargement of the nose; thickening of heel pads; hard and thickened nails

Differential diagnosis
Pachydermoperiostosis; pseudoacromegaloidism; hypothyroidism

Therapy
Transsphenoidal adenomectomy; supervoltage pituitary gland radiation; octreotide 50–500 mcg SC three time daily; bromocriptine 1.25 mg PO daily initially, increased gradually to 20–30 mg PO daily

References
Ben-Shlomo A, Melmed S (2001) Acromegaly. Endocrinology & Metabolism Clinics of North America 30(3):565–583

Acropachy

▶ **Clubbing of the nails**

Acropapulo-vesicular syndrome

▶ **Gianotti-Crosti syndrome**

Acropigmentatio

▶ **Reticulate Acropigmentation of Kitamura**

Acropigmentation of Dohi

Synonym(s)
Symmetrical dyschromatosis of the extremities; acropigmentation symmetrica of Dohi

Definition
Symmetrical, freckle-like pigmentation of the hands and feet, arising in early childhood

Pathogenesis
Autosomal dominant inheritance

Clinical manifestation
Freckle-like hyperpigmented macules on the hands and feet; associated with hypopigmented macules without atrophy

Differential diagnosis
Acromelanosis progressiva; reticulate acropigmentation of Kitamura; universal acquired melanosis

Therapy
None

References
Danese P, Zanca A, Bertazzoni MG (1997) Familial reticulate acropigmentation of Dohi. Journal of the American Academy of Dermatology 37:884–886

Acropigmentation symmetrica of Dohi

▶ **Acropigmentation of Dohi**

Acropustulosis of infancy

Synonym(s)
Infantile acropustulosis

Definition

Pruritic vesiculopustular eruption of the palms and soles, which occurs mostly in black newborns and infants

Pathogenesis

Unknown

Clinical manifestation

Recurrent crops of small vesicles which evolve into pustules; lesions on the palms, soles, and the dorsal aspects of the distal extremities; onset between birth and 2 years; spontaneous permanent remission by 2–3 years of age

Differential diagnosis

Erythema toxicum neonatorum; dyshidrosis; scabies; pyoderma; transient neonatal pustular melanosis; subcorneal pustular dermatosis; pustular psoriasis; cutaneous candidiasis; fire ant bites; hand-foot-and-mouth disease; eosinophilic pustulosis

Therapy

Fluocinonide 0.05% cream applied twice daily; dapsone

References

Wagner A (1997) Distinguishing vesicular and pustular disorders in the neonate. Current Opinion in Pediatrics 9(4):396–405

Acrosclerosis

Definition

Thickening of the skin and subcutaneous tissue of the hands and feet due to swelling and thickening of fibrous connective tissue

References

Hawk A, English JC 3rd (2001) Localized and systemic scleroderma. Seminars in Cutaneous Medicine & Surgery 20(1):27–37

Acrospiroma

▶ Eccrine acrospiroma

Acrospiroma, eccrine

▶ Eccrine acrospiroma

Actinic cheilitis

Synonym(s)

Actinic keratosis of the lip; actinic damage of the lip; solar cheilitis; actinic cheilosis

Definition

A precancerous skin growth usually caused by chronic sun exposure to the lip

Pathogenesis

Chronic sun exposure producing dyskeratotic cell clones which proliferate

Clinical manifestation

Irregular, non-substantive scaly papule or plaque of vermillion portion of the lip

Differential diagnosis

Squamous cell carcinoma; chapped lips; trauma from chronic lip licking; irritant leukoplakia secondary to cigarette smoking, etc.; contact dermatitis; polymorphous light eruption; lupus erythematosus

Therapy

Destruction by liquid nitrogen cryotherapy; fluorouracil cream; photodynamic therapy; laser resurfacing; dermabrasion; surgical excision with mucosal advancement flap

References

Drake LA, Ceilley RI, Cornelison RL (1995) Guidelines of care for actinic keratoses. Committee on Guidelines of Care. Journal of the American Academy of Dermatology 32(1):95–98

Actinic cheilosis

▶ Actinic cheilitis

Actinic damage of the lip

▶ Actinic cheilitis

Actinic dermatitis

▶ Chronic actinic dermatitis

Actinic elastosis

Synonym(s)

Solar elastosis; senile elastosis; dermatoheliosis; sun damage; farmer's neck; sailor's neck

Definition

Histologic degenerative changes in the skin secondary to chronic sun exposure

Pathogenesis

Ultraviolet-induced postinflammatory dermal connective tissue degeneration; relative contribution of UVB and UVA unclear

Clinical manifestation

Yellowish hue to the skin with irregular, firm papules giving the skin a chicken skin-like appearance; dyspigmentation; redundant skin with deep furrows (cutis rhomboidalis nuchae); glistening scaly plaques along the margins of the digits (keratoelastoides marginalis); associated cysts and comedones (syndrome of Favre and Racouchot); discrete semi-translucent papules on the antihelix or helix of the ear; annular plaques with an atrophic center (actinic granuloma); crystalline papules filled with gelatinous material on the forearms and the tips of the ears

Differential diagnosis

Papular mucinosis; pseudoxanthoma elasticum; polymorphous light eruption; lupus erythematosus; basal cell carcinoma; squamous cell carcinoma; granuloma annulare; comedonal acne; epidermoid cysts; aged skin

Therapy

Avoidance of further sun damage; sun protection measures such as sunscreens, protective clothing; tretinoin 0.025% cream; adapalene 0.1% gel; chemical peel; laser resurfacing

References

Fenske NA, Hynes LR, Lober CW (1998) Actinic elastosis (senile elastosis). In: demis DJ (ed) Clinical Dermatology. Lippincott Williams and Wilkins, Philadelphia, Section 1 4–41 pp 1–12

Actinic granuloma

Synonym(s)

Miescher's granulomatosis; annular elastolytic giant-cell granuloma; granulomatosis disciformis chronica et progressiva

Definition

Chronic, plaque-like, and often annular cutaneous photoeruption, with mixed inflammatory dermal infiltrate, numerous multinucleated giant cells, and prominent elastolysis

Pathogenesis
Unclear whether a variant of granuloma annulare in sun-damaged skin or a separate disease entity

Clinical manifestation
Slowly enlarging, asymptomatic, skin-colored or erythematous annular plaque, usually in sun-exposed skin; resolves in months to years without scarring

Differential diagnosis
Granuloma annulare; sarcoidosis; necrobiosis lipoidica; leprosy; syphilis; elastosis perforans serpiginosa; lupus erythematosus; morphea

Therapy
Triamcinolone 5 mg per ml intralesionally

References
O'Brien JP, Regan W (1999) Actinically degenerate elastic tissue is the likely antigenic basis of actinic granuloma of the skin and of temporal arteritis. Journal of the American Academy of Dermatology 40(2 Pt 1):214–222

Actinic keratosis

Synonym(s)
Solar keratosis; senile keratosis

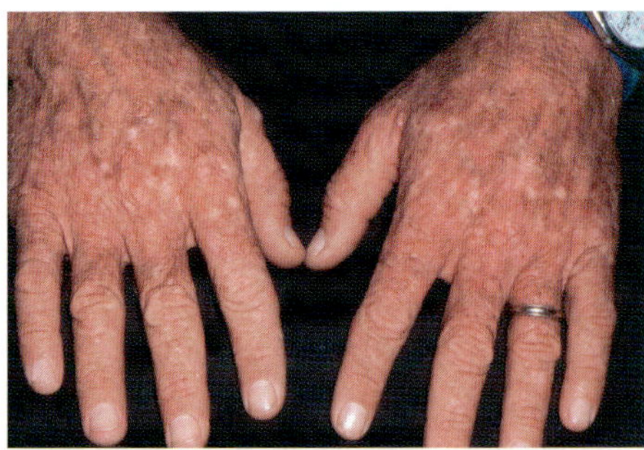

Actinic keratosis. Numerous poorly defined, red, scaly papules on the dorsal aspects of the hands

Definition
A precancerous skin neoplasm usually caused by chronic sun exposure

Pathogenesis
Genetic predisposition; occurrence more frequent in fair, redheaded, or blonde patients that burn frequently and tan poorly; may involve inadequate DNA repair of ultraviolet-light-induced injury

Clinical manifestation
Poorly defined, red, scaly, non-substantive papule on sun-exposed areas of the skin; occurs in the mileau of sun damage (dyspigmentation, telangiectasia, mottling, and solar elastosis)

Differential diagnosis
Squamous cell carcinoma; seborrheic keratosis; wart; lichenoid keratosis; lentigo maligna; Bowen's diseae; cutaneous lupus erythematosus

Therapy
Destruction by liquid nitrogen cryotherapy or electrodesiccation and curettage; fluorouracil 0.5–5% cream; fluorouracil cream plus tretinoin 0.025% cream applied twice daily for 3–6 weeks; photodynamic therapy; tretinoin 0.025% cream; alpha hydroxy acids; dermabrasion; chemical peel

References
Drake LA, Ceilley RI, Cornelison RL (1995) Guidelines of care for actinic keratoses. Committee on Guidelines of Care. Journal of the American Academy of Dermatology 32(1):95–98

Actinic keratosis of the lip

▶ Actinic cheilitis

A

Actinic porokeratosis

▶ Porokeratosis

Actinic prurigo

▶ Polymorphous light eruption

Actinic reticuloid

▶ Chronic actinic dermatitis

Actinophytosis

▶ Botryomycosis

Active junctional nevus

▶ Atypical mole

Acute benign cutaneous leukocytoclastic vasculitis of infancy

▶ Acute hemorrhagic edema of infancy

Acute disseminated epidermal necrosis

▶ Toxic epidermal necrolysis

Acute febrile mucocutaneous lymph node syndrome

▶ Kawasaki disease

Acute febrile neutrophilic dermatosis

Synonym(s)
Sweet syndrome; neutrophilic dermatitis

Definition
Reactive process characterized by the abrupt onset of fever and tender, red-to-purple, circinate papules, nodules, and plaques

Pathogenesis
Hypersensitivity reaction in response to systemic factors, which may include hematologic disease, infection, or drug exposure; neutrophil-mediated process

Clinical manifestation
Erythematous or violaceous papules or nodules; papules often coalescing into circinate or arcuate plaques; pseudovesicular appearance because of subepidermal edema; lesions occasionally studded with pustules

Differential diagnosis

Pyoderma gangrenosum; Behçet's disease; erythema multiforme; bowel-associated dermatitis-arthritis syndrome; neutrophilic rheumatoid dermatitis; leukocytoclastic vasculitis; leukemia cutis; cutaneous metastasis; acute hemorrhagic edema of childhood

Therapy

Prednisone[*]; steroid sparing agents: dapsone; cyclosporine

References

Fett DL, Gibson LE, Su WP (1995) Sweet's Syndrome: systemic signs and symptoms and associated disorders. Mayo Clinic Proceedings 70:234–240

Acute generalized exanthematous pustular dermatitis

Synonym(s)

Acute generalized exanthematous pustulosis

Definition

Generalized eruption of sterile pustules on diffuse erythematous skin, shortly after the administration of a particular drug

Pathogenesis

Hypersensitivity reaction to drug antigen(s); may be a type 3 reaction

Clinical manifestation

Generalized eruption of sterile pustules with diffuse erythema; high fever and peripheral blood leukocytosis

Differential diagnosis

Pustular psoriasis; pustular bacterid; candidiasis; impetigo herpetiformis; pyoderma

Therapy

Cessation of offending medication; prednisone

References

Roujeau JC, Bioulac-Sage P, Bourseau C, Guillaume JC, Bernard P, et al. (1991) Acute generalized exanthematous pustulosis. Analysis of 63 cases. Archives of Dermatology 127:1333–1338

Acute generalized exanthematous pustulosis

▶ Acute generalized exanthematous pustular dermatitis

Acute hemorrhagic edema of infancy

Synonym(s)

Acute infantile hemorrhagic edema; Finkelstein's disease; Seidlmayer syndrome; purpura en cocarde avec oedema; cockade purpura with edema; postinfectious cockade purpura of early childhood; acute benign cutaneous leukocytoclastic vasculitis of infancy

Definition

Cutaneous, small vessel leukocytoclastic vasculitis of young children with large rosetted, annular, or targetoid purpuric lesions

Pathogenesis

Preceded by respiratory tract infections, drug intake, or vaccination; presumably immune complex-mediated

Clinical manifestation

Lesions may begin as urticarial plaques; large, cockade (knot of ribbons appearance), annular, or targetoid purpuric plaques, found primarily on the face, ears, and extremities; acral edema involving the dorsum of the hands and feet

Differential diagnosis
Urticaria, acute febrile neutrophilic dermatosis; erythema multiforme; Henoch-Schönlein purpura; leukemia cutis; meningococcemia or other bacterial septicemia; child abuse

Therapy
None

References
Millard T, Harris A, MacDonald D (1999) Acute infantile hemorrhagic oedema. Journal of the American Academy of Dermatology 41(5 Pt 2): 837–839

Acute infantile hemorrhagic edema

▶ Acute hemorrhagic edema of infancy

Acute infective gangrene

▶ Necrotizing fasciitis

Acute intermittent porphyria

Synonym(s)
AIP

Definition
Defect in the enzyme porphobilinogen-deaminase that results in excessive accumulation of porphyrin precursors which produce distinctive signs and symptoms

Pathogenesis
Accumulation of porphobilinogen and amino-levulinic acid (ALA), which results in neurologic damage that leads to peripheral and autonomic neuropathies and psychiatric manifestations; autosomal dominant disease

Clinical manifestation
Motor neuropathy that is more predominant in the lower extremities; constipation; colicky abdominal pain; vomiting; peripheral neuropathy; seizures; delirium; depression; psychiatric symptoms; cortical blindness; coma

Differential diagnosis
Abdominal diseases such as hernia, appendicitis; abscess, biliary disease, diverticulitis, gastritis; irritable bowel syndrome, aortic dissection, and intestinal obstruction; neurologic-psychiatric diseases such as psychosis, diabetic neuropathy, leprosy, nerve entrapment syndrome, and lead toxicity

Therapy
Glucose, 400 g per day for treatment of mild attacks; hematin 4 mg per kg per day for 4 days in severe attacks

References
Zaider E, Bickers DR (1998) Clinical laboratory methods for diagnosis of the porphyrias. Clinics in Dermatology 16(2):277–293

Acute lupus erythematosus

▶ Lupus erythematosus, acute

Acute miliary tuberculosis of skin

▶ Cutaneous tuberculosis

Acute necrotizing gingivitis

Synonym(s)
Acute necrotizing ulcerative gingivitis; trench mouth

Definition
Acute infectious gingivitis

Pathogenesis
Infection of the gingiva with one of several organisms, including Prevotella intermedia, alpha-hemolytic streptococci, Actinomyces species, or any of a number of different oral spirochetes; emotional stress, smoking, and poor nutrition possibly predisposing factors

Clinical manifestation
Fever; fetid breath; marked gingival edema and ulceration, often with a grayish pseudomembrane; most commonly involving the interdental papillae; may spread to adjacent soft tissues of the mouth

Differential diagnosis
Desquamative gingivitis; pemphigus vulgaris; medication toxicity (cancer chemotherapeutic agents, etc.); aphtous stomatitis; Behçet's syndrome; noma

Therapy
Penicillin VK*; penicillin-allergic patients: erythromycin; topical therapy: chlorhexidine 0.12% oral rinse used for 30 seconds twice daily; lidocaine viscous 2% applied 2–4 times daily as needed

References
Fenesy KE (1998) Periodontal disease: an overview for physicians. Mount Sinai Journal of Medicine 65(5–6):362–369

Acute necrotizing ulcerative gingivitis

▶ Acute necrotizing gingivitis

Acute skin failure

▶ Toxic epidermal necrolysis

Acute sun damage

▶ Sunburn

Acute sunburn reaction

▶ Sunburn

Acyclovir

Trade name(s)
Zovirax

Generic available
Yes

Drug class
Anti-viral

Mechanism of action
DNA polymerase inhibition

Acyclovir. Dermatologic indications and dosage

Disease	Adult dosage	Child dosage
Eczema herpeticum	500 mg IV daily divided into 3 doses for 5 days	15 mg per kg IV daily divided into 3 doses for 5 days
Herpes simplex virus infection, 1st episode	200 mg PO 5 times daily for 10 days	5 mg per kg IV 3 times daily for 5–10 days
Herpes simplex virus infection, prophylaxis	400 mg PO twice daily for up to 1 year	200 mg PO twice daily for up to 1 year
Herpes simplex virus infection, recurrent	200 mg PO 5 times daily for 7 days	5 mg per kg IV 3 times daily for 5–10 days
Herpes zoster	800 mg PO 5 times daily for 7 days	20 mg per kg PO 5 times daily for 7 days
Varicella	800 mg PO 5 times daily for 7 days	20 mg per kg PO 5 times daily for 7 days

Dosage form
200 mg capsule; 400 mg capsule; 800 mg capsule; 200 mg/ml oral suspension powder for IV solution

Dermatologic indications and dosage
See table

Common side effects
Gastrointestinal: nausea; vomiting
Neurologic: headache

Serious side effects
Bone marrow: suppression
Gastrointestinal: hepatitis
Neurologic: seizures; encephalopathy; coma

Drug interactions
Aminoglycoside antibiotics; carboplatin; cidofovir; cisplatin; glyburide; metformin; mycophenolate mofetil; probenecid; nephrotoxic agents

Contraindications/precautions
Hypersensitivity to drug class or component; elderly patients or those with renal failure may need lower dose

References
Brown TJ, Vander Straten M, Tyring T (2001) Antiviral agents. Dermatologic Clinics 19 (1):23–34

ADAM complex

▶ **Amniotic band syndrome**

Adams-Oliver syndrome

Synonym(s)
Scalp and head syndrome

Definition
Congenital absence of scalp skin with hypoplastic or absent distal limbs

Pathogenesis
Unknown; autosomal dominant inheritance in some cases

Clinical manifestation
Solitary or multiple areas of congenital scarring alopecia of the scalp (aplasia cutis); dilated scalp veins; distal limb hypoplasia or aplasia

Differential diagnosis
Focal dermal hypoplasia; congenital absence of skin; constriction from amniotic bands; trisomy 13

Therapy
Surgical correction of scalp defect[*]

References
Beekmans SJ, Wiebe MJ (2001) Surgical treatment
of aplasia cutis in the Adams-Oliver syndrome.
Journal of Craniofacial Surgery 12(6):569–572

Adapalene

Trade name(s)
Differin

Generic available
No

Drug class
Retinoid receptor agonist

Mechanism of action
Binds to retinoid nuclear receptors, which
modulate differentiation, keratinization,
and inflammation

Dosage form
0.1% gel, solution

Dermatologic indications and dosage
See table

Common side effects
Cutaneous: burning sensation; pruritus;
erythema; scaling

Serious side effects
None

Drug interactions
None

Adapalene. Dermatologic indications and dosage

Disease	Adult dosage	Child dosage
Acanthosis nigricans	Apply daily, preferably at bedtime; apply 20–30 minutes after washing and drying skin	Apply daily, preferably at bedtime; apply 20–30 minutes after washing and drying skin
Acne vulgaris	Apply daily, preferably at bedtime; apply 20–30 minutes after washing and drying skin	Apply daily, preferably at bedtime; apply 20–30 minutes after washing and drying skin
Acrokeratoelastoidosis	Apply daily, preferably at bedtime	Apply daily, preferably at bedtime
Acrokeratosis verruciformis	Apply daily, preferably at bedtime; apply 20–30 minutes after washing and drying skin	Apply daily, preferably at bedtime; apply 20–30 minutes after washing and drying skin
Actinic keratosis	Apply daily, preferably at bedtime for up to 3 months	Apply daily, preferably at bedtime for up to 3 months
Melasma	Apply daily, preferably at bedtime; apply 20–30 minutes after washing and drying skin	Apply daily, preferably at bedtime; apply 20–30 minutes after washing and drying skin
Photoaging	Apply daily, preferably at bedtime; apply 20–30 minutes after washing and drying skin	Apply daily, preferably at bedtime; apply 20–30 minutes after washing and drying skin
Post-inflammatory hyperpigmentation	Apply daily, preferably at bedtime; apply 20–30 minutes after washing and drying skin	Apply daily, preferably at bedtime; apply 20–30 minutes after washing and drying skin
Reactive perforating collagenosis	Apply daily, preferably at bedtime; apply 20–30 minutes after washing and drying skin	Apply daily, preferably at bedtime; apply 20–30 minutes after washing and drying skin

Contraindications/precautions
Hypersensitivity to drug class or component; caution in applying to eczematous skin

References
Wolf JE Jr (2002) Potential anti-inflammatory effects of topical retinoids and retinoid analogues. Advances in Therapy 19(3):109–118

Addison disease

▶ Addison's disease

Addison disease-cerebral sclerosis syndrome

▶ Addison-Schilder disease

Addison's disease

Synonym(s)
Addison disease; primary adrenal insufficiency; chronic adrenal insufficiency; hypoadrenalism; hypocorticism; suprarenal insufficiency

Definition
Metabolic disease caused by an inadequate supply or secretion of adrenocortical hormones, mainly mineralocorticoids and cortisol

Pathogenesis
Primary insufficiency caused by inadequate adrenal gland function: infections (viral, tuberculosis, histoplasmosis); autoimmune adrenal gland destruction; malignant disease
Suprarenal insufficiency: occurring after abrupt discontinuance of prolonged systemic corticosteroid therapy; hypopituitarism

Clinical manifestation
Uniform skin hyperpigmentation; malaise; fatigue; dizziness; anorexia; abdominal pain; hypotension; amenorrhea

Differential diagnosis
Acanthosis nigricans; malnutrition; melasma; polyglandular autoimmune disease; depression; hypothyroidism

Therapy
Cortisone 25–300 mg PO per day[*]; fludrocortisone 0.1 mg PO daily[*]

References
Don-Wauchope AC, Toft AD (2000) Diagnosis and management of Addison's disease. Practitioner 244(1614):794–799

Addison-Schilder disease

Synonym(s)
Addison disease-cerebral sclerosis syndrome; Fanconi-Prader syndrome; Schilder-Addison syndrome; Siemerling-Creutzfeldt syndrome; adrenocortical atrophy-cerebral sclerosis syndrome, adrenoleukomyelopathy; adrenomyelopathy; adrenomyeloneuropathy; melanodermic leukodystrophy; adrenoleukodystrophy

Definition
Heritable syndrome which combines the characteristics of Addison's disease (bronze skin disease) and cerebral sclerosis (Schilder disease)

Pathogenesis
X-linked inheritance; disorder of lipid metabolism and particularly the peroxisomes; accumulation of saturated, very long chain fatty acids (VLCFA) resulting in the progressive dysfunction of CNS white matter and the adrenal cortex

Clinical manifestation
Bronze skin color; adrenal insufficiency; extensive demyelination and sclerosis of the brain, causing behavior disturbances and deteriorating mental and motor abnormalities; neurological consequences including blindness, deafness, hemiplegia, quadriplegia, pseudobulbar palsy, and dementia

Differential diagnosis
Addison's disease; Schilder's syndrome

Therapy
Steroid replacement – cortisone acetate 25–300 mg PO every 1–2 days[*]; fludrocortisone 0.1–0.2 mg PO per day[*]; dietary – VLCFA-restricted diet with Lorenzo's oil

References
Gartner J, Braun A, Holzinger A, et al. (1998) Clinical and genetic aspects of X-linked adrenoleukodystrophy. Neuropediatrics 29(1) 3–13

Adenoma hidradenoides

▶ Hidradenoma papilliferum

Adenoma sebaceum

▶ Angiofibroma

Adenomatosis, erosive, of nipple

▶ Erosive adenomatosis of the nipple

Adiponecrosis subcutanea

▶ Rothman-Makai syndrome

Adiposis dolorosa

▶ Dercum's disease

Adrenocortical atrophy-cerebral sclerosis syndrome

▶ Addison-Schilder disease

Adrenoleukodystrophy

▶ Addison-Schilder disease

Adrenoleukomyelopathy

▶ Addison-Schilder disease

Adrenomyeloneuropathy

▶ Addison-Schilder disease

Adrenomyelopathy

▶ Addison-Schilder disease

African river blindness

▶ Filariasis

African trypanosomiasis

Synonym(s)
Sleeping sickness; human African trypanosomiasis; HAT

Definition
Infectious parasitic disease carried by tsetse flies from the Trypanosoma brucei family, characterized by inflammation of the brain and the meninges

Pathogenesis
Humans infected following a tsetse fly bite; reservoir for infection in Africa; trypanosomes developing at skin innoculation site and then invading the blood stream

Clinical manifestation
Early disease: hot, red, tender nodule at innoculation site; regional lymphadenopathy.
Second phase of disease: edema of the extremities and face; transient urticarial or hemorrhagic eruption; behavioral changes, alerations in sleep patterns; extrapyramidal neurologic signs; coma

Differential diagnosis
Malaria; HIV disease; borreliosis; brucellosis; typhoid fever; tuberculosis; bacterial, fungal, or viral meningitis

Therapy
Early disease: Suramin 100–200 mg IV test dose, then 1 g IV on days 1, 3, 7, 14[*]; eflornithine 400 mg per kg per day IV 4 times daily for 14 days[*]
Neurologic (late stage) disease: melarsoprol 2–3.6 mg per kg per day IV for 3 days; after 1 week, 3.6 mg per kg per day for 3 days; after 10–21 days, repeat cycle; eflornithine 400 mg per kg per day IV 4 times daily for 14 days

References
Centers for Disease Control and Prevention Trypanosomiasis Fact Sheet. CDC May, 2000

Aggressive digital papillary adenoma

Synonym(s)
Digital papillary adenoma

Definition
Benign but locally aggressive tumor of the digits

Pathogenesis
Derived from secretory eccrine sweat gland epithelium

Clinical manifestation
Slowly enlarging papule or nodule on one of the digits; occasionally eroding and bleeding; malignant variant (aggressive digital papillary adenocarcinoma) having similar appearance, but with histologic changes of malignancy

Differential diagnosis
Eccrine acrospiroma; chondroid syringoma; papillary eccrine adenoma; aggressive digital papillary adenocarcinoma

Therapy
Wide local excision[*]

References
Smith KJ, Skelton HG, Holland TT (1992) Recent advances and controversies concerning adnexal neoplasms. Dermatologic Clinics 10(1):117–160

Aggressive fibromatosis

▶ Desmoid tumor

AHA revitalizing cream

▶ Alpha hydroxy acids

AHA skin smoothing cream

▶ Alpha hydroxy acids

Ainhum

Synonym(s)
Dactylolysis spontanea; constricting bands of the extremities

Definition
Autoamputation of a digit as a result of a constricting scar in the form of a fibrous band or groove

Pathogenesis
Probably related to trauma to the affected digit, although exact mechanism unclear

Clinical manifestation
Progressive constriction at the base of the toe (usually the 5th toe) with distal edema; toe possibly becoming rotated, distorted at the metatarsophalangeal joint; autoamputation after the band has completely constricted the base of the digit

Differential diagnosis
Pseudoainhum; leprosy; syphilis; endemic syphilis; pityriasis rubra pilaris; morphea; congenital constricting bands of children; pachyonychia congenita

Therapy
Early stages: relaxing incision of the fibrous band
Late stages: surgical amputation

References
Marsden PD (1989) Ainhum. Transactions of the Royal Society of Tropical Medicine & Hygiene 83(6):864

AIP

▶ Acute intermittent porphyria

Albendazole

Trade name(s)
Albenza

Generic available
No

Drug class
Anti-helminthic

Mechanism of action
Most likely works by causing degeneration of cytoplasmic microtubules of organism, with release of proteolytic and hydrolytic enzymes in cytoplasm

Dosage form
200 mg tablet

Dermatologic indications and dosage
See table

Common side effects
Gastrointestinal: abdominal pain, nausea and vomiting, meningeal signs
Neurologic: headache, vertigo
Renal: abnormal liver function tests

Serious side effects
Bone marrow: pancytopenia, granulocytopenia

Drug interactions
Cimetidine; dexamethasone; praziquantel

Contraindications/precautions
Hypersensitivity to drug class or component, specifically benzimidazole class of compounds

Albendazole. Dermatologic indications and dosage

Disease	Adult dosage	Child dosage
Cutaneous larva migrans	400 mg PO daily for 3 days	15 mg per kg PO twice daily for 3 days
Cysticercosis	400 mg PO twice daily; 28–day cycle followed by 14-day rest period, for 3 cycles	< 60 kg – 15 mg per kg PO twice daily; 28–day cycle followed by 14-day rest period, for 3 cycles
Filariasis	400 mg PO as single dose	15 mg per kg PO as single dose
Strongyloidosis	200 mg PO twice daily for 3 days; repeat in 2 weeks if necessary	15 mg per kg PO twice daily for 3 days; repeat in 2 weeks if necessary

References

Horton J (2000) Albendazole: a review of anti-helminthic efficacy and safety in humans. Parasitology 121 Suppl:S113–132

Albenza

▶ Albendazole

Albinism

▶ Oculocutaneous albinism

Albinism-deafness syndrome

▶ Ziprkowski-Margolis syndrome

Albinoidism

Synonym(s)
None

Definition
Mild form of albinism where the pigment dilution is less marked than in other forms; absence of pigment in localized areas; the pigment in the skin, hair and eyes less than normal but not affecting the individual as severely as the oculocutaneous or ocular types of albinism

Pathogenesis
Autosomal dominant or recessive condition

Clinical manifestation
Absence of pigment in localized areas of the skin, hair, and eyes; mild photophobia; vison less than normal but not affecting the individual as severely as the oculocutaneous or ocular types

Differential diagnosis
Oculocutaneous albinism; Hermansky-Pudlak syndrome; phenylketonuria; Chediak-Higashi syndrome; histidinemia; homocystinuria; Menkes steely hair disease; Tietz syndrome; Prader-Willi syndrome; Angelman syndrome

Therapy
Sun protection with protective clothing and sunscreens; corrective lenses for visual impairment

References

Bolognia J, Pawelek JM (1988) Biology of hypopigmentation. Journal of the American Academy of Dermatology 19:217–255

Albright hereditary osteodystrophy

▶ Pseudohypoparathyroidism

Albright syndrome

▶ McCune-Albright syndrome

Albright-Sternberg-McCune syndrome

▶ McCune-Albright syndrome

Albright's syndrome

▶ McCune-Albright syndrome

Alcaptonuria

Synonym(s)
Alkaptonuria; ochronosis; homogentisic acid oxidase deficiency

Definition
Homogentisic acid oxidase deficiency which results in a buildup of polymerized phenols in skin and internal organs

Pathogenesis
Autosomal recessive inheritance; disorder of tyrosine (an amino acid) metabolism resulting from a defect in the enzyme homogentisic acid oxidase; homogentisic acid oxidase deficiency leading to increased tissue levels of homogentisic acid, which polymerizes non-enzymatically; deficient collagen formation because of competitive inhibition by homogentisic acid for ascorbic acid

Clinical manifestation
Slate blue or gray discoloration in the sclerae and ear cartilage; diminished joint mobility; ankylosis; aortic or mitral valvulitis

Differential diagnosis
Aortic stenosis; rheumatoid arthritis, osteoarthritis; mitral stenosis; darkened urine: acute intermittent porphyria; myoglobinuria; hemoglobinuria; blue discoloration: argyria; medication reaction (minocycline, amiodarone, etc); acquired ochronosis from hydroquinone

Therapy
Vitamin C, up to 1 g per day PO

▶ Ochronosis

References
Lubics A, Schneider I, Sebok B, Havass Z (2000) Extensive bluish gray skin pigmentation and severe arthropathy: endogenous ochronosis (alkaptonuria). Archives of Dermatology 136(4):548–549

Aldrich syndrome

▶ Wiskott-Aldrich syndrome

Aleppo oil

▶ Leishmaniasis, cutaneous

Alezzandrini syndrome

▶ Alezzandrini's syndrome

Alezzandrini's syndrome

Synonym(s)
Alezzandrini syndrome

Definition
Disorder consisting of unilateral tapetoretinal degeneration, ipsilateral appearance of facial vitiligo and poliosis, occurring in adolescents and young adults

Pathogenesis
Unknown

Clinical manifestation
Unilateral tapetoretinal degeneration; ipsilateral appearance of facial vitiligo-like pigmentaton; poliosis; occasional ipsilateral perceptual deafness; stable course without spontaneous re-pigmentation

Differential diagnosis
Piebaldism; Waardenburg syndrome; vitiligo; Vogt-Koyanagi-Harada syndrome

Therapy
No specific therapy

References
Hoffman MD, Dudley C (1992) Suspected Alezzandrini's syndrome in a diabetic patient with unilateral retinal detachment and ipsilateral vitiligo and poliosis. Journal of the American Academy of Dermatology 26(3 Pt 2):496–497

Alginates

Trade name(s)
Kaltostat; Sorbsan; Algosteril

Generic available
No

Drug class
Synthetic dressing

Mechanism of action
Absorbant; hemostatic

Dosage form
Sheet

Dermatologic indications and dosage
See table

Common side effects
Pain when removed

Serious side effects
None

Drug interactions
None

Contraindications/precautions
None

References
Thomas S (2000) Alginate dressings in surgery and wound management – Part 1. Journal of Wound Care 9(2):56–60

Alginates. Dermatologic indications and dosage

Disease	Adult dosage	Child dosage
Skin ulceration	Apply directly onto ulcer bed; change when saturated with fluid	Apply directly onto ulcer bed; change when saturated with fluid

Algosteril

▶ **Alginates**

Alkaptonuria

▶ **Alcaptonuria**
▶ **Ochronosis**

Allergic angiitis

▶ **Leukocytoclastic vasculitis**

Allergic angiitis and granulomatosis

▶ **Churg-Strauss syndrome**

Allergic cutaneous vasculitis

▶ **Leukocytoclastic vasculitis**

Allergic granulomatosis

▶ **Churg-Strauss syndrome**

Allylamine

Synonym(s)
None

Definition
Chemical which inhibits squalene epoxidase, an enzyme in the pathway that leads to synthesis of ergosterol, a component of the dermatophyte cell wall

References
Reitberg D (2001) Pharmacokinetics of topical antifungal formulations. Cutis 67(5 Suppl):39–40

Alopecia

Definition
Loss of hair, partial or complete

References
Hogan DJ, Chamberlain M (2000) Male pattern baldness. Southern Medical Journal 93(7):657–662

Alopecia areata

Synonym(s)
Autoimmune alopecia

Definition
Recurrent, non-scarring type of hair loss, most likely caused by autoimmune processes

Pathogenesis
Probably T-cell mediated; occurs in genetically predisposed individuals

Clinical manifestation
Non-scarring, non-inflammatory, patterned alopecia; one or many round-to-oval bald patches; exclamation point hairs (i.e. hairs tapered near proximal end) often present; most commonly occurring in the scalp, but possible in any hair-bearing area

Differential diagnosis

Androgenetic alopecia; tinea capitis; pseudopelade of Brocq; lichen planopilaris; telogen effluvium; trichotillomania; syphilis

Therapy

Localized disease: triamcinolone 2–4 mg per ml intralesional; high potency topical corticosteroids
Widespread disease: prednisone, anthralin; topical immunotherapy with squaric acid; photochemotherapy; cyclosporine

References

Madani S, Shapiro J (2000) Alopecia areata update. Journal of the American Academy of Dermatology 42(4):549–566

Alopecia mucinosa

▶ Follicular mucinosis

Alpha hydroxy acids

Trade name(s)

Aqua Glycolic lotion; Glyderm Plus; Day Cream for dry skin; MD Forte facial cream; AHA Skin Smoothing Cream; AHA Revitalizing Cream

Generic available

No

Drug class

Emollient; keratolytic (chemical exfoliant)

Mechanism of action

Keratolytic at low concentration; epidermolysis at high concentration

Dosage form

Cream, lotion; various concentration/pH combinations

Dermatologic indications and dosage

See table

Alpha hydroxy acids. Dermatologic indications and dosage

Disease	Adult dosage	Child dosage
Acne vulgaris	Apply twice daily	Apply twice daily
Actinic keratosis	Apply twice daily	Apply twice daily
Dermatoheliosis	Apply twice daily	Apply twice daily
Epidermolytic hyperkeratosis	Apply twice daily	Apply twice daily
Ichthyosis vulgaris	Apply twice daily	Apply twice daily
Keratosis pilaris	Apply twice daily	Apply twice daily
Lamellar ichthyosis	Apply twice daily	Apply twice daily
Melasma	Apply twice daily	Apply twice daily
Refsum disease	Apply twice daily	Apply twice daily
Rosacea	Apply twice daily	Apply twice daily
Tylosis	Apply twice daily	Apply twice daily
Ulerythema ophyrogenes	Apply twice daily	Apply twice daily
Xerosis	Apply twice daily	Apply twice daily
X-linked ichthyosis	Apply twice daily	Apply twice daily

Common side effects
Dermatologic: skin peeling; irritation; dyspigmentation

Serious side effects
Herpes simplex virus infection

Drug interactions
Tretinoin; adapalene

Contraindications/precautions
Hypersensitivity to drug class or component

References
Glaser DA, Rogers C (2001) Topical and systemic therapies for the aging face. Facial Plastic Surgery Clinics of North America 9(2):189–196

Alpha interferon

▶ Interferon-α

Alpha-2a interferon

▶ Interferon-α

Alpha-2b interferon

▶ Interferon-α

Alstrom's syndrome

Synonym(s)
None

Definition
Autosomal recessive disorder with insulin resistance, diabetes mellitus, obesity, cone-rod dystrophy, and infantile cardiomyopathy

Pathogenesis
Unknown defect; autosomal recessive inheritance

Clinical manifestation
Acanthosis nigricans; retinitis pigmentosa; cardiomyopathy; deafness; obesity; diabetes mellitus; nephropathy; normal intelligence

Differential diagnosis
Bardet-Biedl syndrome; cone-rod dystrophy; achromatopsia; Leber's congenital amaurosis

Therapy
Treatment of insulin resistance and diabetes mellitus

References
Russell-Eggitt IM, Clayton PT, Coffey R, Kriss A, Taylor DS, Taylor JF (1998) Alstrom syndrome. Report of 22 cases and literature review. Ophthalmology 105(7):1274–1280

Aluminium chloride

Trade name(s)
Drysol; Xerac-AC; Hypercare; Certain-Dri

Generic available
No

Drug class
Antiperspirant; anti-infective

Mechanism of action
Reversible inhibition of eccrine gland secretion

Aluminium chloride. Dermatologic indications and dosage

Disease	Adult dosage	Child dosage
Acne, in cases where sweating is an aggravating factor	Apply daily	Apply daily
Auriculotemporal syndrome	Apply daily until maximum effect is achieved; then apply 2–4 times weekly	Apply daily until maximum effect is achieved; then apply 2–4 times weekly
Hyperhidrosis	Apply daily until maximum effect is achieved; then apply 2–4 times weekly	Apply daily until maximum effect is achieved; then apply 2–4 times weekly
Interdigital maceration	Apply daily until maximum effect is achieved; then apply 2–4 times weekly	Apply daily until maximum effect is achieved; then apply 2–4 times weekly

Dosage form
6.25%–20% solution

Dermatologic indications and dosage
See table

Common side effects
Cutaneous: stinging; burning; pruritus; skin irritation; contact dermatitis (rare)

Serious side effects
None

Drug interactions
None

Contraindications/precautions
Hypersensitivity to drug class or component

References
Benohanian A (2001) Antiperspirants and deodorants. Clinics in Dermatology 19(4):398–405

Aluminium chloride hexahydrate

▶ Aluminium chloride

Aluminium chlorohydrate

Trade name(s)
Ostiderm; Arrid XX; Right Guard Sport; Secret Antiperspirant; Dove Aerosol; Sure Antiperspirant

Generic available
No

Drug class
Antiperspirant; anti-infective

Mechanism of action
Reversible inhibition of eccrine gland secretion

Dosage form
Lotion, cream, roll-on

Dermatologic indications and dosage
See table

Common side effects
Cutaneous: stinging; burning; pruritus; irritation

Serious side effects
None

Aluminium chlorohydrate. Dermatologic indications and dosage

Disease	Adult dosage	Child dosage
Hyperhidrosis	Apply daily	Apply daily

Drug interactions
None

Contraindications/precautions
Hypersensitivity to drug class or component

References
Benohanian A (2001) Antiperspirants and deodorants. Clinics in Dermatology 19(4):398–405

Aluminium granuloma

▶ Aluminium hypersensitivity granuloma

Aluminium hypersensitivity granuloma

Synonym(s)
Aluminium granuloma

Definition
Subcutaneous granuloma formed as a reaction to aluminium-containing injectable material

Pathogenesis
Fine particles of aluminium, producing local immunologic reaction

Clinical manifestation
Pruritic and tender subcutaneous nodules, appearing 2–9 months after injection of vaccine containing aluminium as adsorbing agent

Differential diagnosis
Lupus profundus; polyarteritis nodosa; subcutaneous fungal infection

Therapy
Surgical excision★

References
Fawcett HA, Smith NP (1984) Injection-site granuloma due to aluminium. Archives of Dermatology 120(10):1318–1322

Alveolar soft part sarcoma

Synonym(s)
Malignant organoid granular cell myoblastoma; malignant nonchromaffin paraganglioma

Definition
Malignant soft tissue tumor that has an unclear origin, but distinctive histologic findings

Pathogenesis
Increased risk with Li-Fraumeni syndrome and neurofibromatosis; some association with Epstein Barr virus infection

Clinical manifestation
Slow-growing soft tissue mass, usually in adolescents and young adults; may be pulsitile with bruit

Differential diagnosis
Metastatic disease, particularly melanoma and renal cell carcinoma; granular cell tumor; leiomyosarcoma; rhabdomyosarcoma

Therapy
Surgical excision[*]

References
Nakashima Y, Kotoura Y, Kasakura K, Yamamuro T, Amitani R, Ohdera K (1993) Alveolar soft-part sarcoma. A report of ten cases. Clinical Orthopedics 294:259–266

Amalgam tattoo

Synonym(s)
None

Definition
Implantation of dental amalgam materials into mildly injured or inflamed mucosal tissues

Pathogenesis
Implantation of pigmented material, which fails to evoke an inflammatory response by host

Clinical manifestation
Painless, blue/gray/black macule with no surrounding erythematous reaction; most frequently found on the gingival or alveolar mucosa

Differential diagnosis
Nevus; melanoma; mucosal melanosis; hemangioma; venous lake; Peutz-Jeghers syndrome; medication reaction; hemochromatosis; heavy metal intoxication

Therapy
Q-switched ruby laser; excisional biopsy performed to rule out melanoma or another pigmented lesion

References
Seward GR (1998) Amalgam tattoo. British Dental Journal 184(10):470–471

Ambras syndrome

Synonym(s)
Hypertrichosis universalis congenita, Ambras type

Definition
Congenital hypertrichosis lanuginosa of a distinct pattern with facial dysmorphism

Pathogenesis
Genetic abnormality on chromosome 8 in some patients

Clinical manifestation
Entire body covered with fine long hair, which spares only the palms, soles, and genitalia; shawl-like pattern of excess hair growth over the shoulders; hair of the external auditory canal is long and thick; dental abnormalities; facial dysmorphism

Differential diagnosis
Familial hypertrichosis (normal variant); hypothyroidism; anorexia nervosa; porphyria; mucopolysaccharidoses; GM1 gangliosidosis; medication-induced

Therapy
Laser hair removal; depilatory cream with or without eflornithine 13.9% cream

References
Baumeister FAM, Egger J, Schildhauer MT, Stengel-Rutkowski S (1993) Ambras syndrome: delineation of a unique hypertrichosis universalis congenita and association with a balanced pericentric inversion. Clinical Genetics 44:121–128

Amcinonide

▶ **Corticosteroids, topical, high potency**

Amebiasis

Synonym(s)
Amebic dysentery; intestinal amebiasis

Definition
Protozoal infection caused by the parasite Entamoeba histolytica

Pathogenesis
After colonization of the colonic mucosa, the trophozoite invades intestinal mucosa, thereby gaining access to the circulation, resulting in involvement of the liver, lung, and other sites; genetic susceptibility; factors such as malnutrition, sex, age, and immunocompetence possibly alter the course of the infection

Clinical manifestation
Papules or nodules, which may ulcerate; anogenital location most common cutaneous site; widely disseminated lesions sometimes occur in immunocompromised patients

Differential diagnosis
Inflammatory bowel disease; pyoderma gangrenosum; syphilis; leishmaniasis; chancroid; anogenital carcinoma

Therapy
Metronidazole 750 mg PO three times daily for 10 days; iodoquinol 650 mg PO three times daily for 20 days

References
Torno MS Jr, Babapour R, Gurevitch A, Witt MD (2000) Cutaneous acanthamoebiasis in AIDS. Journal of the American Academy of Dermatology 42(2 Pt 2): 351–354

Amebic dysentery

▶ Amebiasis

American trypanosomiasis

Synonym(s)
Chagas disease; South American trypanosomiasis; New World trypanosomiasis

Definition
Infection due to the flagellate protozoa *Trypanosoma cruzi*, which is transmitted by the feces of blood-sucking insect vectors (reduvid bugs)

Pathogenesis
Epimastigotes invading the skin at bite wound or abrasion; organisms inducing an inflammatory response, cellular lesions, and fibrosis

Clinical manifestation
Red, painful papule or nodule at inoculation site, which sometimes ulcerates (chagoma); conjunctivitis and periorbital edema if the bite is near the eye (Romaña's sign); regional lymphadenopathy
Systemic signs and symptoms 4–12 days after inoculation: fever, headache, malaise, arthralgias, and generalized lymphadenopathy
Chronic phase: congestive heart failure, achalasia, megaesophagus, megacolon

Differential diagnosis
Leishmaniasis; South American blastomycosis; atypical mycobacterial infection; inoculation deep fungal infection; cutaneous tuberculosis; pyoderma

Therapy
Benznidazole 5 mg per kg per day PO divided 2–3 times per day for 60 days

References
Prata A (1994) Chagas' disease. Infectious Disease Clinics of North America 8(1):61–76

Amitriptyline. Dermatologic indications and dosage

Disease	Adult dosage	Child dosage
Burning mouth syndrome	10–25 mg PO daily; increase by 10–15 mg every 2–3 days up to 75 mg daily	Not indicated
Post-herpetic neuralgia	10–25 mg PO daily; increase by 10–15 mg every 2–3 days up to 75 mg daily	Start at 0.1 mg/kg PO daily; increase over 2–3 weeks to 0.5 mg/kg daily

Amitriptyline

Trade name(s)
Elavil; Endep

Generic available
Yes

Drug class
Tricyclic antidepressant

Mechanism of action
Interaction with multiple neurotransmitter sites, including those of norepinephrine and serotonin

Dosage form
10 mg; 25 mg; 50 mg; 75 mg; 100 mg; 150 mg tablet

Dermatologic indications and dosage
See table

Common side effects
Cardiovascular: tachycardia
Cutaneous: dry mouth
Gastrointestinal: increased appetite, constipation
Genitourinary: urinary retention
Neurologic: confusion, dizziness

Serious side effects
Bone marrow: suppression
Neurologic: seizures, cerebrovascular accident

Drug interactions
Acetaminophen/opiate combination drugs; alpha 2 agonists; amphetamines; antiarrhythmics; anticholinergics; other antidepressants; sedating antihistamines

Contraindications/precautions
Hypersensitivity to drug class or component; status immediately post myocardial infarction; MAO inhibitor use within 14 days

References
Tennyson H; Levine N (2001) Neurotropic and psychotropic drugs in dermatology. Dermatologic Clinics 19(1):179–197

Amniotic band syndrome

Synonym(s)
Amniotic constricting band; ADAM complex (amniotic deformity, adhesion, mutilation); Skeeter's syndrome; terminal transverse defects of arm; Streeter's dysplasia

Definition
Defects caused in the limbs or digits by entrapment in fibrous amniotic bands while in utero

Pathogenesis
Fibrous sticky tissues (bands) of the placenta occurring after rupture, entangling the baby, and causing limb anomalies and amputations

Clinical manifestation
Band or indentation around an upper or lower limb or digit; amputation of a digit; facial cleft if band is across the face; abdominal or chest wall defect if band is located there

Differential diagnosis
Genetically-induced congenital anomalies

Therapy
Surgical correction

References
Walter JH Jr, Goss LR, Lazzara AT (1998) Amniotic band syndrome. Journal of Foot & Ankle Surgery 37(4):325–333

Amniotic constricting band

▶ Amniotic band syndrome

Amoxicillin

Trade name(s)
Amoxil; Trimox

Generic available
Yes

Drug class
Penicillins

Mechanism of action
Bacterial cell wall synthesis inhibition

Dosage form
250 mg; 500 mg tablets

Dermatologic indications and dosage
See table

Common side effects
Bone marrow: eosinophilia

Amoxicillin. Dermatologic indications and dosage

Disease	Adult dosage	Child dosage
Acute paronychia	250–500 mg PO 3 times daily for 10 days	250 mg PO 3 times daily for 10 days
Atrophoderma of Pasini and Pierini	250–500 mg PO 3 times daily for 21 days	250 mg PO 3 times daily for 21 days
Cutaneous anthrax	500 mg PO 3 times daily for 7–10 days (60 days in bio terrorism setting	250 mg PO 3 times daily for 7–10 days (60 days in bio terrorism setting)
Glanders	60 mg per kg daily, divided into 3 daily doses for 60–150 days	60 mg per kg daily, divided into 3 daily doses for 60–150 days
Leptospirosis	0.5–1 gm PO 3 times daily for 14–21 days	250–500 mg PO 3 times daily for 14–21 days
Lyme disease	250–500 mg PO 3 times daily for 21 days	20–50 mg per kg PO divided into 3 doses daily for 3 weeks
Melioidosis	60 mg per kg daily, divided into 3 daily doses for 60–150 days	60 mg per kg daily, divided into 3 daily doses for 60–150 days
Pyoderma	250–500 mg PO 3 times daily for 10 days	250 mg PO 3 times daily for 10 days
Salmonellosis	1 gm PO every 8 hours for 10–14 days	250–500 mg PO every 8 hours for 10–14 days

Cutaneous: urticaria or other vascular reaction
Gastrointestinal: nausea and vomiting, diarrhea; elevated liver enzymes

Serious side effects
Bone marrow: suppression
Cutaneous: Stevens-Johnson syndrome, toxic epidermal necrolysis, anaphylaxis
Gastrointestinal: pseudomembranous colitis

Drug interactions
Aminoglycoside antibiotics; allopurinol; oral contraceptives; probenecid; methotrexate

Contraindications/precautions
Hypersensitivity to drug class or component; caution if there is a cephalosporin allergy; caution if patient is suspected of having EB virus infection; caution with impaired renal function

References
Steere AC (1997) Diagnosis and treatment of Lyme arthritis. Medical Clinics of North America 81(1):179–194

Amoxil

▶ Amoxicillin

Ampicillin

Trade name(s)
Omnipen; Principen

Generic available
Yes

Drug class
Penicillins

Mechanism of action
Bacterial cell wall synthesis inhibition

Dosage form
250 mg, 500 mg tablets; 125, 250 mg/5 ml suspension

Dermatologic indications and dosage
See table

Common side effects
Bone marrow: eosinophilia
Cutaneous: urticaria or other vascular reaction
Gastrointestinal: nausea and vomiting, diarrhea, elevated liver enzymes

Serious side effects
Bone marrow: suppression
Cutaneous: Stevens-Johnson syndrome, toxic epidermal necrolysis, anaphylaxis
Gastrointestinal: pseudomembranous colitis

Drug interactions
Aminoglycoside antibiotics; allopurinol; oral contraceptives; probenecid; methotrexate

Contraindications/precautions
Hypersensitivity to drug class or component; caution if there is a cephalosporin allergy; caution if patient is suspected of having EB virus infection; caution with impaired renal function

References
Sadick N (2000) Systemic antibiotic agents. Dermatologic Clinics 19(1):1–21

Amsterdam syndrome

▶ Cornelia de Lange syndrome

Amyloid

▶ Amyloidosis

Ampicillin. Dermatologic indications and dosage

Disease	Adult dosage	Child dosage
Disseminated gonococcal infection	1 gm PO every 6 hours for 7–10 days	500 mg PO every 6 hours for 7–10 days
Pyoderma	250–500 mg PO 4 times daily for 10 days	< 7 years old – 125 mg PO 4 times daily for 10 days

Amyloidosis

Synonym(s)
Amyloid

Definition
Disorder in which insoluble protein fibers are deposited in tissues, causing impaired function

References
Gertz MA, Lacy MQ, Dispenzieri A (1999) Amyloidosis: recognition, confirmation, prognosis, and therapy. Mayo Clinic Proceedings 74(5):490–494

Amyopathic dermatomyositis

▶ Dermatomyositis

Anagen effluvium

Synonym(s)
Chemotherapy-induced alopecia

Definition
Hair loss after any insult to the hair follicle that impairs its mitotic or metabolic activity

Pathogenesis
Inhibition or arrest of cell division in the hair matrix by toxins, resulting in a thin, weakened hair shaft that is susceptible to fracture with minimal trauma or to complete failure of hair formation

Clinical manifestation
Diffuse, non-inflammatory, non-scarring alopecia, which begins 7–14 days after chemotherapy pulse, especially with doxorubicin, the nitrosoureas, and cyclophosphamide

Differential diagnosis
Telogen effluvium; androgenetic alopecia; alopecia mucinosa; traction alopecia; loose anagen syndrome; follicular degeneration syndrome; malnutrition; thyroid disease; diabetes mellitus; Sézary syndrome

Therapy
Minoxidil 5% solution

References
Duvic M, Lemak NA, Valero V, et al. (1996) A randomized trial of minoxidil in chemotherapy-induced alopecia. Journal of the American Academy of Dermatology 35(1):74–78

Anal itching

▶ Pruritus ani

Anaphylactic reaction

▶ Anaphylaxis

Anaphylactoid purpura

▶ Henoch-Schönlein purpura

Anaphylactoid reaction

▶ Anaphylaxis

Anaphylaxis

Synonym(s)
Systemic allergic reaction; anaphylactic reaction; anaphylactoid reaction

Definition
Acute systemic reaction caused by the release of mediators from mast cells and basophils and involving more than one organ system

Pathogenesis
Type I hypersensitivity reaction with mast cell degranulation mediated by antigen binding of specific immunoglobulin E (IgE); released mediators causing smooth muscle spasm in the bronchi and gastrointestinal tract, vasodilation, increased vascular permeability, and stimulation of sensory nerve endings

Clinical manifestation
Cutaneous manifestations: urticaria, angioedema, conjunctival pruritus
Systemic manifestations: tightness, shortness of breath, chest pain, palpitations, syncope, nausea, vomiting, diarrhea

Differential diagnosis
Vasovagal syndrome; mastocytosis; carcinoid syndrome; pheochromocytoma; panic attack

Therapy
Securing of airway; removal of antigenic source, if possible (e.g. bee stinger); tourniquet applied to the extremity with the antigen source, if known; epinephrine 0.3–0.5 mL (0.3–0.5 mg) of 1:1000 solution via subcutaneous or intramuscular route, repeated as needed; diphenhydramine 10–50 mg via either intravenous or intramuscular route every 4 hours as needed; ranitidine 50 mg via either intravenous or intramuscular route every 6–8 hours

References
Ring J, Behrendt H (1999) Anaphylaxis and anaphylactoid reactions. Classification and pathophysiology. Clinical Reviews in Allergy & Immunology 17(4):387–399

Androgenetic alopecia

Synonym(s)
Common baldness; familial baldness; hereditary baldness; male pattern baldness; female pattern baldness; pattern baldness

Definition
Physiologic process in genetically predisposed individuals who develop a patterned scalp hair loss characterized by progressive miniaturization of the follicles and progressive conversion from terminal hair to vellus hair

Pathogenesis
Genetically determined characteristics of hair follicles in the scalp, causing the follicles to be more likely to miniaturize in the presence of androgens, particularly dihydrotestosterone

Clinical manifestation
Progressive, patterned, non-inflammatory, and non-scarring alopecia of the scalp

Differential diagnosis
Telogen effluvium; alopecia areata; anagen effluvium; virilizing disorders in women; thyroid disease; iron deficiency

Therapy
Minoxidil; finasteride (men only)

References
Sinclair RD, Dawber RP (2001) Androgenetic alopecia in men and women. Clinics in Dermatology 19(2):167–178

Anetoderma

Synonym(s)
None

Definition
Localized laxity of the skin with herniation or out-pouching, resulting from abnormal elastic tissues

References
Karrer S, Szeimies RM, Stolz W, Landthaler M (1996) Primary anetoderma in children: report of two cases and literature review. Pediatric Dermatology 13(5):382–385

Angel wing deformity

Definition
Focal destruction of nail matrix in lichen planus, producing central scarred area (pterygium) and peripheral area of preserved nail, simulating angel wings

References
Mirza B, Ashton R (2000) Recognising common nail conditions: a guide. Practitioner 244(1615):873–874, 876–878, 882–883

Angel's kiss

▶ Salmon patch

Angelman syndrome

Synonym(s)
None

Definition
Developmental syndrome of mental retardation, abnormal behavior, and hypopigmentation

Pathogenesis
Chromosomal and molecular changes of the proximal region of chromosome 15

Clinical manifestation
Small stature; developmental delay; no speech; abnormal shape of head; protruding, large tongue; behavioral abnormalities; skin pigment dilution of the skin and eyes

Differential diagnosis
Prader-Willi syndrome; oculocutaneous albinism

Therapy
Sun protection

References
Laan LA, Haeringen A, Brouwer OF (1999) Angelman syndrome: a review of clinical and genetic aspects. Clinical Neurology & Neurosurgery 101(3):161–170

Angio-osteohypertrophy

▶ Klippel-Trenaunay-Weber Syndrome

Angioblastoma

▶ Tufted angioma

Angiocentric lymphoproliferative lesion

▶ Lymphomatoid granulomatosis

Angiodermité de Favre et Chaix

▶ Acroangiodermatitis

Angioedema

Definition
Asymptomatic, non-pitting, and well-circumscribed areas of edema due to increased vascular permeability

References
Kaplan AP (2002) Clinical practice. Chronic urticaria and angioedema. New England Journal of Medicine 346(3):175–179

Angioendotheliomatosis

Synonym(s)
Intravascular lymphomatosis; malignant angioendotheliomatosis; angioendotheliomatosis proliferans systematica; proliferating endotheliosis; angioendo-theliomatosis proliferans; intravascular endothelioma; reactive inflammatory systematized angioendotheliomatosis; reactive angioendotheliomatosis; proliferating systematized endotheliosis

Definition
Benign reactive form: proliferation of cells expressing endothelial cell markers
Malignant form: angiotropic B cell lymphoma

Pathogenesis
Benign reactive form: occlusion of vascular lumina a common feature; associated with systemic infections, paraproteinemias, monoclonal gammopathies, iatrogenic arteriovenous fistulas, antiphospholipid syndrome
Malignant form: vascular occlusion from sludging of the circulating malignant lymphoid cells

Clinical manifestation
Indurated, red, or violaceous papules forming plaques or nodules which may ulcerate; located over the abdominal region, lower extremities, trunk, arms, and face

Differential diagnosis
Angiosarcoma; acroangiodermatitis; tufted angioma; peripheral T-cell lymphoma; cryoglobulinemia; perniosis; vasculitis; bacillary angiomatosis; Kaposi's sarcoma; endovascular papillary angioendothelioma of childhood; angioimmunoblastic lymphadenopathy; angiolymphoid hyperplasia

Therapy
Benign reactive form: no effective therapy
Malignant form: treatment for systemic lymphoma

References
Berger TG. Dawson NA. Angioendotheliomatosis. Journal of the American Academy of Dermatology 18(2 Pt 2):407–412, 1988

Angioendotheliomatosis proliferans

▶ Angioendotheliomatosis

Angioendotheliomatosis proliferans systematica

▶ Angioendotheliomatosis

Angiofibroma

Synonym(s)
Adenoma sebaceum; fibrous papule of the nose and face; pearly penile papules; oral fibroma

Definition
Histologic entity characterized by dermal fibrovascular proliferation

Pathogenesis
Unknown; a cutaneus manifestation of tuberous sclerosis, where it represents a hamartoma

Clinical manifestation
Solitary or multiple firm, discrete, flesh-colored-to-telangiectatic papules

Differential diagnosis
Flat warts; molluscum contagiosum; folliculitis; nevus; basal cell carcinoma; cherry angioma; sarcoidosis; granuloma annulare; acne vulgaris; rosacea; appendageal tumors

Therapy
Shave removal; destruction by electrodesiccation and curettage; laser vaporization; dermabrasion

References
Morelli JG (1998) Use of lasers in pediatric dermatology. Dermatologic Clinics 16(3):489–495

Angioid streak

Definition
Linear, gray or dark red lines with irregular serrated edges lying beneath normal retinal blood vessels, resulting from pathological changes at the level of the Bruch membrane

References
Gurwood AS, Mastrangelo DL (1997) Understanding angioid streaks. Journal of the American Optometric Association 68(5):309–324

Angiokeratoma circumscriptum

Synonym(s)
Corporis circumscriptum naeviforme; angiokeratoma corporis neviform

Definition
Vascular ectasia involving the papillary dermis, producing unilateral hyperkeratotic plaques

Pathogenesis
Unknown mechanism for development, possibly involving altered hemodynamics which produce telangiectatic vessels of the dermis with an overlying reactive epidermal hyperkeratosis

Clinical manifestation
Hyperkeratotic, verrucous, dark red-to-purple, slightly compressible papules or plaques, sometimes in a linear distribution

Differential diagnosis
Angioma corporis diffusum; cherry hemangioma; elastosis perforans serpiginosa; blue

rubber bleb nevus; angioma serpiginosum; lymphangioma circumscriptum; verrucous hemangioma

Therapy
Surgical treatment for cosmesis: surgical excision; flash pump dye or diode laser ablation; destruction by electrodesiccation and curettage; liquid nitrogen cryotherapy

References
Schiller PI, Itin PH (1996) Angiokeratomas: an update. Dermatology 193(4):275–282

Angiokeratoma corporis diffusum

Synonym(s)
Fabry disease; Fabry-Anderson disease; Fabry syndrome

Definition
X-linked, inherited disorder caused by a deficiency of the lysosomal enzyme alpha-galactosidase

Pathogenesis
Defect in the activity of lysosomal alpha-galactosidase, resulting in the storage of two neutral glycosphingolipids, trihexosyl-ceramide and digalactosylceramide; accumulation in many types of cells, including vascular endothelium

Clinical manifestation
Multiple, verrucous, red-to-violaceous papules, with a predilection for the scrotum, penis, lower back, thighs, hips, buttocks, and lips; lesions typically sparing the face, scalp, and ears; progressive neurologic, heart, and kidney disease

Differential diagnosis
Angiokeratoma of the scrotum; adult type beta-galactosidase deficiency; aspartylglucosaminuria; adult onset variant of alpha-N-acetylgalactosaminidase deficiency; fucosidosis; sialidosis

Therapy
No specific therapy for underlying defect; destruction of individual lesions with electrodesiccation and curettage or CO_2 laser vaporization

References
Pastores GM, Lien YH (2002) Biochemical and molecular genetic basis of Fabry disease. Journal of the American Society of Nephrology 13 Suppl 2:S130–133

Angiokeratoma corporis neviform

► Angiokeratoma circumscriptum

Angiokeratoma of Fordyce

► Angiokeratoma of scrotum

Angiokeratoma of Mibelli

Synonym(s)
Naevus a pernione

Definition
Vascular ectasia involving the papillary dermis and producing a hyperkeratotic plaque

Pathogenesis
Unknown

Clinical manifestation
Friable, verrucous, blue-red or gray papule, sometimes with a central crust, occurring in childhood; may involute after minor trauma; associated with acrocyanosis and chilblains

Differential diagnosis
Wart; hemangioma; lymphangioma; pyogenic granuloma; amelanotic melanoma;

seborrheic keratosis; blue rubber bleb nevus

Therapy
Destruction by either liquid nitrogen cryotherapy, electrodessication and curettage, or laser ablation

References
Schiller PI, Itin PH (1996) Angiokeratomas: an update. Dermatology 193(4):275–282

Angiokeratoma of scrotum

Synonym(s)
Angiokeratoma of Fordyce; Fordyce angiokeratoma; angiokeratoma scroti; angiokeratoma of the vulva; angiokeratoma vulvae

Definition
Vascular ectasia involving the papillary dermis and producing unilateral hyperkeratotic papules of the scrotum or vulva

Pathogenesis
Increased venous pressure possible causative factor

Clinical manifestation
Solitary or multiple friable 2–3 mm red-to-blue papules on the scrotum or labia majora

Differential diagnosis
Angiokeratoma corporis diffusum; genital wart; melanoma; pyogenic granuloma; lymphangioma; seborrheic keratosis; blue rubber bleb nevus

Therapy
Destruction by either liquid nitrogen cryotherapy, electrodesiccation and curettage, or laser ablation

References
Schiller PI, Itin PH (1996) Angiokeratomas: an update. Dermatology 193(4):275–282

Angiokeratoma of vulva

► Angiokeratoma of scrotum

Angiokeratoma scroti

► Angiokeratoma of scrotum

Angiokeratoma vulvae

► Angiokeratoma of scrotum

Angiolipoma

Synonym(s)
None

Definition
Benign tumor of subcutaneous fat with an excessive degree of vascular proliferation

Pathogenesis
Unknown

Clinical manifestation
Painful subcutaneous papule or nodule

Differential diagnosis
Lipoma; eccrine spiradenoma; leiomyoma; neuroma; glomus tumor; Dercum's disease; hibernoma; liposarcoma

Therapy
Surgical excision; liposuction

References
Alvi A, Garner C, Thomas W (1998) Angiolipoma of the head and neck. Journal of Otolaryngology 27(2):100–103

Angiolupoid sarcoid

▶ Sarcoidosis

Angiolymphoid hyperplasia with eosinophilia

Synonym(s)
Epithelioid hemangioma; histiocytoid hemangioma; pseudopyogenic granuloma; papular angioplasia; inflammatory angiomatous nodules

Definition
Benign vascular tumor of the head and neck region, often associated with peripheral eosinophilia

Pathogenesis
Unclear, but possibly a reactive process rather than a true neoplasm

Clinical manifestation
Enlarging, dome-shaped, red-to-brown, solitary or multiple papules or nodules, usually in the head and neck area; may be associated with pain or pruritus; peripheral eosinophilia in 20% of cases

Differential diagnosis
Granuloma faciale; hemangioma; lymphoma; pseudolymphoma; Kaposi's sarcoma; angiosarcoma; insect bite reaction; pyogenic granuloma; amelanotic melanoma

Therapy
Surgical excision, to include the arterial and venous segments at the base of the lesion[★]; superificial radiation; intralesional triamcinolone

References
Mariatos G, Gorgoulis VG, Laskaris G, Kittas C (1999) Epithelioid hemangioma (angiolymphoid hyperplasia with eosinophilia) in the oral mucosa. A case report and review of the literature. Oral Oncology 35(4):435–438

Angioma

▶ Hemangioma

Angioma pigmentosum et atrophicum

▶ Xeroderma pigmentosum

Angiosarcoma

Synonym(s)
Malignant angioma; malignant endothelioma

Definition
Malignant neoplasm derived from blood vessels and characterized by rapidly proliferating, extensively infiltrating, anaplastic cells

References
Brown MD (2000) Recognition and management of unusual cutaneous tumors. Dermatologic Clinics 18(3):543–552

Angry back syndrome

Definition
Condition whereby a strongly positive patch test causes increase in the number of positive patch tests at nearby sites

References
Fisher AA (1996) The evolution of the terminology of "crazy" or "angry" back syndrome in

patch testing procedures: Part I. Cutis 58(6):389–390

Anguillulosis

▶ **Strongyloidosis**

Angular cheilitis

Synonym(s)
None

Definition
Inflammation of the skin and mucous membranes of the angles of the mouth

Pathogenesis
Four factors implicated: 1) infections; 2) mechanical factors; 3) nutritional deficiencies; 4) pre-existent skin diseases

Clinical manifestation
Triangular area of erythema, edema, scale, and fissuring at the corners of the mouth; recurrent exudation and crusting; candida a common pathogen

Differential diagnosis
Congenital syphilis; actinic cheilitis

Therapy
Medical: fluconazole; azole antifungal cream; low potency topical corticosteroid; bovine collagen filler injected intradermally to corners of the mouth to restore contour
Non-medical: new dentures to restore facial contour; correction of nutritional deficiencies with multivitamins, etc.

References
Rogers RS 3rd, Bekic M (1997) Diseases of the lips. Seminars in Cutaneous Medicine & Surgery 16(4):328–336

Anhidrosis

Definition
Abnormal lack of sweat in response to heat

References
Leung AK, Cho HY, Choi MC, Chan PY (1999) Hypohidrosis in children. Journal of the Royal Society of Health 119(2):101–107

Anhidrotic ectodermal dysplasia

Synonym(s)
Hypohidrotic ectodermal dysplasia; Christ-Siemens-Touraine syndrome

Definition
Syndrome consisting of anhidrosis or hypohidrosis, defective dentition, and hypotrichosis

Pathogenesis
X-linked disorder, or rarely, autosomal recessive disorder; female carriers mildly affected, possibly because of inactivation of X chromosome

Clinical manifestation
Pyrexia secondary to inadequate sweating; abnormal facies; sparse hair; abnormal nails; skin dryness; markedly dystrophic teeth with early caries

Differential diagnosis
Hidrotic ectodermal dysplasia; Rapp-Hodgkin syndrome; Rosselli-Giulienetti syndrome; ectrodactyly ectodermal dysplasia clefting syndrome

Therapy
Prevention of overheating; regular dental care; emollients for dry skin

References

Vasan N (2000) Management of ectodermal dysplasia in children – an overview. Annals of the Royal Australasian College of Dental Surgeons 15:218–222

Annular

Synonym(s)
None

Definition
Descriptive term of a lesion with an advancing, active margin with central clearing

References

Hsu S, Le EH, Khoshevis MR (2001) Differential diagnosis of annular lesions. American Family Physician 64(2):289–296

Annular elastolytic giant-cell granuloma

▶ Actinic granuloma

Anogenital verrucous carcinoma

▶ Giant condyloma of Buschke and Löwenstein

Anogenital wart

▶ Condyloma acuminatum

Anonychia

Definition
Absence of nails from birth

References

Al Hawsawi K, Al Aboud K, Alfadley A, Al Aboud D (2002) Anonychia congenita totalis: a case report and review of the literature. International Journal of Dermatology 41(7):397–399

Anthralin

Trade name(s)
Anthro-derm; Drithocreme; Dritho-Scalp; Micanol

Generic available
Yes

Drug class
Antimitotic; immunomodulator

Mechanism of action
May work by stimulating monocyte pro-inflammatory activity and/or through antimitotic effects that result from inhibition of DNA synthesis; induces extracellular free radicals

Dosage form
0.1%, 0.25%, 0.5%, 1% cream and ointment;

Dermatologic indications and dosage
See table

Common side effects
Cutaneous: skin irritation; allergic contact dermatitis; erythema
Miscellaneous: discoloration of skin, hair, and nails; staining of clothing, sinks, bathtubs, and furniture

Serious side effects
None

Anthralin. Dermatologic indications and dosage

Disease	Adult dosage	Child dosage
Alopecia areata	Apply for 30 minutes; wash off with warm water without soap; start at low concentration (0.1–0.25%) and titrate upward as tolerated	Apply for 30 minutes; wash off with warm water without soap; start at low concentration (0.1–0.25%) and titrate upward as tolerated
Psoriasis	Apply for 30 minutes; wash off with warm water without soap; start at low concentration (0.1–0.25%) and titrate upward as tolerated	Apply for 30 minutes; wash off with warm water without soap; start at low concentration (0.1–0.25%) and titrate upward as tolerated

Drug interactions
None

Contraindications/precautions
Hypersensitivity to drug class or component; avoid heating lesions on the face, intertriginous areas; use with caution on inflamed skin; to minimize discoloration, rinse the bath/shower with hot water immediately after washing/showering and then use a suitable cleanser to remove any deposit on the surface of the bath or shower

References
Lebwohl M, Ali S (2001) Treatment of psoriasis. Part 1. Topical therapy and phototherapy. Journal of the American Academy of Dermatology 45(4):487–498

Anthrax, cutaneous

Synonym(s)
Malignant pustule; woolsorter's disease; black bane; charbon; murrain; black blood

Definition
Skin disease resulting from exposure to the spores of *Bacillus anthracis*

Pathogenesis
Cutaneous invasion by Bacillus anthracis; may gain access through microscopic or gross breaks in the skin; may occur after handling sick animals or contaminated wool, hair, or animal hides

Clinical manifestation
1–7 days (usually 2–5) incubation period after skin exposure; starts as pruritic papule that enlarges in 24–48 hours to form an ulcer, evolves into a black eschar, and lasts for 7–14 days before separating and leaving a permanent scar; regional lymphadenopathy, which may be present for weeks after the ulceration heals

Differential diagnosis
Bubonic plague; tularemia; syphilis; staphylococcal pyoderma; cat-scratch disease; cowpox; North American blastomycosis; sporotrichosis; atypical mycobacterial infection; orf; milker's nodule; leishmaniasis

Therapy
Penicillin*; doxycycline; ciprofloxacin; amoxicillin

References
Tutrone WD, Scheinfeld NS, Weinberg JM (2002) Cutaneous anthrax: a concise review. Cutis 69(1):27–33

Anticardiolipin antibody syndrome

▶ **Antiphospholipid syndrome**

Anticardiolipin syndrome

▶ Antiphospholipid syndrome

Antihistamines, first generation

Trade name(s)
Generic names in parentheses:
Benadryl, Dermarest, Sominex (diphenhydramine); Pyribenzamine (tripelennamine); Periactin (cyproheptadine); Phenergan (promethazine); Chlor-Trimeton, Comtrex (chlorpheniramine); Polaramine (dexchlorpheniramine); Atarax, Vistaril (hydroxyzine); Dimetane (brompheniramine); Sinequan (doxepin)

Generic available
Yes

Drug class
Antihistamine

Mechanism of action
Competitive inhibitor of histamine at H-1 receptor site

Dosage form
Tablet; elixir; capsule; syrup

Dermatologic indications
See table

Common side effects
Dermatologic: dry mouth
Neurologic: ataxia, dizziness, headache, agitation
Gastrointestinal: diarrhea

Serious side effects
Neurologic: dyskinesia, seizures
Respiratory: wheezing

Drug interactions
Anticholinergics; antidepressants; antipsychotics; barbiturates; opiates; sedative hypnotics

Other interactions
Ethanol

Contraindications/precautions
Hypersensitivity to drug class or component; pregnancy, first trimester; caution in asthmatics

References
Greaves MW (2001) Antihistamines. Dermatologic Clinics 19(1):53–62

Antihistamines, second generation

Trade name(s)
Generic names in parentheses:
Allegra (fexofenadine); Claritin (loratadine); Clarinex (desloratadine); Zyrtec (cetirizine)

Generic available
Yes

Drug class
Antihistamine

Mechanism of action
Competitive inhibitor of histamine at H-1 receptor site

Dosage form
Tablet; capsule; syrup

Dermatologic indications and dosage
See table

Common side effects
Cutaneous: dry mouth

Antihistamines, first generation. Dermatologic indications and dosage

Disease	Adult dosage	Child dosage
Atopic dermatitis	Diphenhydramine 25–50 mg at bedtime for sedation; hydroxyzine 10–25 mg PO at bedtime for sedation. Doxepin 10–50 mg PO at bedtime for sedation	Diphenhydramine 10–25 mg at bedtime for sedation; hydroxyzine 10–25 mg PO at bedtime for sedation. Doxepin 10–25 mg PO at bedtime for sedation
Autoerythrocyte sensitization syndrome	Diphenhydramine 25–50 mg PO 4 times daily; hydroxyzine 10–25 mg PO 4 times daily	Diphenhydramine 5 mg per kg PO daily, divided into 4 doses; hydroxyzine 10–25 mg PO 4 times daily. Doxepin 10–25 mg PO at bedtime for sedation
Cercarial dermatitis	Diphenhydramine 25–50 mg at bedtime for sedation; hydroxyzine 10–25 mg PO at bedtime for sedation. Doxepin 10–50 mg PO at bedtime for sedation	Diphenhydramine 10–25 mg at bedtime for sedation; hydroxyzine 10–25 mg PO at bedtime for sedation. Doxepin 10–25 mg PO at bedtime for sedation
Dermatographism	Diphenhydramine 25–50 mg PO 4 times daily; hydroxyzine 10–25 mg PO 4 times daily. Doxepin 10–50 mg PO at bedtime for sedation	Diphenhydramine 5 mg per kg PO daily, divided into 4 doses; hydroxyzine 10–25 mg PO 4 times daily. Doxepin 10–25 mg PO at bedtime for sedation
Erythema infectiosum	Diphenhydramine 25–50 mg at bedtime for sedation; hydroxyzine 10–25 mg PO at bedtime for sedation. Doxepin 10–50 mg PO at bedtime for sedation	Diphenhydramine 10–25 mg at bedtime for sedation; hydroxyzine 10–25 mg PO at bedtime for sedation. Doxepin 10–25 mg PO at bedtime for sedation
Erythema multiforme	Diphenhydramine 25–50 mg at bedtime for sedation; hydroxyzine 10–25 mg PO at bedtime for sedation. Doxepin 10–50 mg PO at bedtime for sedation	Diphenhydramine 10–25 mg at bedtime for sedation; hydroxyzine 10–25 mg PO at bedtime for sedation. Doxepin 10–25 mg PO at bedtime for sedation
Insect bite reaction	Diphenhydramine 25–50 mg at bedtime for sedation; hydroxyzine 10–25 mg PO at bedtime for sedation. Doxepin 10–50 mg PO at bedtime for sedation	Diphenhydramine 10–25 mg at bedtime for sedation; hydroxyzine 10–25 mg PO at bedtime for sedation. Doxepin 10–25 mg PO at bedtime for sedation

Antihistamines, first generation. Dermatologic indications and dosage (Continued)

Disease	Adult dosage	Child dosage
Lichen simplex chronicus	Diphenhydramine 25–50 mg at bedtime for sedation; hydroxyzine 10–25 mg PO at bedtime for sedation. Doxepin 10–50 mg PO at bedtime for sedation	Diphenhydramine 10–25 mg at bedtime for sedation; hydroxyzine 10–25 mg PO at bedtime for sedation. Doxepin 10–25 mg PO at bedtime for sedation
Mastocytosis	Diphenhydramine 25–50 mg PO 4 times daily; hydroxyzine 10–25 mg PO 4 times daily. Doxepin 10–50 mg PO at bedtime for sedation	Diphenhydramine 5 mg per kg PO daily, divided into 4 doses; hydroxyzine 10–25 mg PO 4 times daily. Doxepin 10–25 mg PO at bedtime for sedation
Pruritus	Diphenhydramine 25–50 mg at bedtime for sedation; hydroxyzine 10–25 mg PO at bedtime for sedation. Doxepin 10–50 mg PO at bedtime for sedation	Diphenhydramine 10–25 mg at bedtime for sedation; hydroxyzine 10–25 mg PO at bedtime for sedation. Doxepin 10–25 mg PO at bedtime for sedation
Seabather's eruption	Diphenhydramine 25–50 mg at bedtime for sedation; hydroxyzine 10–25 mg PO at bedtime for sedation. Doxepin 10–50 mg PO at bedtime for sedation	Diphenhydramine 10–25 mg at bedtime for sedation; hydroxyzine 10–25 mg PO at bedtime for sedation. Doxepin 10–25 mg PO at bedtime for sedation
Serum sickness	Diphenhydramine 25–50 mg PO 4 times daily; hydroxyzine 10–25 mg PO 4 times daily. Doxepin 10–50 mg PO at bedtime for sedation	Diphenhydramine 5 mg per kg PO daily, divided into 4 doses; hydroxyzine 10–25 mg PO 4 times daily. Doxepin 10–25 mg PO at bedtime for sedation
Uremic pruritus	Diphenhydramine 25–50 mg at bedtime for sedation; hydroxyzine 10–25 mg PO at bedtime for sedation. Doxepin 10–50 mg PO at bedtime for sedation	Diphenhydramine 10–25 mg at bedtime for sedation; hydroxyzine 10–25 mg PO at bedtime for sedation. Doxepin 10–25 mg PO at bedtime for sedation
Urticaria	Diphenhydramine 25–50 mg PO 4 times daily; hydroxyzine 10–25 mg PO 4 times daily. Doxepin 10–50 mg PO at bedtime for sedation	Diphenhydramine 5 mg per kg PO daily, divided into 4 doses; hydroxyzine 10–25 mg PO 4 times daily. Doxepin 10–25 mg PO at bedtime for sedation

Antihistamines, first generation. Dermatologic indications and dosage (Continued)

Disease	Adult dosage	Child dosage
Xerosis with pruritus	Diphenhydramine 25–50 mg at bedtime for sedation; hydroxyzine 10–25 mg PO at bedtime for sedation. Doxepin 10–50 mg PO at bedtime for sedation	Diphenhydramine 10–25 mg at bedtime for sedation; hydroxyzine 10–25 mg PO at bedtime for sedation. Doxepin 10–25 mg PO at bedtime for sedation

Gastrointestinal: nausea, diarrhea
Neurologic: somnolence, fatigue, dizziness, agitation, headache

Serious side effects
Respiratory: hypersensitivity reaction, bronchospasm

Drug interactions
Anticholinergics; antidepressants; antipsychotics; barbiturates; opiates; sedative hypnotics

Other interactions
Ethanol

Contraindications/precautions
Hypersensitivity to drug class or component; caution in patients with impaired renal or liver function

References
Greaves MW (2001) Antihistamines. Dermatologic Clinics 19(1):53–62

Antiphospholipid antibody syndrome

▶ Antiphospholipid syndrome

Antiphospholipid syndrome

Synonym(s)
Antiphospholipid antibody syndrome; anticardiolipin syndrome; anticardiolipin antibody syndrome

Antihistamines, second generation. Dermatologic indications and dosage

Disease	Adult dosage	Child dosage
Dermatographism	Fexofenadine 180 mg PO daily; loratadine 10 mg PO daily; desloratadine 5 mg PO daily; cetirizine 10 mg PO daily	Fexofenadine 30 mg PO twice daily; loratadine 5 mg PO daily; cetirizine 2.5 mg PO daily
Mastocytosis	Fexofenadine 180 mg PO daily; loratadine 10 mg PO daily; desloratadine 5 mg PO daily; cetirizine 10 mg PO daily	Fexofenadine 30 mg PO twice daily; loratadine 5 mg PO daily; cetirizine 2.5 mg PO daily
Urticaria	Fexofenadine 180 mg PO daily; loratadine 10 mg PO daily; desloratadine 5 mg PO daily; cetirizine 10 mg PO daily	Fexofenadine 30 mg PO twice daily; loratadine 5 mg PO daily; cetirizine 2.5 mg PO daily

Definition
Disorder characterized by recurrent, venous or arterial thrombosis and/or fetal losses associated with antibodies directed against membrane anionic phospholipids (i.e. anticardiolipin [aCL] antibody, antiphosphatidylserine) or their associated plasma proteins, predominantly beta-2 glycoprotein I (apolipoprotein H), or evidence of a circulating anticoagulant

Pathogenesis
Unclear mechanism, possibly representing a defect in cellular apoptosis, that exposes membrane phospholipids to the binding of various coagulation proteins, which subsequently become the target of autoantibodies; hypercoagulable state resulting in clinical signs and symptoms of disease

Clinical manifestation
History of deep vein thrombosis (DVT), pulmonary embolism, acute ischemia, myocardial infarction, or CVA, often at an early age; frequent miscarriages or premature births; livedo reticularis; superficial thrombophlebitis; leg ulcers; painful purpura; splinter hemorrhages

Differential diagnosis
Endocarditis; disseminated intravascular coagulation; thrombotic thrombocytopenic purpura; hypercoagulable state from other causes such as malignancy; atherosclerotic vascular disease; multiple cholesterol emboli; systemic necrotizing vasculitis

Therapy
Elimination of risk factors, such as oral contraceptives, smoking, hypertension, and hyperlipidemia; aspirin 81 mg PO per day; warfarin: 2–15 mg PO per day; enoxaparin: 1 mg per kg subcutaneously twice daily

References
Gharavi AE (2001) Anticardiolipin syndrome: antiphospholipid syndrome. Clinical Medicine 1(1):14–17

Apert's syndrome

▶ Acrocephalosyndactyly

Aphthae

▶ Aphthous stomatitis

Aphthous stomatitis

Synonym(s)
Aphthae; recurrent aphthous stomatitis; recurrent aphthous ulcers; canker sores; periadenitis mucosa necrotica recurrens

Definition
Benign mouth lesion, presenting as a painful white or yellow ulceration

Pathogenesis
Possible inherited predisposition; possible immune system dysfunction; trauma (dental procedures or aggressive tooth cleaning) precipitates lesions

Clinical manifestation
Aphthae minor: recurrent, discrete, painful, shallow ulcers measuring from 3 mm to < 1 cm occurring on the labial and buccal mucosa and the floor of the mouth; lesions heal without scarring within 7–10 days
Aphthae major: oval-shaped ulcers from 1–3 cm in diameter; multiple lesions often present simultaneously; healing takes up to 6 weeks

Differential diagnosis
Oral cancer; contact dermatitis; erythema multiforme; herpes simplex virus infection; hand-foot-and-mouth disease; lichen planus; lupus erythematosus; pemphigus vulgaris; paraneoplastic pemphigus; Reiter

syndrome; syphilis; traumatic ulceration; drug reaction; Behçet's disease; cyclic neutropenia

Therapy
Topical therapy: Kaopectate applied to ulcer 3–4 times per day; Zilactin gel applied 4–5 times per day; high potency topical corticosteroids; viscous Xylocaine applied as needed; amlexanox 5% paste applied 4 times daily; tetracycline suspension (250 mg capsule contents suspended in 5 ml of water) applied to mouth or genital ulcers 4 times daily
Systemic therapy (used mostly for aphthae major): thalidomide; prednisone; colchicine; azathioprine

References
Porter SR, Hegarty A, Kaliakatsou F, Hodgson TA, Scully C (2000) Recurrent aphthous stomatitis. Clinics in Dermatology 18(5):569–578

Aplasia cutis congenita

Synonym(s)
Congenital ulcer of the newborn; congenital localized absence of skin; Streeter's spots; transient bullous dermolysis of newborn

Definition
Localized, congenital absence of a portion of skin

Pathogenesis
Unclear cause; possibly embryonic arrest in local skin development or intrauterine vascular abnormality or intrauterine trauma; hereditary factors possibly operative

Clinical manifestation
Stellate, linear, or oval, sharply demarcated ulceration, atrophic scar, or bulla, most often over the posterior scalp; multiple lesions occurring over the extremities, trunk, and buttocks; spontaneous healing in 1–3 months; with underlying bony defects, healing in many months

Differential diagnosis
Iatrogenic injury from scalp electrode, etc.; congenital varicella; focal dermal hypoplasia; epidermolysis bullosa; Volkmann's ischemic contracture

Therapy
Surgical reconstruction only for large, nonhealing defects

References
Kruk-Jeromin J, Janik J, Rykala J (1998) Aplasia cutis congenita of the scalp. Report of 16 cases. Dermatologic Surgery 24(5):549–553

Apocrine acne

▶ Hidradenitis suppurativa

Apocrine adenoma

▶ Hidradenoma papilliferum

Apocrine bromhidrosis

▶ Bromhidrosis

Apocrine cystadenoma

▶ Apocrine hidrocystoma

Apocrine hidrocystoma

Synonym(s)
Apocrine cystadenoma; apocrine retention cyst

Definition
Tumor consisting of a cystic proliferation of apocrine secretory glands

Pathogenesis
May be adenomatous cystic proliferation of the apocrine glands

Clinical manifestation
Asymptomatic, solitary, translucent papule or nodule, with a predilection for the eyelid, particularly the inner canthus; cyst containing thin, clear, brownish fluid

Differential diagnosis
Eccrine hidrocystoma; basal cell carcinoma; epidermoid cyst; syringoma; milium

Therapy
Incision and drainage, followed by surgical destruction of the cyst wall by light electrodesiccation and curettage or CO_2 laser vaporization; punch, shave, or elliptical excision

References
Schleicher SM (1998) Multiple translucent facial papules. Apocrine hidrocystoma. Archives of Dermatology 134(12):1627-1628, 1630–1631

Apocrine miliaria

▶ Fox-Fordyce disease

Apocrine poroma

▶ Poroma

Apocrine retention cyst

▶ Apocrine hidrocystoma

Apocrinitis

▶ Hidradenitis suppurativa

Aquagenic pruritus

Synonym(s)
None

Definition
Rare genetic skin disorder causing pruritus upon contact with water or sudden temperature changes

Pathogenesis
Elevated histamine levels during attacks; increased acetyl cholinesterase activity in nerve fibers innervating sweat glands

Clinical manifestation
Intense pruritus, with a pricking quality, which occurs immediately after bathing or swimming; provocation in some patients with change in ambient temperature; symptoms last for 1 hour and may flare with emotional or physical stress; no associated skin signs

Differential diagnosis
Aquagenic urticaria; polycythemia vera-associated pruritus; xerosis-induced pruritus

Therapy
Photochemotherapy; UVB phototherapy; antihistamines, first generation; alkalinization of bath water; intramuscular triamcinolone

References
du Peloux Menage H, Greaves MW (1995) Aquagenic pruritus. Seminars in Dermatology 14(4):313–316

Aquagenic urticaria

Synonym(s)
None

Definition
Rare form of physical urticaria involving hives caused by contact with water

Pathogenesis
Sometimes occurring in patients with dermatographism; acetylcholine and histamine may be mediators

Clinical manifestation
Small urticarial wheals within minutes of contact with either fresh or sea water

Differential diagnosis
Aquagenic pruritus; dermatographism; cold urticaria; cholinergic urticaria

Therapy
Antihistamines, first generation; photochemotherapy; UVB phototherapy

References
Luong KV, Nguyen LT (1998) Aquagenic urticaria: report of a case and review of the literature. Annals of Allergy, Asthma, & Immunology 80(6):483–485

Aqua glycolic lotion

▶ **Alpha hydroxy acids**

Arachnidism

▶ **Brown recluse spider bite**

Arachnodactyly

Definition
Condition involving abnormally long and slender hands and fingers, and often feet and toes may also have similar findings

References
Pyeritz RE (2000) The Marfan syndrome. Annual Review of Medicine 51:481–510

Argyria

Synonym(s)
Argyrosis

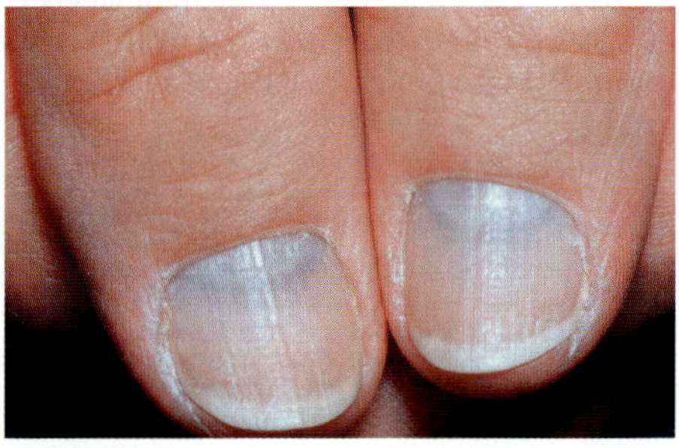

Argyria. Blue lunulae on the thumbs

Definition
Dyspigmentation secondary to silver deposition in the skin

Pathogenesis
Pigmentation secondary to silver deposition in the dermis; metal-induced stimulation of melanogenesis in the epidermis; source of the silver via the oral route or through the skin after topical application

Clinical manifestation
Diffuse, slate-gray pigmentation of the gingiva and oral mucosa, sun-exposed skin, sclera, and nails

Differential diagnosis

Cyanosis; diffuse melanosis from metastatic melanoma; hyperpigmentation from other drugs, such as minocycline, gold, or phenothiazine derivative

Therapy

Discontinuation of exposure to silver; avoidance of sun exposure; chelating agents such as dimercaprol (BAL)

References

Humphreys SD, Routledge PA (1998) The toxicology of silver nitrate. Adverse Drug Reactions & Toxicological Reviews 17(2–3):115–143

Argyrosis

▶ Argyria

Arrid XX

▶ Aluminium chlorohydrate

Arsenical keratosis

Synonym(s)
None

Definition
Punctate keratoses of the palms and soles, occurring after long-term exposure to inorganic trivalent form of arsenic

Pathogenesis
Inorganic arsenic retained in the body for long periods after exposure, because of poor detoxification mechanisms; affecting many enzymes by combining with sulfhydryl groups; acting as a cancer promoter, through its action on chromosomes

Clinical manifestation

Punctate, non-tender, hard, yellowish, often symmetric, corn-like papules, mainly on the palms and soles; pressure points commonly involved; sometimes coalescing to form large, verrucous plaques

Differential diagnosis

Keratosis palmaris et plantaris; clavus; wart; nevoid basal cell carcinoma syndrome; porokeratosis; psoriasis of the palms and soles; lichen planus; Darier disease; Bazex syndrome; pityriasis rubra pilaris

Therapy

Acitretin; destructive modalities such as electrosurgery, liquid nitrogen cryotherapy, and laser vaporization

References

Yerebakan O, Ermis O, Yilmaz E, Basaran E (2002) Treatment of arsenical keratosis and Bowen's disease with acitretin. International Journal of Dermatology 41(2):84–87

Arteriovenous malformation

▶ Vascular malformation

Arteritis cranialis

▶ Temporal arteritis

Arteritis of the aged

▶ Temporal arteritis

Arteritis temporalis

▶ Temporal arteritis

Arthritis urethritica

▶ Reiter syndrome

Ascher syndrome

▶ Ascher's syndrome

Ascher's syndrome

Synonym(s)
Ascher syndrome; double lip and nontoxic thyroid enlargement syndrome; struma-double lips syndrome; thyroid blepharochalasis syndrome; Fuchs' syndrome III; Laffer-Ascher syndrome

Definition
Disorder consisting of blepharochalasis, double lip, and non-toxic goiter

Pathogenesis
Unknown

Clinical manifestation
Blepharochalasis (excessive upper lid skin); duplication of the upper lip; euthyroid goiter

Differential diagnosis
Grave's disease; angioedema

Therapy
Surgical correction of excess eyelid skin and lip

References
Sanchez MR, Lee M, Moy JA, Ostreicher R (1993) Ascher syndrome: a mimicker of acquired angioedema. Journal of the American Academy of Dermatology 29(4):650–651

Ash-leaf macule

Definition
Sharply circumscribed, round-to-oval area of macular hypopigmentation seen at birth in patients with tuberous sclerosis

References
Arbuckle HA, Morelli JG (2000) Pigmentary disorders: update on neurofibromatosis-1 and tuberous sclerosis. Current Opinion in Pediatrics 12(4):354–358

Ashy dermatosis

Synonym(s)
Ashy dermatosis of Ramirez; erythema dyschromicum perstans; dermatosis cenicienta; erythema chronicum figuratum melanodermicum; lichen pigmentosus

Definition
Eruption of gray-blue macules over the trunk; closely linked to lichen planus

Pathogenesis
Unknown

Clinical manifestation
Asymptomatic, gray-blue patches of variable shape and size, distributed symmetrically on the face, trunk, and upper extremities; elevated, erythematous border in the early stages; oral cavity and genitals spared

Differential diagnosis
Lichen planus; lichenoid drug eruption; tuberculoid leprosy; pinta; hemochromatosis

Therapy
Clofazimine 100 mg PO every other day if under 40 kg in weight; clofazimine 100 mg every day if greater than 40 kg in weight; ultraviolet exposure; ultraviolet avoidance; antibiotics; antihistamines; psychotherapy

References
Osswald SS, Proffer LH, Sartori CR (2001) Erythema dyschromicum perstans: a case report and review. Cutis 68(1):25–28

Ashy dermatosis of Ramirez

▶ Ashy dermatosis

Asteatosis

Synonym(s)
Dry skin; xerosis; winter itch

Definition
Irritation caused by lack of moisture in the skin

Pathogenesis
Physiologic process with aging; seen more often in the winter, with cold air outside and heated air inside causing a decrease in humidity

Clinical manifestation
Generalized pruritus, often worse after bathing; most common on the lower legs, arms, flanks, and thighs; may be associated with mild erythema and scaliness

Differential diagnosis
Other causes of generalized pruritus: scabies; atopic dermatitis; drug reaction; obstructive hepatobiliary disease; end-stage renal disease; polycythemia vera; Hodgkin's disease; thyroid disease; hyperparathyroidism; psychogenic pruritus

Therapy
Decreased bathing; use of soap substitutes such as bath gels; application of emollients at least twice daily during the winter months; antihistamines, first generation, for nighttime sedation

▶ Xerosis

References
Beacham BE (1993) Common dermatoses in the elderly. American Family Physician 47(6):1445–1450

Asteatotic dermatitis

▶ Asteatotic eczema

Asteatotic eczema

Synonym(s)
Asteatotic dermatitis; eczema craquelé; eczema craquelatum; xerotic eczema; eczema hiemalis; eczema fendille; etat craquelé

Definition
Pruritic, cracked, and fissured skin occurring most commonly on the shins of elderly patients, caused by lack of moisture in the skin

Pathogenesis
Physiologic process with aging; seen more often in the winter, with cold air outside and heated air inside causing a decrease in humidity; loss of water by stratum corneum causing cells to shrink and creating fine fissures; eczematous changes resulting from patients rubbing and scratching these pruritic areas

Clinical manifestation
Minimally scaly, red, cracked, and or fissured skin, giving the appearance of a "cracked pot"; most commonly involving

the pretibial areas, but also the thighs, hands and trunk; generalized pruritus, often worse after bathing

Differential diagnosis
Ichthyosis; atopic dermatitis; nummular eczema; stasis dermatitis; contact dermatitis; mycosis fungoides; other causes of generalized pruritus: scabies; atopic dermatitis; drug reaction; obstructive hepatobiliary disease; end-stage renal disease; polycythemia vera; Hodgkin's disease; thyroid disease; hyperparathyroidism; psychogenic pruritus

Therapy
Decreased bathing; use of soap substitutes such as bath gels; application of emollients at least twice daily during the winter months; mid potency topical corticosteroid ointment; antihistamines, first generation, for nighttime sedation

References
Beacham BE (1993) Common dermatoses in the elderly. American Family Physician 47(6):1445–1450

Ataxia-telangiectasia

Synonym(s)
Louis-Bar syndrome; Boder-Sedgwick syndrome

Definition
Autosomal, recessive, multisystem disorder characterized by progressive neurological impairment, cerebellar ataxia, variable immunodeficiency, impaired organ maturation, x-ray hypersensitivity, ocular and cutaneous telangiectasia, and a predisposition to malignancy

Pathogenesis
Unclear; possibly associated with dysregulation of the immunoglobulin gene superfamily, which includes genes for T-cell receptors; abnormal sensitivity to x-rays and certain radiomimetic chemicals, possibly leading to chromosomal abnormalities, infections, and malignancies

Clinical manifestation
Ocular and cutaneous telangiectasia; neurological abnormalities, mainly ataxia, abnormal eye movements, and choreoathetosis

Differential diagnosis
Telangiectatic diseases: hereditary hemorrhagic telangiectasia; chronic liver disease; benign essential telangiectasia; sun damage; neurologic disorders; Friedreich disease; cerebral palsy; familial spinocerebellar atrophies; GM1 and GM2 gangliosidoses; progressive rubella panencephalitis; subacute sclerosing panencephalitis; postinfectious encephalomyelitis; cerebellar tumor

Therapy
No effective therapy

References
Gatti RA (1995) Ataxia-telangiectasia. Dermatologic Clinics 13(1):1–6

Atheroma

▶ Epidermoid cyst

Athlete's feet

▶ Tinea pedis

Atopic dermatitis

Synonym(s)
Atopic eczema; infantile eczema; Besnier's prurigo

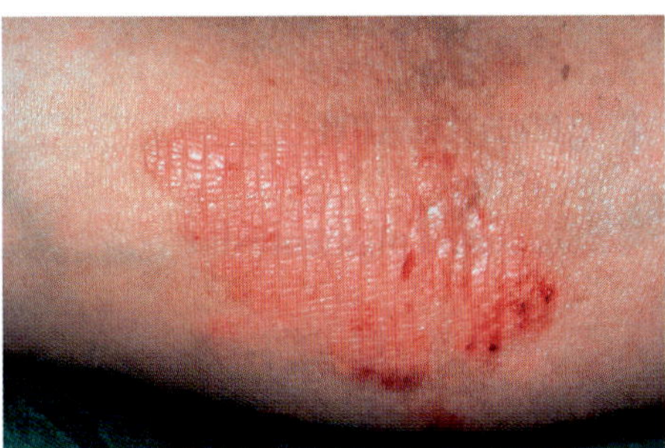

Atopic dermatitis. Lichenified, red plaque with erosions in the antecubital fossa

Definition
Disease starting in early infancy and characterized by pruritus, eczematous lesions, dry skin, and an association with other atopic diseases (asthma, allergic rhinitis, urticaria)

Pathogenesis
Abnormality of T helper type 2 (TH2) cells, resulting in increased production of interleukin 4 (IL-4) and increased IgE; stratum corneum lipid defect, leading to increased transepidermal water loss

Clinical manifestation
Marked pruritus, often starting in the first few months of life; asthma or hay fever or a history of atopic disease in a first-degree relative; dry skin; lichenified plaques with epithelial disruption, occurring on the face in infancy, in the flexural creases, trunk, and diaper area by 1 year of age, and over the distal extremities later in life; scalp involvement, usually after age 3 months

Differential diagnosis
Seborrheic dermatitis; contact dermatitis; stasis dermatitis; nummular eczema; scabies; mycosis fungoides; dermatophytosis

Therapy
Mid potency topical corticosteroids★; prednisone for temporary therapy of severe flares; pimecrolimus 1% cream; tacrolimus 0.3% or 1% ointment; azathioprine; cyclosporine; antihistamines, first generation, for nighttime sedation UVB phototherapy; photochemotherapy (PUVA); evening primrose oil; Chinese herbs; emollients applied at least twice daily, particularly during the winter months

References
Tofte SJ, Hanifin JM (2001) Current management and therapy of atopic dermatitis. Journal of the American Academy of Dermatology 44(1 Suppl):S13–16

Atopic eczema

▶ **Atopic dermatitis**

Atopy

Synonym(s)
None

Definition
Predisposition to develop allergic reactions, often genetically determined and involving the production of IgE antibodies

References
MacLean JA, Eidelman FJ (2001) The genetics of atopy and atopic eczema. Archives of Dermatology 137(11):1474–1476

Atrofodermia idiopatica progressiva

▶ **Atrophoderma of Pasini and Pierini**

Atrophic parapsoriasis

▶ **Large plaque parapsoriasis**

Atrophie brilliante

▶ Confluent and reticulated papillo-matosis

Atrophoderma of Pasini and Pierini

Synonym(s)
Idiopathic atrophoderma of Pasini and Pierini; atrophodermia idiopatica progressiva

Definition
Asymptomatic atrophy of the skin characterized by single or multiple, defined, depressed areas of skin

Pathogenesis
Possibly an end result of morphea; possibly related to spirochete infection (in Europe)

Clinical manifestation
Presenting as asymptomatic, slightly erythematous plaque or plaques on the trunk; lesions developing slate-gray to brown pigmentation, sharp peripheral border, and central depression

Differential diagnosis
Morphea; lichen sclerosus; skin atrophy from steroid injection; anetoderma; post-inflammatory hyperpigmentation

Therapy
Doxycycline; amoxicillin; hyperpigmentation component: Q-switched alexandrite laser

References
Buechner SA, Rufli T (1994) Atrophoderma of Pasini and Pierini. Clinical and histopathologic findings and antibodies to Borrelia burgdorferi in thirty-four patients. Journal of the American Academy of Dermatology 30(3):441–446

Atrophoderma pigmentosum

▶ Xeroderma pigmentosum

Atrophoderma reticulatum

▶ Keratosis pilaris atrophicans

Atrophoderma vermiculatum

▶ Keratosis pilaris atrophicans
▶ Ulerythema ophryogenes

Atypical fibroxanthoma

Synonym(s)
Paradoxical fibrosarcoma; pseudosarcoma; pseudosarcomatous reticulohistiocytoma; pseudosarcomatous dermatofibroma

Definition
Rapidly enlarging tumor, arising in chronically sun-exposed skin, with histologic features suggesting a malignant connective tissue neoplasm, but usually benign clinical course

Pathogenesis
Solar radiation and prior X-irradiation possible predisposing factors

Clinical manifestation
Firm, solitary, eroded or ulcerated papule or nodule on sun-exposed skin, particularly the ear, nose, and cheek; most common in elderly patients

Differential diagnosis

Squamous cell carcinoma; pyogenic granuloma; melanoma; basal cell carcinoma; Merkel cell carcinoma; cutaneous metastasis; leiomyosarcoma; dermatofibrosarcoma protuberans

Therapy

Mohs micrographic surgery[*]; elliptical excision; destruction by electrodesiccation and curettage

References

Davis JL, Randle HW, Zalla MJ, Roenigk RK, Brodland DG (1997) A comparison of Mohs micrographic surgery and wide excision for the treatment of atypical fibroxanthoma. Dermatologic Surgery 23(2):105–110

Atypical lipoma

▶ Liposarcoma

Atypical lipomatous tumors

▶ Liposarcoma

Atypical melanocytic nevus

▶ Atypical mole

Atypical mole

Synonym(s)

Active junctional nevus; atypical melanocytic nevus; B-K mole, Clark's nevus; atypical mole syndrome; dysplastic mole; dysplastic nevus

Definition

Benign melanocytic growth, possibly sharing some of the clinical or microscopic features of melanoma, but not a melanoma

Pathogenesis

Genetic component in some patients (melanoma-prone families; familial atypical mole syndrome); sunlight exposure possibly a factor

Clinical manifestation

Variable features, with some or all of the following: asymmetrical conformation; irregular border which can fade imperceptibly into the surrounding skin; variable coloration, with shades of tan, brown, black; and red; diameter > 6 mm; elevated center and feathered, flat border, giving the lesion the appearance of a fried egg

Differential diagnosis

Melanoma; compound nevus; seborrheic keratosis; dermatofibroma; wart

Therapy

Avoidance of excessive sun exposure; use of sunscreen with a sun protective factor of 15 or greater; evaluation of other family members for evidence of atypical moles; baseline photographs of entire skin surface, if possible

References

Slade J, Marghoob AA, Salopek TG, Rigel DS, Kopf AW, Bart RS (1995) Atypical mole syndrome: risk factor for cutaneous malignant melanoma and implications for management. Journal of the American Academy of Dermatology 32(3):479–494

Atypical mole syndrome

▶ Atypical mole

Audry's glands

▶ Fordyce's disease

Auranofin

Trade name(s)
Ridaura

Generic available
No

Drug class
Anti-rheumatic

Mechanism of action
Inhibition of complement and lysosomal enzymes; normalization of defective Langerhans cell antigen presentation

Dosage form
3 mg tablet

Dermatologic indications and dosage
See table

Common side effects
Cutaneous: skin eruption, stomatitis, pruritus, glossitis
Gastrointestinal: diarrhea, abdominal pain
Laboratory: anemia, leukopenia, proteinuria
Neurologic: change in taste sensation
Ocular: keratitis

Serious side effects
Bone marrow: agranulocytosis
Neurologic: seizures
Pulmonary: pneumonitis
Renal: renal failure, nephrotic syndrome

Drug interactions
Atovaquone/proguanil

Auranofin. Dermatologic indications and dosage

Disease	Adult dosage	Child dosage
Cicatricial pemphigoid	3 mg PO twice daily	Initial: 0.1 mg per kg daily in 1–2 divided doses; usual maintenance: 0.15 mg/kg/day in 1–2 divided doses; maximum: 0.2 mg/kg/day in 1–2 divided doses
Epidermolysis bullosa acquisita	3 mg PO twice daily	Initial: 0.1 mg per kg daily; usual maintenance: 0.15 mg/kg/day in 1–2 divided doses; maximum: 0.2 mg/kg/day in 1–2 divided doses
Lupus erythematosus	3 mg PO twice daily	Initial: 0.1 mg per kg daily in 1–2 divided doses; usual maintenance: 0.15 mg/kg/day in 1–2 divided doses; maximum: 0.2 mg/kg/day in 1–2 divided doses
Pemphigus vulgaris	3 mg PO twice daily	Initial: 0.1 mg per kg daily in 1–2 divided doses; usual maintenance: 0.15 mg/kg/day in 1–2 divided doses; maximum: 0.2 mg/kg/day in 1–2 divided doses

Contraindications/precautions
Hypersensitivity to drug class or component; pulmonary fibrosis; bone marrow aplasia; caution with impaired liver or renal function

References
Papp KA, Shear NH (1991) Systemic gold therapy. Clinics in Dermatology 9(4):535–551

Auriculotemporal syndrome

Synonym(s)
Frey's syndrome; Baillarger's syndrome; Dupuy's syndrome; salivosudoriparous syndrome; sweating gustatory syndrome; gustatory sweating

Definition
Gustatory sweating secondary to auriculotemporal nerve injury

Pathogenesis
Misdirection of parasympathetic fibers, which migrate into the postganglionic sympathetic fibers to innervate the sweat glands

Clinical manifestation
Flushing or sweating on one side of the face when certain foods are eaten

Differential diagnosis
Gustatory sweating from diabetic neuropathy or post-herpetic neuralgia; Horner's syndrome; lacrimal sweating; harlequin syndrome

Therapy
Surgical: tympanic neurectomy for severe symptoms; perineural alcohol injection
Medical: scopolamine 3–5% cream applied twice daily; aluminium chloride

▶ Gustatory sweating

References
Kaddu S, Smolle J, Komericki P, Kerl H (2000) Auriculotemporal (Frey) syndrome in late childhood: an unusual variant presenting as gustatory flushing mimicking food allergy. Pediatric Dermatology 17(2):126–128

Aurothioglucose

Trade name(s)
Solganol

Generic available
No

Drug class
Anti-rheumatic

Mechanism of action
Inhibition of complement and lysosomal enzymes; normalization of defective Langerhans cell antigen presentation

Dosage form
Intramuscular injection

Dermatologic indications and dosage
See table

Common side effects
Cutaneous: stomatitis, glossitis, skin eruption, pruritus
Gastrointestinal: diarrhea, abdominal pain, dyspepsia, change in taste sensation
Laboratory: proteinuria, anemia, leukopenia
Neurologic: change in taste sensation
Ocular: keratitis

Serious side effects
Laboratory: agranulocytosis
Neurologic: seizures
Pulmonary: pneumonitis
Renal: renal failure, nephrotic syndrome

Drug interactions
Atovaquone/proguanil

Aurothioglucose. Dermatologic indications and dosage

Disease	Adult dosage	Child dosage
Cicatricial pemphigoid	25–50 mg IM once weekly	Initial – 0.25 mg per kg per dose first week; increment at 0.25 mg per kg per dose increasing with each weekly dose; maintenance – 0.75–1 mg per kg per dose weekly, not to exceed 25 mg per dose
Epidermolysis bullosa acquisita	25–50 mg IM once weekly	Initial – 0.25 mg per kg per dose first week; increment at 0.25 mg per kg per dose increasing with each weekly dose; maintenance – 0.75–1 mg per kg per dose weekly, not to exceed 25 mg per dose
Lupus erythematosus; pemphigus vulgaris; cicatricial pemphigoid; epidermolysis bullosa acquisita	25–50 mg IM once weekly	Initial – 0.25 mg per kg per dose first week; increment at 0.25 mg per kg per dose increasing with each weekly dose; maintenance – 0.75–1 mg per kg per dose weekly, not to exceed 25 mg per dose
Pemphigus vulgaris	25–50 mg IM once weekly	Initial – 0.25 mg per kg per dose first week; increment at 0.25 mg per kg per dose increasing with each weekly dose; maintenance – 0.75–1 mg per kg per dose weekly, not to exceed 25 mg per dose

Contraindications/precautions

Hypersensitivity to drug class or component; pulmonary fibrosis; bone marrow aplasia; caution with impaired liver or renal function

References

Papp KA, Shear NH (1991) Systemic gold therapy. Clinics in Dermatology 9(4):535–551

Auspitz sign

Definition

Bleeding points appearing when overlying scale removed physically from a lesion of psoriasis

References

Bernhard JD (1997) Clinical pearl: auspitz sign in psoriasis scale. Journal of the American Academy of Dermatology 36(4):621

Autoeczematization

▶ Id reaction

Autoerythrocyte sensitization

▶ Autoerythrocyte sensitization syndrome

Autoerythrocyte sensitization syndrome

Synonym(s)
Gardner-Diamond syndrome; autoerythrocyte sensitization; psychogenic purpura; purpura autoerythrocytica

Definition
Purpuric disorder in women, characterized by painful ecchymotic patches, unrelated to vascular or clotting abnormalities

Pathogenesis
Possibly an immune-mediated reaction; psychological issues in the patients possibly the main causative factor

Clinical manifestation
Painful ecchymoses, often appearing after minor trauma, usually over the extremities and trunk; lesions appearing in crops, and lasting for weeks to months

Differential diagnosis
Anaphylactoid purpura; Ehlers-Danlos syndrome; child abuse; factitial purpura; amyloidosis; thrombotic thrombocytopenic purpura; solar purpura; leukemia

Therapy
Medroxyprogesterone acetate 10 mg PO per day or 150 mg intramuscularly once per month; prednisone; antihistamines, first generation

References
Berman DA, Roenigk HH, Green D (1992) Autoerythrocyte sensitization syndrome (psychogenic purpura). Journal of the American Academy of Dermatology 27(5 Pt 2):829–832

Autoimmune alopecia

▶ **Alopecia areata**

Autoimmune dermatosis of pregnancy

▶ **Herpes gestationis**

Autosensitization

▶ **Id reaction**

Autosomal dominant ichthyosis

▶ **Ichthyosis vulgaris**

Autumnal fever

▶ **Leptospirosis**

Axillary freckling

Definition
Brown macules in the axillary vault, present in more than 90 percent of people with neurofibromatosis, type 1

References
Wainer S (2002) A child with axillary freckling and cafe au lait spots. Canadian Medical Association Journal 167(3):282–283

Azathioprine

Trade name(s)
Imuran

Azathioprine. Dermatologic indications and dosage

Disease	Adult dosage	Child dosage
Atopic dermatitis	2–3 mg per kg PO daily	2–3 mg per kg PO daily
Behçet's disease	Corticosteroid sparing function; 2–3 mg per kg PO daily	Corticosteroid sparing function; 2–3 mg per kg PO daily
Bullous pemphigoid	Corticosteroid sparing function; 2–3 mg per kg PO daily	Corticosteroid sparing function; 2–3 mg per kg PO daily
Chronic actinic dermatitis	Corticosteroid sparing function; 2–3 mg per kg PO daily	Corticosteroid sparing function; 2–3 mg per kg PO daily
Cicatricial pemphigoid	Corticosteroid sparing function; 2–3 mg per kg PO daily	Corticosteroid sparing function; 2–3 mg per kg PO daily
Fogo selvagem	2–3 mg per kg PO daily	2–3 mg per kg PO daily
Leukocytoclastic vasculitis	Corticosteroid sparing function; 2–3 mg per kg PO daily	Corticosteroid sparing function; 2–3 mg per kg PO daily
Lupus erythematosus, acute	Corticosteroid sparing function; 2–3 mg per kg PO daily	Corticosteroid sparing function; 2–3 mg per kg PO daily
Mixed connective tissue disease	2–3 mg per kg PO daily	2–3 mg per kg PO daily
Paraneoplastic pemphigus	Corticosteroid sparing function; 2–3 mg per kg PO daily	Corticosteroid sparing function; 2–3 mg per kg PO daily
Pemphigus foliaceus	2–3 mg per kg PO daily	2–3 mg per kg PO daily
Pemphigus vulgaris	Corticosteroid sparing function; 2–3 mg per kg PO daily	Corticosteroid sparing function; 2–3 mg per kg PO daily
Persistent light reaction	Corticosteroid sparing function; 2–3 mg per kg PO daily	Corticosteroid sparing function; 2–3 mg per kg PO daily
Polyarteritis nodosa	Corticosteroid sparing function; 2–3 mg per kg PO daily	Corticosteroid sparing function; 2–3 mg per kg PO daily
Pyoderma gangrenosum	Corticosteroid sparing function; 2–3 mg per kg PO daily	Corticosteroid sparing function; 2–3 mg per kg PO daily
Relapsing polychondritis	2–3 mg per kg PO daily	2–3 mg per kg PO daily
Sarcoidosis	2–3 mg per kg PO daily	2–3 mg per kg PO daily
Sulzberger-Garbe syndrome	2–3 mg per kg PO daily	2–3 mg per kg PO daily
Weber-Christian disease	2–3 mg per kg PO daily	2–3 mg per kg PO daily
Wegener's granulomatosis	Corticosteroid sparing function; 2–3 mg per kg PO daily	Corticosteroid sparing function; 2–3 mg per kg PO daily

Generic available
Yes

Drug class
Antimetabolite; immunosuppressant

Mechanism of action
Active metabolite is purine analog, which inhibits DNA and RNA synthesis and has immunosuppressive activity

Dosage form
50 mg tablet

Dermatologic indications and dosage
See table

Common side effects
Cutaneous: alopecia, skin eruption
Gastrointestinal: nausea and vomiting, diarrhea, dyspepsia
Laboratory: elevated liver enzymes

Serious side effects
Cutaneous: hypersensitivity reaction
Gastrointestinal: hepatotoxicity, pancreatitis
Immune: immunosuppression
Neoplastic: increased risk of neoplasm, particularly lymphoma

Drug interactions
ACE inhibitors; allopurinol; cisplatin; cytotoxic chemotherapeutic agents; interferon alfa 2a; interferon beta; mycophenolate mofetil; warfarin; zidovudine

Contraindications/precautions
Hypersensitivity to drug class or component; pregnancy; caution if patient has low levels or lacks thiopurine methyltransferase (measure enzyme level before starting therapy); caution if impaired liver function

References
Silvis NG (2001) Antimetabolites and cytotoxic drugs. Dermatologic Clinics 19(1):105–118

Azelaic acid

A

Trade name(s)
Azelex; Finacea

Generic available
No

Drug class
Anti-acne; anti-rosacea

Mechanism of action
May be related to antimicrobial effects

Dosage form
15% cream, 20% cream

Dermatologic indications and dosage
See table

Common side effects
Cutaneous: pruritus, burning sensation, dryness, skin eruption

Serious side effects
None

Drug interactions
None

Contraindications/precautions
Hypersensitivity to drug class or component

Azelaic acid. Dermatologic indications and dosage

Disease	Adult dosage	Child dosage
Acne vulgaris	Apply twice daily	Apply twice daily
Melasma	Apply twice daily	Apply twice daily
Postinflammatory hyperpigmentation	Apply twice daily	Apply twice daily
Rosacea	Apply twice daily	Apply twice daily

References

Nguyen QH, Bui TP (1995) Azelaic acid: pharmacokinetic and pharmacodynamic properties and its therapeutic role in hyperpigmentary disorders and acne. International Journal of Dermatology 34(2):75–84

Azithromycin

Trade name(s)
Zithromax

Generic available
No

Drug class
Macrolide antibiotic

Mechanism of action
Inhibits protein synthesis of sensitive bacterial organisms

Dosage form
250 mg, 500 mg tablet; powder for oral suspension

Dermatologic indications and dosage
See table

Common side effects
Cutaneous: skin eruption, vaginitis
Gastrointestinal: nausea, vomiting, abdominal pain, diarrhea, anorexia

Serious side effects
Cutaneous: anaphylaxis, Stevens-Johnson syndrome, toxic epidermal necrolysis
Gastrointestinal: pseudomembranous colitis, cholestatic jaundice

Drug interactions
Antacids; oral contraceptives; warfarin; digoxin

Azithromycin. Dermatologic indications and dosage

Disease	Adult dosage	Child dosage
Bacillary angiomatosis	500 mg PO on day 1; 250 mg PO on days 2–5	Not indicated in those < 45 kg in weight; 500 mg PO on day 1; 250 mg PO on days 2–5
Bartonellosis	500 mg PO on day 1; 250 mg PO on days 2–5	Not indicated in those < 45 kg in weight; 500 mg PO on day 1; 250 mg PO on days 2–5
Cellulitis	500 mg PO on day 1; 250 mg PO on days 2–5	Not indicated in those < 45 kg in weight; 500 mg PO on day 1; 250 mg PO on days 2–5
Chancroid	1 gm PO for 1 dose	Not indicated in those < 45 kg in weight; 20 mg per kg PO for 1 dose
Ecthyma	500 mg PO on day 1; 250 mg PO on days 2–5	Not indicated in those < 45 kg in weight; 500 mg PO on day 1; 250 mg PO on days 2–5
Furuncle	500 mg PO on day 1; 250 mg PO on days 2–5	Not indicated in those < 45 kg in weight; 500 mg PO on day 1; 250 mg PO on days 2–5
Impetigo	500 mg PO on day 1; 250 mg PO on days 2–5	Not indicated in those < 45 kg in weight; 500 mg PO on day 1; 250 mg PO on days 2–5
Trench fever	250-500 mg PO for 4 weeks	Not indicated in those < 45 kg; 250 mg PO daily for 4 weeks

Azole antifungal agents. Dermatologic indications and dosage

Disease	Adult dosage	Child dosage
Angular cheilitis	Apply twice daily for 2–4 weeks	Apply twice daily for 2–4 weeks
Cutaneous candidiasis	Apply twice daily for 2–4 weeks	Apply twice daily for 2–4 weeks
Majocchi granuloma	Apply twice daily for 4–8 weeks	Apply twice daily for 4–8 weeks
Onychomycosis	Apply twice daily for 2–4 weeks	Apply twice daily for 2–4 weeks
Tinea corporis	Apply twice daily for 2–4 weeks	Apply twice daily for 2–4 weeks
Tinea cruris	Apply twice daily for 2–4 weeks	Apply twice daily for 2–4 weeks
Tinea faciei	Apply twice daily for 2–4 weeks	Apply twice daily for 2–4 weeks
Tinea nigra	Apply twice daily for 2–4 weeks	Apply twice daily for 2–4 weeks
Tinea pedis	Apply twice daily for 2–4 weeks	Apply twice daily for 2–4 weeks
Tinea versicolor	Apply twice daily for 2–4 weeks	Apply twice daily for 2–4 weeks
White piedra	Apply twice daily for 2–4 weeks	Apply twice daily for 2–4 weeks

Contraindications/precautions

Hypersensitivity to drug class or component; caution in those with impaired liver function; do not use concomitantly with terfenadine or astemizole

References

Alvarez-Elcoro S, Enzler MJ (1999) The macrolides: erythromycin, clarithromycin, and azithromycin. Mayo Clinic Proceedings 74(6):613–634

Azole antifungal agents

Trade name(s)

Generic in parentheses:
Exelderm (sulconazole); Lamisil AT (terbinafine); Lotrimin; Mycelex (clotrimazole); Micatin (miconazole); Nizoral (ketoconazole); Oxistat (oxiconazole); Spectazole (econazole)

Generic available

Yes

Drug class

Azole antifungal agents

Mechanism of action

Cell wall ergosterol inhibition secondary to blockade of 14α-demethlyation of lanosterol

Dosage form

Cream; solution; lotion

Dermatologic indications and dosage

See table

Common side effects

Cutaneous: skin eruption, pruritus

Serious side effects

None

Drug interactions

None

Contraindications/precautions

Hypersensitivity to drug class or component

References

Weinstein A, Berman B (2002) Topical treatment of common superficial tinea infections. American Family Physician 65(10):2095–2102

Azul

▶ Pinta

B-K mole

▶ Atypical mole

Bacillary ailuronosis

▶ Bacillary angiomatosis

Bacillary angiomatosis

Synonym(s)
Epithelioid angiomatosis; bartonellosis; bacillary ailuronosis; disseminated cat-scratch disease

Definition
Infection caused by closely related gram-negative bacteria, Bartonella henselae and Bartonella quintana, occurring mostly in immunocompromised patients

Pathogenesis
Gram-negative bacillary infection results from exposure to flea-infested cats with *B* henselae and the human body louse for *B* quintana

Clinical manifestation
Globular angiomatous papules or nodules resembling pyogenic granulomas; violaceous nodules resembling Kaposi's sarcoma; lichenoid violaceous plaques; subcutaneous papules or nodules, with or without ulceration

Differential diagnosis
Kaposi's sarcoma; glomangioma; verruga peruana; angiokeratoma; hemangioma; pyogenic granuloma; gram-positive bacterial abscess; nodal myofibromatosis; melanoma

Therapy
Erythromycin*; azithromycin; clarithromycin; doxycycline

References
Manders SM (1996) Bacillary angiomatosis. Clinics in Dermatology 14(3):295–299

Bacillary peliosis

▶ Bartonellosis

Bacitracin

Trade name(s)
Bacitracin as single agent: Baciguent; bacitracin as one component of a multi-agent preparation: Betadine antibiotic ointment; Gold Bond Triple Action; Mycitracin; Neosporin; Polysporin; Spectrocin Plus

Bacitracin. Dermatologic indications and dosage

Disease	Adult dosage	Child dosage
Impetigo	Apply twice per day for 7 days	Apply twice per day for 7 days
Postoperative wound infection prophylaxis	Apply twice per day for 7 days	Apply twice per day for 7 days

Generic available
Yes

Drug class
Antibiotic

Mechanism of action
Inhibits bacterial cell wall synthesis

Dosage form
Cream; ointment

Dermatologic indications and dosage
See table

Common side effects
Cutaneous: contact dermatitis

Serious side effects
None

Drug interactions
None

Contraindications/precautions
Hypersensitivity to drug class or component

References
Bass, JW, Chan DS, Creamer KM, Thompson MW, Malone FJ, Becker TM, Marks SN (1997) Comparison of oral cephalexin, topical mupirocin and topical bacitracin for treatment of impetigo. Pediatric Infectious Disease Journal 16(7):708–710

Bagdad boil

▶ **Leishmaniasis, cutaneous**

Baillarger's syndrome

▶ **Auriculotemporal syndrome**

Balanitis

Synonym(s)
Balanoposthitis

Definition
Inflammation of the foreskin and head of the penis

References
Bunker CB (2001) Topics in penile dermatology. Clinical & Experimental Dermatology 26(6):469–479

Balanitis circumscripta plasmacellularis

▶ **Zoon balanitis**

Balanitis xerotica obliterans

Synonym(s)
Lichen sclerosus of the penis; male genital lichen sclerosus; lichen sclerosus et atrophicus of the penis; penile lichen sclerosus

Definition
Chronic, progressive, sclerosing, inflammatory dermatosis of the penis and prepuce

Pathogenesis
Unknown; minor relationship with autoimmune disorders

Clinical manifestation
Presents with soreness, burning sensation, mild erythema and hypopigmentation; as disease progresses, single or multiple discrete erythematous papules or macules coalescing into atrophic ivory, white, or purple-white patches or plaques, which may erode; possible development of vesiculation; possible phimosis occurring in uncircumcised men; occasional signs of lichen sclerosus at other skin sites

Differential diagnosis
Plasma cell balanitis; candidiasis; lichen planus; psoriasis; vitiligo; Reiter syndrome; erythroplasia of Queyrat

Therapy
Surgical therapy: circumcision; laser vaporization
Medical therapy: superpotent topical corticosteroids; testosterone propionate 1% ointment applied twice daily; acitretin

▶ **Lichen sclerosus**

References
Das S, Tunuguntla HS (2000) Balanitis xerotica obliterans – A review. World Journal of Urology 18(6):382–387

Balanoposthitis

▶ **Balanitis**

Baldness

▶ **Alopecia**

Bamboo hair

▶ **Trichorrhexis invaginata**

Bancroftian filariasis

▶ **Filariasis**

Bannayan syndrome

▶ **Bannayan-Riley-Ruvalcaba syndrome**

Bannayan-Riley-Ruvalcaba syndrome

Synonym(s)
Bannayan-Zonana syndrome; Riley-Smith syndrome; Ruvalcaba-Myhre syndrome; Ruvalcaba-Myhre-Smith syndrome; Bannayan syndrome; Cowden/Bannayan-Riley-Ruvalcaba overlap syndrome; PTEN hamartoma tumor syndrome; macrocephaly; pseudopapilledema; multiple hemangiomata syndrome; multiple lipomas

Definition
Disease characterized by hamartomatous polyps of the small and large intestine, macrocephaly, lipomas, hemangiomas, thyroid abnormalities, and freckling of the penis

Pathogenesis
Autosomal dominant inheritance; mutation in the tumor suppressor gene, PTEN

Clinical manifestation
Hamartomatous polyps of the small and large intestine; macrocephaly; lipomas; hemangiomas; thyroid abnormalities; penile freckling; developmental delay; increased risk for both benign and malignant tumors

Differential diagnosis
Cowden's syndrome; Gardner's syndrome; multiple lentigines syndrome

Therapy
Increased breast, thyroid, and colon cancer surveillance; surgical excision of lipomas and hemangiomas for cosmetic purposes only

References
Fargnoli MC, Orlow SJ, Semel-Concepcion J, Bolognia JL (1996) Clinicopathologic findings in the Bannayan-Riley-Ruvalcaba syndrome. Archives of Dermatology 132(10):1214–1218

Bannayan-Zonana syndrome

▶ Bannayan-Riley-Ruvalcaba syndrome

Barber's itch

▶ Sycosis barbae

Barber-Say syndrome

Synonym(s)
Say syndrome

Definition
Disease entity consisting of hypertrichosis, xerosis, cutis laxa, dysmorphic facial features, and eye changes

Pathogenesis
Autosomal recessive inheritance

Clinical manifestation
Hypertrichosis over the upper trunk and face; xerosis; generalized cutis laxa; macrostomia; opacification of the corneas; variable nystagmus

Differential diagnosis
Cone-rod congenital amaurosis; ablepharon-macrostomia syndrome; Turner's syndrome; Brachmann-de Lange syndrome; Sanfilippo syndrome; Hunter's syndrome; leprechaunism

Therapy
No effective therapy

References
Martinez Santana S, Perez Alvarez F, Frias JL, Martinez-Frias ML (1993) Hypertrichosis, atrophic skin, ectropion, and macrostomia (Barber-Say syndrome): report of a new case. American Journal of Medical Genetics 47(1):20–23

Barlow's disease

Synonym(s)
Möller-Barlow disease; Barlow's syndrome; Cheadle-Möller-Barlow syndrome; Moeller's disease; infantile scurvy; vitamin C deficiency syndrome

Definition
Vitamin C deficiency disease in children, manifested by gingival lesions, hemorrhage, arthralgia, loss of appetite, and listlessness

Pathogenesis
Vitamin C deficiency, after at least 3 months of severe or total lack of vitamin C, resulting in defective collagen synthesis and defective folic acid and iron utilization

Clinical manifestation
Perifollicular hyperkeratotic papules, surrounded by a hemorrhagic halo; hairs twisted like corkscrews and possibly fragmented; submucosal gingival bleeding, subperiosteal hemorrhage, arthralgia; anorexia; listlessness; exophthalmos and conjunctival hemorrhage; poor wound healing

Differential diagnosis
Vasculitis; child abuse; coagulation abnormalities with leukemia; platelet abnormalities, etc.; deep vein thrombosis; thrombophlebitis

Therapy
Ascorbic acid 150–300 mg per day for 1 month

References
Ghorbani AJ, Eichler C (1994) Scurvy. Journal of the American Academy of Dermatology 30(5 Pt 2):881–883

Barlow's syndrome

▶ Barlow's disease

Barraquer-Simons disease

▶ Progressive lipodystrophy

Barraquer-Simons syndrome

▶ Progressive lipodystrophy

Bartonellosis

Synonym(s)
Cat scratch disease; catscratch disease; trench fever; urban trench fever; bacillary peliosis; Parinaud oculoglandular syndrome; Parinaud's oculoglandular syndrome; Oroya fever; Carrión disease; Carrión's disease; verruga peruana; benign lymphoreticulosis

Definition
Infections caused by species belonging to the bacterial genus Bartonella

Pathogenesis
Bartonella henselae found in association with both domestic and feral cats and presumably passed from cat to human; Bartonella quintana spread via human body louse

Clinical manifestation
Cat scratch disease: papule or pustule developing 5–10 days after exposure; fever; malaise; lymphadenopathy
Oroya fever (verruga peruana): onset of fever 3–12 weeks after a sand fly bite; crops of small papules enlarging and healing by fibrosis over several months

Differential diagnosis
Lymphoma; leukemia; deep fungal infection; tuberculosis; plague; lymphogranuloma venereum; AIDS; syphilis; dengue fever; malaria; babesiosis

Therapy
Doxycycline; erythromycin; azithromycin; clarithromycin

▶ Bacillary angiomatosis

References
Maguina C, Gotuzzo E (2000) Bartonellosis: new and old. Infectious Disease Clinics of North America 14(1):1–22

Bart's syndrome

Synonym(s)
None

Definition
Subtype of dominant dystrophic epidermolysis bullosa with congenital localized absence of skin, nail abnormalities, and blistering

Pathogenesis
Mutation of the COLA7A1 gene, resulting in the production of poorly formed anchoring fibrils at the skin's basement membrane zone

Clinical manifestation
Congenital erosions of the lower extremities, which heal with hairless scars; trauma-induced blistering; absent or dystrophic nails; mucous membrane erosions only in early life

Differential diagnosis
Aplasia cutis congenita; epidermolysis bullosa simplex; junctional epidermolysis bullosa; child abuse

Therapy
Hydrocolloid dressings to erosions; petrolatum between toes to minimize scarring

References
Amichai B, Metzker A (1994) Bart's syndrome. International Journal of Dermatology 33(3):161–163

Basal cell carcinoma

Synonym(s)
Basal cell epithelioma; basalioma; Jacob's ulcer; rodent ulcer

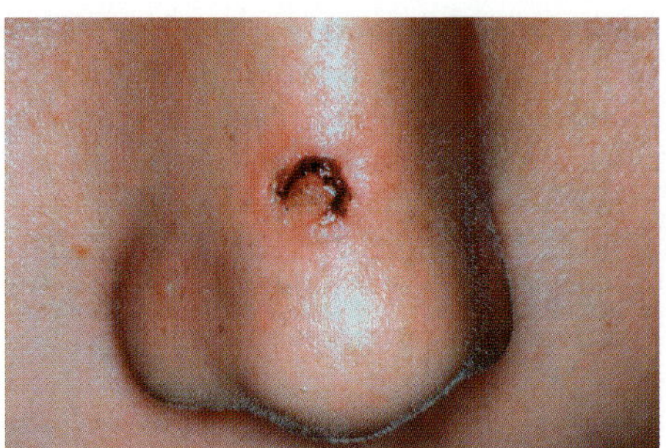

Basal cell carcinoma. Papule with rolled margins and central erosion on the nasal bridge

Definition
Cutaneous neoplasm arising from pluripotential cells of the epidermis or its appendages

Pathogenesis
Early, intense sun exposure possibly causing p53 tumor suppressor gene mutations, allowing unrestricted proliferation

Clinical manifestation
Nodular variant: pearly, translucent papule with central depression, erosion, or ulceration; rolled borders; telangiectasia on the surface
Pigmented variant: flecks of gray or blue pigment in addition to features described for nodular variant
Superficial variant: pink-to-brown, scaly plaque or papule, often with annular configuration
Morpheaform variant: poorly demarcated, sclerotic plaque or papule

Differential diagnosis
Squamous cell carcinoma; nevus; fibrous papule; wart; appendage tumor; seborrheic keratosis; sebaceous gland hyperplasia; Bowen's disease

Therapy
Primary tumor in anatomically insensitive sites: destruction by electrodesiccation and curettage; elliptical excision; cryotherapy; orthovoltage radiation therapy; fluorouracil cream

Recurrent tumor or tumors in anatomically sensitive sites: Mohs micrographic surgery[*]

References

Thissen MR, Neumann MH, Schouten LJ (1999) A systematic review of treatment modalities for primary basal cell carcinomas. Archives of Dermatology 135(10):1177–1183

Basal cell epithelioma

▶ Basal cell carcinoma

Basal cell nevus syndrome

Synonym(s)

Nevoid basal cell carcinoma syndrome; Gorlin syndrome; Gorlin-Goltz syndrome; bifid-rib basal-cell nevus syndrome

Definition

Inherited group of defects involving the skin, nervous system, eyes, endocrine glands, and bones, producing an unusual facial appearance and a predisposition for skin cancers

Pathogenesis

Chromosomal mutation of the PTC gene, a tumor suppressor gene; inactivation of this gene associated with development of basal cell carcinoma, other tumors, and developmental errors

Clinical manifestation

Pitting of the palms or soles; multiple basal cell carcinomas, often early in life; jaw cysts; cleft palate; coarse facies with milia, frontal bossing, widened nasal bridge, and mandibular prognathia; strabismus; dystrophic canthorum; ocular hypertelorism; calcification of the falx cerebri; spine and rib abnormalities; high arched eyebrows and palate; kidney anomalies; hypogonadism in males

Differential diagnosis

Non-syndromic basal cell carcinoma; Bazex syndrome; linear unilateral basal cell nevus with comedones; Rasmussen syndrome; Rombo syndrome

Therapy

Medical therapy: fluorouracil cream; isotretinoin; radiation therapy
Surgical therapy: primary tumor in anatomically insensitive sites – destruction by electrodesiccation and curettage; elliptical excision; cryotherapy; fluorouracil cream; recurrent tumor or those in anatomically sensitive sites: Mohs micrographic surgery[*]

References

Gorlin RJ (1987) Nevoid basal-cell carcinoma syndrome. Medicine 66(2):98–113

Basal cell papilloma

▶ Seborrheic keratosis

Basalioma

▶ Basal cell carcinoma

Basan syndrome

Synonym(s)

Ectodermal dysplasia absent dermatoglyphics

Definition

Autosomal dominant syndrome consisting of ectodermal dysplasia, absent dermatoglyphic pattern, nail abnormalities, and a simian crease

Pathogenesis

Inherited; mutation site unknown

Clinical manifestation
Thin skin; simian crease; multiple dental caries; absent or decreased eyebrows; nail dystrophy; sparse or absent scalp hair; decreased sweating; photophobia; absent dermatoglyphic pattern

Differential diagnosis
Anhidrotic ectodermal dysplasia; hidrotic ectodermal dysplasia; focal dermal hypoplasia; Down's syndrome; progeria

Therapy
No effective therapy

References
Masse JF, Perusse R (1994) Ectodermal dysplasia. Archives of Disease in Childhood 71(1):1–2

Bather's itch

▶ Cercarial dermatitis

Bazin's disease

▶ Nodular vasculitis

Beals' arachnodactyly

▶ Beals-Hecht syndrome

Beals' syndrome

▶ Beals-Hecht syndrome

Beals-Hecht syndrome

Synonym(s)
Beals' arachnodactyly; Beals' syndrome; Hecht-Beals syndrome; congenital contractural arachnodactyly syndrome

Definition
Heritable disorder of connective tissue, present from birth, combining features of Marfan's syndrome with arthrogryposis

Pathogenesis
Unknown; autosomal dominant inheritance

Clinical manifestation
Multiple, congenital, joint contractures; arachnodactyly; dolichostenomelia; kyphoscoliosis; changes of the ear muscle, producing crumpled-appearing ears

Differential diagnosis
Marfan's syndrome; Stickler's syndrome

Therapy
None

References
Jones JL, Lane JE, Logan JJ, Vanegas ME (2002) Beals-Hecht syndrome. Southern Medical Journal 95(7):753–755

Bean syndrome

▶ Blue rubber bleb nevus syndrome

Bean-Walsh angioma

▶ Venous lake

Beau's lines

Definition
Transverse grooves or lines seen on finger-nails following systemic illness, local trauma, or skin disease involving the fingertips

References
De Berker D (1994) What do Beau's lines mean? International Journal of Dermatology 33(8):545–546

Becker melanosis

▶ Becker's nevus

Becker nevus

▶ Becker's nevus

Becker pigmented hairy nevus

▶ Becker's nevus

Becker's nevus

Synonym(s)
Becker melanosis; Becker nevus; Becker's pigmented hairy nevus; Becker pigmented hairy nevus; nevus spilus tardus; pigmented hairy epidermal nevus

Definition
Acquired melanosis and hypertrichosis in a unilateral distribution

Pathogenesis
Androgens possibly a factor in growth of the lesion

Clinical manifestation
Asymptomatic, irregular, tan-to-brown patch, most commonly located over the chest, shoulder, or back; often at the time of puberty; thick, brown-to-black hairs develops both within and in close proximity to the patch; possibly associated with underlying smooth muscle hamartoma

Differential diagnosis
Melanoma; café au lait macule; Albright's syndrome; congenital melanocytic nevus; nevus spilus; postinflammatory hyperpigmentation

Therapy
Treatment for cosmetic reasons only – surgical excision; Q-switched ruby laser ablation; Q-switched neodymium: yttrium-aluminium-garnet (YAG) laser

References
Goldman MP, Fitzpatrick RE (1994) Treatment of benign pigmented cutaneous lesions. Cutaneous Laser Surgery 106–141

Becker's pigmented hairy nevus

▶ Becker's nevus

Beckwith-Wiedemann syndrome

Synonym(s)
None

Definition
Disorder consisting of macroglossia, visceromegaly, large body size, umbilical hernia or omphalocele, neonatal hypoglycemia

Pathogenesis
Sometimes occurring with chromosome 11 defect

Clinical manifestation
Large at birth; abdominal wall defect, such as an umbilical hernia or omphalocele; distinctive facial appearance with a gaping mouth and large tongue; increased incidence of childhood tumors, such as Wilms tumor or adrenal carcinoma

Differential diagnosis
Children presenting with overgrowth: Simpson-Golabi-Behmel syndrome; Perlman syndrome; Costello syndrome; proteus syndrome; Klippel-Trenaunay-Weber syndrome; neurofibromatosis

Therapy
Neonatal hypoglycemia: intravenous glucose; defects of the abdominal wall: surgical repair

References
Weng EY, Mortier GR, Graham JM Jr (1995) Beckwith-Wiedemann syndrome. An update and review for the primary pediatrician. Clinical Pediatrics 34(6):317–326

Bed sore

▶ Decubitus ulcer

Bednar tumor

▶ Dermatofibrosarcoma protuberans

Bee sting

▶ Hymenoptera sting

Behçet disease

▶ Behçet's disease

Behçet's disease

Synonym(s)
Behçet disease; Behçet's syndrome

Definition
Chronic, inflammatory disorder of blood vessels, resulting in recurrent oral ulcers, genital ulcers, eye inflammation, and internal organ involvement

Pathogenesis
Unknown; immune reactions involving blood vessels cause many of the signs and symptoms

Clinical manifestation
Mucocutaneous lesions: erythema nodosum; subcutaneous thrombophlebitis; folliculitis; acne-like lesions; cutaneous hypersensitivity (pathergy); recurrent oral and genital aphthae
Eye lesions: anterior or posterior uveitis; chorioretinitis; arthritis without deformity or ankylosis
Gastrointestinal lesions: ileocecal ulcers; epididymitis; central nervous system symptoms

Differential diagnosis
Aphthous stomatitis; pemphigus vulgaris; herpes simplex virus infection; lichen planus; acute neutrophilic dermatosis; inflammatory bowel disease; Stevens-Johnson syndrome; lupus erythematosus

Therapy
Local therapy: tetracycline suspension (250 mg capsule contents suspended in 5 ml of water) applied to mouth or genital ulcers 4 times daily; high potency topical corticosteroid gel; Kaopectate applied to ulcer 3–4

times per day; Zilactin gel applied 4–5 times per day; viscous lidocaine applied as needed; amlexanox 5% paste applied 4 times daily
Systemic therapy: thalidomide; prednisone; azathioprine; cyclosporine; colchicine

References

Lee LA (2001) Behcet disease. Seminars in Cutaneous Medicine & Surgery 20(1):53–57

Behçet's syndrome

▶ **Behçet's disease**

Bejel

Synonym(s)

Non-venereal syphilis of children; endemic syphilis

Definition

Non-venereal disease caused by Treponema endemicum, transmitted chiefly by direct contact, among children living in tropical and subtropical climates

Pathogenesis

Organism invades through traumatized cutaneous or mucosal surfaces that come in contact with a draining open sore of the index case; subsequent spread from original site either locally by scratching or by the hematogenous route

Clinical manifestation

Primary stage: painless ulcers within the oral cavity; sometimes also appearing as a nipple ulceration of a mother with a suckling infected child
Secondary stage: eroded plaques on the lips, tongue, and tonsils; angular stomatitis vitamin B deficiency; condyloma lata-like lesions in the anogenital area; generalized lymphadenopathy; painful osteoperiostitis in the long bones
Tertiary (late) stage: gummas which destroy bone and cartilage, particularly of the nose, causing saddle nose deformity

Differential diagnosis

Syphilis; yaws; pinta; atopic dermatitis; dermatophytosis; psoriasis; leprosy; herpes simplex virus infection; perlèche; condylomata acuminata; lupus vulgaris; lupus erythematosus; squamous cell carcinoma

Therapy

Penicillin G benzathine[*]; tetracycline; erythromycin

References

Koff AB, Rosen T (1993) Nonvenereal treponematoses: yaws, endemic syphilis, and pinta. Journal of the American Academy of Dermatology 29(4):519–535

Benign calcifying epithelioma

▶ **Pilomatricoma**

Benign calcifying epithelioma of Malherbe

▶ **Pilomatricoma**

Benign chronic T-cell infiltrative disorder

▶ **Jessner lymphocytic infiltration of skin**

Benign lichenoid keratosis

▶ Lichenoid keratosis

Benign lymphoreticulosis

▶ Bartonellosis

Benign migratory glossitis

Synonym(s)
Geographic tongue; stomatitis areata migrans, erythema areata migrans

Definition
Map-like appearance of the tongue resulting from irregular migratory denuded plaques on its surface

Pathogenesis
Unknown; results from the loss of papillae of tongue, giving areas of the tongue a flat surface, and the subsequent geographic appearance; may be related to local trauma or irritants

Clinical manifestation
Irregular, smooth, red plaques on the dorsal surface of the tongue, rapidly changing in pattern; surrounding the area of erythema and loss of filiform papillae is a well-defined hyperkeratotic yellow-white border with an irregular outline; often associated with burning sensation

Differential diagnosis
Lingua plicata; contact stomatitis; candidiasis; psoriasis; lichen planus

Therapy
No therapy indicated

References
Delaney JE (1995) Periodontal and soft-tissue abnormalities. Dental Clinics of North America 39(4):837–850

Benign mixed tumor of melanocytes and malpighian cells

▶ Melanoacanthoma

Benign mucous membrane pemphigoid

▶ Cicatricial pemphigoid

Benign nerve sheath tumor

▶ Neurothekeoma

Benign papillomatosis of nipple

▶ Erosive adenomatosis of the nipple

Benign parapsoriasis

▶ Small plaque parapsoriasis

Benign pigmented purpura

Synonym(s)
Pigmented purpuric dermatitis; pigmented purpuric eruption; subgroups: Schamberg disease (progressive pigmentary dermatosis); itching purpura of Loewenthal; eczematid-like purpura of Doucas and Kapetanakis; pigmented purpuric lichenoid dermatosis of Gougerot and Blum; lichen aureus; purpura annularis telangiectoides (Majocchi disease)

Definition
Group of chronic diseases characterized by extravasation of erythrocytes in the skin with marked hemosiderin deposition

Pathogenesis
Venous hypertension, exercise, and gravitational dependency possible cofactors

Clinical manifestation
Reddish-brown, speckled discoloration in patches or plaques
Schamberg variant: cayenne pepper-like punctate petechial macules in a larger purpuric patch
Lichen aureus variant: golden-yellow patch, most commonly on the leg
Majocchi variant: annular patches of purpura with telangiectasia
Gougerot and Blum variant: lichenoid surface change

Differential diagnosis
Thrombocytopenia; cryoglobulinemia; cutaneous T-cell lymphoma; clotting disorders; stasis pigmentation; scurvy; leukocytoclastic vasculitis; drug hypersensitivity reaction

Therapy
Topical corticosteroid, mid potency

References
Piette WW (1994) The differential diagnosis of purpura from a morphologic perspective. Advances in Dermatology 9:3–23

Benign schwannoma

▶ Neurilemmoma

Benign symmetric lipomatosis

Synonym(s)
Madelung's disease; cervical lipomatosis; Launois-Bensaude syndrome; multiple symmetrical lipomatosis; horse-collar neck

Definition
Progressive, symmetric deposition of adipose tissue around the postauricular area, neck, and shoulders

Pathogenesis
Sympathetic denervation locally may be an etiologic factor

Clinical manifestation
Diffuse and symmetrical fat deposition in a "horse-collar" distribution around the neck; occasional fat deposition at other sites

Differential diagnosis
Obesity; Dercum's disease; multiple hereditary lipomatosis; lymphadenopathy; soft tissue neoplasms

Therapy
Liposuction; surgical excision

References
Ruzicka T, Vieluf D, Landthaler M, Braun-Falco O (1987) Benign symmetric lipomatosis Launois-

Bensaude. Report of ten cases and review of the literature. Journal of the American Academy of Dermatology 17(4):663–674

Benzoyl peroxide

Trade name(s)
Benoxyl; Benzac AC; Benza-Gel; Brevoxyl; Desquam-E; PanOxyl; Persa-Gel; Triaz; combination benzoyl peroxide products: Benzamycin; BenzaClin; Duac

Generic available
Yes

Drug class
Antibiotic

Mechanism of action
Free-radical, oxygen-mediated bacterio-cidal effects on P. acnes in sebaceous follicles

Dosage form
2.5 %, 4%, 5%, 8%, 10% cream, gel, lotion

Dermatologic indications and dosage
See table

Common side effects
Cutaneous: dryness, erythema, peeling, contact dermatitis

Serious side effects
None

Drug interactions
Isotretinoin

Other interactions
Fabrics: may cause color bleaching

Contraindications/precautions
Hypersensitivity to drug class or component

References
Basak PY, Gultekin F, Kilinc I, Delibas N (2002) The effect of benzoyl peroxide and benzoyl peroxide/erythromycin combination on the anti-oxidative defence system in papulopustular acne. European Journal of Dermatology 12(1):53–57

Bequez Cesar syndrome

▶ Chédiak-Higashi syndrome

Berardinelli syndrome

▶ Berardinelli-Seip syndrome

Berardinelli-Seip syndrome

Synonym(s)
Berardinelli syndrome; Berardinelli-Seip-Lawrence syndrome; Miescher syndrome 2; Seip syndrome; generalized lipodystrophy

Definition
Acquired complex of acanthosis nigricans, generalized lipodystrophy, diabetes mellitus, and hyperlipemia

Pathogenesis
Monogenic defect, type unknown

Benzoyl peroxide. Dermatologic indications and dosage

Disease	Adult dosage	Child dosage
Acne vulgaris	Apply twice per day	Apply twice per day

Clinical manifestation
Often preceded by an illness; absence of fat clinically evident by age 15 years; acanthosis nigricans; diabetes mellitus; associated autoimmune disorders; prone to infection

Differential diagnosis
Lawrence-Seip syndrome; progressive partial lipodystrophy; post-traumatic partial lipodystrophy

Therapy
Dietary fish oil supplementation; acitretin

References
Seip M, Trygstad O (1996) Generalized lipodystrophy, congenital and acquired (lipoatrophy). Acta Paediatrica Suppl413:2

Berardinelli-Seip-Lawrence syndrome

▶ Berardinelli-Seip syndrome

Bergamot phototoxicity

▶ Berloque dermatitis

Bergapten phototoxicity

▶ Berloque dermatitis

Berkshire neck

▶ Poikiloderma of Civatte

Berlock dermatitis

▶ Berloque dermatitis

Berloque dermatitis

Synonym(s)
Berlock dermatitis; perfume phototoxicity; bergapten phototoxicity; bergamot phototoxicity; photodermatitis pigmentaria; dermite pigmentée en forme de coulée

Definition
Phototoxic reaction induced by the effect of long-wave ultraviolet (UVA) radiation on bergapten (5-methoxypsoralen), a photoactive component of bergamot oil

Pathogenesis
Photoactivation of bergapten by UVA radiation, causing phototoxicity and melanocyte stimulation to produce melanin; distribution of melanosomes in keratinocyte changing from the aggregate to disaggregated form, similar to that seen in skin of black individuals

Clinical manifestation
Erythema; edema; vesiculation; desquamation; pendant-like hyperpigmentation at sites of oil of bergamot application, often on the lateral neck

Differential diagnosis
Contact dermatitis; Riehl melanosis; melasma; postinflammatory hyperpigmentation; acanthosis nigricans

Therapy
Avoidance of bergamot oil-containing perfumes; minimized exposure to the sun (sunscreens, etc.); hydroquinone

References
None

Besnier-Boeck-Schaumann disease

▶ Sarcoidosis

Besnier's prurigo

▶ Atopic dermatitis

Betamethasone

▶ Corticosteroids, topical, medium potency

Betamethasone dipropionate

▶ Corticosteroids, topical, high potency

Betamethasone valerate

▶ Corticosteroids, topical, medium potency

Beurmann's disease

▶ Sporotrichosis

Bifid-rib basal-cell nevus syndrome

▶ Basal cell nevus syndrome

Biskra button

▶ Leishmaniasis, cutaneous

Black bane

▶ Anthrax, cutaneous

Black blood

▶ Anthrax, cutaneous

Black dot ringworm

Definition
Appearance of punctate black dots representing broken hairs at sites of tinea capitis, caused by the fungal pathogen, T. tonsurans

References
Elewski BE (2000) Tinea capitis: A current perspective. Journal of the American Academy of Dermatology 42(1 Pt 1):1–20

Black hairy tongue

▶ Hairy tongue

Black heel

Synonym(s)
Talon noir; tennis heel; hyperkeratosis haemorrhagica; pseudochromhidrosis plantaris; calcaneal petechiae

Definition
Self-limited, asymptomatic, trauma-induced darkening of the posterior or posterolateral aspect of the heel occurring after minor trauma, mostly from athletic pursuits

Pathogenesis
Lateral shearing force of the epidermis sliding over the rete pegs of the papillary dermis, resulting in hemorrhage

Clinical manifestation
Multiple asymptomatic petechiae centrally aggregated with a few scattered satellite patches, located over posterior and posterolateral heel

Differential diagnosis
Melanoma; wart; nevus; lentigo

Therapy
Paring of lesion with a scalpel blade; protective heel pad for prophylaxis

References
Levine N, Baron J (2000) Black Heel in: James WD, Elston D (Chief eds.) eMedicine Dermatology St. Petersburg: eMedicine Corporation

Black piedra

▶ Piedra

Blaschkitis

▶ Lichen striatus

Blaschko linear acquired inflammatory skin eruption

▶ Lichen striatus

Blastomycosis

▶ North American blastomycosis

Blennorrheal idiopathic arthritis

▶ Reiter syndrome

Blepharochalasis

▶ Dermatochalasis

Blinding filariasis

▶ Filariasis

Blistering dactylitis

▶ Blistering distal dactylitis

Blistering distal dactylitis

Synonym(s)
Blistering dactylitis

Definition
Superficial infection of the anterior fat pad of distal phalanx, usually caused by β-hemolytic streptococcal pathogens

Pathogenesis
S. pyogenes colonizes normal skin surfaces for extended periods; following acquisition on the normal skin, minor trauma may be a prerequisite for initiating infection

Clinical manifestation
Tender vesicle or bulla on an erythematous base, covering the volar surface of the affected digit

Differential diagnosis
Herpetic whitlow; friction blister; epidermolysis bullosa; burn trauma

Therapy
Penicillin G benzathine; penicillin VK; incision and drainage

References
Ney AC, English JC 3rd, Greer KE (2002) Coexistent infections on a child's distal phalanx: blistering dactylitis and herpetic whitlow. Cutis 69(1):46–48

Bloch-Siemens syndrome

▶ Incontinentia pigmenti

Bloch-Sulzberger syndrome

▶ Incontinentia pigmenti

Bloom syndrome

▶ Bloom's syndrome

Bloom's syndrome

Synonym(s)
Bloom syndrome; congenital telangiectatic erythema

Definition
Autosomal recessive disorder characterized by telangiectases and photosensitivity, growth deficiency, a variable degree of immunodeficiency, and increased susceptibility to neoplasms

Pathogenesis
Mutation in the gene designated BLM, on 15q26.1; protein encoded by the normal gene has DNA helicase activity and functions in the maintenance of genomic stability; mutation likely responsible for the phenotype and the cancer predisposition

Clinical manifestation
Telangiectatic erythema in photodistributed pattern; cheilitis; café au lait macules; bird-like facies; malar hypoplasia, small mandible; large, protruding ears; growth delay; short stature; malignancies, such as acute leukemia, lymphoma, and gastrointestinal adenocarcinoma

Differential diagnosis
Cockayne syndrome; Rothmund-Thomson syndrome; lupus erythematosus; erythropoietic protoporphyria

Therapy
No specific treatment; sun protection

References
German J (1995) Bloom's syndrome. Dermatologic Clinics 13(1):7–18

Blue neuronevus

▶ Blue nevus

Blue nevus

Synonym(s)
Nevus of Jadassohn and Tieche; blue neuronevus; dermal melanocytoma

Definition
Blue or blue-black skin lesion produced by a collection of functioning deep dermal melanocytes

Pathogenesis
Dermal arrest in fetal migration of melanocytes of neural crest origin results in failure to reach the epidermis

Clinical manifestation
Smooth-surfaced, dome-shaped blue or blue-gray papules; common blue nevi less than 1 cm; cellular variant sometimes larger than 1 cm

Differential diagnosis
Melanoma; traumatic tattoo; seborrheic keratosis; dermatofibroma; nevus of Ota/Ito; cherry hemangioma

Therapy
Diagnostic biopsy if melanoma seriously considered; simple excision for cosmetic reasons*

References
Schaffer JV, Bolognia JL (2000) The clinical spectrum of pigmented lesions. Clinics in Plastic Surgery 27(3):391–408

Blue rubber bleb nevus syndrome

Synonym(s)
Bean syndrome

Definition
Disorder characterized by multiple cutaneous venous malformations with visceral lesions most commonly affecting the gastrointestinal tract

Pathogenesis
Unknown

Clinical manifestation
Multiple, protuberant, dark blue, compressible nodules; large, cavernous lesions that may compress vital structures; irregular blue macules or patches; multiple gastrointestinal hemangiomas which may bleed, cause intussusception, volvulus, or bowel infarction; other extra-cutaneous sites, including skull, central nervous system, thyroid, parotid gland, eyes, oral cavity, lungs, pleura, pericardium, musculoskeletal system, peritoneal cavity, mesentery, kidney, liver, spleen, penis, vulva, and bladder

Differential diagnosis
Arteriovenous malformation; Kaposi's sarcoma; Mafucci syndrome; Klippel-Trenaunay-Weber syndrome

Therapy
Destruction by electrodesiccation and curettage, liquid nitrogen cryotherapy; surgical excision; CO_2 laser vaporization

References
Moodley M, Ramdial P (1993) Blue rubber bleb nevus syndrome: case report and review of the literature. Pediatrics 92(1):160–162

Boder-Sedgwick syndrome

▶ **Ataxia-telangiectasia**

Boeck's sarcoid

▶ **Sarcoidosis**

Boil

▶ Furuncle

Bonnet-Dechaume-Blanc syndrome

▶ Wyburn-Mason syndrome

Bonnevie-Ullrich syndrome

▶ Turner syndrome

Böök syndrome

Synonym(s)
Böök's syndrome

Definition
Syndrome consisting of premature graying of the hair, tooth development abnormalities, and palmoplantar hyperhidrosis

Pathogenesis
Autosomal dominant inheritance; unknown genetic defect

Clinical manifestation
Graying of the hair before age 14 years, mostly in the scalp hair; bicuspid aplasia; hyperhidrosis of the palms and soles

Differential diagnosis
Ectodermal dysplasia; essential hyperhidrosis

Therapy
None

References
Böök JA (1950) Clinical and genetical studies of hypodontia. Premolar aplasia, hyperhidrosis, and canities prematura: A new hereditary syndrome in man. American Journal of Human Genetics 2:240–263

Böök's syndrome

▶ Böök syndrome

Boston exanthem

Synonym(s)
Echovirus 16 infection

Definition
Skin eruption caused by an infection with echovirus 16

Pathogenesis
Echovirus 16 infection acquired by the oral or respiratory route

Clinical manifestation
Prodrome of fever and anorexia after 3–8 day incubation period; exanthem begins on the face and chest and quickly generalizes; enanthem occasionally present; posterior auricular lymphadenopathy

Differential diagnosis
Roseola; other viral exanthems; meningococcal infection; medication reaction

Therapy
None; no specific isolation needed

References
Cherry JD (1983) Viral exanthems. Current Problems in Pediatrics 13(6):1–44

Botryomycosis

Synonym(s)
Granular bacteriosis; actinophytosis

Definition
Chronic, purulent, bacterial infection with formation of granules

Pathogenesis
Most cases caused by Staphylococcus aureus; may represent suboptimal host response to bacterial organism

Clinical manifestation
Cutaneous or subcutaneous doughy nodules with ulcerations and draining sinuses; grainy material extruding from the lesions

Differential diagnosis
Mycetoma; actinomycosis; kerion; subcutaneous granuloma annulare; Kaposi's sarcoma; lymphoma

Therapy
Surgical therapy: debridement; surgical excision; laser vaporization
Medical therapy: dicloxacillin; cephalexin

References
Bonifaz A, Carrasco E (1996) Botryomycosis. International Journal of Dermatology 35(6):381–388

Bouba

▶ Yaws

Bourneville disease

▶ Tuberous sclerosis

Boutonneuse fever

Synonym(s)
Mediterranean spotted fever; Carducci fever; tick typhus; South African tick typhus; Indian tick typhus; tick bite fever

Definition
Rickettsial disease caused by Rickettsia conorii occurring in the Mediterranean basin

Pathogenesis
Organism introduced through a tick bite; invasion and proliferation in the endothelial cells of small vessels

Clinical manifestation
History of recent travel in endemic area; fever; erythematous papules, mainly on the lower extremities; eschar at the site of the tick bite; localized or generalized purpura

Differential diagnosis
Viral exanthem; Rocky Mountain spotted fever; rubeola; Lyme disease; medication reaction; Kawasaki disease; aseptic acute arthritis; leukocytoclastic vasculitis

Therapy
Doxycycline; ciprofloxacin 250–500 mg PO twice daily for 7–14 days

References
Cascio A, Dones P, Romano A (1998) Clinical and laboratory findings of boutonneuse fever in Sicilian children. European Journal of Pediatrics 157(6):482–486

Bowen disease

▶ Bowen's disease

Bowen's carcinoma

▶ Bowen's disease

Bowen's disease

Synonym(s)
Squamous cell carcinoma in-situ; Bowen disease; Bowen's carcinoma

Definition
Cutaneous squamous cell carcinoma with full thickness dysplasia of the epidermis without dermal invasion

Pathogenesis
Chronic solar damage, inorganic arsenic ingestion, and certain human papilloma virus subtypes (12, 13, 16 and 34) implicated as etiologic factors

Clinical manifestation
Red, scaly, non-substantive papule or plaque, most often occurring on the head and neck, but sometimes appearing on other sun-exposed areas or the trunk

Differential diagnosis
Actinic keratosis; superficial basal cell carcinoma; seborrheic keratosis; lichenoid keratosis; extramammary Paget's disease; psoriasis; tinea corporis; lupus erythematosus

Therapy
Destruction by electrodesiccation and curettage or liquid nitrogen cryotherapy; surgical excision; fluorouracil cream; photodynamic therapy

References
Fitzgerald DA (1998) Cancer precursors. Seminars in Cutaneous Medicine & Surgery 17(2):108–113

Bowenoid papulosis

Synonym(s)
Viral keratoses; bowenoid papulosis of the penis; bowenoid papulosis of the genitalia

Definition
Human papillomavirus (HPV)-induced wart with histologic features of Bowen's disease

Pathogenesis
HPV type 16 most common causative agent; sometimes also occurring with viral types 18, 31, 32, 33, 34, 35, 39, 42, 48, 51, 52, 53, and 54

Clinical manifestation
Solitary or multiple, pigmented papules with a flat-to-velvety surface; lesions sometimes coalescing into plaques; occur most commonly on the penile shaft or the external genitalia of females

Differential diagnosis
Seborrheic keratosis; squamous cell carcinoma; melanocytic nevus; lichen planus

Therapy
Local excision; destruction by electrodesiccation and curettage, cryosurgery, CO_2 laser ablation; tretinoin; podofilox; 5-fluorouracil cream

References
Schwartz RA, Janniger CK (1991) Bowenoid papulosis. Journal of the American Academy of Dermatology 24(2 Pt 1):261–264

Bowenoid papulosis of the genitalia

▶ Bowenoid papulosis

Bowenoid papulosis of the penis

▶ Bowenoid papulosis

Brachmann-de Lange syndrome

▶ Cornelia de Lange syndrome

Branchial cleft cyst

Synonym(s)
Branchial cyst; lateral cervical cyst; branchiogenic cyst; branchioma

Definition
Epithelial cyst arising on the lateral neck from a failure of obliteration of the second branchial cleft during embryonic life

Pathogenesis
Branchial arch clefts, which normally involute by week 7 of embryonic development, become ectoderm-lined cavities; with incomplete involution, entrapped remnant forms an epithelium-lined cyst

Clinical manifestation
Asymptomatic, fluctuant nodule, occurring along the lower portion of the anteromedial border of the sternocleidomastoid muscle between the muscle and overlying skin; sometimes becomes tender if secondarily inflamed or infected; with a sinus tract, occasional mucoid or purulent exudate

Differential diagnosis
Lymphadenopathy; vascular malformation; hemangioma; carotid body tumor; cystic hygroma; ectopic salivary or thyroid tissue

Therapy
Surgical excision, usually after age 3 months*; incision and drainage if abscess forms

References
Brown RL, Azizkhan RG (1998) Pediatric head and neck lesions. Pediatric Clinics of North America 45(4):889–905

Branchial cyst

▶ Branchial cleft cyst

Branchiogenic cyst

▶ Branchial cleft cyst

Branchioma

▶ Branchial cleft cyst

Brauer's syndrome

Synonym(s)
Focal facial dysplasia; hereditary symmetrical aplastic nevi of the temples

Definition
Hereditary, focal pigmented nevi of the forehead and chin associated with either the absence of eyelashes or double rows of eyelashes and absence of sweat glands in the lesions

Pathogenesis
Unknown; autosomal dominant inheritance

Clinical manifestation
Hereditary, focal pigmented nevi, similar to forceps marks; located on the forehead and chin; absence of eyelashes or double rows of eyelashes and aplasia of the sweat glands in the lesions; protuberant nose

Differential diagnosis
Hypohidrotic ectodermal dysplasia

Therapy
None

References
Pinheiro M, Freire-Maia N (1994) Ectodermal dysplasias: A clinical classification and a causal review. American Journal of Medical Genetics 53(2):153–162

Brazilian blastomycosis

▶ South American blastomycosis

Brazilian pemphigus

▶ Fogo selvagem

Brazilian pemphigus foliaceus

▶ Fogo selvagem

Brill-Zinsser disease

▶ Typhus

Brocq pseudopelade

▶ Pseudopelade

Brocq's disease

▶ Small plaque parapsoriasis

Broken capillaries

▶ Varicose and telangiectatic leg veins

Bromhidrosis

Synonym(s)
Apocrine bromhidrosis; osmidrosis; bromidrosis

Definition
Condition of abnormal or offensive body odor

Pathogenesis
Odor as a consequence of apocrine gland secretion; bacterial decomposition of apocrine secretion yields short-chain fatty acids with characteristic odors; other odor-inducing situations include metabolic disorders, ingestion of foods or drugs, or toxic materials, or contact with certain xenobiotics

Clinical manifestation
Appearance normal except when associated with other unrelated conditions, such as erythrasma or intertrigo

Differential diagnosis
Fish odor syndrome (trimethylaminuria); organic brain lesions (tumors, etc.); body dysmorphic disorder

B

Therapy
Hygienic measures: adequate washing of the axillary vault; drying powders; frequent clothing changes
Diet: omission of certain foods (e.g. certain spices, garlic, alcohol) in instances when contributory
Surgical: superficial liposuction to remove apocrine glands

References
Lockman DS (1981) Olfactory diagnosis. Cutis 27(6):645–647

Bromidrosis

▶ Bromhidrosis

Bromoderma

▶ Halogenoderma

Brompheniramine

▶ Antihistamines, first generation

Bronze baby syndrome

Synonym(s)
Brown baby syndrome

Definition
Complication of neonatal phototherapy in infants with hepatic disease, with skin taking on a bronze color

Pathogenesis
Proposed mechanisms including photodestruction of porphyrin and deposition in the skin or a deposition of a photo-isomer of bilirubin the skin

Clinical manifestation
Dark gray-brown discoloration of the entire skin surface, fading approximately 6 weeks after stopping phototherapy

Differential diagnosis
Gray baby syndrome (chloramphenicol overdosage); cyanosis

Therapy
Evaluation and treatment of underlying hyperbilirubinemia

References
Rubaltelli FF, Da Riol R, D'Amore ES, Jori G (1996) The bronze baby syndrome: evidence of increased tissue concentration of copper porphyrins. Acta Paediatrica 85(3):381–384

Bronze diabetes

▶ Hemochromatosis

Brooke tumor

▶ Trichoepithelioma

Brown baby syndrome

▶ Bronze baby syndrome

Brown recluse spider bite

Synonym(s)
Necrotic arachnidism; arachnidism; loxoscelism; latrodectism

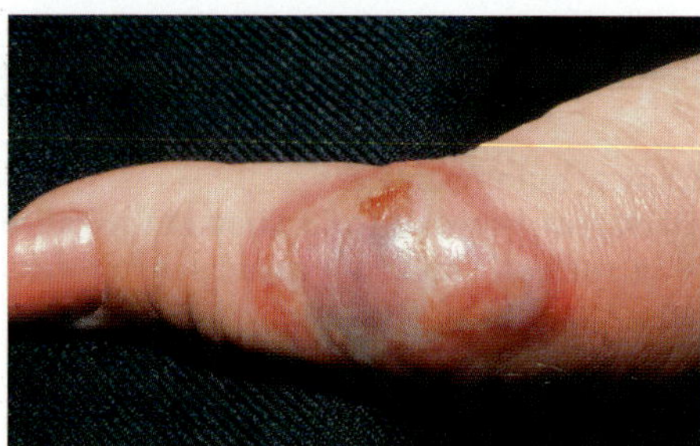

Brown recluse spider bite. Plaque with early necrosis in the center and an erythematous border

Definition
Skin necrosis and sloughing secondary to the bite of the brown recluse spider

Pathogenesis
Envenomation from brown recluse spider (Loxosceles reclusa); phospholipase D main toxic factor

Clinical manifestation
Bite minimally symptomatic; fewer than 10% of bites result in severe skin necrosis; signs of progression within 48–72 hours of the bite; mild-to-severe pain beginning 2–8 hours after bite; central papule and associated erythema occur 6–12 hours after bite; purple vesicle sometimes ulcerates; stellate necrotic area sometimes ensues.
Constitutional signs and symptoms: hemolysis; hemoglobinuria; thrombocytopenia; disseminated intravascular coagulation; fever; headache; malaise; arthralgia; nausea; vomiting

Differential diagnosis
Pyoderma gangrenosum; ecthyma; herpes simplex virus infection; insect bite reaction; squamous cell carcinoma; coumarin necrosis; vasculitis; vascular insufficiency; necrotizing fasciitis; factitial ulceration; thromboembolic phenomenon; skin trauma; thromboangiitis obliterans; neuropathic ulceration; tularemia; mucormycosis

Therapy
Local therapy: cleansing of the bite site; cold compresses; simple analgesics; elevation of an affected extremity; intralesional corticosteroids
Systemic therapy: dapsone; prednisone for systemic signs and symptoms
Surgical therapy: excision of necrotic area only after 6 weeks if healing not progressing

References
Sams HH, Dunnick CA, Smith ML, King LE Jr (2001) Necrotic arachnidism. Journal of the American Academy of Dermatology 44(4):561–573

Brown spot syndrome

▶ McCune-Albright syndrome

Brugian filariasis

▶ Filariasis

Brunaur-Fuhs-Siemens syndrome

▶ Striate keratoderma

Bulldog scalp

▶ Cutis verticis gyrata

Bullous congenital ichthyosiform erythroderma

▶ Epidermolytic hyperkeratosis

Bullous diabeticorum

▶ Bullous eruption of diabetes mellitus

Bullous disease of diabetes mellitus

▶ Bullous eruption of diabetes mellitus

Bullous eruption of diabetes mellitus

Synonym(s)
Bullous disease of diabetes mellitus; bullous diabeticorum; diabetic bullae

Definition
Non-inflammatory, blistering condition of acral skin in patients with diabetes mellitus

Pathogenesis
Possibly related to diabetic neuropathy or nephropathy; possibly associated with defect in anchoring fibrils

Clinical manifestation
Non-inflammatory vesicles and bullae, most commonly on the hands and lower legs

Differential diagnosis
Bullous pemphigoid; epidermolysis bullosa acquisita; porphyria cutanea tarda; burn; friction blister; blistering distal dactylitis

Therapy
No specific therapy

References
Basarab T, Munn SE, McGrath J, Russell Jones R (1995) Bullosis diabeticorum. A case report and literature review. Clinical & Experimental Dermatology 20(3):218–220

Bullous ichthyosiform erythroderma

▶ Epidermolytic hyperkeratosis

Bullous ichthyotic erythroderma

▶ Epidermolytic hyperkeratosis

Bullous pemphigoid

Synonym(s)
Pemphigoid; pemphigoid vegetans

Definition
Autoimmune, blistering disease characterized by the presence of IgG autoantibodies specific for the hemi-desmosomal antigens

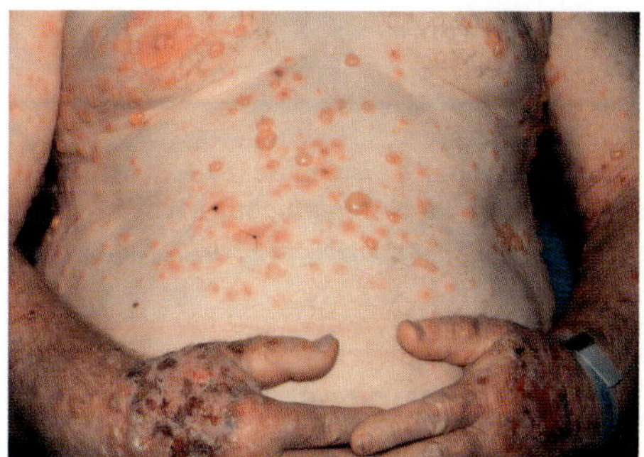

Bullous pemphigoid. Numerous tense vesicles and bullae, many of which arise from normal-appearing skin

Pathogenesis

IgG autoantibodies specific for the hemi-desmosomal bullous pemphigoid antigens BP230 (BPAg1) and BP180 (BPAg2); binding of antibodies at the basement membrane, activating complement and inflammatory mediators and producing injury at the basement membrane zone

Clinical manifestation

Tense vesicles and bullae, with a predilection for the flexor areas of the skin; oral and ocular mucosa involvement seldom occurs; bullae clinically either inflammatory or non-inflammatory; blisters usually heal without scarring or milia formation; localized form with blisters confined to the extremities; lesions sometimes urticarial without vesiculation

Differential diagnosis

Cicatricial pemphigoid; herpes gestationis; linear IgA bullous dermatosis; dermatitis herpetiformis; chronic bullous dermatosis of childhood; dyshidrosis; bullous lupus erythematosus; pemphigus vegetans; urticaria

Therapy

Mild to moderate disease: high potency topical corticosteroids; combination of tetracycline and niacinamide 500 mg PO 2-3 times daily
Severe disease: prednisone; steroid-sparing medications: azathioprine; cyclophosphamide; mycophenolate mofetil; dapsone; methotrexate

References

Khumalo NP, Murrell DF, Wojnarowska F, Kirtschig G (2002) A systematic review of treatments for bullous pemphigoid. Archives of Dermatology 138(3):385–389

Bullous photosensitivity, drug- or therapy-induced

▶ **Pseudoporphyria**

Burning mouth syndrome

Synonym(s)

None

Definition

Sensation of burning or pain in the mouth without an identifiable visible pathologic process responsible for the symptom

Pathogenesis

Possible etiologic factors: nutritional deficiency (e.g. B vitamin deficiency), major depression; increased taste sensation; menopause (90% of affected women postmenopausal); trigeminal nerve neuropathy

Clinical manifestation

Burning pain affecting oropharynx; onset in the morning; peak symptoms in the late afternoon; lower lip mucosa, anterior tongue, anterior hard palate affected; pain relief with eating; associated with dry mouth and taste disturbance; no evident lesions

Differential diagnosis

Tobacco abuse; atrophic glossitis; menopausal glossitis; heavy metal poisoning; vitamin deficiency; leukemia; lichen planus; uremia; medication reaction

Therapy

Capsaicin: starting with hot pepper diluted 1:2 with water; rinsing of mouth with 1 teaspoon; decreasing dilution to 1:1 as tolerated; amitriptyline; gabapentin: starting with 300 mg PO at bedtime, titrating up to a maximum of 1800 mg per day; serotonin reuptake inhibitor

References

Muzyka BC, De Rossi SS (1999) A review of burning mouth syndrome. Cutis 64(1):29–35

Buruli ulcer

Synonym(s)
Mycobacterium ulcerans infection

Definition
Chronic, necrotizing disease of the skin due to Mycobacterium ulcerans

Pathogenesis
Inoculation of Mycobacterium ulcerans into the skin occurring via trauma; organism produces mycolactone, an immunosuppressive, soluble, polyketide toxin with cytotoxic properties

Clinical manifestation
Presenting as firm, nontender subcutaneous nodule; within the next 1 to 2 months, area becomes fluctuant and forms a painless, undermined ulceration; lesions with a scalloped border and a sloughing, necrotic base; spontaneous healing after many months

Differential diagnosis
Tropical phagedenic ulcer; cutaneous tuberculosis; deep fungal infection; leishmaniasis; pyoderma gangrenosum; squamous cell carcinoma; vasculitis

Therapy
Surgical therapy: excision of ulcer[*]
Medical therapy: rifampin 600 mg PO per day

References
van der Werf TS, van der Graaf WT, Tappero JW, Asiedu K (1999) Mycobacterium ulcerans infection. Lancet 354(9183):1013–1018

Buschke-Löwenstein tumor

▶ Giant condyloma of Buschke and Löwenstein

Buschke-Ollendorff syndrome

Synonym(s)
Dermatofibrosis lenticularis; disseminated lenticular dermatofibrosis; dermatofibrosis lenticularis disseminata with osteopoikilosis

Definition
Ectodermal dysplasia of connective tissue, consisting of osteopoikilosis and connective tissue nevi

Pathogenesis
Possibly resulting from abnormal regulation of extracellular matrix, leading to increased accumulation of elastin in the dermis

Clinical manifestation
Asymptomatic, slightly elevated, yellowish papules and nodules coalescing to form plaques; arising over several years; osteopoikilosis of the epiphysis and the metaphysis of long bones

Differential diagnosis
Pseudoxanthoma elasticum; tuberous sclerosis; connective tissue nevus; morphea

Therapy
Surgical excision of skin lesions for cosmetic purposes

References
Woodrow SL, Pope FM, Handfield-Jones SE (2001) The Buschke-Ollendorff syndrome presenting as familial elastic tissue naevi. British Journal of Dermatology 144(4):890–893

Busse-Buschke disease

▶ Cryptococcosis

Café au lait macule

Synonym(s)
Café au lait spot; hypermelanotic macule

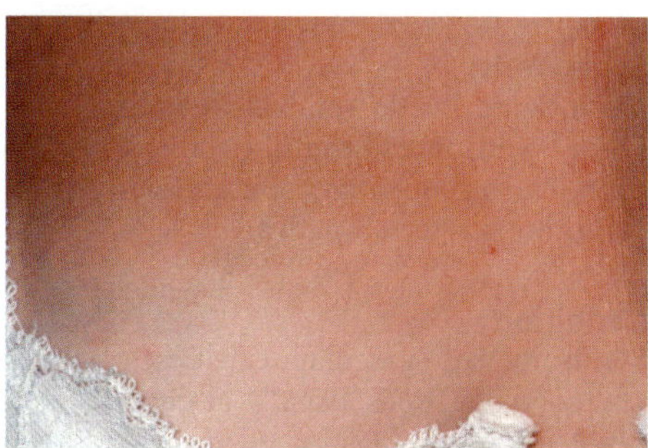

Café au lait macule. Tan-brown patch on the chest wall

Definition
Discrete, tan-brown macule with irregular margins

Pathogenesis
Possibly represents increased melanocyte size or increased melanosome production

Clinical manifestation
Asymptomatic, 2–20 mm discrete tan-brown macule or patch; occurring in patients with neurofibromatosis, McCune-Albright syndrome, Watson's syndrome, proteus syndrome, Bloom's syndrome, piebaldism, and Fanconi's anemia

Differential diagnosis
Lentigo; seborrheic keratosis; nevocellular nevus; nevus spilus; multiple lentigines syndrome

Therapy
Q-switched Nd:YAG or Q-switched ruby laser ablation; hydroquinone

References
Landau M, Krafchik BR (1999) The diagnostic value of cafe-au-lait macules. Journal of the American Academy of Dermatology 40(6 Pt 1):877–890

Café au lait spot

▶ Café au lait macule

Café-au-lait spots syndrome

▶ Watson syndrome

Calcaneal petechiae

▶ Black heel

Calcific uremic arteriolopathy

▶ Calciphylaxis

Calcifying epithelioma of Malherbe

▶ Pilomatricoma

Calcinosis cutis

Synonym(s)
Cutaneous calcinosis; cutaneous calculi

Definition
A group of disorders in which calcium salts, consisting primarily of hydroxyapatite crystals or amorphous calcium phosphate, are deposited in the skin

Pathogenesis
Unclear; involves both metabolic and physical factors; in the setting of hypercalcemia and/or hyperphosphatemia, calcium deposition occurring without preceding tissue damage; damaged tissue possibly allows an influx of calcium ions, leading to calcium precipitation

Clinical manifestation
Multiple, asymptomatic, firm, whitish papules, plaques, or nodules in the dermis and/or subcutis; sometimes spontaneously ulcerating and extruding a chalky white material; dystrophic calcinosis cutis: deposits at the site of trauma; metastatic calcification: widespread calcinosis, often around large joints; common in children with dermatomyositis and in those with CREST syndrome

Differential diagnosis
Gouty tophus; granuloma annulare; xanthoma; foreign body granuloma; milium; osteoma cutis

Therapy
Surgical excision; sodium etidronate and diphosphonates; colchicine; warfarin; intralesional triamcinolone 3–4 mg per ml

References
Rodriguez-Cano L, Garcia-Patos V, Creus M. Bastida P, Ortega JJ, Castells A (1996) Childhood calcinosis cutis. Pediatric Dermatology 13(2):114–117

Calciphylaxis

Synonym(s)
Necrotizing livedo reticularis; uremic gangrene syndrome; uremic necrosis; calcific uremic arteriolopathy; obliterative calcific-thrombotic arteriolopathy

Definition
Syndrome of vascular calcification with cutaneous necrosis, usually in patients with renal failure

Pathogenesis
Pathogenic factors possibly include chronic renal failure, hypercalcemia, hyperphosphatemia, an elevated calcium-phosphate product, and secondary hyperparathyroidism

Clinical manifestation
Presents as livedo reticularis or as erythematous papules or plaques, mostly on the lower extremities, evolving into stellate purpuric ulcerations with central necrosis; extreme pain and tenderness in lesions

Differential diagnosis
Polyarteritis nodosa; pyoderma gangrenosum; Wegener's granulomatosis; lupus erythematosus; cryoglobulinemia; coumarin

necrosis; protein C or protein S deficiency; antiphospholipid syndrome; atherosclerotic peripheral vascular disease; pancreatic panniculitis; cholesterol emboli; disseminated intravascular coagulation

Therapy
Total or subtotal parathyroidectomy only with evidence of hyperparathyroidism; aggressive wound care and debridement of necrotic tissue; dietary alteration with phosphate binders and low calcium-bath dialysis to decrease serum calcium and phosphate concentrations

References
Oh DH, Eulau D, Tokugawa DA, McGuire JS, Kohler S (1999) Five cases of calciphylaxis and a review of the literature. Journal of the American Academy of Dermatology 40(6 Pt 1):979–987

Calcipotriene

Trade name(s)
Dovonex

Generic available
No

Drug class
Vitamin D3 derivative

Mechanism of action
Acts through the vitamin D nuclear receptor to regulate growth, differentiation, and immune functions

Dosage form
0.005% cream, ointment, lotion

Dermatologic indications and dosage
See table

Common side effects
Cutaneous: pruritus; irritant contact dermatitis; erythema

Serious side effects
Hematologic: hypercalcemia

Drug interactions
None

Contraindications/precautions
Hypersensitivity to drug class or component

References
Lebwohl M, Ali S (2001) Treatment of psoriasis. Part 1. Topical therapy and phototherapy. Journal of the American Academy of Dermatology 45(4):487–98

Calcipotriene. Dermatologic indications and dosage

Disease	Adult dosage	Child dosage
Epidermolytic hyperkeratosis	Apply twice daily	Apply twice daily
Grover's disease	Apply twice daily	Apply twice daily
Inflammatory linear verrucous nevus	Apply twice daily	Apply twice daily
Morphea	Apply twice daily	Apply twice daily
Porokeratosis	Apply twice daily	Apply twice daily
Psoriasis	Apply twice daily	Apply twice daily
Reiter syndrome	Apply twice daily	Apply twice daily
Vitiligo	Apply twice daily	Apply twice daily

Callosity

▶ Clavus

Callous

▶ Clavus

Callus

▶ Clavus

Campbell de Morgan spots

▶ Cherry hemangioma

Candidiasis

Synonym(s)
Moniliasis; candidosis; thrush

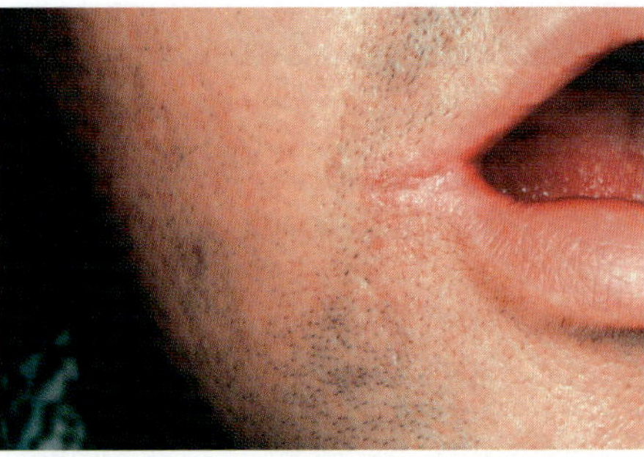

Candidiasis. Red, fissured plaque at the corner of the mouth

Definition
Skin and mucous membrane infections caused by Candida species

Pathogenesis
Warm, moist parts of the body susceptible to infection; host factors such as oral hygiene important in intraoral infection (thrush); primary immune defects in mucocutaneous candidiasis; endocrinopathies such as diabetes mellitus, Cushing's syndrome, Addison's disease, hypoparathyroidism associated with recurrent infections

Clinical manifestation
Thrush: discrete or confluent white plaques on oral mucosa common on the tongue; erythema and fissures at the corners of the mouth
Candida intertrigo: red macerated intertriginous areas with satellite pustules
Vulvovaginitis: pruritic, white, cheesy discharge; beefy red vulva
Chronic mucocutaneous variant: white adherent plaques of thrush or the angular cheilitis of perlèche; oral involvement may extend to the esophagus; nails are thickened, fragmented, and discolored, with significant edema and erythema of the surrounding periungual tissue; skin lesions often are acral or in the scalp, with erythematous, hyperkeratotic, serpiginous plaques
Interdigital involvement (erosio interdigitalis blastomycetica): erythema, scale, and satellite papules and pustules, most commonly in the space between the long finger and ring finger

Differential diagnosis
Thrush: Fordyce spots; hairy leukoplakia; lichen planus; aphthous stomatitis; pemphigus vulgaris; herpes simplex virus infection
Candida intertrigo : tinea cruris; contact dermatitis; seborrheic dermatitis
Inverse psoriasis mucocutaneous variant: acrodermatitis enteropathica; immunodeficiency diseases such as HIV infection, DiGeorge syndrome, Nezelof syndrome or

severe combined immunodeficiency; nutritional deficiency

Therapy
Thrush: clotrimazole 10 mg troche taken 3 times daily for 7–10 days; fluconazole; itraconazole

Candida intertrigo: fluconazole; azole antifungal agents; Zeasorb AF powder used twice daily as prophylaxis

Mucocutaneous variant: fluconazole; clotrimazole 10 mg troche taken 3 times daily for 7–10 days; cimetidine 400 mg PO 4 times daily indefinitely

References
Zuber TJ, Baddam K (2001) Superficial fungal infection of the skin. Where and how it appears help determine therapy. Postgraduate Medicine 109(1):117–120,123–126,131–132

Candidosis

▶ Candidiasis

Cane-cutter fever

▶ Leptospirosis

Canicola fever

▶ Leptospirosis

Canities

Definition
Graying or whitening of hair

References
Tobin DJ, Paus R (2001) Graying: gerontobiology of the hair follicle pigmentary unit. Experimental Gerontology 36(1):29–54

Canker sore

▶ Aphthous stomatitis

Cannon's disease

▶ White sponge nevus

Cantharidin

Trade name(s)
Canthacur

Generic available
No

Drug class
Vesicating agent

Mechanism of action
Interferes with mitochondria, which leads to epidermal cell necrosis

Dosage form
Colloidal solution

Dermatologic indications and dosage
See table

Common side effects
Cutaneous: irritant dermatitis, pain at site of application

Cantharidin. Dermatologic indications and dosage

Disease	Adult dosage	Child dosage
Molluscum contagiosum	Apply once under tape occlusion for 24 hours	Apply once under tape occlusion for 24 hours
Wart	Apply once under tape occlusion for 24 hours	Apply once under tape occlusion for 24 hours

Serious side effects
None

Drug interactions
None

Contraindications/precautions
Hypersensitivity to drug class or component

References
Moed L, Shwayder TA, Chang MW (2001) Cantharidin revisited: A blistering defense of an ancient medicine. Archives of Dermatology 137(10):1357–1360

Cantu syndrome

Synonym(s)
Hypertrichotic osteochondrodysplasia

Definition
Hereditary syndrome consisting of congenital hypertrichosis; osteochondrodysplasia leading to multiple skeletal defects and cardiomegaly

Pathogenesis
Unknown

Clinical manifestation
Congenital hypertrichosis; macrosomia at birth; narrow thorax; cardiomegaly; wide ribs; hypoplastic ischiopubic branches; small obturator foramen; bilateral coxa valga; enlarged medullary canal; Erlenmeyer-flask-like long bones; generalized osteopenia

Differential diagnosis
Costello syndrome

Therapy
None

References
Lazalde B, Sanchez-Urbina R, Nuno-Arana I, Bitar WE, de Lourdes Ramirez-Duenas M (2000) Autosomal dominant inheritance in Cantu syndrome (congenital hypertrichosis, osteochondrodysplasia, and cardiomegaly). American Journal of Medical Genetics 94(5):421–427

Capillary angioma

▶ Capillary hemangioma

Capillary hemangioma

Synonym(s)
Strawberry hemangioma; strawberry mark; raspberry lesion; infantile hemangioma; capillary angioma

Definition
Benign vascular neoplasm, consisting of proliferating endothelial cells, with early proliferation, usually followed by spontaneous involution

Pathogenesis
May involve abnormal release of angiogenic factors; possible role of estrogens

Clinical manifestation

Early lesion (up to 6 weeks of age): blanching of the involved skin; development of fine telangiectasias; formation of a red or violaceous macule or papule, often surrounded by a faint whitish halo

Proliferative stage (up to 12 months): dome-shaped, multilobular papule or nodule; may develop central erosion or ulceration; firm, rubbery consistency; expands with increased intravascular pressure

Involution stage: shrinks centrifugally from the center of the lesion; lesion becomes less red, with a dusky maroon to purple color; eventually regains normal flesh tones ("graying")

Cavernous variant: deep dermal and subcutaneous red-to-violaceous nodule; regression is often incomplete

Differential diagnosis

Nevus flammeus; blue rubber bleb nevus syndrome; Mafucci syndrome; angiosarcoma arteriovenous malformation; infantile fibrosarcoma; infantile myofibromatosis; pseudo-Kaposi's hemangioendothelioma; lymphatic malformation; teratoma; Gorham syndrome; Riley-Smith syndrome

Therapy

Ulcerated hemangiomas and thin superficial hemangiomas – flash lamp-pumped pulsed dye laser; lesions compromising function (e.g. larynx or eyelid) – prednisolone 2–5 mg per kg per day PO

References

Richards KA, Garden JM (2000) The pulsed dye laser for cutaneous vascular and nonvascular lesions. Seminars in Cutaneous Medicine & Surgery 19(4):276–286

Capsaicin

Trade name(s)
Zostrix; Zostrix HP

Generic available
Yes

Drug class
Analgesic

Mechanism of action
Depletes substance P and prevents re-accumulation in peripheral neurons

Dosage form
0.025% cream, gel, lotion; roll-on; 0.075% cream, gel, lotion; roll-on

Dermatologic indications and dosage
See table

Common side effects
Cutaneous: burning sensation; erythema

Serious side effects
None

Capsaicin. Dermatologic indications and dosage

Disease	Adult dosage	Child dosage
Brachioradial pruritus	Apply 4–5 times daily for first 1–3 weeks; then taper as per therapeutic response	Apply 4–5 times daily for first 1–3 weeks; then taper as per therapeutic response
Notalgia paresthetica	Apply 4–5 times daily for first 1–3 weeks; then taper as per therapeutic response	Apply 4–5 times daily for first 1–3 weeks; then taper as per therapeutic response
Post herpetic neuralgia	Apply 4–5 times daily for first 1–3 weeks; then taper as per therapeutic response	Apply 4–5 times daily for first 1–3 weeks; then taper as per therapeutic response

Drug interactions
None

Contraindications/precautions
Hypersensitivity to drug class or component

References
Sugeng MW, Yosipovitch G, Leok GC (2001) Post herpetic neuralgia and the dermatologist. International Journal of Dermatology 40(1):6–11>

Carate

▶ Pinta

Carbon baby

▶ Universal acquired melanosis

Carbuncle

▶ Furuncle

Carcinoid syndrome

▶ Malignant carcinoid syndrome

Carcinoma cuniculatum

▶ Verrucous carcinoma

Carcinoma in situ

▶ Bowen's disease

Carcinoma in situ of the penis

▶ Erythroplasia of Queyrat

Cardiocutaneous lentiginosis syndrome

▶ LEOPARD syndrome

Cardiocutaneous syndrome

▶ LEOPARD syndrome

Carducci fever

▶ Boutonneuse fever

Carney myxoma-endocrine complex

▶ Carney's syndrome

Carney's syndrome

Synonym(s)
Carney myxoma-endocrine complex; myxoma-spotty pigmentation-endocrine overactivity

Definition
Familial multiple neoplasia and lentiginosis syndrome with primary pigmented nodular adrenocortical disease (PPNAD); primary adrenal form of hypercortisolism, lentigines, ephelides, and blue nevi of the skin and mucosae and a variety of endocrine and other types of tumors

Pathogenesis
Autosomal dominant trait; two genetically distinct forms: one type mapped to chromosome 17 (CNC type 1); second type mapped to chromosome 2

Clinical manifestation
Lentigines; nevocellular nevi; freckling; hamartomas of the oral cavity; striae; kyphosis; easy bruising; sparse or absent hair; atrial and skin myxomas
Endocrinopathies: Cushing syndrome; acromegaly; hyperparathyroidism; prolactin-secreting tumor; multiple thyroid nodules

Differential diagnosis
Nevi; lentigines; McCune-Albright syndrome; neurofibromatosis; ephelides

Therapy
Treatment of the endocrine overactivity; surgical excision of symptomatic myxomas

References
Kiryu T, Kawaguchi S, Matsui E, Hoshi H, Kokubo M, Shimokawa K (1999) Multiple chondromatous hamartomas of the lung: A case report and review of the literature with special reference to Carney syndrome. Cancer 85(12):2557–2261

Carotenemia

Synonym(s)
None

Definition
Increased carotenoid pigments from ingestion of foodstuffs containing these nutrients

Pathogenesis
Deposition of yellow-orange pigments in the stratum corneum after the prolonged or excessive consumption of carotene-rich foods

Clinical manifestation
Asymptomatic, yellow-orange discoloration, particularly at sites with a thick stratum corneum, such as the palms and soles; no change in scleral pigmentation

Differential diagnosis
Jaundice; lycopenemia (orange-yellow skin discoloration due to the ingestion of large amounts of tomatoes); riboflavinemia; Addison's disease; drug reaction (e.g. quinicrine)

Therapy
Decreased ingestion of carotene-rich foods

References
Leung AK (1987) Carotenemia. Advances in Pediatrics 34:223–248

Carrión disease

▶ Bartonellosis

Carrión's disease

▶ Bartonellosis

Cat-scratch disease

► Bartonellosis

Cavernous hemangioma

► Capillary hemangioma

Cavernous lymphangioma

► Lymphangioma

CD30+ cutaneous large T-cell lymphoma

► Cutaneous CD30+ (Ki-1) anaplastic large-cell lymphoma

Cellulite

Definition
Fat deposits under the skin outwardly giving the skin a dimpled or orange-peel-like appearance

References
Draelos ZD, Marenus KD (1997) Cellulite. Etiology and purported treatment. Dermatologic Surgery 23(12):1177–1181

Cellulitis

Synonym(s)
None

Definition
Purulent inflammation of the deep dermis and subcutaneous tissue, most often secondary to a bacterial infection

Pathogenesis
Immune reaction to invading bacteria with an inflammatory response in the dermis and subcutaneous tissues, resulting in signs of inflammation

Clinical manifestation
Four signs of infection: erythema, pain, swelling, and warmth; imprecise margins of infection; areas of edema and erythema blending into the surrounding normal skin; systemic symptoms (e.g. fever, malaise); signs of lymphangitis with red lines extending proximal from the area of inflammation; regional lymphadenopathy; crepitus with anaerobic organisms

Differential diagnosis
Panniculitis; stasis dermatitis; contact dermatitis; arthropod envenomation; burns; septic joints; erysipelas; ecthyma; gas gangrene

Therapy
Oral antibiotic: dicloxacillin; cephalexin; azithromycin; clarithromycin
Systemic antibiotic: nafcillin: adults – 0.5–1.5 gm IV every 4 hours for 3–7 days; children – 10–20 mg per kg IV every 4 hours for 3–7 days
Cefotaxime: adults – 1 gm IV every 12 hours for 3–7 days; children – 12.5–45 mg per kg IV every 6 hours for 3–7 days

References
Danik SB, Schwartz RA, Oleske JM (1999) Cellulitis. Cutis 64(3):157–160,163–164

Central papillary atrophy

► Median rhomboid glossitis

Centrofacial lentiginosis

▶ **LEOPARD syndrome**

Cephalexin

Trade name(s)
Keflex; Keftab; Biocef

Generic available
Yes

Drug class
Cephalosporin antibiotic

Mechanism of action
Inhibition of penicillin-binding proteins, which results in defective bacterial cell wall synthesis

Dosage form
250 mg, 500 mg tablet; 125 mg per 5 ml, 250 mg per 5 ml suspension

Dermatologic indications and dosage
See table

Common side effects
Cutaneous: skin eruption

Gastrointestinal: nausea, vomiting, diarrhea
Laboratory: eosinophilia, elevated liver enzymes
Neurologic: headache, dizziness

Serious side effects
Bone marrow: thrombocytopenia, neutropenia
Gastrointestinal: pseudomembranous colitis
Immunologic: anaphylaxis

Drug interactions
Aminoglycoside antibiotics; oral contraceptives; probenecid

Contraindications/precautions
Hypersensitivity to drug class or component; caution if there is a history of penicillin allergy; caution with impaired renal function or if patient is lactating

References
Sadick N (2001) Systemic antibiotics. Dermatologic Clinics 19(1):1–24>

Cephalothoracic dystrophy

▶ **Progressive lipodystrophy**

Cephalexin. Dermatologic indications and dosage

Disease	Adult dosage	Child dosage
Cellulitis	250–500 mg PO 4 times daily for 7 days	25–100 mg per kg daily, divided into 4 doses for 7–10 days
Ecthyma	250–500 mg PO 4 times daily for 7 days	25–100 mg per kg daily, divided into 4 doses for 7–10 days
Erysipelas	250–500 mg PO 4 times daily for 7 days	25–100 mg per kg daily, divided into 4 doses for 7–10 days
Impetigo	250–500 mg PO 4 times daily for 7 days	25–100 mg per kg daily, divided into 4 doses for 7–10 days
Scarlet fever	250–500 mg PO 4 times daily for 7 days	25–100 mg per kg daily, divided into 4 doses for 7–10 days

Cercarial dermatitis

Synonym(s)
Swimmer's itch; bather's itch; clam digger's itch; silt itch; swamp itch; sedge pool itch

Definition
Pruritic eruption from an inflammatory reaction to schistosomal cercariae at the point of entry

Pathogenesis
Snail as primary host for schistosomal cercariae; free-swimming organisms penetrate into human skin and fail to complete life cycle; inflammatory reaction to the organism causes inflammation

Clinical manifestation
Localized pruritus followed by red macules and papules; occurring mainly in exposed parts of the skin; inflammatory response peaking at 2–3 days and subsiding in 1–2 weeks

Differential diagnosis
Seabather's eruption; insect bite reaction; harvest mite infestation; creeping eruption

Therapy
Ice compresses applied for 15–20 minutes 2–4 times per day; mid potency topical corticosteroids; antihistamines, first generation, for nighttime sedation

References
Folster-Holst R, Disko R, Rowert J, Bockeler W, Kreiselmaier I, Christophers E (2001) Cercarial dermatitis contracted via contact with an aquarium: case report and review. British Journal of Dermatology 145(4):638–640

Chagas disease

▶ **American trypanosomiasis**

Chalazion

Synonym(s)
Meibomian cyst

Definition
Granuloma of either meibomian gland or Zeis gland of the eyelid

Pathogenesis
Lipid-breakdown products from retained glandular secretions resulting in granulation tissue and inflammation; bacterial enzyme actions possibly part of the process

Clinical manifestation
Firm, red papule of the lid; associated with seborrheic dermatitis, chronic blepharitis, and rosacea

Differential diagnosis
Hordeolum; sebaceous neoplasm; orbital cellulitis; marginal cyst; mucocele; hydrocystoma; oncocytoma

Therapy
Medical therapy: moist heat applied twice daily for 15–30 minutes
Surgical therapy: incision and drainage of fluctuant lesions; drainage via a transconjunctival incision and curettage

References
Lederman C, Miller M (1999) Hordeola and chalazia. Pediatrics in Review 20(8):283–284

Cervical lipomatosis

▶ **Benign symmetric lipomatosis**

Chanarin Dorfman disease

▶ **Chanarin-Dorfman syndrome**

Chanarin-Dorfman syndrome

Synonym(s)
Chanarin Dorfman disease; Dorfman Chanarin syndrome; ichthyosiform erythroderma with vacuolation; ichthyotic neutral lipid storage disease; neutral lipid storage disease; triglyceride storage disease

Definition
Hereditary disorder of lipid metabolism, characterized by ichthyosis, myopathy, and abnormal white blood cells with vacuoles filled with lipids

Pathogenesis
Precise defect unknown; autosomal recessive trait; inability to break down intracellular triglycerides

Clinical manifestation
Moderate, generalized erythema and scale; myopathy; psychomotor delay; cataracts; decreased hearing

Differential diagnosis
Congenital ichthyosiform erythroderma; Refsum's disease

Therapy
Alpha hydroxy acids

References
Wessalowski R, Schroten H, Neuen-Jacob E, Reichmann H, Melnik BC, Lenard HG, Voit T (1994) Multisystem triglyceride storage disorder without ichthyosis in two siblings. Acta Paediatrica 83(1):93–98

Chancre

Definition
Painless ulcer characterizing primary syphilis

References
Goens JL, Janniger CK, De Wolf K (1994) Dermatologic and systemic manifestations of syphilis. American Family Physician 50(5):1013–1020

Chancroid

Synonym(s)
Soft chancre

Definition
Sexually transmitted genital disease, caused by the gram-negative bacillus Haemophilus ducreyi, characterized by painful genital ulcers and inflammatory inguinal adenopathy

Pathogenesis
Caused by gram-negative bacillus Haemophilus ducreyi; organism produces a potent distending toxin, probably contributing to the production and slow healing of ulcers

Clinical manifestation
Disease in men: painful, erythematous papules at the site of recent sexual contact; foreskin most common site of infection, but occasionally occurring on the shaft, glans, or meatus of the penis; lesions become pustular and then ulcerate; associated with regional lymphadenopathy; constitutional symptoms, such as malaise and low-grade fevers
Disease in women: ulcers most commonly occur on the labia majora but sometimes also on the labia minora, thigh, perineum, or cervix; lesions usually less symptomatic than in men

Differential diagnosis
Syphilis; lymphogranuloma venereum; herpes simplex virus infection; traumatic ulceration; aphthae; Behçet's disease; Crohn's disease; fixed drug reaction

Therapy
Azithromycin; ciprofloxacin; ceftriaxone 250 mg IM for 1 dose

References

Brown TJ, Yen-Moore A, Tyring SK (1999) An overview of sexually transmitted diseases. Part I. Journal of the American Academy of Dermatology 41(4):511–532

Charbon

▶ **Anthrax, cutaneous**

Cheadle-Möller-Barlow syndrome

▶ **Barlow's disease**

Chédiak-Higashi syndrome

Synonym(s)

Bequez Cesar syndrome, Chédiak-Steinbrinck-Higashi syndrome

Definition

Disorder characterized by immune deficiency, partial oculocutaneous albinism, easy bruising, and bleeding, as a result of deficient platelets and recurrent infections

Pathogenesis

Autosomal recessive trait; gene mutation affecting the synthesis and/or maintenance of storage/secretory granules in various types of cells, including melanocytes and neutrophils; abnormal intracellular protein transport

Clinical manifestation

Lack of skin pigmentation, similar to albinos, but in patchy distribution; blonde hair; blue eyes; photophobia; gingivitis and oral mucosal ulceration; frequent and severe pyogenic infections; neurologic dysfunction

Differential diagnosis

Oculocutaneous albinism; Griscelli syndrome; postinflammatory hypopigmentation; poliosis; piebaldism

Therapy

Bone marrow transplantation★

References

Stolz W, Graubner U, Gerstmeier J, Burg G, Belohradsky BH (1989) Chediak-Higashi syndrome: Approaches in diagnosis and treatment. Current Problems in Dermatology 18:93–100

Chédiak-Steinbrinck-Higashi syndrome

▶ **Chédiak-Higashi syndrome**

Cheilitis

Definition

Dryness, chapping, and fissuring of the lip

References

Kaugars GE, Pillion T, Svirsky JA, Page DG, Burns JC, Abbey LM (1999) Actinic cheilitis: A review of 152 cases. Oral Surgery Oral Medicine Oral Pathology Oral Radiology & Endodontics 88(2):181–186

Cheilitis, actinic

▶ **Actinic cheilitis**

Cheilitis, angular

▶ **Angular cheilitis**

Cheilitis granulomatosa

Synonym(s)
Miescher-Melkersson-Rosenthal syndrome; granulomatous cheilitis; orofacial granulomatosis; Miescher's cheilitis granulomatosa

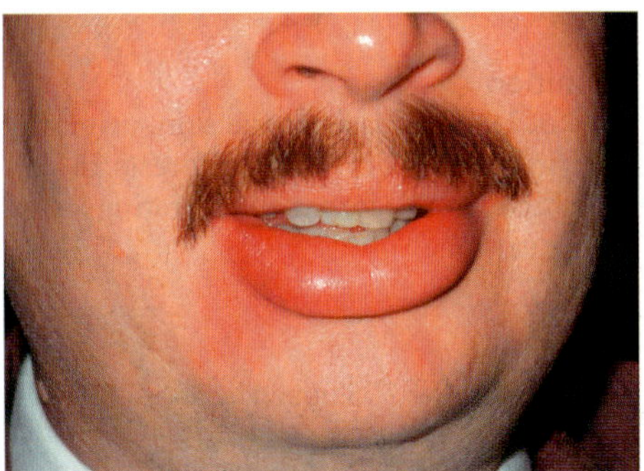

Cheilitis granulomatosa. Infiltrated lower vermillion portion of the lip, with secondary irritant dermatitis of the cutaneous portion of the lip

Definition
Chronic, non-tender swelling of the lip due to granulomatous inflammation; Melkersson-Rosenthal syndrome: chronic swelling of the lip, facial palsy, and lingua plicata

Pathogenesis
Unknown stimulus to granuloma formation; swelling secondary to edema and granulomas in the lamina propria

Clinical manifestation
First episode of edema resolves completely in hours or days; after recurrent attacks, occasional constitutional symptoms with attacks; swelling sometimes persists and becomes permanent; recurrences common from days to years; affected lip cracks and fissures, with reddish-brown discoloration and scaling; slow regression over several years

Differential diagnosis
Sarcoidosis; dental abscess; angioedema; lip trauma; insect bite reaction; Crohn's disease

Therapy
Triamcinolone 3–4 mg per ml intralesional; clofazimine 100 mg PO twice daily for 10 days, then twice weekly for 4 months; metronidazole 500 mg PO twice daily

References
Ridder GJ, Fradis M, Lohle E (1997) Cheilitis granulomatosa Miescher: treatment with clofazimine and review of the literature. Annals of Otology, Rhinology & Laryngology 110(10):964–967

Cheiloid

▶ **Keloid**

Cheilosis

▶ **Cheilitis**

Chemotherapy-induced alopecia

▶ **Anagen effluvium**

Cherry angioma

▶ **Cherry hemangioma**

Cherry hemangioma

Synonym(s)
Cherry angioma; Campbell de Morgan spots; senile angioma

Definition
Benign growth of the skin formed by a proliferation of dilated venules

Pathogenesis
Unknown

Clinical manifestation
Small, red-to-violaceous macule, or a larger dome-shaped or polypoid papule; occurs on all body sites except mucous membranes; increases in number and size with advancing age

Differential diagnosis
Angiokeratoma; petechiae; thrombocytopenia; Kaposi's sarcoma; bacillary angiomatosis; vasculitis; benign pigmented purpura; insect bite reaction; blue rubber bleb nevus syndrome

Therapy
Destruction by electrodesiccation and curettage; liquid nitrogen cryotherapy; pulse dye laser ablation; CO_2 laser vaporization

References
Sala F, Crosti C, Menni S, Piccinno R (1984) Cherry hemangioma: An SEM study. Journal of Cutaneous Pathology 11(6):531–533

Cheveux incoiffables

▶ **Uncombable hair syndrome**

Chickenpox

▶ **Varicella**

Chiclero's ulcer

Definition
Type of leishmaniasis of the skin, primarily affecting men who visit the forests to collect chicle (gum); forms an ulcerating lesion on the ear lobe

References
Andrade-Narvaez FJ, Simmonds-Diaz E, Rico-Aguilar S, Andrade-Narveez M, Palomo-Cetina A, Canto-Lara SB, Garcia-Miss MR, Madera-Sevilla M, Albertos-Alpuche N (1990) Incidence of localized cutaneous leishmaniasis (chiclero's ulcer) in Mexico. Transactions of the Royal Society of Tropical Medicine & Hygiene 84(2):219–220

Chilblains

Synonym(s)
Pernio; perniosis

Definition
Inflammatory skin condition presenting as pruritic and/or painful acral lesions after exposure to cold

Pathogenesis
Abnormal vascular response to cold exposure

Clinical manifestation
Recurrent, painful and/or pruritic, red-to-violaceous papules or nodules on the fin-

gers and/or toes; sometimes vesiculating or ulcerating; occurs 12–24 hours after cold exposure; sometimes occurs in association with systemic diseases, including chronic myelomonocytic leukemia, anorexia nervosa, dysproteinemias, macroglobulinemia, cryoglobulinemia, cryofibrinogenemia, cold agglutinins, antiphospholipid antibody syndrome, or Raynaud disease

Differential diagnosis
Vasculitis; sarcoidosis; erythema multiforme; acrocyanosis; septic or cholesterol emboli; erythromelalgia; polycythemia vera; purple toe syndrome secondary to coumarin; Raynaud phenomenon

Therapy
Prophylactic warming of acral areas with minimization of cold exposure; UVB phototherapy

References
Carruthers R (1988) Chilblains (perniosis). Australian Family Physician 17(11):968–969

CHILD syndrome

Synonym(s)
Congenital hemidysplasia; ichthyosiform nevus

Definition
Variant of ichthyosiform erythroderma characterized by congenital hemidysplasia, unilateral ichthyosiform erythroderma, and limb defects

Pathogenesis
Suggestion that peroxisomal deficiency in involved skin leads to accumulation of PGE2, resulting in keratinocyte growth and epidermal hyperproliferation; mosaicism possibly accounts for unilateral distribution

Clinical manifestation
Unilateral, scaly, erythematous plaques with a sharp midline demarcation, usually present at birth or early infancy; nail dystrophy; ipsilateral limb defects; ipsilateral hypoplasia of the brain, lung, thyroid and reproductive tract

Differential diagnosis
Congenital ichthyosiform erythroderma; inflammatory linear verrucous epidermal nevus (ILVEN); epidermal (organoid) nevus syndrome (Schimmelpfennig-Feuerstein-Mims); phacomatosis pigmentokeratotica

Therapy
Alpha hydroxy acids

References
Happle R, Mittag H, Kuster W (1995) The CHILD nevus: A distinct skin disorder. Dermatology 191(3):210–216

Chloasma

▶ Melasma

Chloracne

Synonym(s)
Occupational acne

Definition
Acneform eruption, with a preponderance of comedones, after exposure to chlorinated hydrocarbons, found in herbicide manufacturing and cable splicing, and polychlorinated biphenyls

Pathogenesis
Unknown

Clinical manifestation
Small, flesh-colored cysts and comedones, associated with pruritus, involving the face, postauricular region, and angles of the jaw; but sparing the nose and malar regions

Differential diagnosis
Acne vulgaris; syndrome of Favre-Racouchot; acne cosmetica; steroid-induced acne; pomade acne; tropical acne; radiation acne; gram negative folliculitis

Therapy
Isotretinoin[*]; tretinoin; tetracycline; incision and drainage; avoidance of agents containing chlorinated hydrocarbons

References
Rosas Vazquez E, Campos Macias P, Ochoa Tirado JG, Garcia Solana C, Casanova A, Palomino Moncada JF (1996) Chloracne in the 1990s. International Journal of Dermatology 35(9):643–645

Chlorpheniramine

▶ Antihistamines, first generation

Chondrodermatitis nodularis chronica antihelicis

▶ Chondrodermatitis nodularis helicis

Chondrodermatitis nodularis chronica helicis

▶ Chondrodermatitis nodularis helicis

Chondrodermatitis nodularis helicis

Synonym(s)
Chondrodermatitis nodularis chronica helicis; chondrodermatitis nodularis chronica antihelicis

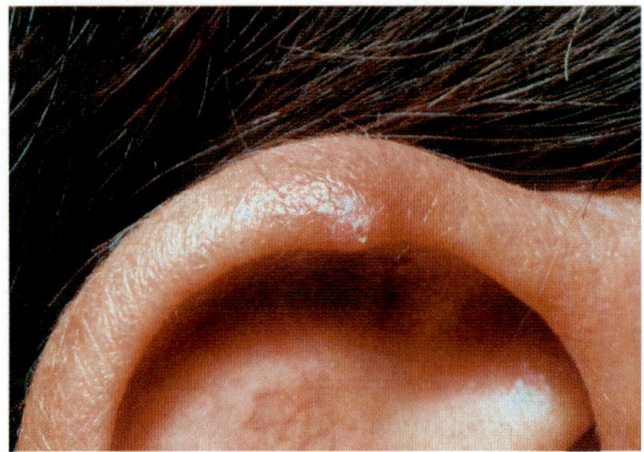

Chondrodermatitis nodularis helicis. Flesh-colored papule with punctate central erosion on the underside of the pinna of the ear

Definition
Inflammatory condition of the ear producing painful papules and nodules

Pathogenesis
Possibly involves dermal inflammation from trauma, cold, actinic damage, or pressure

Clinical manifestation
Firm, tender, well demarcated papule, with a raised, rolled edge and central erosion or ulceration; develops on the most prominent projection of the ear, most commonly on the apex of the helix; distribution on the antihelix more common in women

Differential diagnosis
Actinic keratosis; basal cell carcinoma; squamous cell carcinoma; keratoacanthoma; tophus; rheumatoid nodule; colloid milium; endochondral pseudocyst

Therapy
Cryotherapy; triamcinolone 3–5 mg per ml intralesional; surgical excision; CNH pillow to relieve pressure

References
Beck MH (1985) Treatment of chondrodermatitis nodularis helicis and conventional wisdom? British Journal of Dermatology 113(4):504–505

Chondrodysplasia punctata

▶ Conradi disease

Chondrodystrophia calcificans congenita

▶ Conradi disease

Choristoma

▶ Dermoid cyst

Christ-Siemens-Touraine syndrome

▶ Anhidrotic ectodermal dysplasia

Chromhidrosis

Synonym(s)
Ephidrosis tincta; eccrine chromhidrosis

Definition
Condition characterized by colored sweat, mostly secondary to colored apocrine secretions

Pathogenesis
Elevated levels of lipofuscins possibly involved; substance P possibly an important neurotransmitter; extrinsic contributing factors include dyes, chromogenic bacteria, and chemical contactants

Clinical manifestation
Turbid, yellow, red, blue, or green apocrine secretion; color accentuated in the pores

Differential diagnosis
Hyperbilirubinemia; pseudomonas infection; poisoning; alkaptonuria; bleeding diathesis (red sweat, hematohidrosis); copper exposure (blue sweat)

Therapy
Capsaicin 0.025% cream applied 4–5 times per day

References
Marks JG Jr (1989) Treatment of apocrine chromhidrosis with topical capsaicin. Journal of the American Academy of Dermatology 21(2 Pt 2):418–420

Chromoblastomycosis

Synonym(s)
Chromomycosis; verrucous dermatitis; phaeohyphomycosis; cystic chromomycosis

Definition
Chronic skin and subcutaneous fungal infection caused by one of multiple fungal pathogens

Pathogenesis
Inoculation by one of the following: Hormodendrum pedrosoi, H. compactum, or

Phialophora verrucosa; organisms isolated from wood and soil

Clinical manifestation
Asymptomatic, verrucous papule, slowly enlarging to large plaque or thick nodule; lesions often ulcerate; satellite lesions produced by autoinoculation

Differential diagnosis
North American blastomycosis; South American blastomycosis; tuberculosis; leishmaniasis; syphilis; yaws; squamous cell carcinoma; atypical mycobacterial infection; sporotrichosis; nocardiosis

Therapy
Itraconazole; terbinafine; flucytosine with or without localized hyperthermia; cryotherapy; surgical excision for small lesions

References
Rivitti EA, Aoki V (1999) Deep fungal infections in tropical countries. Clinics in Dermatology 17(2):171–190

Chromomycosis

▶ Chromoblastomycosis

Chromophytosis

▶ Tinea versicolor

Chronic actinic dermatitis

Synonym(s)
Actinic reticuloid; persistent light reactivity; photosensitive eczema; photosensitivity dermatitis; persistent light reaction

Definition
Persistent eczematous eruption in the sun-exposed areas of greater than 3 months' duration, with abnormal sensitivity to either ultraviolet or visible light

Pathogenesis
Delayed type hypersensitivity reaction involving a light-induced immune response

Clinical manifestation
Eczematous and infiltrated plaques that involve mostly exposed skin, but may generalize to erythroderma

Differential diagnosis
Polymorphous light eruption; allergic contact dermatitis; photocontact dermatitis; solar urticaria; actinic prurigo; atopic dermatitis; lupus erythematosus; cutaneous T cell lymphoma

Therapy
Protection from sunlight; photochemotherapy; azathioprine; hydroxychloroquine sulfate; cyclosporine

References
Lim HW, Morison WL, Kamide R, Buchness MR, Harris R, Soter NA (1994) Chronic actinic dermatitis. An analysis of 51 patients evaluated in the United States and Japan. Archives of Dermatology 130(10):1284–1289

Chronic adrenal insufficiency

▶ Addison's disease

Chronic atrophic acrodermatitis

▶ Acrodermatitis chronica atrophicans

Chronic atrophic polychondritis

▶ Relapsing polychondritis

Chronic bullous dermatosis of childhood

▶ Linear IgA dermatosis

Chronic bullous disease of childhood

▶ Linear IgA dermatosis

Chronic cutaneous lupus erythematosus

▶ Lupus erythematosus, discoid

Chronic erythema nodosum

▶ Subacute nodular migratory panniculitis

Chronic granulomatous disease

Synonym(s)

Chronic granulomatous disease of childhood; fatal granulomatosis of childhood; progressive septic granulomatosis; X-linked chronic granulomatous disease

Definition

Inherited disorder of phagocytic cells, leading to recurrent, life-threatening bacterial and fungal infections

Pathogenesis

Failure of phagocytes to generate sufficient quantities of reactive oxygen species; molecular defect represents a mutation in the gene encoding the *b* subunit of cytochrome $b558$ (*CYBB*), located on the X chromosome

Clinical manifestation

Early onset of severe recurrent bacterial and fungal infections, often involving the skin; lungs most common site of infection; other involved sites include gastrointestinal tract, lymph nodes, liver, and spleen

Differential diagnosis

Bruton agammaglobulinemia; common variable immunodeficiency; severe combined immunodeficiency; HIV infection; complement deficiency; leukocyte adhesion deficiency; Wiskott-Aldrich syndrome

Therapy

Prophylaxis of bacterial infections with trimethoprim-sulfamethoxazole 5 mg per kg per day PO divided into 2 doses; bone marrow transplantation★

References

Goldblatt D, Thrasher AJ, Chronic granulomatous disease. Clinical & Experimental Immunology 122(1):1–9

Chronic granulomatous disease of childhood

▶ Chronic granulomatous disease

Chronic hair pulling

▶ Trichotillomania

Chronic papulopustular facial dermatitis

▶ Perioral dermatitis

Chronic superficial dermatitis

▶ Small plaque parapsoriasis

Chrysiasis

Synonym(s)
Chrysoderma

Definition
Development of a blue-gray pigmentation in skin and mucous membranes, caused by exposure to gold compounds

Pathogenesis
Deposition of gold salts in the dermis; increased melanin production in the epidermis

Clinical manifestation
Blue-gray or violaceous hue to sun-exposed skin and sclerae; mucous membranes spared; pigmentation usually permanent; occurs only after a cumulative dose of at least 50 mg per kg

Differential diagnosis
Argyria; other drug-induced pigmentation (e.g. minocycline; amiodarone); Addison's disease; hemosiderosis; jaundice; carotenemia; hemochromatosis

Therapy
No effective therapy

References
Smith RW, Cawley MI (1997) Chrysiasis. British Journal of Rheumatology 36(1):3–5

Chrysoderma

▶ Chrysiasis

Churg-Strauss disease

▶ Churg-Strauss syndrome

Churg-Strauss granulomatosis syndrome

▶ Churg-Strauss syndrome

Churg-Strauss syndrome

Synonym(s)
Allergic granulomatosis; allergic angiitis and granulomatosis; eosinophilic granulomatous vasculitis; Churg-Strauss granulomatosis syndrome; granulomatous vasculitis with asthma

Definition
Disorder characterized by asthma, transient pulmonary infiltrates, eosinophilia, and systemic vasculitis

Pathogenesis
Activated eosinophils possibly pathogenic

Clinical manifestation
Cutaneous findings: red papules and macules; palpable purpuric papules and plaques; cutaneous and subcutaneous papules and nodules
Respiratory tract findings: allergic rhinitis; asthma; transient pulmonary infiltrates
Vasculitis target organs: kidney, heart, central nervous system, gastrointestinal tract

Differential diagnosis
Henoch-Schönlein purpura; lupus erythematosus; bronchopulmonary aspergillosis; lymphoma; Loeffler syndrome; lymphomatoid granulomatosis; polyarteritis nodosa; rheumatoid arthritis

Therapy
Prednisone*; steroid-sparing agents: methotrexate; azathioprine 100–150 mg PO per day; cyclosporine; cyclophosamide pulse therapy 0.6 gm per m^2 IV monthly for up to 1 year

References
Gross WL (2002) Churg-Strauss syndrome: update on recent developments. Current Opinion in Rheumatology 14(1):11–14

Cicatricial pemphigoid

Synonym(s)
Benign mucous membrane pemphigoid; scarring pemphigoid; mucosal pemphigoid

Definition
Autoimmune vesiculobullous disease predominately affecting mucous membranes

Pathogenesis
IgG antibodies against antigens in basement zone; major antigens associated are BPAG2 and epiligrin (laminin 5); immune reaction causes loss of adhesion at the dermal-epidermal junction and blisters

Clinical manifestation
Persistent, painful erosions on mucous membranes, often healing with scarring; ocular involvement: pain or the sensation of grittiness in the eye; conjunctival inflammation and erosions; keratinization of the conjunctiva and shortening of the fornices; entropion with subsequent trichiasis; skin: tense vesicles or bullae, sometimes hemorrhagic, sometimes healing with scarring or milia; scalp involvement leads to alopecia

Differential diagnosis
Bullous pemphigoid; linear IgA dermatosis; erythema multiforme; Stevens-Johnson syndrome; epidermolysis bullosa; epidermolysis bullosa acquisita; dermatitis herpetiformis; impetigo; pemphigus foliaceus; pemphigus vulgaris; herpes simplex virus infection; herpes zoster

Therapy
Limited disease: mid potency topical corticosteroid gel for mucous membranes
Extensive disease: prednisone, dapsone; cyclophosphamide; azathioprine

References
Fleming TE, Korman NJ (2000) Cicatricial pemphigoid. Journal of the American Academy of Dermatology 43(4):571–591

Ciclopirox

Trade name(s)
Loprox; Penlac

Generic available
No

Drug class
Topical antifungal agent

Mechanism of action
Affects synthesis of fungal cell wall

Dosage form
0.77% cream, gel, lotion; 8% nail lacquer

Dermatologic indications and dosage
See table

Common side effects
Cutaneous: burning, itching, redness, swelling

Serious side effects
None

Drug interactions
None

Contraindications/precautions
Hypersensitivity to drug class or component

References
Gupta AK, Baran R (2000) Ciclopirox nail lacquer solution 8% in the 21st century. Journal of the American Academy of Dermatology 43(4 Supplement):S96–102

Ciprofloxacin

Trade name(s)
Cipro

Generic available
No

Drug class
Fluoroquinolone antibiotic

Mechanism of action
Inhibition of bacterial DNA gyrase, which results in interference with DNA replication

Dosage form
100 mg, 250 mg, 500 mg, 750 mg tablet; 250, 500 mg per 5 ml for intravenous infusion

Dermatologic indications and dosage
See table

Common side effects
Cutaneous: photosensitivity, urticaria, or other vascular reaction
Gastrointestinal: nausea and vomiting, diarrhea, abdominal pain
Neurologic: agitation, confusion, insomnia, headache, dizziness, restlessness

Serious side effects
Gastrointestinal: pseudomembranous colitis
Neurologic: toxic psychosis, seizures

Drug interactions
Antacids; caffeine; calcium salts; clozapine; oral contraceptives; cyclosporine; glyburide/metformin; iron salts; non-steroidal anti-inflammatory drugs; olanzapine; phenytoin; probenecid; theophylline; warfarin

Ciclopirox. Dermatologic indications and dosage

Disease	Adult dosage	Child dosage
Onychomycosis	Apply Penlac once daily for up to 48 weeks	Apply Penlac once daily for up to 48 weeks
Tinea corporis	Apply Loprox twice daily	Apply Loprox twice daily
Tinea cruris	Apply Loprox twice daily	Apply Loprox twice daily
Tinea faciei	Apply Loprox twice daily	Apply Loprox twice daily
Tinea nigra	Apply Loprox twice daily	Apply Loprox twice daily
Tinea pedis	Apply Loprox twice daily	Apply Loprox twice daily
White piedra	Apply Loprox twice daily	Apply Loprox twice daily

Ciprofloxacin. Dermatologic indications and dosage

Disease	Adult dosage	Child dosage
Cellulitis	250–500 mg PO twice daily for 7–21 days, depending on response	Not indicated
Chancroid	500 mg PO twice daily for 3 days	Not indicated
Malakoplakia	250–500 mg PO for 7–14 days	Not indicated
Mycobacterium marinum infection	500 mg 1–2 times daily for 4–6 weeks	Not indicated
Rhinoscleroma	250–500 mg PO twice daily for months to years	Not indicated
Rickettsialpox	250–500 mg PO daily for 5 days	Not indicated
Salmonellosis	500 mg IV twice daily, then switch to PO when tolerated for a total course of 10–14 days	Not indicated

Contraindications/precautions
Hypersensitivity to drug class or component; safety not established for patients < 18 years old; caution in those with impaired renal or liver function; caution in those with seizures

References
Sadick N (2000) Systemic antibiotic agents. Dermatologic Clinics 19(1):1–21

Circumscribed neurodermatitis

▶ Lichen simplex chronicus

Circumscribed scleroderma

▶ Morphea

Clam digger's itch

▶ Cercarial dermatitis

Clarithromycin

Trade name(s)
Biaxin

Generic available
No

Drug class
Macrolide antibiotic

Mechanism of action
Inhibits protein synthesis of sensitive bacterial organisms

Dosage form
250 mg, 500 mg tablet

Dermatologic indications and dosage
See table

Common side effects
Cutaneous: skin eruption, vaginitis
Gastrointestinal: nausea, vomiting, abdominal pain, diarrhea, anorexia

Serious side effects
Cutaneous: anaphylaxis, Stevens-Johnson syndrome, toxic epidermal necrolysis
Gastrointestinal: pseudomembranous colitis, cholestatic jaundice

Clarithromycin. Dermatologic indications and dosage

Disease	Adult dosage	Child dosage
Atypical mycobacterial infection	500 mg PO twice daily for 6–12 weeks after clinical remission	> 45 kg weight; 7.5 mg per kg PO twice daily for 6–12 weeks after clinical remission
Bacillary angiomatosis	250 mg PO twice daily for 3 weeks	> 45 kg weight; 7.5 mg per kg PO twice daily for 3 weeks
Bartonellosis	250 mg PO twice daily for 3 weeks	> 45 kg weight; 7.5 mg per kg PO twice daily for 3 weeks
Cellulitis	250 mg PO twice daily for 5–7 days	> 45 kg weight; 7.5 mg per kg PO twice daily for 5–7 days
Ecthyma	250 mg PO twice daily for 5–7 days	> 45 kg weight; 7.5 mg per kg PO twice daily for 5–7 days
Erythrasma	1 gm PO for 1 dose	> 45 kg weight; 7.5 mg per kg PO for 1 dose
Impetigo	250 mg PO twice daily for 5–7 days	> 45 kg weight; 7.5 mg per kg PO twice daily for 5–7 days
Mycobacterium marinum infection	500 mg PO twice daily for 6–12 weeks	15 mg per kg PO divided into 2 doses daily for 6–12 weeks

Drug interactions

Amiodarone; antacids; budesonide; buspirone; carbamazepine; clozapine; oral contraceptives; cyclosporine; digoxin; ergot alkaloids; methadone; phenytoin; pimozide; protease inhibitors; quinidine; statins; tacrolimus; theophylline; valproic acid; vinca alkaloids; warfarin

Contraindications/precautions

Hypersensitivity to drug class or component; caution in those with impaired liver function; do not use concomitantly with terfenadine or astemizole

References

Alvarez-Elcoro S, Enzler MJ (1999) The macrolides: erythromycin, clarithromycin, and azithromycin. Mayo Clinic Proceedings 74(6):613–634

Clark's nevus

▶ **Atypical mole**

Classic typhus

▶ **Epidemic typhus**

Clavus

Synonym(s)

Callus; callosity; corn, heloma, callous

Definition

Thickening of the skin due to intermittent pressure and frictional forces

Pathogenesis

Inappropriate distribution of pressure onto a specific site, producing increased frictional forces and reactive skin thickening

Clinical manifestation

Thickened skin, with retained skin dermatoglyphics, most commonly on the foot; occasional secondary maceration and fungal or bacterial infection

Differential diagnosis

Wart; gout; lichen planus; interdigital neuroma; lichen simplex chronicus; palmoplantar keratoderma; keratosis punctata; porokeratosis plantaris

Therapy

Mechanical pressure redistribution: orthotics; well-fitted shoes; protective pads on pressure points; skin-surface paring for symptomatic lesions

References

Freeman DB (2002) Corns and calluses resulting from mechanical hyperkeratosis. American Family Physician 65(11):2277–2280

Clear cell acanthoma

Synonym(s)

Clear cell acanthoma of Degos; Degos' acanthoma; acanthome à cellules claires

Definition

Skin tumor with accumulation of clear, glycogen-containing cells

Pathogenesis

Unknown

Clinical manifestation

Solitary, dome-shaped papule or nodule, with a peripheral scale; occurring most commonly on the lower extremities

Differential diagnosis

Histiocytoma; seborrheic keratosis; lichenoid keratosis; pyogenic granuloma; amelanotic melanoma

Therapy

Surgical excision*

References

Degos R, Civatte J (1970) Clear-cell acanthoma. Experience of 8 years. British Journal of Dermatology 83(2):248–254

Clear cell acanthoma of Degos

▶ Clear cell acanthoma

Clear cell adenoma

▶ Eccrine acrospiroma

Clear cell hidradenoma

▶ Eccrine acrospiroma

Clear cell myoepithelioma

▶ Eccrine hidradenoma

Climatic bubo

▶ Lymphogranuloma venereum

Clindamycin, systemic

Trade name(s)

Cleocin

Generic available

Yes

Drug class

Lincosamide antibiotic

Mechanism of action

Binds to bacterial 50S ribosomal subunit, interfering with protein synthesis

Clindamycin, systemic. Dermatologic indications and dosage

Disease	Adult dosage	Child dosage
Acne vulgaris	150 mg PO 2–3 times daily	Not indicated
Gas gangrene	15 mg per kg IV daily divided into 3 doses	10 mg per kg daily IV divided into 3 doses
Necrotizing fasciitis	600–900 mg IV every 6–12 hours	25–40 mg per kg IV divided into 3–4 doses daily
Paronychia, acute	150 mg PO 3 times daily for 7–10 days	Not indicated
Streptococcal toxic shock-like syndrome	600–900 mg IV every 6–12 hours	25–40 mg per kg IV divided into 3–4 doses daily

Dosage form
75 mg, 150 mg tablet; intramuscular preparation; solution for intravenous injection

Dermatologic indications and dosage
See table

Common side effects
Cutaneous: skin eruption, pruritus
Gastrointestinal: nausea, vomiting, diarrhea, abdominal pain, jaundice

Serious side effects,
Bone marrow: thrombocytopenia; granulocytopenia
Cutaneous: anaphylaxis, Stevens-Johnson syndrome
Gastrointestinal: pseudomembranous colitis, esophagitis

Drug interactions
Oral contraceptives; neuromuscular blockers

Contraindications/precautions
Hypersensitivity to drug class or component; history of ulcerative colitis; caution with renal or hepatic impairment

References
Weingarten-Arams J, Adam HM (2002) Clindamycin. Pediatrics in Review 23(4):149–150

Clostridial myonecrosis

▶ Gas gangrene

Clouston's disease

▶ Hidrotic ectodermal dysplasia

Clubbing of the nails

Definition
A broadening and thickening of the fingers or toes, with increased lengthwise curvature and curvature of the tip of the nail, and flattening of the angle between the cuticle and nail

References
Collins KP, Burkhart CG (1985) Clubbing of the fingers. International Journal of Dermatology 24(5):296–297

Cobb syndrome

Synonym(s)
Cutaneomeningospinal angiomatosis

Definition
Association of spinal angiomas or arteriovenous malformations with congenital cutaneous vascular lesions in the same dermatome

Pathogenesis
Apparently a developmental abnormality of the vessels of the spinal cord and skin

Clinical manifestation
Vascular abnormalities, including asymptomatic port wine stain, angiokeratoma, or hemangioma; various neurologic findings depending on level of the vascular abnormality; associated scoliosis or kyphoscoliosis

Differential diagnosis
Nevus flammeus; infantile hemangioma; Sturge-Weber syndrome; Wyburn-Mason syndrome; Klippel-Trenaunay-Weber syndrome; angiokeratoma corporis diffusum

Therapy
Neurosurgical evaluation

References
Shim JH, Lee DW, Cho BK (1996) A case of Cobb syndrome associated with lymphangioma circumscriptum. Dermatology 193(1):45–47

Coccidioidomycosis

Synonym(s)
Valley fever, San Joaquin Valley fever; desert rheumatism; coccidiosis

Definition
Disease caused by the spores of the fungus, Coccidioides immitis

Pathogenesis
Inhalation of arthroconidia from the organism C. immitis; sometimes spreading within the lungs or via the bloodstream; rare direct skin inoculation of C immitis

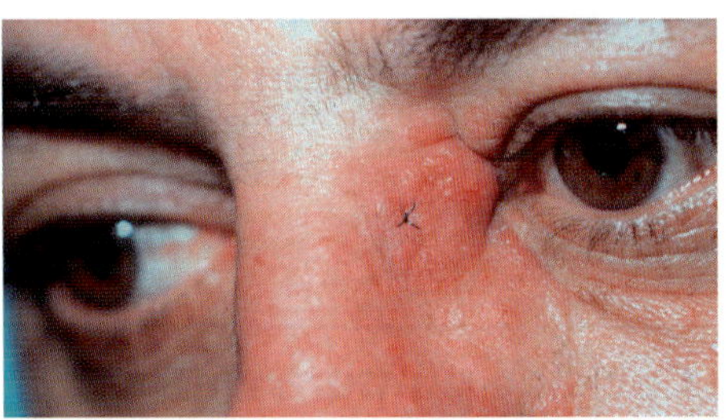

Coccidioidomycosis. Erythematous, edematous plaque on the upper nasal bridge

Clinical manifestation
Prodrome of fever, weight loss, malaise, and headache; acute or subacute pneumonic illness most common clinical presentation, with cough and inspiratory chest pain
Non-specific skin findings: erythema nodosum; erythema multiforme
Specific skin findings: superficial papules; keratotic nodules; verrucous ulcers; subcutaneous fluctuant abscesses
Other organs of dissemination: bones and joints; adrenal glands; central nervous system; liver

Differential diagnosis
Rosacea; tuberculosis; sarcoidosis; actinomycosis; leishmaniasis; Wegener's granulomatosis; vasculitis; syphilis; tinea faciei; sporotrichosis; chromoblastomycosis; parapsoriasis; mycosis fungoides; lichen planus

Therapy
Disseminated disease: Amphotericin B 0.3–1 mg per kg per day IV; start with 0.25 mg per kg per day and increased by 5–10 mg per day; fluconazole; itraconazole

References
Galgiani JN (1997) Coccidioidomycosis. Current Clinical Topics in Infectious Diseases 17:188–204

Coccidiosis

► Coccidioidomycosis

Cochin China diarrhea

▶ Strongyloidosis

Cockade purpura with edema

▶ Acute hemorrhagic edema of infancy

Cockayne syndrome

Synonym(s)
Cockayne's syndrome; dwarfism with retinal atrophy and deafness

Definition
Disorder characterized by sunlight sensitivity, short stature, neurologic abnormalities, cataracts, and the appearance of premature aging

Pathogenesis
Defective DNA repair, specifically transcription-coupled repair; two defective genes, CSA and CSB, coding for proteins that interact with components of the transcriptional machinery and with DNA repair proteins

Clinical manifestation
Growth failure; aged appearance; extreme photosensitivity; dental abnormalities; progressive neurologic abnormalities, including mental retardation and deafness; degenerative retinal pigmentary abnormalities

Differential diagnosis
Xeroderma pigmentosum, particularly the DeSanctis-Cacchione variant; Bloom's syndrome; progeria; Werner's syndrome; Rothmund-Thompson syndrome; ataxia-telangiectasia

Therapy
Strict sunlight avoidance

References
Nance MA, Berry SA (1992) Cockayne syndrome: review of 140 cases. American Journal of Medical Genetics 42:68–84

Cockayne's syndrome

▶ Cockayne syndrome

Colchicine

Trade name(s)
None

Generic available
Yes

Drug class
Anti-inflammatory

Mechanism of action
Binds to dimers of tubulin, preventing microtubule assembly

Dosage form
0.5 mg, 0.6 mg tablet

Dermatologic indications and dosage
See table

Common side effects
Cutaneous: skin eruption, alopecia
Gastrointestinal: diarrhea, nausea, vomiting, abdominal pain
Hematologic: anemia, thrombophlebitis

Serious side effects
Cutaneous: cellulitis
Hematologic: agranulocytosis, aplastic anemia, neutropenia
Neurologic: myoneuropathy

Colchicine. Dermatologic indications and dosage

Disease	Adult dosage	Child dosage
Acute neutrophilic dermatosis	0.6–1.8 mg PO daily	Not established
Aphthous stomatitis	0.6–1.8 mg PO daily	Not established
Behçet's disease	0.6–1.8 mg PO daily	Not established
Calcinosis cutis	0.6–1.8 mg PO daily	Not established
Dermatomyositis	0.6–1.8 mg PO daily	Not established
Leukocytoclastic vasculitis	0.6–1.8 mg PO daily	Not established
Linear IgA bullous dermatosis	0.6–1.8 mg PO daily	Not established
Pachydermoperiostosis	0.6–1.8 mg PO daily	Not established
Relapsing polychondritis	0.6–1.8 mg PO daily	Not established
Urticarial vasculitis	0.6–1.8 mg PO daily	Not established

Drug interactions
Cyclosporine

Contraindications/precautions
Hypersensitivity to drug class or component; blood dyscrasias; pregnancy; caution in serious gastrointestinal disorders

References
Ritter S, George R, Serwatka LM, Elston DM (2002) Long-term suppression of chronic Sweet's syndrome with colchicine. Journal of the American Academy of Dermatology 47(2):323–324

Cold panniculitis

Synonym(s)
Popsicle panniculitis; Haxthausen's disease

Definition
Acute, nodular, erythematous eruption at skin sites exposed to the cold

Pathogenesis
Localized cold injury leading to inflammation of the subcutaneous adipose tissue; infants possibly at greater risk because of increased fatty acid content in adipose tissue

Clinical manifestation
Beginning 1–3 days after a cold injury to exposed or poorly protected areas; painful, firm, red or cyanotic, indurated nodules with ill-defined margins; in obese patients, buttocks, thighs, arms, and area under the chin are most commonly affected; in small children, is the site of involvement often cheeks

Differential diagnosis
Subcutaneous fat necrosis of the newborn; sclerema neonatorum; poststeroid panniculitis; erythema infectiosum; atopic dermatitis; cellulitis

Therapy
None

References
Ter Poorten JC, Hebert AA, Ilkiw R (1995) Cold panniculitis in a neonate. Journal of the American Academy of Dermatology 33(2 Pt 2):383–385

Cold urticaria

Synonym(s)
None

Definition
Physical urticaria characterized by erythematous papules and plaques arising when the body temperature cools

Pathogenesis
Familial type: autosomal dominant trait; unknown cause
Acquired type: unknown cause

Clinical manifestation
Pruritus, erythema, and urticaria precipitated by exposure to cold objects, cold air, or cold water; sometimes associated with constitutional signs and symptoms, such as fever, chills, headache, myalgia, loss of consciousness; symptoms often disappear in a few months in the acquired type

Differential diagnosis
Aquagenic urticaria; dermatographism; anaphylaxis from foods, medications, etc.; cholinergic urticaria

Therapy
Antihistamines, first generation, especially cyproheptadine

References
Claudy A (2001) Cold urticaria. Journal of Investigative Dermatology Symposium Proceedings 6(2):141–142

Collagenoma

▶ **Connective tissue nevus**

Collagenoma perforant verruciforme

▶ **Reactive perforating collagenosis**

Collodion baby

Definition
Newborn infant enveloped in a shiny, smooth collodion-like membrane, which may deform the facial features and distal extremities

References
Frenk E, de Techtermann F (1992) Self-healing collodion baby: evidence for autosomal recessive inheritance. Pediatric Dermatology 9(2):95–97

Colloid degeneration

Synonym(s)
Colloid milium; colloid pseudomilium; colloid degeneration of the skin; elastosis colloidalis conglomerata

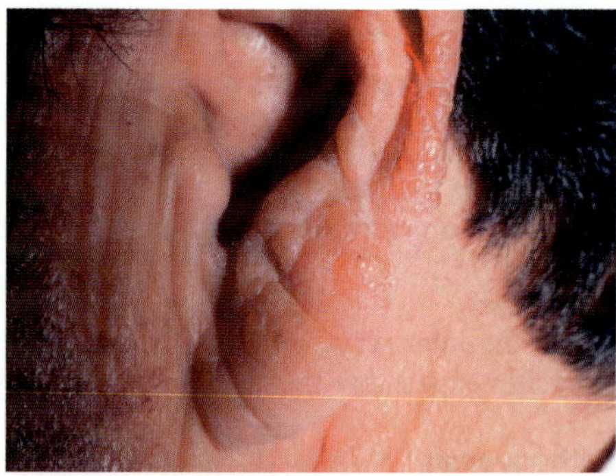

Colloid degeneration. Multiple translucent papules on the ear

Definition
Deposition of amorphous material (colloid) in the dermis

Pathogenesis
Related to excessive sun exposure; juvenile form inherited; origin of colloid unclear; possibly formed from degeneration of elastic fibers or synthesized from ultraviolet light-transformed keratinocytes

Clinical manifestation
Adult type: multiple, discrete, shiny, translucent papules in sun-exposed areas of face and ears; sometimes gelatinous material extruded

Juvenile type: onset before puberty; numerous, yellow-to-brown, waxy papules, mainly on the face; possibly related to severe sunburn

Nodular type: one or a few large, pink-to-brown, smooth nodules on the face

Differential diagnosis
Nodular amyloidosis; sarcoidosis; epidermoid cyst; syndrome of Favre-Racouchot; sebaceous hyperplasia; xanthoma; tuberous sclerosis; porphyria cutanea tarda

Therapy
Cryotherapy; dermabrasion

References
Touart DM, Sau P (1998) Cutaneous deposition diseases. Part I. Journal of the American Academy of Dermatology 39(2 Pt 1):149–171

Colloid degeneration of the skin

▶ Colloid degeneration

Colloid milium

▶ Colloid degeneration

Colloid pseudomilium

▶ Colloid degeneration

Com

▶ Clavus

Coma blister

Synonym(s)
None

Definition
Bullae arising over pressure points in patients who experience prolonged periods of unconsciousness

Pathogenesis
Unclear; several theories proposed: pressure necrosis; direct toxic action of a drug, such as a barbiturate or illicit drugs; drug-induced hyperthermia

Clinical manifestation
One or a few vesicles or bullae over pressure points, such as fingers, heels, or knees, may involve two limbs apposing one another for long periods during an unconscious state

Differential diagnosis
Fixed drug eruption; insect bite reaction; localized bullous pemphigoid; herpes simplex virus infection; bullous impetigo; porphyria cutanea tarda; epidermolysis bullosa acquisita

Therapy
None

References
Mehregan DR, Daoud M, Rogers RS 3rd (1992) Coma blisters in a patient with diabetic ketoac-

idosis. Journal of the American Academy of Dermatology 27(2 Pt 1):269–270

Comedone

Definition
Small, flesh-colored, white, or dark concretion found at the opening of a sebaceous follicle; also known as whitehead or blackhead

References
Thiboutot DM (1996) An overview of acne and its treatment. Cutis 57(1 Suppl):8–12

Còmel-Netherton syndrome

▶ Netherton syndrome

Common baldness

▶ Androgenetic alopecia

Common ichthyosis

▶ Ichthyosis vulgaris

Compulsive hair pulling

▶ Trichotillomania

Condyloma acuminata

▶ Condyloma acuminatum

Condyloma acuminatum

Synonym(s)
Genital wart; anogenital wart; condyloma acuminata

Definition
Viral disease characterized by a soft, wart-like growth on the genital skin

Pathogenesis
Human papilloma virus (HPV); acquired by inoculation of the virus into the epidermis via defects in the epithelium or by autoinoculation

Clinical manifestation
Pink-to-brown, verrucous, soft papules or nodules of the genitalia, perineum, crural folds, and anus, often forming large, exophytic, cauliflower-like tumors

Differential diagnosis
Syphilis; verrucous carcinoma of genitalia (giant condyloma of Buschke-Löwenstein); bowenoid papulosis; seborrheic keratosis; anogenital carcinoma; erythroplasia of Queyrat; lichen planus; Reiter syndrome; pearly penile papules

Therapy
Cryotherapy; imiquimod; podofilox; keratolytic agents, such as salicylic acid; destruction by electrodesiccation and curettage or laser ablation; surgical excision of large tumors

References
Krogh G von (2001) Management of anogenital warts (condylomata acuminata). European Journal of Dermatology 11(6):598–603

Condyloma lata

Definition
Skin lesions associated with secondary syphilis, characterized by flat-topped,

necrotic papules clustering in intertriginous sites and secreting a seropurulent fluid

References
Rosen T, Hwong H (2001) Pedal interdigital condylomata lata: A rare sign of secondary syphilis. Sexually Transmitted Diseases 28(3):184–186

Confluent and reticular papillomatosis

▶ Confluent and reticulated papillomatosis

Confluent and reticulate papillomatosis

▶ Confluent and reticulated papillomatosis

Confluent and reticulated papillomatosis

Synonym(s)
Cutaneous papillomatosis; Gougerot-Carteaud papillomatosis; Gougerot-Carteaud syndrome; atrophie brilliante; confluent and reticular papillomatosis; confluent and reticulate papillomatosis; erythrokeratodermia papillaris et reticularis; parakeratose brilliante; pigmented reticular dermatosis of the flexures

Definition
Disorder characterized by chronic, persistent, verrucous papules, with a reticulated pattern and a tendency to become confluent

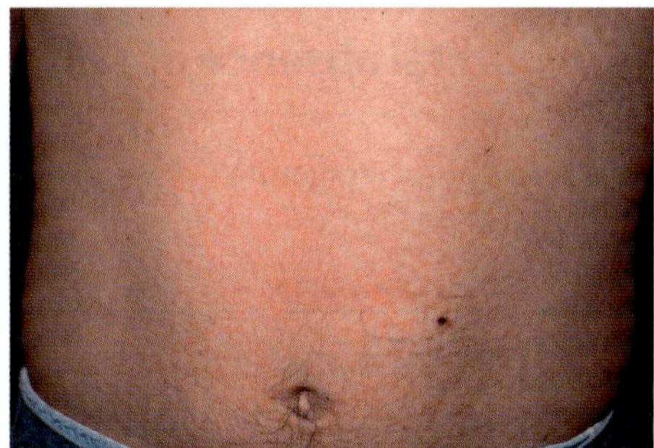
Confluent and reticulated papillomatosis. Reddish-brown, scaly papules coalescing into reticulated plaques

Pathogenesis
Possibly involves abnormal keratinocyte differentiation and maturation

Clinical manifestation
Beginning as small, grayish-brown, hyperkeratotic papules, enlarging and coalescing to form a reticular pattern peripherally and confluent plaques centrally; most commonly occurring on the trunk, face, and neck, and sparing the mucous membranes

Differential diagnosis
Tinea versicolor; erythrokeratoderma variabilis; epidermodysplasia verruciformis; pityriasis rubra pilaris; acanthosis nigricans; dermatopathic pigmentosa reticularis; dyschromatosis universalis; epidermal nevus; Naegeli-Franceschetti-Jadassohn syndrome; flat warts

Therapy
Minocycline*; isotretinoin; keratolytics; vitamin A; sodium thiosulphate; oral contraceptives; tretinoin; ultraviolet light; propylene glycol; calcipotriene

References
Jang HS, Oh CK, Cha JH, Cho SH, Kwon KS (2001) Six cases of confluent and reticulated papillomatosis alleviated by various antibiotics. Journal of the American Academy of Dermatology 44(4):652–655

Congenital absence of skin

▶ **Aplasia cutis congenita**

Congenital contractural arachnodactyly syndrome

▶ **Beals-Hecht syndrome**

Congenital dermal melanocytosis

▶ **Mongolian spot**

Congenital erythropoietic porphyria

Synonym(s)
Gunther's disease; erythropoietic porphyria; congenital porphyria; porphyria erythropoietica; congenital hematoporphyria; erythropoietic uroporphyria

Definition
Inborn error of porphyrin-heme synthesis involving mutation of a gene encoding the enzyme uroporphyrinogen III synthase, which leads to accumulation of porphyrins of the isomer I type, that causes cutaneous photosensitivity

Pathogenesis
Disorder of bone marrow heme synthesis; deficient uroporphyrinogen III synthase activity in erythrocyte precursor cells causes a shift away from the isomer III porphyrinogen production that affects the end-product heme; isomer I porphyrinogens are overproduced; interaction of excess porphyrins in the skin and light radiation causes photo-oxidative damage of biomolecular targets, manifested as mechanical fragility and blistering

Clinical manifestation
Blistering and fragility of light-exposed skin; hypertrichosis; teeth have a reddish color; blepharitis, cicatricial ectropion, and conjunctivitis; hemolytic anemia can cause secondary hypersplenism

Differential diagnosis
Erythropoietic protoporphyria; porphyria cutanea tarda; variegate porphyria; pseudoporphyria; polymorphous light eruption; xeroderma pigmentosum; Bloom's syndrome

Therapy
Strict sun avoidance; erythrocyte transfusion; bone marrow transplantation; beta-carotene 120–300 mg PO per day in divided doses; activated charcoal; cholestyramine; alpha-tocopherol; ascorbic acid

References
Desnick RJ, Astrin KH (2002) Congenital erythropoietic porphyria: Advances in pathogenesis and treatment. British Journal of Haematology 117(4):779–795

Congenital erythropoietic protoporphyria

▶ **Erythropoietic protoporphyria**

Congenital hematoporphyria

▶ **Congenital erythropoietic porphyria**

Congenital hemidysplasia

▶ CHILD syndrome

Congenital histiocytosis X

▶ Congenital self-healing Langerhans cell histiocytosis

Congenital hypertrichosis

Synonym(s)
None

Definition
Excess hair growth present in the newborn period which persists beyond the neonatal period

References
Schnur RE (1996) Congenital hypertrichosis. In: demis DJ (ed) Clinical Dermatology. Lippincott Williams & Wilkins, Philadelphia, Volume 1 Section 2–26

Congenital keratoma of the palms and soles

▶ Unna-Thost palmoplantar keratoderma

Congenital, localized absence of skin

▶ Aplasia cutis congenita

Congenital palmoplantar and periorificial keratoderma

▶ Olmsted Syndrome

Congenital porphyria

▶ Congenital erythropoietic porphyria
▶ Erythropoietic porphyria

Congenital punctate chondrodystrophy

▶ Conradi disease

Congenital self-healing Langerhans cell histiocytosis

Synonym(s)
Congenital self-healing Langerhans cell reticulohistiocytosis; congenital histiocytosis X; Hashimoto-Pritzker disease

Definition
Heterogeneous eruption, with the histological appearance of Langerhans cell histiocytosis, occurring at birth or in infancy and healing spontaneously

Pathogenesis
Considered a benign variant of Langerhans cell histiocytosis

Clinical manifestation
Macules, papules, and nodules of varying color, some hemorrhagic; resolves in 2–3 months, sometimes with recurrences; usually no systemic involvement

Differential diagnosis
Other forms of Langerhans cell histiocytosis; mastocytosis; lymphoma; juvenile xanthogranuloma; benign cephalic histiocytosis

Therapy
None indicated

References
Larralde M, Rositto A, Giardelli M, Gatti CF, Santos Munoz A (1999) Congenital self-healing histiocytosis (Hashimoto-Pritzker). International Journal of Dermatology 38(9):693–696

Congenital self-healing Langerhans cell reticulohistiocytosis

▶ Congenital self-healing Langerhans cell histiocytosis

Congenital telangiectatic erythema

▶ Bloom's syndrome

Congenital ulcer of the newborn

▶ Aplasia cutis congenita

Congenital xanthoma tuberosum

▶ Juvenile xanthogranuloma

Conglobate acne

▶ Acne conglobata

Conjunctivitis

Definition
Inflammation or infection of the membrane lining the eyelids

References
Shields SR (2000) Managing eye disease in primary care. Part 2. How to recognize and treat common eye problems. Postgraduate Medicine 108(5):83–86, 91–96

Connective tissue nevus

Synonym(s)
Collagenoma; elastoma; nevus mucinosis

Definition
Hamartomatous proliferation of one or more connective tissue elements in the dermis

Pathogenesis
Unknown

Clinical manifestation
Multiple, indurated, cutaneous papules or nodules often over the upper two-thirds of the back, associated with multiple endocrine neoplasia (MEN) type I; shagreen patch – connective tissue nevus in a patient with tuberous sclerosis; nevus mucinosis (Hunter syndrome): small, firm papules on the arms, chest, and over the scapular region, with coarse facial features, mental retardation, and deafness

Differential diagnosis
Milia; morphea; scar; athlete's nodules (knuckle pads, etc.); Cowden disease

Therapy
Surgical excision for cosmetic reasons only

References
Sears JK, Stone MS, Argenyi Z (1988) Papular elastorrhexis: A variant of connective tissue nevus. Case reports and review of the literature. Journal of the American Academy of Dermatology 19(2 Pt 2):409–414

Conradi disease

Synonym(s)
Conradi Hunermann syndrome; congenital punctate chondrodystrophy; chondrodystrophia calcificans congenita; dysplasia epiphysialis punctata; chondrodysplasia punctata, X-linked dominant type

Definition
Form of chondrodysplasia punctata, characterized by punctate opacities within the growing ends of long bones and other regions, dysmorphic facial features, cataracts, sparse, coarse scalp hair, and/or abnormal thickening, dryness, and scaling of the skin

Pathogenesis
Unknown; X-linked dominant trait

Clinical manifestation
Sparse, coarse scalp hair; thickening, dryness, and scaling of the skin; mild-to-moderate growth deficiency; disproportionate shortening of long bones, particularly those of the humeri and the femora; short stature; kyphoscoliosis; prominent forehead with midfacial hypoplasia and a low nasal bridge; cataracts

Differential diagnosis
Epidermal nevus; incontinentia pigmenti; ichthyosis vulgaris; X-linked ichthyosis

Therapy
None

References
O'Brien TJ (1990) Chondrodysplasia punctata (Conradi disease). International Journal of Dermatology 29(7):472–476

Conradi Hunermann syndrome

▶ Conradi disease

Constricting bands of the extremities

▶ Ainhum

Consumptive thrombocytopenia

▶ Kasabach-Merritt syndrome

Contact dermatitis

Synonym(s)
Dermatitis venenata; contact eczema

Definition
Inflammation of the skin caused by direct contact with an irritating or allergy-causing substance

Pathogenesis
Irritant variant: caused by direct injury of the skin by an agent capable of producing

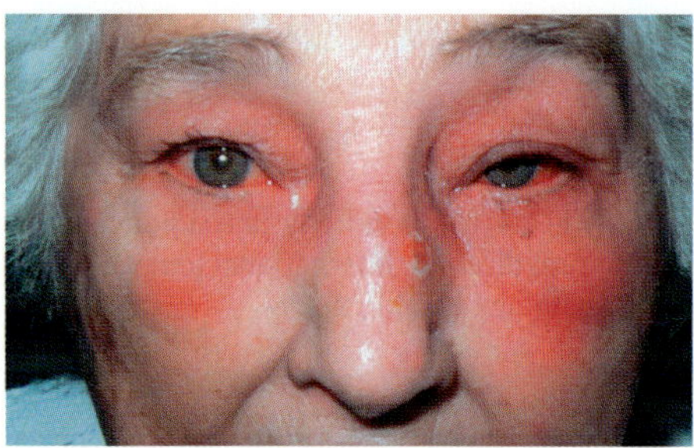

Contact dermatitis. Erythematous, edematous plaques around the eyes in a patient with an allergic contact dermatitis to a topical eye medication

cell damage in any individual if applied for sufficient time and in sufficient concentration

Allergic variant: type IV hypersensitivity reaction only affecting previously sensitized individuals

Contact urticaria variant: possibly immunologic in some cases

Photocontact variant: irradiation of certain substances by light resulting in the transformation of the substance into full antigens (photoallergic) or irritants (phototoxic)

Clinical manifestation
Acute contact stage: red and edematous skin; vesicles or bullae sometimes develop; weeping and oozing as vesicles rupture

Subacute stage: less edematous and erythematous; scaling and punctate crusts from scratching (excoriations) often present

Chronic stage: scaling, fissuring, and lichenification with minimal edema

Contact urticaria variant: urticarial wheals at site of contact

Phototoxic variant: appearance of an exaggerated sunburn

Differential diagnosis
Atopic dermatitis; dyshidrotic eczema; sunburn; chemical burn; seborrheic dermatitis; insect bites; erysipelas; erythema multiforme; nummular eczema; lichen simplex chronicus; asteatotic eczema; bullous pemphigoid; pemphigus vulgaris; epidermolysis bullosa; dermatophyte infection; candidiasis; impetigo; scabies

Therapy
Removal of source of dermatitis

Mild-to-moderate disease: corticosteroids, topical, mid potency or high potency; aluminium acetate 5% compresses applied 15–30 minutes 2–4 times daily

Severe disease: prednisone*; antihistamines, first generation, for sedation

References
Bruckner AL, Weston WL (2001) Beyond poison ivy: understanding allergic contact dermatitis in children. Pediatric Annals 30(4):203–206

Moore DE (2002) Drug-induced cutaneous photosensitivity: incidence, mechanism, prevention and management. Drug Safety 25(5):345–372

Wakelin SH (2001) Contact urticaria. Clinical & Experimental Dermatology 26(2):132–136

Contact eczema

▶ Contact dermatitis

Contact stomatitis

▶ Contact dermatitis

Contagious ecthyma

▶ Orf

Contagious pustular dermatitis

▶ Orf

Corn

▶ Clavus

Cornelia de Lange syndrome

Synonym(s)
Brachmann-de Lange syndrome; de Lange syndrome; Amsterdam syndrome; typus degenerativus amstelodamensis

Definition
Syndrome characterized by a distinctive facial appearance, prenatal and postnatal growth deficiency, feeding difficulties, psychomotor delay, behavioral problems; malformations mainly involve the upper extremities

Pathogenesis
Unknown; few cases transmitted in autosomal dominant pattern

Clinical manifestation
Short stature; microcephaly; facial features: confluent eyebrows, long curly eyelashes, low anterior and posterior hairline, underdeveloped orbital arches, anteverted nares, down-turned angles of the mouth, thin lips, low-set ears, depressed nasal bridge, micrognathia; hypertrichosis; micromelia; behavioral abnormalities

Differential diagnosis
Fetal alcohol syndrome; Coffin-Siris syndrome

Therapy
No specific therapy

References
Opitz JM, Brachmann-de Lange syndrome (1994) A continuing enigma. Archives of Pediatrics & Adolescent Medicine 148(11):1206–1208

Corporis circumscriptum naeviforme

▶ Angiokeratoma circumscriptum

Corpus callosum agenesis-facial anomalies-Robin sequence syndrome

▶ Toriello-Carey syndrome

Corrugated skin

▶ Cutis verticis gyrata

Corticosteroids, topical, high potency

Trade name(s)
Generic in parentheses:
Cyclocort (amcinonide); Lidex, Lidex-E, Licon (fluocinonide); Topicort (desoximetasone); Diprosone, Maxivate, Alphatrex (betamethasone dipropionate); Halog, Halog-E (halcinonide)

Generic available
Yes

Drug class
Glucocorticoid

Mechanism of action
Anti-inflammatory; anti-proliferative; atrophy causing

Dosage form
Cream; ointment; lotion; gel

Corticosteroids, topical, high potency. Dermatologic indications and dosage

Disease	Adult dosage	Child dosage
Atopic dermatitis	Apply twice daily	Apply twice daily
Bullous pemphigoid	Apply twice daily	Apply twice daily
Contact dermatitis	Apply twice daily	Apply twice daily
Dyshidrotic eczema;	Apply twice daily	Apply twice daily
Erythema annulare centrifugum	Apply twice daily	Apply twice daily
Follicular mucinosis	Apply twice daily	Apply twice daily
Herpes gestationis	Apply twice daily	Apply twice daily
Jessner's lymphocytic infiltration of skin	Apply twice daily	Apply twice daily
Langerhans cell histiocytosis	Apply twice daily	Apply twice daily
Lichen planus	Apply twice daily	Apply twice daily
Lichen simplex chronicus	Apply twice daily	Apply twice daily
Lichen striatus	Apply twice daily	Apply twice daily
Lupus erythematosus, subacute systemic	Apply twice daily	Apply twice daily
Nummular eczema	Apply twice daily	Apply twice daily
Pemphigus vulgaris	Apply twice daily	Apply twice daily
Pityriasis lichenoides	Apply twice daily	Apply twice daily
Polymorphous light eruption	Apply twice daily	Apply twice daily
Pruritic urticarial papules and plaques of pregnancy	Apply twice daily	Apply twice daily
Psoriasis	Apply twice daily	Apply twice daily
Seabather's eruption	Apply twice daily	Apply twice daily
Seborrheic dermatitis	Apply twice daily	Apply twice daily
Subcorneal pustular dermatosis	Apply twice daily	Apply twice daily
T cell lymphoma	Apply twice daily	Apply twice daily
Xerotic dermatitis	Apply twice daily	Apply twice daily

Dermatologic indications and dosage
See table

Common side effects
Cutaneous: skin atrophy; steroid addiction (rebound flare after discontinuing the medication); tachyphylaxis; increased susceptibility to local infection; perioral dermatitis; delayed wound healing; hypopigmentation; acneform eruption; striae

Serious side effects
Miscellaneous: adrenal insufficiency

Drug interactions
None

Corticosteroid, topical, low potency. Dermatologic indications and dosage

Disease	Adult dosage	Child dosage
Atopic dermatitis	Apply twice daily	Apply twice daily
Contact dermatitis	Apply twice daily	Apply twice daily
Dyshidrosis	Apply twice daily	Apply twice daily
Netherton syndrome	Apply twice daily	Apply twice daily
Nummular eczema	Apply twice daily	Apply twice daily
Pityriasis alba	Apply twice daily	Apply twice daily
Seborrheic dermatitis	Apply twice daily	Apply twice daily
Xerotic eczema	Apply twice daily	Apply twice daily

Contraindications/precautions
Hypersensitivity to drug class or component; avoid use on the face for more than 14 days; avoid getting in the eye; do not apply in intertriginous areas for more than 1 week at a time

References
Brazzini B, Pimpinelli N (2002) New and established topical corticosteroids in dermatology: clinical pharmacology and therapeutic use. American Journal of Clinical Dermatology 3(1):47–58

Corticosteroids, topical, low potency

Trade name(s)
Generic in parentheses:
Hydrocortisone 1% (Hytone; Cortef; Cortaid; Texacort); alclometasone 0.05% (Aclovate); desonide 0.05% (Tridesilon; DesOwen)

Generic available
Yes

Drug class
Glucocorticoid

Mechanism of action
Anti-inflammatory; antiproliferative; atrophy-causing

Dosage form
Cream; ointment; lotion; gel

Dermatologic indications and dosage
See table

Common side effects
Cutaneous: skin atrophy; steroid addiction (rebound flare after discontinuing the medication); tachyphylaxis; increased susceptibility to local infection; perioral dermatitis; delayed wound healing; hypopigmentation; acneform eruption; striae

Serious side effects
Miscellaneous: adrenal insufficiency

Drug interactions
None

Contraindications/precautions
Hypersensitivity to drug class or component; avoid placing drug in the eye

References
Brazzini B, Pimpinelli N (2002) New and established topical corticosteroids in dermatology: clinical pharmacology and therapeutic use. American Journal of Clinical Dermatology 3(1):47–58

Corticosteroids, topical, medium potency

Trade name(s)
Generic in parentheses:
Kenalog, Aristocort (triamcinolone); Valisone, Betatrex, Luxiq (betamethasone valerate); Cloderm (clocortolone); Cordran (flurandrenolide); Cutivate (fluticasone); Dermatop (prednicarbate); Synalar, Derma-Smoothe (fluocinolone); Elocon (mometasone); Locoid (hydrocortisone butyrate); Uticort (betamethasone benzoate); Westcort (hydrocortisone valerate)

Generic available
Yes

Drug class
Glucocorticoid

Mechanism of action
Anti-inflammatory; anti-proliferative; atrophy-causing

Dosage form
Cream; ointment; lotion; gel; foam

Dermatologic indications and dosage
See table

Common side effects
Cutaneous: skin atrophy; steroid addiction (rebound flare after discontinuing the medication); tachyphylaxis; increased susceptibility to local infection; perioral dermatitis; delayed wound healing; hypopigmentation; acneform eruption; striae

Serious side effects
Miscellaneous: adrenal insufficiency

Corticosteroids, topical, medium potency. Dermatologic indications and dosage

Disease	Adult dosage	Child dosage
Atopic dermatitis	Apply twice daily	Apply twice daily
Benign pigmented purpura;	Apply twice daily	Apply twice daily
Cercarial dermatitis	Apply twice daily	Apply twice daily
Contact dermatitis	Apply twice daily	Apply twice daily
Dyshidrosis	Apply twice daily	Apply twice daily
Id reaction	Apply twice daily	Apply twice daily
Idiopathic guttate hypomelanosis	Apply twice daily	Apply twice daily
Keratosis pilaris	Apply twice daily	Apply twice daily
Nummular eczema	Apply twice daily	Apply twice daily
Pityriasis lichenoides	Apply twice daily	Apply twice daily
Prurigo of pregnancy	Apply twice daily	Apply twice daily
Psoriasis	Apply twice daily	Apply twice daily
Seborrheic dermatitis	Apply twice daily	Apply twice daily
Stasis dermatitis	Apply twice daily	Apply twice daily
Sunburn	Apply twice daily	Apply twice daily
Wiskott-Aldrich syndrome	Apply twice daily	Apply twice daily
Xerotic eczema	Apply twice daily	Apply twice daily

Drug interactions
None

Contraindications/precautions
Hypersensitivity to drug class or component; avoid use on the face for more than 14 days; avoid getting in the eye; do not apply in intertriginous areas for more than 2 weeks at a time

References
Brazzini B, Pimpinelli N (2002) New and established topical corticosteroids in dermatology: clinical pharmacology and therapeutic use. American Journal of Clinical Dermatology 3(1):47–58

Corticosteroids, topical, super potency

Trade name(s)
Generic in parentheses:
Temovate, Olux, Cormax, Embeline (clobetasol); Ultravate (halobetasol); Diprolene AF (augmented betamethasone dipropionate); Psorcon, Maxiflor, Florone (diflorasone diacetate); Cordran Tape (flurandrenolide tape)

Generic available
Yes

Drug class
Glucocorticoid

Mechanism of action
Anti-inflammatory; anti-proliferative; atrophy-causing

Dosage form
Cream; ointment; lotion; gel; foam; tape

Dermatologic indications and dosage
See table

Common side effects
Cutaneous: skin atrophy; steroid addiction (rebound flare after discontinuing the med-

ication); tachyphylaxis; increased susceptibility to local infection; perioral dermatitis; delayed wound healing; hypopigmentation; acneform eruption; striae

Serious side effects
Miscellaneous: adrenal insufficiency

Drug interactions
None

Contraindications/precautions
Hypersensitivity to drug class or component; avoid use on the face; do not apply in intertriginous areas for more than one week at a time

References
Brazzini B, Pimpinelli N (2002) New and established topical corticosteroids in dermatology: clinical pharmacology and therapeutic use. American Journal of Clinical Dermatology 3(1):47–58

Coumarin necrosis

Synonym(s)
Coumarin skin necrosis; warfarin skin necrosis

Definition
Rapid onset of localized skin necrosis associated with recent onset of coumarin therapy

Pathogenesis
Low constitutive levels of protein C; in the presence of coumarin, levels of protein C fall more rapidly than do procoagulant factors IX, X and prothrombin, producing a transient hypercoagulable state and local thrombosis of dermal vessels

Clinical manifestation
Signs and symptoms beginning 3–5 days after initiation of coumarin; single or multiple areas of painful erythema rapidly ulcer-

Corticosteroids, topical, super potency. Dermatologic indications and dosage

Disease	Adult dosage	Child dosage
Alopecia areata	Apply twice daily for up to 2 weeks; 1 week rest period before reuse	Apply twice daily for up to 2 weeks; 1 week rest period before reuse
Atopic dermatitis	Apply twice daily for up to 2 weeks; 1 week rest period before reuse	Apply twice daily for up to 2 weeks; 1 week rest period before reuse
Contact dermatitis	Apply twice daily for up to 2 weeks; 1 week rest period before reuse	Apply twice daily for up to 2 weeks; 1 week rest period before reuse
Dyshidrosis	Apply twice daily for up to 2 weeks; 1 week rest period before reuse	Apply twice daily for up to 2 weeks; 1 week rest period before reuse
Eosinophilic pustular folliculitis	Apply twice daily for up to 2 weeks; 1 week rest period before reuse	Apply twice daily for up to 2 weeks; 1 week rest period before reuse
Inflammatory epidermal nevus	Apply twice daily for up to 2 weeks; 1 week rest period before reuse	Apply twice daily for up to 2 weeks; 1 week rest period before reuse
Lichen nitidus	Apply twice daily for up to 2 weeks; 1 week rest period before reuse	Apply twice daily for up to 2 weeks; 1 week rest period before reuse
Lichen planus	Apply twice daily for up to 2 weeks; 1 week rest period before reuse	Apply twice daily for up to 2 weeks; 1 week rest period before reuse
Lichen simplex chronicus	Apply twice daily for up to 2 weeks; 1 week rest period before reuse	Apply twice daily for up to 2 weeks; 1 week rest period before reuse
Lupus erythematosus, discoid	Apply twice daily for up to 2 weeks; 1 week rest period before reuse	Apply twice daily for up to 2 weeks; 1 week rest period before reuse
Lupus erythematosus, subacute systemic	Apply twice daily for up to 2 weeks; 1 week rest period before reuse	Apply twice daily for up to 2 weeks; 1 week rest period before reuse
Mastocytosis	Apply twice daily for up to 2 weeks; 1 week rest period before reuse	Apply twice daily for up to 2 weeks; 1 week rest period before reuse
Nummular eczema	Apply twice daily for up to 2 weeks; 1 week rest period before reuse	Apply twice daily for up to 2 weeks; 1 week rest period before reuse
Pemphigus foliaceus	Apply twice daily for up to 2 weeks; 1 week rest period before reuse	Apply twice daily for up to 2 weeks; 1 week rest period before reuse
Pityriasis lichenoides	Apply twice daily for up to 2 weeks; 1 week rest period before reuse	Apply twice daily for up to 2 weeks; 1 week rest period before reuse
Psoriasis	Apply twice daily for up to 2 weeks; 1 week rest period before reuse	Apply twice daily for up to 2 weeks; 1 week rest period before reuse
Reiter syndrome	Apply twice daily for up to 2 weeks; 1 week rest period before reuse	Apply twice daily for up to 2 weeks; 1 week rest period before reuse
Seborrheic dermatitis	Apply twice daily for up to 2 weeks; 1 week rest period before reuse	Apply twice daily for up to 2 weeks; 1 week rest period before reuse
Vitiligo	Apply twice daily	Apply twice daily
Xerotic eczema	Apply twice daily for up to 2 weeks; 1 week rest period before reuse	Apply twice daily for up to 2 weeks; 1 week rest period before reuse

ating and developing a blue-black eschar; most common areas of involvement: thighs, breasts, and buttocks; most likely occurring in patients in whom large initial doses of coumarin initiated in the absence of heparin anticoagulation

Differential diagnosis
Other coagulopathies; heparin necrosis; spider bite reaction; pyoderma gangrenosum; vasculitis; cutaneous anthrax; traumatic ulceration; calciphylaxis; necrotizing soft tissue infection

Therapy
Medical therapy: continued coumarin therapy
Surgical therapy: hydrocolloid dressings; skin grafting if healing markedly delayed

References
Cole MS, Minifee PK, Wolma FJ (1988) Coumarin necrosis – A review of the literature. Surgery 103(3):271–277

Coumarin skin necrosis

▶ **Coumarin necrosis**

Cowden disease

Synonym(s)
Cowden's syndrome; Cowden syndrome; multiple hamartoma syndrome

Definition
Hamartomatous neoplasms of the skin and mucosa, gastrointestinal tract, bones, central nervous system, eyes, and genitourinary tract

Pathogenesis
Mutation in the *PTEN* tumor suppressor gene on chromosome 10q23 regulating the function of other proteins by removing phosphate groups from those molecules; mutation causing loss of the protein's function and allowing over-proliferation of cells, resulting in hamartomatous growths

Clinical manifestation
Flesh-colored, flat-topped, lichenoid or elongated, verrucous papules of the face; oral cavity papules with a smooth surface and a whitish color; sometimes coalescing into cobblestone-like plaques; acral keratotic papules, including palmoplantar keratotic papules; thyroid abnormalities; fibrocystic disease and fibroadenomas of the breast; increased incidence of breast carcinoma; gastrointestinal polyps; ovarian cysts; uterine leiomyomas

Differential diagnosis
Wart; sebaceous hyperplasia; milia; xanthoma; trichilemmoma; trichoepithelioma; Darier disease; syringoma; fibrofolliculoma; multiple benign fibromas; multiple endocrine neoplasia; tuberous sclerosis; lipoid proteinosis; Goltz syndrome; florid oral papillomatosis

Therapy
Surgical therapy: chemical peel; laser resurfacing; excisional surgery

References
Hildenbrand C, Burgdorf WH, Lautenschlager S (2001) Cowden syndrome-Diagnostic skin signs. Dermatology 202(4):362–366

Cowden syndrome

▶ **Cowden disease**

Cowden's syndrome

▶ **Cowden disease**

Cowden/Bannayan-Riley-Ruvalcaba overlap syndrome

▶ **Bannayan-Riley-Ruvalcaba syndrome**

Creeping eruption

▶ Cutaneous larva migrans

Crocker syndrome

▶ Niemann-Pick disease

Crocker's syndrome

▶ Niemann-Pick disease

Crocker-Farber syndrome

▶ Niemann-Pick disease

Cronkhite Canada syndrome

Synonym(s)
Gastrointestinal polyposis syndrome, generalized, associated with hyperpigmentation, alopecia, and nail atrophy

Definition
Association of generalized gastrointestinal polyps, cutaneous pigmentation, alopecia, and onychodystrophy

Pathogenesis
Unknown

Clinical manifestation
Onset of constant or episodic pain in the lower or upper abdomen, with weight loss; alopecia simultaneously from the scalp, eyebrows, face, axillae, pubic areas, and extremities; lentigo-like macules and/or diffuse hyperpigmentation, including the buccal mucosa; nail dystrophy; peripheral or generalized edema; multiple gastrointestinal polyps, with increased incidence of colon carcinoma

Differential diagnosis
Gardner's syndrome; Peutz-Jeghers syndrome; Bandler syndrome; Ménétrier disease; familial polyposis

Therapy
No therapy for cutaneous manifestations; close follow-up for gastrointestinal problems

References
Finan MC, Ray MK (1989) Gastrointestinal polyposis syndromes. Dermatologic Clinics 7(3):419–434

Crotch rot

▶ Tinea cruris

Crow-Fukase syndrome

▶ POEMS Syndrome

Cryofibrinogenemia

Synonym(s)
None

Definition
Presence of the cryoprotein, cryofibrinogen, in serum, with resultant cutaneous manifestations

Pathogenesis
Unknown

Clinical manifestation
Primary (essential) form: unassociated with underlying disease; secondary form: associated most commonly with internal malignancies and thromboembolic disease, but also with rheumatic diseases, diabetes mellitus, and pregnancy; purpura; ecchymoses; cutaneous gangrene; persistent, painful ulcerations, with surrounding livedo reticularis

Differential diagnosis
Cryoglobulinemia; benign pigmented purpura; antiphospholipid antibody syndrome; Churg-Strauss syndrome; polyarteritis nodosa; serum sickness; Waldenström hyperglobulinemia; septic vasculitis; systemic lupus erythematosus; sarcoidosis

Therapy
Stanozolol: 4–8 mg PO daily; plasmapheresis

References
Helfman T, Falanga V (1995) Stanozolol as a novel therapeutic agent in dermatology. Journal of the American Academy of Dermatology 33(2 Pt 1):254–258

Cryoglobulinemia

Synonym(s)
Cryoproteinemia

Definition
Presence of abnormal proteins in the bloodstream, which thicken or gel on exposure to cold

Pathogenesis
Some of the sequelae of cryoglobulinemia related to immune-complex disease; other sequelae related to cryoprecipitation in vivo, including plugging and thrombosis of small arteries and capillaries; some cases in otherwise normal patients (essential mixed cryoglobulinemia)

Clinical manifestation
Skin findings: palpable purpura; distal necrosis; urticaria, and ischemic necrosis leading to ulceration; cold-induced urticaria; acrocyanosis

Internal manifestations: pulmonary; renal; joints; central nervous system; sometimes present in mycoplasma pneumonia, viral hepatitis, multiple myeloma, certain leukemias, primary macroglobulinemia, and some autoimmune diseases, such as systemic lupus erythematosus and rheumatoid arthritis

Differential diagnosis
Antiphospholipid antibody syndrome; Churg-Strauss syndrome; polyarteritis nodosa; serum sickness; Waldenström hyperglobulinemia; septic vasculitis; systemic lupus erythematosus; sarcoidosis

Therapy
No therapy indicated for asymptomatic disease

Symptomatic disease: nonsteroidal anti-inflammatory drugs; prednisone

Steroid-sparing medications: azathioprine; cyclophosphamide

Plasmapheresis for life-threatening disease; interferon-α for cryoglobulinemia associated with hepatitis C infection

References
Cacoub P, Costedoat-Chalumeau N, Lidove O, Alric L (2002) Cryoglobulinemia vasculitis. Current Opinion in Rheumatology 14(1):29–35

Cryoproteinemia

▶ Cryoglobulinemia

Cryptococcosis

Synonym(s)
Busse-Buschke disease; European blastomycosis; torulosis

Definition
Fungal infection caused by the inhalation of the fungus, Cryptococcus neoformans

Pathogenesis
Human disease associated only with Cryptococcus neoformans; following inhalation of the organism, alveolar macrophages ingest the yeast; cryptococcal polysaccharide capsule has antiphagocytic properties and may be immunosuppressive; antiphagocytic properties of the capsule block recognition of the yeast by phagocytes and inhibit leukocyte migration into the area of fungal replication; decreased host immunity main element in susceptibility to clinical infection; organ damage primarily from tissue distortion secondary to increasing fungal burden

Clinical manifestation
Pre-existing medical problems, such as systemic steroid use, malignant disease, organ transplantation, or HIV infection.
Skin findings: papules, sometimes umbilicated; pustules; nodules; ulcers; draining sinuses; rarely occurs as a primary inoculation disease
Internal organ involvement: pulmonary – variable, ranging from asymptomatic airway colonization to acute respiratory distress syndrome
Central nervous system: usually meningitis or meningoencephalitis

Differential diagnosis
Pyogenic abscess; nocardia, aspergillosis; lymphoma; meningeal metastases; tuberculosis; histoplasmosis; acne; molluscum contagiosum; syphilis; toxoplasmosis

Therapy
Non-AIDS-related: amphotericin B 0.5–1 mg per kg per day IV; total cumulative dose of 3 gm*; fluconazole
AIDS-related infection: initially, amphotericin B for 2 weeks, with or without 2 weeks of flucytosine, followed by fluconazole for a minimum of 10 weeks*

References
Thomas I, Schwartz RA (2001) Cutaneous manifestations of systemic cryptococcosis in immunosuppressed patients. Journal of Medicine 32(5-6):259–266

Cushing syndrome

Synonym(s)
Hypercorticalism; Cushing's syndrome

Definition
Hormonal disorder caused by prolonged exposure of the body's tissues to high levels of cortisol

Pathogenesis
Excess levels of either exogenously administrated glucocorticoids or endogenous overproduction of cortisol from tumors or adrenal gland hyperplasia, lead to signs and symptoms of hypercorticalism

Clinical manifestation
Skin changes: facial plethora; striae; ecchymoses and purpura; telangiectasias; skin atrophy; hirsutism and male pattern balding in women; increased lanugo facial hair; steroid acne; acanthosis nigricans
Central obesity; increased adipose tissue in the face (moon facies), upper back at the base of neck (buffalo hump), and above the clavicles
Endocrine abnormalities: hypothyroidism; galactorrhea; polyuria and nocturia from diabetes insipidus
Menstrual irregularities, amenorrhea, and infertility
Other organ system abnormalities: cardiovascular; musculoskeletal; gastroenterologic; neuropsychological

Differential diagnosis
Exogenous obesity; anorexia nervosa; alcoholism; drug effects from phenobarbital phenytoin or rifampin; psychiatric illness

Therapy

Medical therapy: ketoconazole*
Surgical therapy: surgical resection of the causative tumor, if present, either by transsphenoidal surgery for pituitary tumors or adrenalectomy for adrenal tumors*; pituitary irradiation when transsphenoidal surgery not successful or not possible

References

Norton JA, Li M. Gillary J, Le HN (2001) Cushing's syndrome. Current Problems in Surgery 38(7):488–545

Cushing's syndrome

▶ Cushing syndrome

Cutaneomeningospinal angiomatosis

▶ Cobb syndrome

Cutaneous aspergillosis

Synonym(s)

None

Definition

Cutaneous manifestation of disseminated infection with the fungus Aspergillus

Pathogenesis

Caused by infection with soil- and water-dwelling saprophytes of the Aspergillus genus; initial infection of the pulmonary system via inhalation of fungal spores; hematogenous dissemination leads to skin involvement

Clinical manifestation

Begins as a febrile illness, pneumonia, or sinusitis; asymptomatic or tender, solitary or multiple, erythematous or violaceous indurated papules or plaques, sometimes at the sites of an intravenous catheter or a venipuncture; rapid evolution into pustules and hemorrhagic vesicles, producing eschars

Differential diagnosis

Ecthyma; mucormycosis; cryptococcosis; phaeohyphomycosis; ecthyma gangrenosum; Sweet's syndrome; pyoderma gangrenosum

Therapy

Amphotericin B 3–5 mg per kg per day intravenously, increasing dose as tolerated*; itraconazole

References

van Burik JA, Colven R, Spach DH (1998) Cutaneous aspergillosis. Journal of Clinical Microbiology 36(11):3115–3121

Cutaneous calcinosis

▶ Calcinosis cutis

Cutaneous calculi

▶ Calcinosis cutis

Cutaneous CD30+ (Ki-1) anaplastic large-cell lymphoma

Synonym(s)

Regressing atypical histiocytosis; CD30+ cutaneous large T-cell lymphoma, pseudo-Hodgkin disease

Definition
Heterogeneous neoplastic disorder, characterized by either primary cutaneous form without extracutaneous involvement or systemic form with secondary skin involvement at onset of disease activity

Pathogenesis
Neoplastic cells are CD30 positive and usually have T-helper phenotype; systemic form related to novel fusion protein (NPM-ALK)

Clinical manifestation
Primary cutaneous form: solitary or few, reddish-brown, indurated, ulcerative nodules or tumors; sometimes spontaneously regressing; involvement of draining regional lymph nodes; good prognosis
Systemic form: skin and systemic lesions at presentation; poor prognosis

Differential diagnosis
Lymphomatoid papulosis; CD30 negative lymphoma; Hodgkin's disease; Jessner's benign lymphocytic infiltration; granuloma faciale; metastasis; Merkel cell carcinoma; melanoma; squamous cell carcinoma; basal cell carcinoma

Therapy
Solitary or localized cutaneous disease: radiation therapy*; methotrexate; surgical excision
Systemic disease: multidrug cancer chemotherapy

References
LeBoit PE (1996) Lymphomatoid papulosis and cutaneous CD30+ lymphoma. American Journal of Dermatopathology 18(3):221–23

Cutaneous ciliated cyst

▶ Cutaneous columnar cyst

Cutaneous columnar cyst

Synonym(s)
Cutaneous ciliated cyst

Definition
Developmental cyst with columnar epithelial lining

Pathogenesis
Derived from embryological vestiges, such as the branchial arch cleft, thyroglossal duct, tracheobronchial bud, urogenital sinus, and Müllerian structures; represents incomplete involution of embryologic vestigial structures

Clinical manifestation
Thyroglossal cyst: occurring anywhere along thyroglossal duct, from base of tongue to the anterior neck; asymptomatic, gradually enlarging, near-midline nodule that moves with swallowing; drainage of clear or purulent fluid
Thymic cyst: found in the mediastinum or neck; ill-defined painless swelling in children
Bronchogenic cyst: present at birth or in neonatal period in suprasternal notch, neck, scapular area, and chin; sometimes forming sinuses and drains mucoid fluid
Cutaneous ciliated cyst: occurs primarily on the leg in women; ill-defined subcutaneous swelling without central pore
Median raphe cyst: midline developmental cyst on ventral penis or scrotum, on raphe connecting external urethral meatus to anus

Differential diagnosis
Benign tumor of adnexal structure; lipoma; epidermoid cyst; dermoid cyst; eruptive vellus hair cyst; basal cell carcinoma; melanocytic nevus; steatocystoma multiplex

Therapy
Surgical excision*

References
Enepekides DJ (2001) Management of congenital anomalies of the neck. Facial Plastic Surgery Clinics of North America 9(1):131–145

Cutaneous horn

Definition
Conical projection above the surface of the skin, resembling a miniature animal horn, occurring in conjunction with underlying dermatoses such as wart, actinic keratosis, seborrheic keratosis, basal cell carcinoma, squamous cell carcinoma, and keratoacanthoma

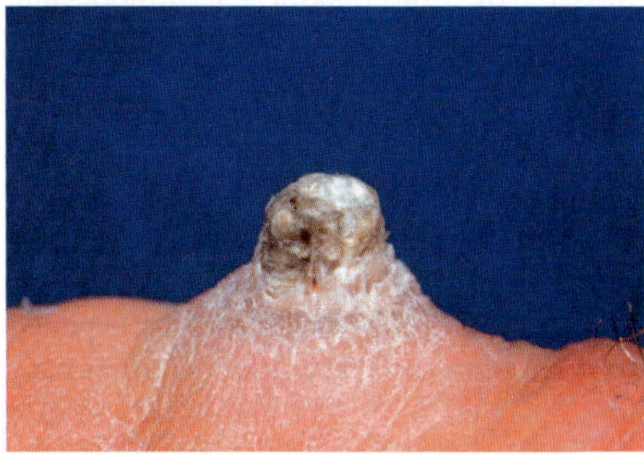

Cutaneous horn. Keratotic horn arising from the center of a papule on the upper extremity

References
Thappa DM, Garg BR, Thadeus J, Ratnakar C (1997) Cutaneous horn: A brief review and report of a case. Journal of Dermatology 24(1):34–37

Cutaneous larva migrans

Synonym(s)
Creeping eruption; larva migrans; plumber's itch; sandworm disease

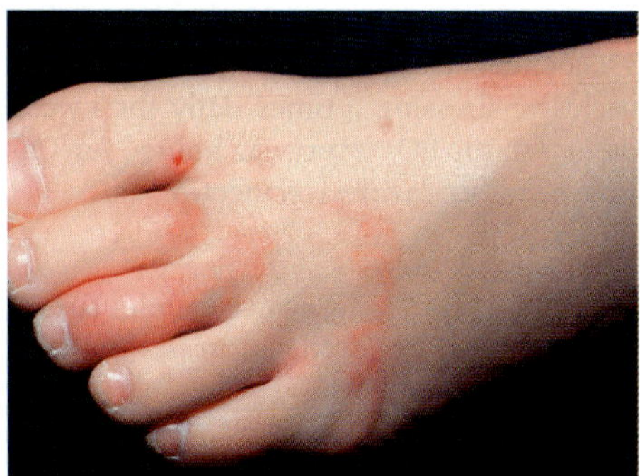

Cutaneous larva migrans. Serpiginous, linear, red-brown plaque on the foot

Definition
Disorder characterized by percutaneous penetration and subsequent migration of larvae of various nematode parasites

Pathogenesis
Ancylostoma braziliense (hookworm of wild and domestic dogs and cats) most common cause; in humans (accidental hosts), larvae lack enzymes required to invade through the dermis, so disease limited to the skin

Clinical manifestation
Often associated with history of sunbathing or walking barefoot on the beach; tingling/prickling, pruritus at site of exposure within 30 minutes of larvae penetration; advancing, erythematous, often linear lesions, occurring on dorsa of feet, interdigital spaces of toes, anogenital region, buttocks, hands, and knees; 2–3-mm-wide, serpiginous, slightly elevated, erythematous tunnels, tracking 3–4 cm from penetration site; vesicles with serous fluid; occasional secondary impetiginization; systemic signs: peripheral eosinophilia and increased IgE levels

Differential diagnosis
Scabies; insect bite reaction; foreign body granuloma; dermatophytosis; erythema migrans; myiasis; photoallergic dermatitis; larva currens

Therapy
Thiabendazole: 10–15% suspension under occlusive dressing 4 times daily for 1 week or 25–50 mg PO every 12 hours for 2–5 days★; albendazole; ivermectin

References
Caumes E (2000) Treatment of cutaneous larva migrans. Clinical Infectious Diseases 30(5):811–814

Cutaneous lymphangioma

▶ Lymphangioma

Cutaneous lymphomatous hyperplasia

▶ Pseudolymphoma

Cutaneous lymphoplasia

▶ Pseudolymphoma

Cutaneous papillomatosis

▶ Confluent and reticulated papillomatosis

Cutaneous periarteritis nodosa

▶ Polyarteritis nodosa

Cutaneous strongyloidiasis

▶ Strongyloidosis

Cutaneous TB

▶ Cutaneous tuberculosis

Cutaneous tuberculosis

Synonym(s)
Cutaneous TB; tuberculous chancre; tuberculosis verrucosa cutis; miliary tuberculosis of the skin; scrofuloderma; tuberculous gumma; tuberculosis cutis orificialis; lupus vulgaris; lichen scrofulosorum

Definition
Cutaneous manifestations of an airborne communicable disease that occurs after inhalation of infectious droplets expelled from patients with laryngeal or pulmonary TB

Pathogenesis
Systemic spread of a pulmonary infection, often in a host with poor immunity; direct innoculation into the skin of the tubercule bacillus

Clinical manifestation
Primary inoculation TB (tuberculous chancre): chronic, shallow, nontender, undermined ulcer; painless regional lymphadenopathy
TB verrucosa cutis: slow growing verrucous papule; may show central involution with an atrophic scar; fissures with purulent and keratinous material
Miliary TB of the skin: small red macules or papules with purpura, vesicles, and central

necrosis in a patient with fulminant tuberculosis

Scrofuloderma: firm, painless, subcutaneous nodules that enlarge and suppurate, forming ulcers and sinus tracts in overlying skin

TB cutis orificialis: affects orificial sites such as tip and lateral margins of the tongue, hard and soft palate, perianal skin, the vulva, the urinary meatus, and the glans penis; lesions present as red papules that evolve into painful, soft, punched-out, shallow ulcers

Lupus vulgaris: solitary, small, sharply marginated, red-brown papules of the head and neck, which slowly evolve by peripheral extension and central atrophy into large plaques

Lichen scrofulosorum: asymptomatic, grouped, closely set, small, perifollicular, lichenoid papules; occur in children and young adults with TB

Differential diagnosis
Sarcoidosis; disseminated deep fungal infection; sporotrichosis; squamous cell carcinoma; pyoderma gangrenosum; lymphoma; pseudolymphoma; leprosy; leishmaniasis; syphilis; actinomycosis; tularemia; Langerhans cell histiocytosis

Therapy
First 2 months of therapy: isoniazid 5 mg per kg per day in adults; 10–20 mg per kg per day in children; rifampin 10 mg per kg per day in adults; 10–20 mg per kg per day in children; pyrazinamide 15–30 mg per kg per day in adults and children; ethambutol 15–25 mg per kg per day in adults and children or streptomycin 15 mg per kg per day in adults; 20–40 mg per kg per day in children

Next 4 months of therapy: isoniazid and rifampin if isolates are sensitive

References
Small PM, Fujiwara PI (2001) Management of tuberculosis in the United States. New England Journal of Medicine 345(3):189–200

Cutis hyperelastica

▶ Ehlers Danlos syndrome

Cutis laxa

Synonym(s)
Cutis pendula; dermatochalasis; elastolysis; dermatomegaly; elastolysis cutis laxa

Definition
Connective tissue disorder in which skin loses its elasticity and hangs in folds

Pathogenesis
Possibly due to abnormal elastin metabolism, resulting in markedly reduced dermal elastin content and degenerative changes in elastic fibers; biochemical basis of the disorder may be heterogeneous

Clinical manifestation
Skin loose, inelastic, hanging in folds, and demonstrating decreased elastic recoil on stretching; patient looks much older than chronologic age

Internal organ involvement: gastrointestinal tract: diverticula of small and large bowel; rectal prolapse; umbilical, inguinal, and hiatal hernias

Pulmonary: bronchiectasis, emphysema, cor pulmonale

Cardiovascular: cardiomegaly; congestive heart failure; murmurs; aortic aneurysms

Skeletal: dislocation of hips; osteoporosis; growth retardation; delayed fontanelle closure; ligamentous laxity

Differential diagnosis
Costello syndrome; Ehlers-Danlos syndrome; granulomatous slack skin variant of peripheral T cell lymphoma; Marfan syndrome; mid-dermal elastolysis; pseudoxanthoma elasticum; anetoderma; atrophoderma of Pasini and Pierini

Therapy
No effective therapy

References
DeAngelis DD, Carter SR, Seiff SR (2002) Dermatochalasis. International Ophthalmology Clinics 42(2):89–101

Cutis pendula

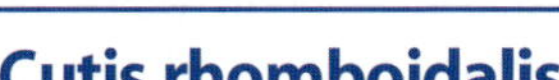

▶ Cutis laxa

Cutis rhomboidalis

Definition
Deep furrows in a rhomboid geometric pattern on the posterior neck, as a sign of advanced sun damage

References
Goldberg LH, Altman A (1984) Benign skin changes associated with chronic sunlight exposure. Cutis 34(1):33–38,40

Cutis sulcata

▶ Cutis verticis gyrata

Cutis verticis gyrata

Synonym(s)
Robert-Unna syndrome; bulldog scalp; cutis sulcata; corrugated skin; cutis verticis plicata; pachydermia verticis gyrata

Definition
Scalp condition characterized by convoluted folds and furrows formed by thickened skin

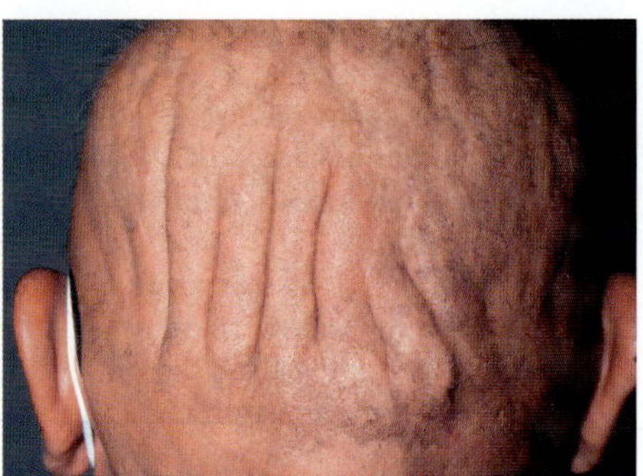

Cutis verticis gyrata. Soft, spongy folds of skin on the posterior scalp

Pathogenesis
Primary form: unknown etiology; possible factor, is increased peripheral use of testosterone.
Secondary form: depends on the underlying process (e.g. systemic diseases, inflammatory dermatoses, underlying nevoid abnormalities, and trauma)

Clinical manifestation
Primary form: only scalp involvement; symmetrical, soft, and spongy folds developing after puberty, usually in vertex and occipital region
Secondary form: sometimes present at birth
Both forms: hair over the folds sometimes sparse but normal in the furrows; maceration and unpleasant smell sometimes present in cases with secondary infection in the furrows

Differential diagnosis
Acromegaly; cutis laxa; pachydermoperiostosis; congenital nevus; cylindroma

Therapy
Surgical resection for psychological or esthetic reasons

References
Snyder MC, Johnson PJ, Hollins RR (2002) Congenital primary cutis verticis gyrata. Plastic & Reconstructive Surgery 110(3):818–821

Cutis verticis plicata

▶ Cutis verticis gyrata

Cyclophosphamide

Trade name(s)
Cytoxan; Neosar

Generic available
No

Drug class
Alkylating agent; immunosuppressant

Mechanism of action
Cell-cycle nonspecific suppression of B cells and T cells; forms DNA cross-links

Dosage form
25 mg, 50 mg tablets; 100 mg, 200 mg, 300 mg vials for intravenous injection

Dermatologic indications and dosage
See table

Common side effects
Cutaneous: alopecia, stomatitis, dyspigmentation of skin and nails, skin eruption
Gastrointestinal: nausea and vomiting, diarrhea
Genitourinary: cystitis

Serious side effects
Bone marrow: suppression
Cardiovascular: congestive failure, cardiomyopathy
Cutaneous: anaphylaxis
Genitourinary: hemorrhagic cystitis, sterility; increased risk of cancer

Drug interactions
Bone marrow suppressants; allopurinol; doxorubicin; zidovudine

Contraindications/precautions
Hypersensitivity to drug class or component; bone marrow depression; caution in impaired renal or liver function; caution in leukopenia or thrombocytopenia

References
Silvis NG (2001) Antimetabolites and cytotoxic drugs. Dermatologic Clinics 19(1):105–118

Cyclosporine

Trade name(s)
Neoral; Sandimmune; SangCya

Generic available
Yes

Drug class
Immunosuppressive

Mechanism of action
Calcineurin inhibition causes decreased IL-2 production; leads to decline in activated T lymphocytes

Dosage form
Neoral: 25 mg, 100 mg capsule; 100 mg per ml oral solution.
Sandimmune: 25 mg, 50 mg, 100 mg capsule; 100 mg per ml oral solution; 50 mg per ml for IV infusion

Dermatologic indications and dosage
See table

Common side effects
Cutaneous: hypertrichosis, acne, gingival hyperplasia
Gastrointestinal: nausea and vomiting, diarrhea, abdominal pain
Laboratory: elevated liver function tests, elevated BUN and creatinine, hyperkalemia, hyperuricemia, hypomagnesemia hyperglycemia

Cyclophosphamide. Dermatologic indications and dosage

Disease	Adult dosage	Child dosage
Acute febrile neutrophilic dermatosis	50–200 mg PO daily	Not indicated
Behçet's disease	50–200 mg PO daily	Not indicated
Bullous pemphigoid	50–200 mg PO daily	Not indicated
Cicatricial pemphigoid	50–200 mg PO daily	Not indicated
Cryoglobulinemia	50–200 mg PO daily	Not indicated
Dermatomyositis	50–200 mg PO daily	Not indicated
Epidermolysis bullosa acquisita	50–200 mg PO daily	Not indicated
Fogo selvagem	50–200 mg PO daily	Not indicated
Lichen myxedematosus	50–200 mg PO daily	Not indicated
Lupus erythematosus	50–200 mg PO daily	Not indicated
Mixed connective tissue disease	50–200 mg PO daily	Not indicated
Paraneoplastic pemphigus	50–200 mg PO daily	Not indicated
Pemphigus foliaceus	50–200 mg PO daily	Not indicated
Pemphigus vulgaris	50–200 mg PO daily	Not indicated
Polyarteritis nodosa	50–200 mg PO daily	Not indicated
Pyoderma gangrenosum	50–200 mg PO daily	Not indicated
Relapsing polychondritis	50–200 mg PO daily	Not indicated
Scleroderma	50–200 mg PO daily	Not indicated
Vasculitis	50–200 mg PO daily	Not indicated
Weber-Christian disease	50–200 mg PO daily	Not indicated
Wegener's granulomatosis	2 mg per kg PO daily or 0.5 g per m^2 IV every month for 6 months	Not indicated

Serious side effects

Bone marrow: suppression
Cutaneous: anaphylaxis
Neurologic: seizures
Renal: nephrotoxicity

Drug interactions

Antifungal agents; barbiturates; carbamazepine; carboplatin; cimetidine; ciprofloxacin; colchicine; oral contraceptives; diltiazem; systemic corticosteroids; erythromycin; lovastatin; glyburide/metformin; metronidazole; nafcillin; non-steroidal anti-inflammatory agents; phenytoin; pimozide; potassium salts; pravastatin; protease inhibitors; rifampin; simvastatin; verapamil; vinca alkaloids

Cyclosporine. Dermatologic indications and dosage

Disease	Adult dosage	Child dosage
Alopecia areata	3–5 mg per kg PO daily, divided into 2 doses	3–5 mg per kg PO daily, divided into 2 doses
Atopic dermatitis	3–5 mg per kg PO daily, divided into 2 doses	3–5 mg per kg PO daily, divided into 2 doses
Behçet's disease	3–5 mg per kg PO daily, divided into 2 doses	3–5 mg per kg PO daily, divided into 2 doses
Bullous pemphigoid	3–5 mg per kg PO daily, divided into 2 doses	3–5 mg per kg PO daily, divided into 2 doses
Chronic actinic dermatitis	3–5 mg per kg PO daily, divided into 2 doses	3–5 mg per kg PO daily, divided into 2 doses
Dermatomyositis	3–5 mg per kg PO daily, divided into 2 doses	3–5 mg per kg PO daily, divided into 2 doses
Epidermolysis bullosa acquisita	3–5 mg per kg PO daily, divided into 2 doses	3–5 mg per kg PO daily, divided into 2 doses
Hyperimmunoglobulin E syndrome	3 mg per kg daily for 6 months	3 mg per kg daily for 6 months
Lichen amyloidosis	3–5 mg per kg PO daily, divided into 2 doses	Not indicated
Lichen planus, erosive	Oral solution applied to erosions 3–4 times daily	Oral solution applied to erosions 3–4 times daily
Lupus erythematosus, acute	3–5 mg per kg PO daily, divided into 2 doses	3–5 mg per kg PO daily, divided into 2 doses
Mycosis fungoides	3–5 mg per kg PO daily, divided into 2 doses	3–5 mg per kg PO daily, divided into 2 doses
Pemphigus vulgaris	3–5 mg per kg PO daily, divided into 2 doses	3–5 mg per kg PO daily, divided into 2 doses
Pityriasis rubra pilaris	3–5 mg per kg PO daily, divided into 2 doses	3–5 mg per kg PO daily, divided into 2 doses
Psoriasis	3–5 mg per kg PO daily, divided into 2 doses	Not indicated
Pyoderma gangrenosum	3–5 mg per kg PO daily, divided into 2 doses	3–5 mg per kg PO daily, divided into 2 doses
Reiter syndrome	3–5 mg per kg PO daily, divided into 2 doses	Not indicated
Relapsing polychondritis	3–5 mg per kg PO daily, divided into 2 doses	3–5 mg per kg PO daily, divided into 2 doses
Scleroderma	3–5 mg per kg PO daily, divided into 2 doses	Not indicated
Sézary's syndrome	3–5 mg per kg PO daily, divided into 2 doses	3–5 mg per kg PO daily, divided into 2 doses
Urticaria	3–5 mg per kg PO daily for no longer than 3 months; to be used only for severe, recalcitrant disease	3–5 mg per kg PO daily for no longer than 3 months; to be used only for severe, recalcitrant disease

Cyclosporine. Dermatologic indications and dosage (Continued)

Disease	Adult dosage	Child dosage
Weber-Christian disease	3–5 mg per kg PO daily, divided into 2 doses	Not indicated

Contraindications/precautions
Hypersensitivity to drug class or component; caution with impaired renal or hepatic function; caution with other potentially nephrotoxic drugs

References
Cather J, Abramovits W, Menter A (2000) Cyclosporine and tacrolimus in dermatology. Dermatologic Clinics 19(1);119–138

Cylindroma

Synonym(s)
Turban tumor; tomato tumor

Definition
Primitive, benign, sweat gland tumor, most commonly occurring on the head, neck, and scalp

Pathogenesis
Solitary tumor variant: unknown; tumor differentiation toward either the eccrine or apocrine line
Multiple tumor variant: autosomal dominant trait

Clinical manifestation
Solitary tumor variant: firm, rubbery, red-to-blue papule or nodule, located on scalp, head, or neck; rare malignant transformation
Multiple tumor variant: numerous masses of pink, red, or blue papules or nodules, sometimes resembling bunches of small tomatoes; located on the head and neck region, trunk, or extremities

Differential diagnosis
Pilar cyst; eccrine spiradenoma; metastases; cutis verticis gyrata

Therapy
Solitary or multiple small tumors: simple excision or CO2 laser ablation
Multiple clustered tumors: extensive excisions with reconstruction

References
Gerretsen AL, van der Putte SC, Deenstra W, van Vloten WA (1993) Cutaneous cylindroma with malignant transformation. Cancer 72(5):1618–1623

Cyst

Synonym(s)
None

Definition
A sac or capsule filled with fluid, mucinous, or keratinous material

References
Langley RG, Walsh N, Ross JB (1997) Multiple eruptive milia: report of a case, review of the literature, and a classification. Journal of the American Academy of Dermatology 37(2 Pt 2):353–356

Cyst, dermoid

▶ Dermoid cyst

Cyst, epidermoid

▶ Epidermoid cyst

Cyst, mucinous

▶ Digital mucous cyst

Cyst, myxoid

▶ Digital mucous cyst

Cystadenoma, apocrine

▶ Apocrine hidrocystoma

Cystic chromomycosis

▶ Chromoblastomycosis

Cystic hidradenoma

▶ Eccrine acrospiroma

Cystic hygroma

▶ Lymphangioma

Cysticercosis

Synonym(s)
Neurocysticercosis; Taenia solium infestation

Definition
Systemic illness caused by dissemination of the larval form of the pork tapeworm, Taenia solium

Pathogenesis
Intermediate host (normally pigs) ingests eggs in contaminated food or water; T solium embryos penetrate GI mucosa of the pig and are hematogenously disseminated to peripheral tissues, with formation of larval cysts (cysticerci); with consumption of undercooked pork, intestinal tapeworm again formed, completing the life cycle of the worm; cyst dissemination in humans cause signs and symptoms of disease

Clinical manifestation
Skin findings: subcutaneous nodules resembling epidermoid cysts
Neurologic findings: papilledema and decreased retinal venous pulsations; meningismus; hyperreflexia; nystagmus or visual deficits
Musculoskeletal findings: muscular pseudohypertrophy

Differential diagnosis
Toxoplasmosis; coccidioidomycosis; tuberculosis; meningitis; encephalitis; brain abscess; cerebrovascular accident; sarcoidosis; brain tumor

Therapy
Albendazole 15 mg per kg per day PO divided into 2 or 3 doses for 2 weeks; praziquantel 50 mg per kg per day PO divided into 3 doses for 2 weeks

References
Garcia HH, Del Brutto OH (2000) Taenia solium cysticercosis. Infectious Disease Clinics of North America 14(1):97–119

Cystomata

▶ Digital mucous cyst

Cytophagic histiocytic panniculitis

Synonym(s)
None

Definition
Proliferative disorder of histiocytes, characterized by fever, subcutaneous nodules, and abnormal liver function

Pathogenesis
Unknown

Clinical manifestation
Tender, red, subcutaneous nodules, sometimes ulcerating; mucous membrane ulcerations; enlarged liver and spleen; lymphadenopathy; prolonged clinical course, usually ending with pancytopenia and hepatosplenomegaly

Differential diagnosis
Weber-Christian disease; lymphoma; nodular vasculitis; polyarteritis nodosa; lupus profundus; traumatic panniculitis; pancreatic panniculitis; alpha-1 anti-trypsin deficiency; factitial disease; pyoderma gangrenosum; Sweet's syndrome

Therapy
Prednisone; cyclosporine

References
Requena L, Sanchez Yus E (2001) Panniculitis. Part II. Mostly lobular panniculitis. Journal of the American Academy of Dermatology 45(3):325–361

D

Dabska tumor

▶ Endovascular papillary angioendothelioma of childhood

Dactylitis

Definition
Inflammation of the fingers and/or toes

References
Rhody C (2000) Bacterial infections of the skin.
Primary Care: clinics in Office Practice
27(2):459–473

Dactylolysis spontanea

▶ Ainhum

Danbolt-Closs syndrome

▶ Acrodermatitis enteropathica

Dandruff

▶ Seborrheic dermatitis

Dapsone

Trade name(s)
None

Generic available
Yes

Drug class
Sulfone

Mechanism of action
Leprosy: folic acid pathway inhibition
Inflammatory disorders: effects on neutrophils, including inhibition of myeloper-
oxidase and inhibition of neutrophil chemotaxis

Dosage form
25 mg, 100 mg tablet

Dermatologic indications and dosage
See table

Common side effects
Cutaneous: skin eruption, including urticaria; photosensitivity

Dapsone. Dermatologic indications and dosage

Disease	Adult dosage	Child dosage
Acropustulosis of infancy	Start at 100 mg PO daily; titrate as per therapeutic response	2 mg per kg PO daily
Acute febrile neutrophilic dermatosis	Start at 100 mg PO daily; titrate as per therapeutic response	2 mg per kg PO daily
Behçet's disease	Start at 100 mg PO daily; titrate as per therapeutic response	2 mg per kg PO daily
Brown recluse spider bite	Start at 100 mg PO daily; titrate as per therapeutic response	2 mg per kg PO daily
Bullous pemphigoid	Start at 100 mg PO daily; titrate as per therapeutic response	2 mg per kg PO daily
Cicatricial pemphigoid	Start at 100 mg PO daily; titrate as per therapeutic response	2 mg per kg PO daily
Dermatitis herpetiformis	Start at 100 mg PO daily; titrate as per therapeutic response	2 mg per kg PO daily
Eosinophilic pustular folliculitis and other forms of folliculitis	Start at 100 mg PO daily; titrate as per therapeutic response	2 mg per kg PO daily
Epidermolysis bullosa acquisita	Start at 100 mg PO daily; titrate as per therapeutic response	2 mg per kg PO daily
Erythema elevatum diutinum	Start at 100 mg PO daily; titrate as per therapeutic response	2 mg per kg PO daily
Eumycetoma	50–200 mg PO daily for months to years	25–50 mg PO daily for months to years
Granuloma annulare	Start at 100 mg PO daily; titrate as per therapeutic response	2 mg per kg PO daily
Granuloma faciale	Start at 100 mg PO daily; titrate as per therapeutic response	2 mg per kg PO daily
Hidradenitis suppurativa	Start at 100 mg PO daily; titrate as per therapeutic response	2 mg per kg PO daily
Leprosy	Start at 100 mg PO daily; titrate as per therapeutic response	2 mg per kg PO daily
Linear IgA dermatosis	25–100 mg PO daily initially; if blistering is not controlled, use 50 mg increments every 1–2 weeks	1–2 mg per kg PO daily
Lupus erythematosus, bullous	Start at 100 mg PO daily; titrate as per therapeutic response	2 mg per kg PO daily
Pemphigus foliaceus	Start at 100 mg PO daily; titrate as per therapeutic response	2 mg per kg PO daily
Pemphigus vulgaris	Start at 100 mg PO daily; titrate as per therapeutic response	2 mg per kg PO daily
Pyoderma gangrenosum	Start at 100 mg PO daily; titrate as per therapeutic response	2 mg per kg PO daily

Dapsone. Dermatologic indications and dosage (Continued)

Disease	Adult dosage	Child dosage
Relapsing polychondritis	Start at 100 mg PO daily; titrate as per therapeutic response	2 mg per kg PO daily
Subacute nodular migratory panniculitis	Start at 100 mg PO daily; titrate as per therapeutic response	2 mg per kg PO daily
Subcorneal pustular dermatosis	Start at 100 mg PO daily; titrate as per therapeutic response	2 mg per kg PO daily
Urticaria	50–100 mg PO daily for no longer than 3 months; to be used only for severe, recalcitrant disease	Not indicated
Vasculitis, including urticarial vasculitis	Start at 100 mg PO daily; titrate as per therapeutic response	2 mg per kg PO daily

Gastrointestinal: nausea, vomiting, abdominal pain, pancreatitis
General: malaise
Neurologic: dizziness, peripheral neuropathy

Serious side effects
Cutaneous: dapsone hypersensitivity syndrome, exfoliative dermatitis, toxic epidermal necrolysis
Gastrointestinal: hepatotoxicity
Hematologic: agranulocytosis; leukopenia; methemoglobinemia
Renal: acute tubular necrosis

Drug interactions
Antacids; bone marrow suppressants; clozapine; cytotoxic chemotherapeutic agents; interferon; probenecid; trimethoprim; zidovudine

Contraindications/precautions
Hypersensitivity to drug class or component; caution in G6PD deficiency, impaired renal function, or decreased liver function

References
Paniker U, Levine N (2000) Dapsone and sulfapyridine. Dermatologic Clinics 19(1):79–86

Darier disease

Synonym(s)
Darier's disease; Darier-White disease; keratosis follicularis

Definition
Dominantly inherited disease characterized by hyperkeratotic papules in seborrheic regions and nail abnormalities

Pathogenesis
Abnormal cell-cell adhesion and aberrant epidermal keratinization; mutations in the gene ATP2A2, which encodes a calcium pump; calcium-dependent signaling pathway in desmosomal assembly and cell-cell adhesion; defects cause alterations of cytosolic calcium level, influencing adhesion between keratinocytes and cellular differentiation in the epidermis

Clinical manifestation
Yellowish-brown, greasy, verrucous papules, most common in the seborrheic areas, such as forehead, scalp, nasolabial folds, ears, chest and back; mucosal surfaces with white papules with central

depression; heat, humidity, stress, sunlight, and UVB rays exacerbate the condition; lesions on palms, including punctate keratosis, palmar pits, and hemorrhagic macules; verrucous papules present on the backs of the hands; nail changes, including white and red longitudinal bands, longitudinal nail ridges, and splits

Differential diagnosis
Transient acantholytic dermatosis (Grover's disease); Hailey-Hailey disease; pemphigus foliaceus; seborrheic dermatitis; acrokeratosis verruciformis of Hopf; pityriasis lichenoides chronica; folliculitis; follicular eczema

Therapy
Isotretinoin; tretinoin; tazarotene

References
Burge S (1999) Management of Darier's disease. Clinical & Experimental Dermatology 24(2):53–56

Darier-White disease

▶ Darier disease

Darier's disease

▶ Darier disease

Dark dot disease

▶ Reticulate pigmented anomaly

Darling's disease

▶ Histoplasmosis

Day cream for dry skin

▶ Alpha hydroxy acids

De Lange syndrome

▶ Cornelia de Lange syndrome

De Sanctis-Cacchione syndrome

▶ Xeroderma pigmentosum

Decubitus

▶ Decubitus ulcer

Decubitus ulcer

Synonym(s)
Decubitus; pressure sore; pressure ulcer; ischemic ulcer; bed sore

Definition
Localized area of devitalized tissue secondary to vascular occlusion from prolonged external pressure against an internal body prominence, such as the sacrum or heel

Pathogenesis
Microcirculatory occlusion as pressures rise above capillary filling pressure, resulting in ischemia, causing inflammation and tissue anoxia, leading to cell death, tissue necrosis, and ulceration; paralysis result in muscle and soft tissue atrophy, decreasing the bulk over which bony prominences are supported; sensory loss, malnutrition, hypo-

proteinemia, and anemia can be contributing factors in prolonged healing time

Clinical manifestation
Stage 1: intact skin with signs of impending ulceration, with blanching erythema from reactive hyperemia
Stage 2: partial-thickness loss of skin involving epidermis and some dermis; sometimes presenting as an abrasion, blister, or superficial ulceration
Stage 3: full-thickness loss of skin with extension into subcutaneous tissue but not through the underlying fascia
Stage 4: full-thickness loss of skin and subcutaneous tissue and extension into muscle, bone, tendon, or joint capsule

Differential diagnosis
Pyoderma gangrenosum; squamous cell carcinoma; factitial ulcer; burn; contact dermatitis; bullous pemphigoid; spider bite; stasis ulcer; vasculitis

Therapy
Reduction or elimination of the source of external pressure, with frequent turning, protective pads, special mattresses, etc*; stage 2: hydrocolloid dressings; stages 3 and 4: wet dressings; silver sulfadiazine cream; hydrogels; xerogels; daily whirlpool use

References
Walker P (2001) Management of pressure ulcers. Oncology 15(11):1499–1508, 1511

Deep fibromatosis

▶ Desmoid tumor

Deer-fly fever

▶ Tularemia

Degos' acanthoma

▶ Clear cell acanthoma

Degos' disease

▶ Malignant atrophic papulosis

Degos' syndrome

▶ Malignant atrophic papulosis

Delhi boil

▶ Leishmaniasis, cutaneous

Dental abscess

▶ Oral cutaneous fistula

Dental abscess with sinus tract formation

▶ Oral cutaneous fistula

Dental sinus

▶ Oral cutaneous fistula

Depilatories, chemical. Dermatologic indications and dosage

Disease	Adult dosage	Child dosage
Hirsutism	Apply as needed	Apply as needed
Hypertrichosis	Apply as needed	Apply as needed
Pseudofolliculitis barbae	Apply as needed	Apply as needed

Depilatories, chemical

Trade name(s)
Nair; Neet; Nudit; Magic Shaving Powder; Royal Crown Shaving Powder

Generic available
No

Drug class
Chemical depilatory agent

Mechanism of action
Hydrolysis of hair disulfide bonds

Dosage form
Cream, powder

Dermatologic indications and dosage
See table

Common side effects
Cutaneous: skin irritation

Serious side effects
None

Drug interactions
None

Contraindications/precautions
Hypersensitivity to drug class or component

References
Ramos-e-Silva M, de Castro MC, Carneiro LV Jr (2001) Hair removal. Clinics in Dermatology 19(4):437–444

Dercum disease

▶ Dercum's disease

Dercum's disease

Synonym(s)
Dercum's syndrome; Dercum disease; adiposis dolorosa

Definition
Disorder in which there are fatty deposits that apply pressure to the underlying nerves, resulting in weakness and pain

Pathogenesis
Unknown; autosomal dominant inheritance

Clinical manifestation
Painful, nodular fatty deposits; general obesity, fatigability, weakness; emotional disturbances, such as depression and confusion; dementia

Differential diagnosis
Neurofibromatosis; proteus syndrome; progressive lipodystrophy; familial multiple lipomatosis; fibromyalgia; Weber-Christian disease; multiple symmetrical lipomatosis (Madelung syndrome)

Therapy
Liposuction; surgical excision of painful lipomas

References

Brodovsky S, Westreich M, Leibowitz A, Schwartz Y (1994) Adiposis dolorosa (Dercum's disease): 10-year follow-up. Annals of Plastic Surgery 33(6) 664–668

Dercum's syndrome

▶ Dercum's disease

Dermal dendrocytoma

▶ Dermatofibroma

Dermal duct tumor

▶ Poroma

Dermal melanocytoma

▶ Blue nevus

Dermatitis artefacta

Synonym(s)
Factitial dermatitis

Definition
Physical or psychological symptoms and signs intentionally produced or feigned to assume a sick role

Pathogenesis
External trauma, producing skin lesions

Clinical manifestation
Multiple, irregularly shaped, eroded or ulcerated papules, usually in a distribution within easy reach of the dominant hand; blistering sometimes occurring after burns; morphology and distribution not consistent with any other dermatosis

Differential diagnosis
Atopic dermatitis; scabies; bacterial pyoderma; herpes simplex virus infection; herpes zoster; insect bite reaction; polyarteritis nodosa; Wegener's granulomatosis; septic vasculitis; Weber-Christian disease; nodular vasculitis

Therapy
Unna boot covering to extremity, if involved; careful evaluation to determine if secondary gain something other than psychological (monetary, etc); psychiatric consultation, if necessary

References
Koblenzer CS (2000) Dermatitis artefacta. Clinical features and approaches to treatment. American Journal of Clinical Dermatology 1(1):47–55

Dermatitis, Berloque

▶ Berloque dermatitis

Dermatitis contusiformis

▶ Erythema nodosum

Dermatitis, diaper

▶ Diaper dermatitis

Dermatitis, exfoliative

▸ **Exfoliative dermatitis**

Dermatitis herpetiformis

Synonym(s)
Dühring's disease; Dühring-Bloch disease; hydroa herpetiformis; pemphigus circinatus

Definition
Immune-mediated, blistering skin disease with an associated gluten-sensitive enteropathy

Pathogenesis
Gluten main factor in both bowel and skin disease; strong HLA associations (HLA-A1, HLA-B8, HLA DR3, HLA DQw2); unclear pathogenic significance of granular deposition of IgA at the dermal-epidermal junction of the skin

Clinical manifestation
Tense vesicles on an erythematous base, occurring in tight clusters (herpetiform pattern), symmetrically distributed over extensor surfaces, including elbows, knees, buttocks, shoulders, and the posterior scalp; occasional occurrence of erosions and crusts in the absence of vesicles; symptoms include burning, stinging, and intense pruritus; oral mucosa lesions occur infrequently; palms and soles usually spared; gastrointestinal symptoms usually mild or absent

Differential diagnosis
Bullous pemphigoid; erythema multiforme; epidermolysis bullosa; epidermolysis bullosa acquisita; linear IgA dermatosis; impetigo; pemphigus foliaceus; pemphigus vulgaris; herpes simplex virus infection; herpes zoster

Therapy
Dapsone*; sulfapyridine 500–1000 mg PO twice daily; gluten-free diet; prednisone

References
Reunala TL (2001) Dermatitis herpetiformis. Clinics in Dermatology 19(6):728–736

Dermatitis venenata

▸ **Contact dermatitis**

Dermatochalasis

Synonym(s)
Blepharochalasis; steatoblepharon

Definition
Redundant and lax eyelid skin and muscle

References
DeAngelis DD, Carter SR, Seiff SR (2002) Dermatochalasis. International Ophthalmology Clinics 42(2):89–101

Dermatofibroma

Synonym(s)
Dermal dendrocytoma; dermatofibroma lenticulare; fibroma durum; fibroma simplex; histiocytoma; histiocytoma cutis; nodular subepidermal fibrosis; sclerosing angioma; sclerosing hemangioma

Definition
Benign dermal lesion formed by the proliferation of histiocytes or fibroblasts

Pathogenesis
Probably a reactive tissue change rather than a true neoplasm

Clinical manifestation

Solitary, flesh-colored-to-brown, firm, asymptomatic or mildly tender papule; tethering of the overlying epidermis to the underlying lesion with lateral compression (dimple or button sign); most common on the extremities; may be multiple lesions

Differential diagnosis

Nevus; melanoma; seborrheic keratosis; basal cell carcinoma; dermatofibrosarcoma protuberans; wart; epidermoid cyst; scar; keloid; prurigo nodularis; desmoplastic trichoepithelioma; foreign body granuloma; mastocytoma; metastasis; juvenile xanthogranuloma

Therapy

Surgical excision; shave removal; cryotherapy

References

Pariser RJ (1998) Benign neoplasms of the skin. Medical Clinics of North America 82(6):1285–1307

Dermatofibroma lenticulare

▶ Dermatofibroma

Dermatofibrosarcoma protuberans

Synonym(s)

Bednar tumor; hypertrophic morphea; progressive and recurring dermatofibroma; fibrosarcoma of the skin

Definition

Low-grade, locally invasive sarcoma of the skin

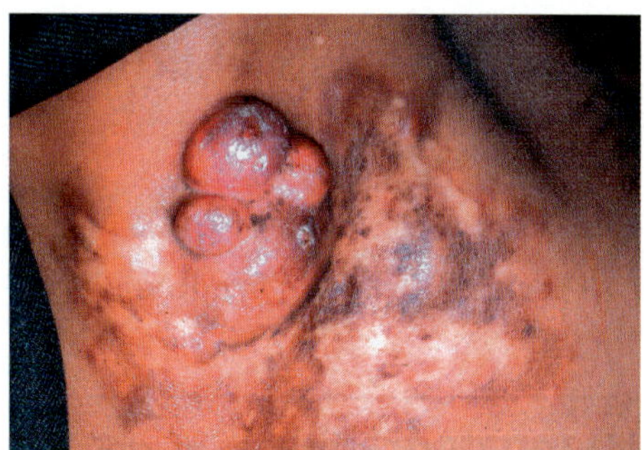

Dermatofibrosarcoma protuberans. Indurated plaque with irregular nodules

Pathogenesis

Cell of origin unclear; possibly fibroblastic, histiocytic, or neuroectodermal

Clinical manifestation

Begins as small, asymptomatic papule, most commonly on the trunk or proximal upper extremities; slowly enlarges into indurated plaque, composed of firm, irregular nodules, varying from flesh-colored to reddish-brown in color

Differential diagnosis

Dermatofibroma; melanoma; keloid; morphea; cutaneous metastasis; lymphoma

Therapy

Mohs micrographic surgery*; wide, local excision

References

Gloster HM Jr, Harris KR, Roenigk RK (1996) A comparison between Mohs micrographic surgery and wide surgical excision for the treatment of dermatofibrosarcoma protuberans. Journal of the American Academy of Dermatology 35(1):82–87

Dermatofibrosis lenticularis

▶ Buschke-Ollendorff syndrome

Dermatofibrosis lenticularis disseminata with osteopoikilosis

▶ Buschke-Ollendorff syndrome

Dermatographism

Synonym(s)
Dermographism; factitious urticaria; skin writing

Definition
Linear, urticarial wheal which occurs within minutes of vigorously stroking the skin with an object

Pathogenesis
Unclear; skin trauma possibly releases an antigen that interacts with the membrane-bound immunoglobulin E (IgE) of mast cells, releasing inflammatory mediators, particularly histamine, resulting leakage in small blood vessels; no association with systemic diseases, food allergies, or ingested medications

Clinical manifestation
Urticarial wheals develop within 5 minutes of stroking the skin and persist for 15–30 minutes; resolve without residua

Differential diagnosis
Chronic urticaria; contact urticaria; insect bite reaction; mastocytosis

Therapy
Antihistamines, second generation*

References
Lee EE, Maibach HI (2001) Treatment of urticaria. An evidence-based evaluation of antihistamines. American Journal of Clinical Dermatology 2(1):27–32

Dermatoheliosis

▶ Actinic elastosis

Dermatomegaly

▶ Cutis laxa

Dermatomycosis furfuracea

▶ Tinea versicolor

Dermatomycosis nigricans

▶ Tinea nigra

Dermatomyofibroma

Synonym(s)
Plaque-like dermal fibromatosis

Definition
Benign dermal proliferation consisting of fibroblasts and myofibroblasts

Pathogenesis
Unknown

Clinical manifestation
Solitary, asymptomatic, slow growing, flesh-colored-to-red, firm plaque, occurring in women, often around the axilla

Differential diagnosis
Morphea; lichen sclerosus; dermatofibroma; scar; keloid; dermatofibrosarcoma protuberans; desmoid; leiomyoma; myofi-

broma; neurofibroma; granuloma annulare; sarcoidosis

Therapy
Surgical excision[*]

References
Rose C, Brocker EB (1999) Dermatomyofibroma: case report and review. Pediatric Dermatology 16(6):456–459

Dermatomyositis

Synonym(s)
Idiopathic inflammatory myopathy; dermatomyositis sine myositis; amyopathic dermatomyositis

Definition
Inflammatory myopathy with characteristic cutaneous findings

Pathogenesis
Possible etiologic factors: genetic predisposition; immunologic abnormalities; infections; concomitant medication use

Clinical manifestation
Skin disease sometimes initial or sole manifestation; muscle disease occurring concurrently, sometimes preceding skin disease or following skin disease by weeks to years; eruption photodistributed and photo-exacerbated; violaceous-to-dusky, erythematous plaques with or without edema in a symmetrical distribution involving periorbital skin; central facial erythema
Scalp involvement: erythematous to violaceous, psoriasiform plaques; slightly elevated, violaceous papules and plaques; Gottron papules over bony prominences, particularly the metacarpophalangeal joints, the proximal interphalangeal joints, and/or the distal interphalangeal joints
Similar lesions overly the elbows, knees, and/or feet; periungual telangiectases; irregular, ragged cuticles with hypertrophy and hemorrhagic infarcts; calcinosis of the skin or muscle common in children or adolescents
Muscle disease: proximal symmetrical muscle weakness; associated with internal malignancies in patients older than 50 years old

Differential diagnosis
Lupus erythematosus; psoriasis; lichen planus; scleroderma; seborrheic dermatitis; pemphigus foliaceus; polymorphous light eruption; dermatophytosis; parapsoriasis; rosacea; sarcoidosis

Therapy
Prednisone[*]; steroid-sparing drugs – methotrexate; azathioprine; cyclophosphamide; cyclosporine, mycophenolate mofetil; hydroxychloroquine; methotrexate; IVIG 1 gm IV on 2 successive days, repeated every 4–6 weeks as needed; calcinosis cutis: surgical excision of symptomatic lesions

References
Olsen NJ, Park JH, King LE Jr (2001) Amyopathic dermatomyositis. Current Rheumatology Reports 3(4):346–351

Dermatomyositis sine myositis

▶ Dermatomyositis

Dermatosis cenicienta

▶ Ashy dermatosis

Dermatosis papulosa nigra

Synonym(s)
None

Definition

Skin condition characterized by multiple, small, hyperpigmented papules on the face of adult blacks

Pathogenesis

Probably genetically determined; hamartomatous developmental defect of the pilosebaceous follicle

Clinical manifestation

Multiple, firm, smooth, dark-brown-to-black, flattened papules, mainly on the malar area of the face and the forehead; first appear after puberty; new lesions occur throughout life

Differential diagnosis

Wart; nevus; acrochordon; adenoma sebaceum; seborrheic keratosis

Therapy

Light electrodesiccation and curettage; cryotherapy

References

Kauh YC, McDonald JW, Rapaport JA, Ruschak PJ, Luscombe HA (1983) A surgical approach for dermatosis papulosa nigra. International Journal of Dermatology 22(10):590–592

Dermite pigmentée en forme de coulée

▶ Berloque dermatitis

Dermographism

▶ Dermatographism

Dermoid

▶ Dermoid cyst

Dermoid cyst

Synonym(s)

Choristoma; dermoid; lipodermoid

Definition

Subcutaneous cysts of ectodermal origin, arising along embryonic fusion planes

Pathogenesis

Sequestrations of cutaneous epithilium during fetal development

Clinical manifestation

Occur most commonly on the head and neck, particularly over the supraorbital region, glabella, upper eyelid and scalp; appear as subcutaneous masses, sometimes with a dimple or sinus tract; with deeper extension, lesion feel bound to underlying periosteum; sometimes contain nails, dental structures, cartilage-like and bone-like material, and fat

Differential diagnosis

Epidermoid cyst; pilomatricoma; metastasis; meningocele; encephalocele; nevus sebaceous; thyroglossal duct cyst; cutaneous ectopic brain; lymph node

Therapy

Surgical excision[*]

References

Ogle RF, Jauniaux E (1999) Fetal scalp cysts–dilemmas in diagnosis. Prenatal Diagnosis 19(12):1157–1159

Dermolytic pemphigoid

▶ Epidermolysis bullosa acquisita

Desert rheumatism

▶ Coccidioidomycosis

Desmoid

▶ Desmoid tumor

Desmoid tumor

Synonym(s)
Desmoid; musculoaponeurotic fibromatosis; aggressive fibromatosis; deep fibromatosis; non-metastasizing fibrosarcoma

Definition
Benign fibrous neoplasm, related to fibromatosis, originating from the musculoaponeurotic structures, usually on the abdominal wall

Pathogenesis
Uncertain; possibly related to genetic factors, trauma, or hormonal factors; myofibroblast is the cell responsible for tumor growth

Clinical manifestation
Solitary, slow-growing, firm, smooth, mobile mass, most commonly in the anterior abdominal wall and shoulder girdle; history of trauma (often surgical) to the site of tumor development; often adherent to surrounding structures; locally invasive, but not metastatic; overlying skin usually unaffected

Differential diagnosis
Dermatofibrosarcoma protuberans; metastasis; leiomyosarcoma; Gardner syndrome

Therapy
Wide surgical resection*; radiation therapy

References
Shields CJ, Winter DC, Kirwan WO, Redmond HP (2001) Desmoid tumours. European Journal of Surgical Oncology 27(8):701–706

Desonide

▶ Corticosteroids, topical, low potency

Desoximetasone

▶ Corticosteroids, topical, high potency

Desquamative gingivitis

Definition
Inflammation of the outermost soft tissue of the gums, which become red, form superficial erosions, lose their normal shape, and bleed easily; most often seen in patients with cicatricial pemphigoid

References
Fleming TE, Korman NJ (2000) Cicatricial pemphigoid. Journal of the American Academy of Dermatology 43(4):571–591

Dexamethasone

▶ Corticosteroids, topical, low potency

Diabetic bulla

▶ Bullous eruption of diabetes mellitus

Diabetic bullae

▶ Bullous eruption of diabetes mellitus

Diabetic dermopathy

Synonym(s)
Shin spots; pigmented pretibial patches; diabetic microangiopathy; spotted leg syndrome

Definition
Hyperpigmented, atrophic lesions on the legs of patients with diabetes mellitus

Pathogenesis
Uncertain; possibly microangiopathy; trauma with poor wound healing

Clinical manifestation
Small, brown, atrophic papules on the anterior legs, appearing singly or in groups

Differential diagnosis
Lupus erythematosus; lichen planus; posttraumatic scars; benign pigmented purpura; lichen sclerosus; morphea

Therapy
None

References
Romano G, Moretti G, Di Benedetto A, Giofre C, Di Cesare E, Russo G, Califano L, Cucinotta D (1998) Skin lesions in diabetes mellitus: prevalence and clinical correlations. Diabetes Research & Clinical Practice – Supplement 39(2):101–106

Diabetic microangiopathy

▶ Diabetic dermopathy

Diaper dermatitis

Synonym(s)
Diaper rash, perianal dermatitis

Definition
Irritant contact dermatitis caused by overhydration of the skin, maceration, prolonged contact with urine and feces, retained diaper soaps, and irritating topical preparations

Pathogenesis
Increased wetness makes the skin more susceptible to damage by physical, chemical, and enzymatic mechanisms; urease enzyme found in the stratum corneum liberates ammonia from cutaneous bacteria; lipases and proteases in feces mix with urine on eroded skin, and cause an alkaline surface pH; bile salts in the stools enhance activity of fecal enzymes; Candida albicans possible cause or effect of eruption; children with history of atopic dermatitis possibly more susceptible

Clinical manifestation
Erythematous scaly diaper area, often with fissures and erosions; sometimes patchy or confluent; affects the abdomen from the umbilicus to the thighs, encompassing the genitalia, perineum, and buttocks; genitocrural folds spared

Differential diagnosis
Psoriasis; atopic dermatitis; allergic contact dermatitis; biotin deficiency; acrodermatitis enteropathica; candidiasis; scabies; Langerhans cell histiocytosis; child abuse

Therapy
Changing of diapers frequently and/or leaving inflamed area uncovered for as long as possible between diaper changes[*]; zinc oxide paste; white petrolatum

References
Wolf R, Wolf D, Tuzun B, Tuzun Y (2000) Diaper dermatitis. Clinics in Dermatology 18(6):657–660

Diaper rash

► Diaper dermatitis

Dicloxacillin

Trade name(s)
Dynapen

Generic available
Yes

Drug class
Penicillin antibiotic

Mechanism of action
Inhibition of penicillin-binding proteins causes blockade of bacterial cell wall synthesis

Dosage form
250 mg, 500 mg tablet

Dermatologic indications and dosage
See table

Common side effects
Cutaneous: urticaria and other skin eruptions
Gastrointestinal: nausea, vomiting, diarrhea

Serious side effects
Bone marrow: thrombocytopenia
Cutaneous: anaphylaxis, Stevens-Johnson syndrome, toxic epidermal necrolysis
Gastrointestinal: pseudomembranous colitis
Renal: interstitial nephritis

Drug interactions
Aminoglycosides; oral contraceptives; methotrexate; probenecid

Contraindications/precautions
Hypersensitivity to drug class or component; use with caution in patients with

Dicloxacillin. Dermatologic indications and dosage

Disease	Adult dosage	Child dosage
Cellulitis	250–500 mg PO 4 times daily for 7–10 days	25–50 mg per kg PO 4 times daily for 7–10 days
Ecthyma	250–500 mg PO 4 times daily for 7–10 days	25–50 mg per kg PO 4 times daily for 7–10 days
Erysipelas	250–500 mg PO 4 times daily for 7–10 days	25–50 mg per kg PO 4 times daily for 7–10 days
Impetigo	250–500 mg PO 4 times daily for 7–10 days	25–50 mg per kg PO 4 times daily for 7–10 days
Staphylococcal scalded skin syndrome	250–500 mg PO 4 times daily for 7–10 days	< 40 kg – 12.5 mg per kg daily PO divided into 4 doses; > 40 kg – 125 mg PO 4 times daily

cephalosporin allergy, seizure disorder, impaired renal function

References
Salkind AR, Cuddy PG Foxworth JW (2001) The rational clinical examination. Is this patient allergic to penicillin? An evidence-based analysis of the likelihood of penicillin allergy. Journal of the American Medical Association 285(19):2498–2950

Diffuse nonepidermolytic palmoplantar keratoderma

▶ Unna-Thost palmoplantar keratoderma

Diffuse systemic sclerosis

▶ Progressive systemic sclerosus

Diflorasone diacetate

▶ Corticosteroids, topical, super potency

Digital duplication

▶ Supernumerary digit

Digital fibrokeratoma, acquired

▶ Acquired digital fibrokeratoma

Digital fibrous tumor of childhood

▶ Infantile digital fibromatosis

Digital mucinous pseudocyst

▶ Digital mucous cyst

Digital mucoid cyst

▶ Digital mucous cyst

Digital mucous cyst

Synonym(s)
Cystomata; myxomatous cutaneous cyst; myxomatous degenerative cyst; mucous cyst; myxoid cyst; synovial cyst; digital mucoid cyst; digital myxoid cyst; digital mucinous pseudocyst

Definition
Soft, cystic papule of the digits, containing mucinous material

Pathogenesis
Arises from mucoid degeneration of connective tissue; osteophytes in those with osteoarthritis possibly a stimulus

Clinical manifestation
Solitary, round-to-oval, dome-shaped, papule, with normal overlying skin; contains a viscous, gelatinous, clear or yellow-tinged fluid

Differential diagnosis
Epidermoid cyst; fibrokeratoma; giant-cell tendon sheath tumor; Heberden node; myxoid malignant fibrous histiocytoma; myxoid variant of liposarcoma; rheumatoid nodule; gouty tophus; subcutaneous granuloma annulare

Therapy
Intralesional triamcinolone 3–5 mg per ml; cryotherapy; incision and drainage; destruction by electrodesiccation; surgical excision

References
de Berker D, Goettman S, Baran R (2002) Subungual myxoid cysts: clinical manifestations and response to therapy. Journal of the American Academy of Dermatology 46(3):394–398

Digital myxoid cyst

▶ Digital mucous cyst

Digital papillary adenoma

▶ Aggressive digital papillary adenoma

Digitate dermatitis

▶ Small plaque parapsoriasis

Digitate dermatosis

▶ Small plaque parapsoriasis

Dilated pore

Synonym(s)
Winer's pore; Winer's dilated pore; dilated pore of Winer; giant follicle; enlarged solitary comedone

Definition
Hair structure anomaly appearing as an enlarged, solitary comedone

Pathogenesis
Unknown; neoplasm of the intraepidermal follicle and infundibulum of pilosebaceous apparatus

Clinical manifestation
Solitary large comedone on the face or trunk, most commonly the back; lateral pressure yields keratinous material

Differential diagnosis
Epidermoid cyst; trichoepithelioma; solar comedone; pilar sheath acanthoma; sebaceous trichofolliculoma

Therapy
Expression of comedone contents, followed by electrodesiccation of the base; surgical excision

References
Toshitani A; Imayama S, Urabe A, Kiryu H, Hori Y (1996) Hair cortex comedo. American Journal of Dermatopathology 18(3):322–325

Dilated pore of Winer

▶ Dilated pore

Diphtheria, cutaneous

Synonym(s)
None

Definition
Acute, toxin-mediated disease caused by Corynebacterium diphtheriae

Pathogenesis
C. diphtheriae (causative organism) an aerobic, toxin-producing, gram-positive bacillus; toxin production only when the bacillus infected by a specific virus carrying the genetic information for the toxin; only toxigenic strains cause severe disease; toxin inhibiting cellular protein synthesis responsible for local tissue destruction and membrane formation; toxin produced at the site of the membrane absorbed into the bloodstream and disseminated

Clinical manifestation
Skin findings: seen mainly in homeless persons; erythematous scaling plaques; ulcers with an overlying membrane and demarcated edges; mucous membranes sometimes involved

Differential diagnosis
Other bacterial pyodermas; erythema multiforme; tropical ulcer; pyoderma gangrenosum; Majocchi's granuloma; atypical mycobacterial infection; nocardiosis; aspergillosis; syphilis; granuloma inguinale; chancroid

Therapy
Erythromycin; procaine penicillin G; diphtheria antitoxin 20,000–50,000 units IM*

References
Efstratiou A, Roure C (2000) The European Laboratory Working Group on diphtheria: A global microbiologic network. Journal of Infectious Diseases 181 Suppl 1:S146–151

Discoid eczema

▶ Nummular eczema

Discoid lupus erythematosus

▶ Lupus erythematosus, discoid

Discrete keratoderma

▶ Knuckle pads

Dissecting cellulitis

▶ Dissecting cellulitis of scalp

Dissecting cellulitis of scalp

Synonym(s)
Dissecting cellulitis; perifolliculitis capitis abscedens et suffodiens; Hoffman's disease

Definition
Chronic inflammatory disease characterized by painful suppurating lesions of the scalp, leading to scarring alopecia

Pathogenesis
Associated with acne conglobata, hidradenitis suppurativa, and pilonidal cysts, all of which have follicular blockage as the common mechanism; retained material dilates and causes follicular rupture; keratin and organisms from the damaged hair follicles initiate neutrophilic and granulomatous response; bacterial infection secondary event

Clinical manifestation
Perifollicular pustules; tender nodules (some discharging pus or gelatinous material); intercommunicating sinuses between nodules; patchy alopecia with scarring ; frequent recurrences over many years

Differential diagnosis
Folliculitis keloidalis; folliculitis decalvans; kerion; pseudopelade of Brocq; lichen planopilaris; bacterial pyoderma

Therapy
Isotretinoin; dapsone; intralesional triamcinolone 5 mg per ml; laser hair removal; wide local excision

References
Sullivan JR, Kossard S (1999) Acquired scalp alopecia. Part II: A review. Australasian Journal of Dermatology 40(2):61–70

Disseminated cat-scratch disease

▶ Bacillary angiomatosis

Disseminated gonococcal infection

▶ Gonococcemia

Disseminated lenticular dermatofibrosis

▶ Buschke-Ollendorff syndrome

Disseminated superficial actinic porokeratosis

▶ Porokeratosis

Donohue syndrome

▶ Leprechaunism

Donovanosis

▶ Granuloma inguinale

Dorfman Chanarin syndrome

▶ Chanarin-Dorfman syndrome

Double lip and nontoxic thyroid enlargement syndrome

▶ Ascher's syndrome

Dove aerosol

▶ Aluminium chlorohydrate

Dowling Degos Ossipowski disease

▶ Reticulate pigmented anomaly

Dowling-Degos disease

▶ Reticulate pigmented anomaly

Doxepin

▶ Antihistamines, first generation

Doxycycline

Trade name(s)
Vibramycin; Doryx; Vibra-Tabs; Monodox

Generic available
Yes

Drug class
Tetracycline

Mechanism of action
Antibiotic activity: protein synthesis inhibition by binding to the 30S ribosomal subunit; anti-inflammatory activity: unclear mechanisms

Dosage form
50 mg, 100 mg tablets

Dermatologic indications and dosage
See table

Common side effects
Cutaneous: photosensitivity, stomatitis, oral candidiasis, urticaria or other vascular reaction
Gastrointestinal: nausea and vomiting, diarrhea, esophagitis
Neurologic: tinnitus, dizziness, drowsiness, headache, ataxia

Serious side effects
Gastrointestinal: pseudomembranous colitis, hepatotoxicity
Hematologic: neutropenia, thrombocytopenia
Neurologic: pseudotumor cerebri

Drug interactions
Antacids; calcium salts; oral contraceptives; digoxin; iron salts; isotretinoin; magnesium salts; warfarin

Contraindications/precautions
Hypersensitivity to drug class or component; pregnancy; patient < 8 years old; caution if impaired renal or liver function

References
Sadick N (2000) Systemic antibiotic agents. Dermatologic Clinics 19(1):1–22

Drug-induced bullous photosensitivity

▶ Pseudoporphyria

Dry skin

▶ Asteatosis
▶ Xerosis

Dryness of skin

▶ Xerosis

Doxycycline. Dermatologic indications and dosage

Disease	Adult dosage	Child dosage
Acne vulgaris	50–100 mg PO twice daily	> 8 years old – 50–100 mg PO twice daily
Anthrax	100 mg PO twice daily for 60 days in bioterrorism situation	> 8 years old – 50 mg PO twice daily for 60 days in bioterrorism situation
Atrophoderma of Pasini-Pierini	50–100 mg PO twice daily	> 8 years old – 50 mg PO twice daily
Bacillary angiomatosis	100 mg PO twice daily for 3 weeks	> 8 years old – 100 mg PO twice daily for 3 weeks
Bartonellosis	100 mg PO twice daily for 3 weeks	> 8 years old – 50 mg PO twice daily for 3 weeks
Boutonneuse fever	200 mg PO or IV immediately and at bedtime, followed by 100 mg PO twice daily for 3 days	> 8 years old – 2–5 mg per kg PO daily for 7–10 days
Bullous pemphigoid	50–100 mg PO twice daily	> 8 years old – 50 mg PO twice daily
Dermatitis herpetiformis	50–100 mg PO twice daily	> 8 years old – 50 mg PO twice daily
Epidemic typhus	200 mg PO or IV twice daily for 3 days, then 100 mg PO of IV daily until 48–72 hours after patient becomes afebrile	> 8 years old – 200 mg PO or IV twice daily for 3 days, then maintenance dose 100 mg PO or IV twice daily until 48–72 hours after patient becomes afebrile
Folliculitis	50–100 mg PO twice daily	> 8 years old – 50 mg PO twice daily
Leptospirosis	100 mg PO twice daily for 3 weeks	> 8 years old – 50 mg PO twice daily for 3 weeks
Linear IgA bullous dermatosis	50–100 mg PO twice daily	> 8 years old – 50 mg PO twice daily
Lyme disease	100 mg PO twice daily for 21 days; prophylaxis after tick bite – 200 mg PO for 1 dose	> 8 years old – 50 mg PO twice daily for 3 weeks
Lymphogranuloma venereum	100 mg PO twice daily for 3 weeks	> 8 years old – 50 mg PO twice daily for 3 weeks
Perioral dermatitis	100 mg PO twice daily for at least 30 days	> 8 years old – 50–100 mg PO twice daily for at least 30 days
Relapsing fever	100 mg PO twice daily for 7 days	> 8 years old – 50 mg PO twice daily for 7 days
Rickettsialpox	100 mg PO twice daily for 5 days	> 8 years old – 50 mg PO twice daily for 5 days
Rocky Mountain spotted fever	100 mg PO twice daily for 7–10 days	> 8 years old – 2 mg per kg PO or IV loading dose, followed by 1 mg per kg PO or IV every 12 hours for 7 days and for at least 48 hours after defervescence
Rosacea	100 mg PO twice daily for at least 30 days	> 8 years old – 50–100 mg PO twice daily for at least 30 days

Doxycycline. Dermatologic indications and dosage (Continued)

Disease	Adult dosage	Child dosage
Scrub typhus	100 mg PO twice daily for 7–14 days	> 8 years old – 50 mg PO twice daily for 14 days
Trench fever	100 mg PO twice daily for 4 weeks	> 8 years old – 50 mg PO twice daily for 4 weeks
Tularemia	100 mg PO twice daily for 7–14 days or until patient is afebrile for 5–7 days	> 8 years old – 50 mg PO twice daily for 7–14 days or until patient is afebrile for 5–7 days
Yaws	100 mg PO twice daily for 15 days	> 8 years old – 2–5 mg per kg PO divided into 2 doses daily for 15 days

Drysol

▶ **Aluminium chloride**

DSAP

▶ **Porokeratosis**

Dühring-Bloch disease

▶ **Dermatitis herpetiformis**

Dühring's disease

▶ **Dermatitis herpetiformis**

Dupuy's syndrome

▶ **Auriculotemporal syndrome**

Dupuytren's contracture

Synonym(s)
Palmoplantar fibromatosis; Dupuytren's disease, palmar fasciitis; Viking disease

Definition
Disorder characterized by subcutaneous fascia thickening and shortening, causing the fingers to retract down towards the palm of the hand

Pathogenesis
Unclear; dominant genetic inheritance; often involves individuals of northern European descent; trauma sometimes initiates or accelerates the process; associated with alcoholism, diabetes mellitus, smoking, epilepsy, pulmonary disease

Clinical manifestation
Asymptomatic, palmar skin nodule, generally within the distal aspect of the palm, often with puckering of the skin above the nodularity; overlying skin sometimes adherent to the fascia, and fibrous cord sometimes extending into the finger; ring finger most commonly involved site, followed by the small finger

Differential diagnosis
Trigger finger

Therapy
Physical therapy in early stages*; intralesional triamcinolone 3–5 mg per ml; partial surgical fasciectomy for a patient with significant functional disability

References
Saar JD, Grothaus PC (2000) Dupuytren's disease: An overview. Plastic & Reconstructive Surgery 106(1):125–134

Dupuytren's disease

▶ Dupuytren's contracture

Dwarfism with retinal atrophy and deafness

▶ Cockayne syndrome

Dyschondrodysplasia with hemangiomas

▶ Maffucci syndrome

Dyshidrosis

▶ Dyshidrotic eczema

Dyshidrotic eczema

Synonym(s)
Dyshidrosis; pompholyx; vesicular palmoplantar eczema; vesicular eczema of palms and soles

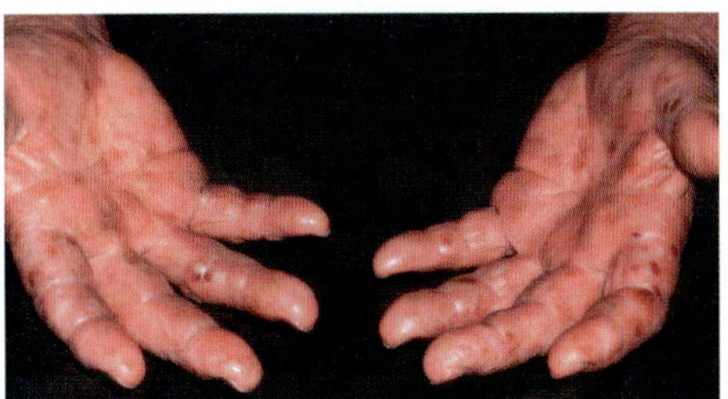

Dyshidrotic eczema. Multiple vesicles on the hands, with concentration along the sides of the digits

Definition
Recurrent or chronic relapsing form of vesicular palmoplantar dermatitis

Pathogenesis
Occurring commonly in atopic individuals; associated with stress, infection, exogenous contactants, climate changes

Clinical manifestation
Symmetric crops of clear vesicles and/or bullae on the palms and lateral aspects of fingers and feet; vesicles deep seated, with a tapioca-like appearance, and sometimes becoming confluent to form bullae; may develop crusting, scaling, and fissuring after persistent scratching

Differential diagnosis
Contact dermatitis; vesicular tinea pedis; tinea manus; palmoplantar pustular psoriasis; autosensitization reaction (id reaction)

Therapy
Corticosteroid, topical, high potency*; severe flare: prednisone; triamcinolone 40–80 mg IM as single dose.
Chronic persistent disease: azathioprine; local photochemotherapy; disulfiram 250–500 mg PO per day in nickel-sensitive patients; aluminium acetate 5% solution soaks

References
Landow K (1998) Hand dermatitis. The perennial scourge. Postgraduate Medicine 103(1):141–142, 145–148, 151–152

Dyskeratoma, warty

▶ **Warty dyskeratoma**

Dyskeratosis congenita

Synonym(s)
Zinsser-Engman-Cole syndrome; Zinsser-Cole-Engman syndrome

Definition
Genodermatosis characterized by reticulated hyperpigmentation, nail dystrophy, premalignant leukoplakia of the oral mucosa, and progressive pancytopenia

Pathogenesis
Mutations in *DKC1* cause X-linked recessive form; involved in the regulation of the proliferative capacity of the cell; defect in maintenance of telomeres results in chromosomal instability, telomeric rearrangements, and cancer progression; etiology of autosomal dominant and autosomal recessive forms unknown

Clinical manifestation
Cutaneous manifestations developing between 5 and 15 years of age; tan-to-gray, hyperpigmented or hypopigmented macules and patches in a mottled, or reticulated pattern, sometimes with poikiloderma; located on the upper trunk, neck, and face, often with involvement of sun-exposed areas; scalp alopecia; mucosal leukoplakia on the buccal mucosa, tongue, oropharynx, esophagus, urethral meatus, glans penis, lacrimal duct, conjunctiva, vagina, anus; dental caries; progressive nail dystrophy; increased incidence of malignant neoplasms, particularly squamous cell carcinoma of the skin, mouth, nasopharynx, esophagus, rectum, vagina, and cervix; late bone marrow failure; pulmonary complications

Differential diagnosis
Graft versus host disease; Fanconi syndrome; Rothmund-Thompson syndrome; ataxia telangiectasia

Therapy
No therapy for skin disease; bone marrow transplantation

References
Dokal I (2000) Dyskeratosis congenita in all its forms. British Journal of Haematology 110(4):768–779

Dysplasia epiphysialis punctata

▶ **Conradi disease**

Dysplastic mole

▶ **Atypical mole**

Dysplastic nevus

▶ **Atypical mole**

Dystrophic epidermolysis bullosa

▶ **Epidermolysis bullosa**

E

Early-onset prurigo of pregnancy

▶ Prurigo of pregnancy

Eccrine acrospiroma

Synonym(s)
Acrospiroma; myoepithelioma; clear cell hidradenoma; clear cell adenoma; cystic hidradenoma; sweat gland adenoma; eccrine sweat gland adenoma

Definition
Tumor of eccrine sweat gland origin, with a predominance of clear cells

Pathogenesis
Unknown

Clinical manifestation
Onset after minor trauma; solitary, flesh-colored dermal papule; occurring most commonly on the scalp, face, and trunk; tendency for central ulceration; occasional malignant degeneration

Differential diagnosis
Basal cell carcinoma; lymphangioma; hemangioma; squamous cell carcinoma

Therapy
Surgical excision[★]

References
Ishikawa M, Nakanishi Y, Yamazaki N, Yamamoto A (2001) Malignant eccrine spiradenoma: A case report and review of the literature. Dermatologic Surgery 27(1):67–70

Eccrine adenocarcinoma

▶ Eccrine carcinoma

Eccrine bromhidrosis

▶ Bromhidrosis

Eccrine carcinoma

Synonym(s)
Eccrine adenocarcinoma; malignant tumor with eccrine differentiation

Definition
Neoplasm of eccrine sweat gland with potential for destructive local tissue infiltration and metastasis; sometimes subdivided into tumors arising de novo in normal skin and tumors originating from pre-existing, benign, sweat gland tumors

Pathogenesis
Derived from any portion of the eccrine apparatus or resulting from the malignant transformation of an existing benign eccrine tumor

Clinical manifestation
Non-specific solitary nodule or plaque with occasional ulceration, on the head, extremities, or trunk

Differential diagnosis
Basal cell carcinoma; squamous cell carcinoma; Merkel cell carcinoma; cutaneous metastasis; eccrine acrospiroma; microcystic adnexal carcinoma; eccrine porocarcinoma; cutaneous adenoid cystic carcinoma

Therapy
Wide local excision; Mohs micrographic surgery; radiation therapy

References
Katzman BM, Caligiuri DA, Klein DM, DiMaio TM, Gorup JM (1997) Eccrine carcinoma of the hand: a case report. Journal of Hand Surgery – American Volume 22(4):737–739

Eccrine chromhidrosis

► Chromhidrosis

Eccrine cystadenoma

► Eccrine hidrocystoma

Eccrine hidradenoma

Synonym(s)
Clear cell hidradenoma; clear cell myoepithelioma; solid cystic hidradenoma

Definition
Skin tumor of sweat gland origin with distinctive histologic appearance

Pathogenesis
Unknown

Clinical manifestation
Solitary, dome-shaped papule or nodule, often attached to the overlying epidermis; associated epidermal thickening or ulceration; most common over scalp, face, and trunk

Differential diagnosis
Basal cell carcinoma; squamous cell carcinoma; dermatofibroma; epidermoid cyst

Therapy
Surgical excision★

References
Hernández-Perez E, Cestoni-Parducci R (1985) Nodular hidradenoma and hidradenocarcinoma. Journal of the American Academy of Dermatology 12:15–20

Eccrine hidrocystoma

Synonym(s)
Eccrine cystadenoma; eccrine syringocystadenoma; syringectasia

Definition
Tumor consisting of a cystic proliferation of eccrine secretory elements

Pathogenesis
Possibly adenomatous cystic proliferations of the eccrine glands or retention cysts of the eccrine sweat apparatus

Clinical manifestation
Asymptomatic, solitary, translucent-to-bluish papule, with a predilection for the periorbital area

Differential diagnosis
Apocrine hidrocystoma; basal cell carcinoma; epidermoid cyst; mucous cyst; syringoma; milium; steatocystoma multiplex

Therapy
Incision and drainage, followed by surgical destruction of the cyst wall by light electrodesiccation and curettage; punch, shave, or elliptical excision

References
Alfadley A, Al Aboud K, Tulba A, Mourad MM (2001) Multiple eccrine hidrocystomas of the face. International Journal of Dermatology 40(2):125–129

Eccrine poroma

▶ Poroma

Eccrine spiradenoma

▶ Spiradenoma

Eccrine sweat gland adenoma

▶ Eccrine acrospiroma

Eccrine syringocystadenoma

▶ Eccrine hidrocystoma

Echovirus 16 infection

▶ Boston exanthem

Econazole

▶ Azole antifungal agents

Ecthyma

Synonym(s)
Pyoderma

Definition
Skin infection that invades into the dermis, most often caused by organism Streptococcus

Pathogenesis
Caused by bacterial infection, usually Streptococcus but sometimes Staphylococcus; predisposing factors: previous tissue injury, immunocompromised state; environmental factors: high temperature and humidity, crowded living conditions, poor hygiene

Clinical manifestation
Begins as a vesicle or pustule, ulcerating and producing a yellowish crust with erythematous, indurated borders

Differential diagnosis
Herpes simplex virus infection; atypical mycobacterial infection; nocardia infection; sporotrichosis; trauma; insect or spider bite reaction; pyoderma gangrenosum

Therapy
Mupirocin ointment applied 3 times daily for 7–10 days; dicloxacillin; cephalexin; known Streptococcal infection: penicillin[*]

References

Mancini AJ (2000) Bacterial skin infections in children: the common and the not so common. Pediatric Annals 29(1):26–35

Ecthyma contagiosum

▶ Orf

Ecthyma gangrenosum

Synonym(s)
None

Definition
Cutaneous manifestation of Pseudomonas aeruginosa bacteremia, usually occurring in patients who are critically ill and/or immunocompromised

Pathogenesis
Caused by Pseudomonas aeruginosa, a gram negative bacterial pathogen which disseminates in patients with impaired cellular or humoral immunity or those with severe underlying illnesses such as severe burns, malnutrition, recent chemotherapy, immunosuppressive therapy, or diabetes mellitus

Clinical manifestation
Appears as edematous, well-circumscribed plaques, rapidly evolving into hemorrhagic bullae, spreading peripherally, and eventually turning into a black necrotic ulcer with an erythematous rim; commonly occurs in the gluteal or perineal region or extremities; sign of widespread dissemination of infection

Differential diagnosis
Ecthyma; herpes simplex virus infection; atypical tuberculosis; nocardiosis; sporotrichosis; trauma; gram negative folliculitis; pyoderma gangrenosum; septicemia from other infectious agents; cryoglobulinemia; polyarteritis nodosa; necrotizing fasciitis; vasculitis

Therapy
Initial therapy: antipseudomonal penicillin (piperacillin) with an aminoglycoside (gentamicin).
Subsequent therapy based on culture sensitivity

References

Khan MO, Montecalvo MA, Davis I, Wormser GP (2000) Ecthyma gangrenosum in patients with acquired immunodeficiency syndrome. Cutis 66(2):121–123

Ecthyma infectiosum

▶ Orf

Ectodermal dysplasia absent dermatoglyphics

▶ Basan syndrome

Ectodermal dysplasia, anhidrotic

▶ Anhidrotic ectodermal dysplasia

Ectodermal dysplasia, hidrotic

▶ Hidrotic ectodermal dysplasia

Ectodermal dysplasia, hypohidrotic

▶ Anhidrotic ectodermal dysplasia

Eczema craquelatum

▶ Asteatotic eczema

Eczema craquelé

▶ Asteatotic eczema

Eczema fendille

▶ Asteatotic eczema

Eczema herpeticum

Synonym(s)
Kaposi varicelliform eruption; eczema vaccinatum

Definition
Eruption caused by herpes simplex virus (HSV)-1, herpes simplex virus (HSV)-2, Coxsackie A16 virus, or vaccinia virus that infects a preexisting dermatosis, most commonly atopic dermatitis

Pathogenesis
Caused by herpes simplex virus (HSV)-1, herpes simplex virus (HSV)-2, Coxsackie A16 virus, or vaccinia virus infecting a preexisting dermatosis; possibly associated with local T-cell immune defect, low NK cells, and/or a low antibody titer against the infective organism

Clinical manifestation
Presents as clusters of umbilicated vesiculopustules in areas where the skin has been affected by a preexistent dermatitis; umbilicated vesiculopustules progress to erosions, usually over the upper trunk and head; vesicles often become hemorrhagic and crusted, coalescing to form large, denuded plaques that bleed and sometimes become secondarily infected with bacteria

Differential diagnosis
Impetigo; varicella; contact dermatitis; bullous pemphigoid; dermatitis herpetiformis; erythema multiforme; pemphigus

Therapy
Acyclovir; valacyclovir

References
Mooney MA, Janniger CK, Schwartz RA (1994) Kaposi's varicelliform eruption. Cutis 53(5):243–245

Eczema hiemalis

▶ Asteatotic eczema

Eczema marginatum

▶ Tinea cruris

Eczema vaccinatum

▶ Eczema herpeticum

Eczematidlike purpura of Doucas and Kapetanakis

▶ Benign pigmented purpura

Eflornithine. Dermatologic indications and dosage

Disease	Adult dosage	Child dosage
Hypertrichosis	Apply twice daily	Apply twice daily

Eczematoid epitheliomatous dermatosis

▶ Paget's disease

Effluvium, anagen

▶ Anagen effluvium

Effluvium, telogen

▶ Telogen effluvium

Eflornithine

Trade name(s)
Vaniqa

Generic available
No

Drug class
Ornithine decarboxylase inhibitor

Mechanism of action
Possibly related to ornithine decarboxylase inhibition, which decreases hair growth

Dosage form
13.9% cream

Dermatologic indications and dosage
See table

Common side effects
Cutaneous: stinging; burning sensation, irritant contact dermatitis, acneform eruption, pseudofolliculitis barbae

Serious side effects
None

Drug interactions
None

Contraindications/precautions
Hypersensitivity to drug class or component

References
Hickman JG, Huber F, Palmisano M (2001) Human dermal safety studies with eflornithine HCl 13.9% cream (Vaniqa), a novel treatment for excessive facial hair. Current Medical Research & Opinion 16(4):235–244

Ehlers Danlos syndrome

Synonym(s)
Cutis hyperelastica

Definition
Heterogeneous group of inherited connective tissue disorders characterized by joint hypermobility, skin fragility, and hyperextensibility

Pathogenesis
Specific collagen defect has been identified in 6 of the 11 types: Type IV – decreased

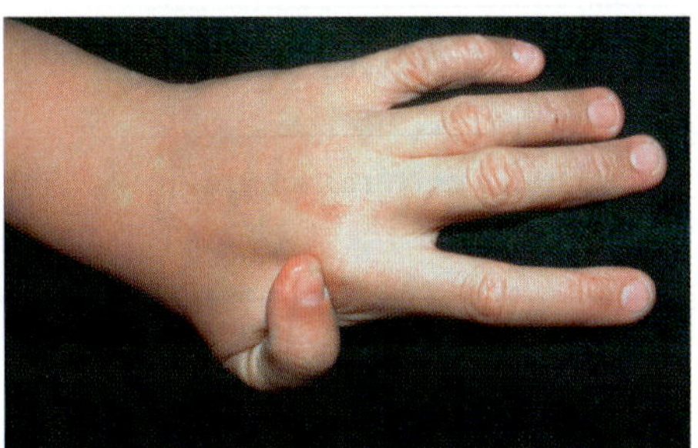

Ehlers Danlos syndrome. Marked joint hypermobility of digits

type III collagen; types V and VI – deficiencies in hydroxylase and lysyl oxidase; type VII – amino-terminal procollagen peptidase deficiency; type IX – abnormal copper metabolism; type X – nonfunctioning plasma fibronectin

Clinical manifestation
Findings common to all subtypes: skin hyperextensible, doughy, white, and soft, with underlying vessels sometimes visible; small, spongy tumors (molluscoid pseudotumors) over scars and pressure points; smaller palpable, and movable calcified nodules in subcutaneous tissue; nodules in arms and over tibias; skin fragility, with frequent bruises, lacerations, and poor wound healing; hyperextensible joints, with frequent dislocations

Differential diagnosis
Pseudoxanthoma elasticum; cartilage-hair syndrome; cutis laxa; Turner's syndrome; Marfan syndrome

Therapy
None; avoidance of surgery, if possible, because of poor-healing wounds

References
Germain DP (2002) Clinical and genetic features of vascular Ehlers-Danlos syndrome. Annals of Vascular Surgery 16(3):391–397

Elastofibroma

Synonym(s)
Elastofibroma dorsi

Definition
Benign, slow growing, connective tissue tumor, occurring most often in the subscapular area in elderly women

Pathogenesis
Possibly related to trauma by mechanical friction of the scapula against the ribs in some cases

Clinical manifestation
Well-circumscribed, painless or slightly tender tumor in the subscapular area in elderly women

Differential diagnosis
Lipoma; cyst; leiomyoma; sarcoma; metastasis; fibromatosis

Therapy
Surgical excision in symptomatic patients

References
Bieger AK, Varma SK, Timmons MJ (1994) Elastofibroma dorsi: case report and brief review. Annals of Plastic Surgery 32(5):548–549

Elastofibroma dorsi

▶ Elastofibroma

Elastolysis

▶ Cutis laxa

Elastolysis cutis laxa

▶ Cutis laxa

Elastoma

▶ Connective tissue nevus

Elastoma intrapapillare perforans

▶ Elastosis perforans serpiginosa

Elastoma intrapapillare perforans verruciformis

▶ Elastosis perforans serpiginosa

Elastoma verruciform perforans

▶ Elastosis perforans serpiginosa

Elastosis colloidalis conglomerata

▶ Colloid degeneration

Elastosis intrapapillare

▶ Elastosis perforans serpiginosa

Elastosis perforans

▶ Elastosis perforans serpiginosa

Elastosis perforans serpiginosa

Synonym(s)
Elastosis perforans serpiginosum; elastosis intrapapillare; elastoma intrapapillare perforans; elastoma intrapapillare perforans verruciformis; elastosis perforans; elastoma verruciform perforans; keratosis follicularis et parafollicularis serpiginosa; keratosis follicularis serpiginosa; reactive perforating elastosis

Definition
Skin condition with abnormal dermal elastic tissue fibers and other connective tissue elements expelled via trans-epidermal elimination

Pathogenesis
Granulomatous inflammation displaying an atypical method for removing elastic tissue from the area of involvement

Clinical manifestation
Three subtypes:
Reactive form: associated with other diseases such as Down syndrome, Ehlers-Danlos syndrome, Marfan syndrome, osteogenesis imperfecta, scleroderma, acrogeria, pseudoxanthoma elasticum
Drug-induced form: associated with penicillamine use
Idiopathic form (most common variety): flesh-colored or pale red, umbilicated papules grouped in linear, arciform, circular, or serpiginous patterns; most commonly occurring over the nape of the neck

Differential diagnosis

Reactive perforating collagenosis; perforating folliculitis; Kyrle's disease; folliculitis; prurigo nodularis; granuloma annulare; tinea corporis; lupus erythematosus

Therapy

Tretinoin; isotretinoin; cryotherapy; electrodessication and curettage

References

Mehta RK, Burrows NP, Payne CM, Mendelsohn SS, Pope FM, Rytina E (2001) Elastosis perforans serpiginosa and associated disorders. Clinical & Experimental Dermatology 26(6):521–524

Elastosis perforans serpiginosum

▶ Elastosis perforans serpiginosa

Elavil

▶ Amitriptyline

Elephantiasis

Definition

Visible enlargement of the arms, legs, or genitals to elephantoid size, usually secondary to chronic lymphedema

References

McGuinness CL, Burnand KG (2001) Lymphoedema. Tropical Doctor 31(1):2–7

Elephantiasis nostras verrucosa

Definition

In later stages of chronic lymphedema, affected skin becomes indurated and develops verrucous papules and plaques with scale

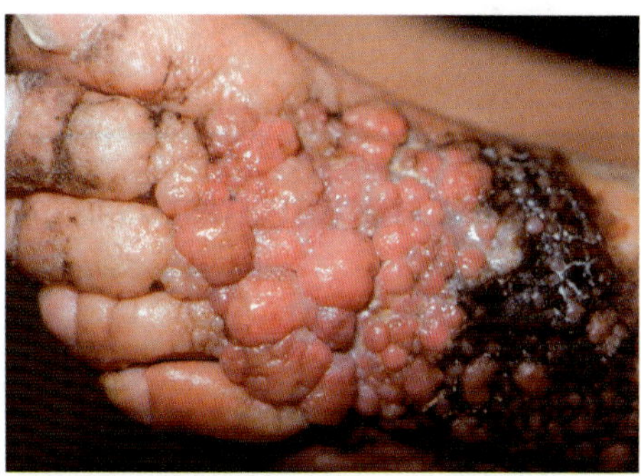

Elephantiasis nostras verrucosa. Plaque consisting of multiple nodules on the distal lower extremity

References

Brantley D, Thompson EC, Brown MF (1995) Elephantiasis nostras verrucosa. Journal of the Louisiana State Medical Society 147(7):325–327

Enchondromatosis

▶ Maffucci syndrome

Enchondromatosis with multiple cavernous hemangiomas

▶ Maffucci syndrome

Endemic pemphigus foliaceus

▸ Fogo selvagem

Endemic syphilis

▸ Bejel

Endemic treponematosis

▸ Pinta

Endep

▸ Amitriptyline

Endovascular papillary angioendothelioma of childhood

Synonym(s)
Dabska tumor; malignant endovascular papillary angioendothelioma; papillary intralymphatic angioendothelioma

Definition
Low-grade angiosarcoma of the skin of children, with a distinctive histologic architecture of anastomosing vascular channels with intravascular papillary outpouchings

Pathogenesis
Unclear cell of origin, but tumor marker studies suggest resemblance to lymphangioma

Clinical manifestation
Slow-growing, intradermal nodule that is violaceous, pink, or bluish-black in color

Differential diagnosis
Reactive angioendotheliomatosis; benign intravascular endothelial hyperplasia; retiform hemangioendothelioma; glomeruloid hemangioma; infantile hemangioma; Kaposi's sarcoma; angiolymphoid hyperplasia

Therapy
Surgical excision; lymph node dissection if regional nodes are involved

References
Schwartz RA, Dabski C, Dabska M (2000) The Dabska tumor: a thirty-year retrospect. Dermatology 201(1):1–5

Enlarged solitary comedone

▸ Dilated pore

Eosinophilia-myalgia syndrome

Synonym(s)
L-tryptophan-induced eosinophilia-myalgia syndrome; sclerodermoid myalgia; sclerodermoid fasciitis

Definition
Multisystem disease with prominent eosinophilia and generalized myalgia, usually associated with L-tryptophan ingestion

Pathogenesis
Cell-mediated immune response causing widespread tissue injury; skin and connective tissue fibrosis pervading muscles, nerves, and other organs; L-tryptophan involvement in process, but mechanism unclear

Clinical manifestation
Acute episode: shortness of breath, cough, fever; fatigue, arthralgias, paresthesias, severe weakness, muscle cramps, periorbital and peripheral edema, generalized erythematous eruption
Chronic signs and symptoms: generalized myalgias, skin tightening; fingers and toes usually spared; Raynaud phenomenon usually absent; scalp alopecia; cutaneous hyperesthesia

Differential diagnosis
Progressive systemic sclerosis; toxic oil syndrome; dermatomyositis; polymyositis; eosinophilic fasciitis; mixed connective disease

Therapy
Discontinuance of all products containing L-tryptophan*; prednisone*

References
Blackburn WD Jr. (1997) Eosinophilia myalgia syndrome. Seminars in Arthritis & Rheumatism 26(6):788–793

Eosinophilic cellulitis

Synonym(s)
Wells syndrome; recurrent granulomatous dermatitis with eosinophilia, Wells' syndrome, Well's syndrome

Definition
Cellulitis-like eruption with typical histology, including flame figures and marked dermal infiltrate of eosinophils

Pathogenesis
Association with insect bites in some cases

Clinical manifestation
Pruritus and burning sensation, followed by cellulitis-like eruption; large, indurated plaques of edema and erythema, with violaceous edges; occasionally also annular plaques, papules, and urticarial-like wheals; recurrent episodes common

Differential diagnosis
Cellulitis; erysipelas; urticaria; insect bite reaction; Lyme disease; hypereosinophilic syndrome; inflammatory metastasis; granuloma annulare; Churg-Strauss syndrome

Therapy
High potency topical corticosteroids; prednisone

References
Weiss G, Shemer A, Confino Y, Kaplan B, Trau H (2001) Wells' syndrome: report of a case and review of the literature. International Journal of Dermatology 40(2):148–152

Eosinophilic folliculitis

▶ Eosinophilic pustular folliculitis

Eosinophilic granuloma

▶ Langerhans cell histiocytosis

Eosinophilic granuloma of soft tissue

▶ Kimura's disease

Eosinophilic granulomatous vasculitis

▶ Churg-Strauss syndrome

Eosinophilic hyperplastic lymphogranuloma

▶ Kimura's disease

Eosinophilic lymphofollicular granuloma

▶ Kimura's disease

Eosinophilic lymphofolliculosis

▶ Kimura's disease

Eosinophilic lymphoid granuloma

▶ Kimura's disease

Eosinophilic pustular dermatosis

▶ Eosinophilic pustular folliculitis

Eosinophilic pustular folliculitis

Synonym(s)
Ofuji's disease; Ofuji disease; eosinophilic folliculitis; HIV-associated eosinophilic folliculitis; HIV-related eosinophilic folliculitis, sterile eosinophilic pustulosis; eosinophilic pustular dermatosis; infantile/childhood eosinophilic pustulosis of the scalp

Definition
Recurrent follicular and non-follicular papules associated with tissue and peripheral eosinophilia

Pathogenesis
Unclear; possibly abnormal immunologic reaction to follicular pathogens

Clinical manifestation
Follicular-based erythematous papules and pustules, with or without coalescence into plaques; face, back, and extensor surfaces of the upper extremities most commonly involved in adults; scalp most common site in children; increased incidence in HIV-infected patients; peripheral eosinophilia often present

Differential diagnosis
Other forms of folliculitis, including bacterial and fungal varieties; pustular psoriasis; acne; rosacea; perioral dermatitis; scabies; candidiasis; folliculitis decalvans; insect bite reaction; Langerhans cell histiocytosis; follicular mucinosis; superficial pemphigus

Therapy
Dapsone; super potent topical corticosteroids; prednisone; isotretinoin; itraconazole; UVB phototherapy; photochemotherapy

References
Lazarov A, Wolach B, Cordoba M, Abraham D, Vardy D (1996) Eosinophilic pustular folliculitis (Ofuji disease) in a child. Cutis 58(2):135–138

Ephelides

Synonym(s)
Freckles

Definition
Tan macules which darken after sun exposure and fade in the winter months

Pathogenesis
Autosomal dominant trait; possibly somatic mutations in epidermal melanocytes that promote increased melanogenesis

Clinical manifestation
Multiple, small, uniformly tan macules on sun-exposed skin; sometimes coalescing into patches; most common in individuals with fair skin and/or blond or red hair

Differential diagnosis
Lentigo; seborrheic keratosis; nevus; café au lait spot; tinea versicolor

Therapy
Sun avoidance

References
Ortonne JP (1990) The effects of ultraviolet exposure on skin melanin pigmentation. Journal of International Medical Research 18 Suppl 3:8C–17C

Ephelis ab igne

▶ Erythema ab igne

Ephidrosis tincta

▶ Chromhidrosis

Epidemic arthritic erythema

▶ Rat-bite fever

Epidemic typhus

Synonym(s)
Louse-borne typhus; classic typhus

Definition
Acute, febrile, infectious illness caused by Rickettsia prowazekii, characterized by rash, lymphadenopathy, and systemic signs and symptoms

Pathogenesis
Caused by Rickettsia prowazekii; louse infected after feeding on rickettsemic person with typhus or during a recrudescent case; bites human to engage in blood meal and causes pruritic reaction on host skin; scratching by host causes crushing of lice and Rickettsia-laden excrement inoculated into wound

Clinical manifestation
Painless papule at site of chigger bite; subsequently undergoes central necrosis with formation of eschar; fever; headache; regional or generalized lymphadenopathy; rigors; myalgias; malaise; CNS symptoms; recrudescent form (Brill-Zinser disease): months to decades after treatment, organisms reemerge and cause recurrence of typhus

Differential diagnosis
Tularemia; leptospirosis; typhoid fever; other rickettsial infections; viral exanthem; dengue fever; anthrax; ehrlichiosis; infectious mononucleosis; Kawasaki disease; malaria; meningococcemia; relapsing fever; toxic shock syndrome; rubella; rubeola

Therapy
Doxycycline*; chloramphenicol – 0.5–1 gm IV every 6 hours until 48–72 hours after patient becomes afebrile; pediatric dose – 80–100 mg per kg per day IV divided into 4 doses until 48–72 hours after patient becomes afebrile

References
Baxter JD (1996) The typhus group. Clinics in Dermatology 14(3):271–278

Epidermal cyst

▶ Epidermoid cyst

Epidermal inclusion cyst

▶ Epidermoid cyst

Epidermal nevus

Synonym(s)
Organoid nevus; epithelial nevus

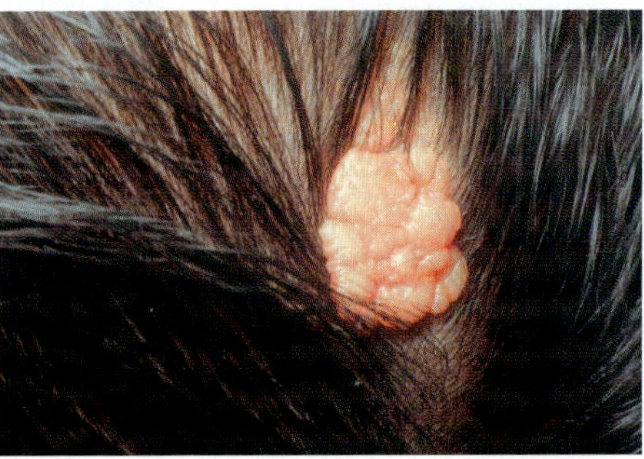

Epidermal nevus. Flesh-colored verrucous nodule on the scalp

Definition
Congenital hamartoma of embryonal ecto-dermal origin, classified on the basis of its main component, which may be keratinoc-ytic, sebaceous, sweat gland, or follicular

Pathogenesis
Probable somatic mutation, which may reflect genetic mosaicism; arises from pluripotential germinative cells of the basal layer of the embryonic epidermis; possible dermal effect on growth

Clinical manifestation
Nevus verrucosus (verucous epidermal nevus): usually present at birth or early childhood; solitary or multiple, linear or S-shaped, verrucous or velvety plaques, never crossing the midline; flexural lesions some-times macerated and foul-smelling; lesions with sebaceous or apocrine elements may enlarge at puberty
Inflammatory epidermal nevus (ILVN): usually present in the first 5 years of life; pruritic, linear, erythematous, scaly plaques, most commonly on the leg; nevus comedonicus (comedo nevus): confluent clusters of dilated follicular orifices plugged with keratin, giving the appearance of aggregated open comedones; often arranged in a linear, arcuate, or zosteri-form pattern; occasionally paralleling the lines of Voigt or the lines of Blaschko
Nevus unius lateris (linear epidermal nevus): solitary linear verrucous plaque, present at birth or in early infancy
Nevus sebaceous (sebaceous nevus): usu-ally present at birth; well-circumscribed, pink-to-yellow, smooth or velvety plaques, almost always on the head and neck area; enlarges and thickens at puberty; small risk of malignant degeneration to basal cell car-cinoma
Epidermal nevus syndrome: one or more epidermal nevi and involvement of the nervous, ophthalmologic, and/or skeletal systems; mental retardation, seizures, movement disorders; intracranial and/or intraspinal lipomas

Differential diagnosis
Proteus syndrome; CHILD syndrome; wart; Darier disease; lichen striatus; incontinen-tia pigmenti; psoriasis; syndrome of Favre-Racouchot; acne vulgaris; mastocytoma; juvenile xanthogranuloma; xanthoma

Therapy
Nevus verrucosus: surgical excision[*]; tretinoin; acetretin; inflammatory epider-mal nevus: super potent topical corticoster-

oids; cryotherapy; surgical excision; nevus comedonicus: tretinoin; surgical excision; nevus sebaceous: surgical excision*; epidermal nevus syndrome: as above for individual variants

References

Losee JE, Serletti JM, Pennino RP (1999) Epidermal nevus syndrome: a review and case report. Annals of Plastic Surgery 43(2):211-214

Epidermodysplasia verruciformis

Synonym(s)
None

Definition
Inherited disorder characterized by widespread and persistent human papilloma virus (HPV) infection and malignant degeneration of the virally induced tumors

Pathogenesis
Autosomal recessive trait; impaired cellular immunity to specific wart virus subtypes; co-factors: ultraviolet light and X-rays

Clinical manifestation
Polymorphic, verrucous or flat-topped papules resembling flat warts; macules and reddish-brown plaques with slightly scaly surfaces and irregular borders; localized mostly on sun-exposed regions, palms, soles, in the axillae, and on external genitalia; mucous membranes rarely affected; malignant tumors typically appears during the fourth and fifth decades of life

Differential diagnosis
Verruca plana; squamous cell carcinoma; tinea versicolor; trichoepithelioma; basal cell carcinoma; papular mucinosis; solar elastosis

Therapy
Cryotherapy; electrodessication and curettage; sun avoidance

References

Majewski S, Jablonska S, Orth G (1997) Epidermodysplasia verruciformis. Immunological and nonimmunological surveillance mechanisms: role in tumor progression. Clinics in Dermatology 15(3):321–334

Epidermoid carcinoma

▶ Squamous cell carcinoma

Epidermoid cyst

Synonym(s)
Epidermal cyst; epidermal inclusion cyst; wen; atheroma; steatoma; sebaceous cyst

Definition
Cyst with a stratified squamous lining, which produces keratin

Pathogenesis
Derived from follicular infundibulum; often occurring at site of previous trauma (inflammatory acne, etc.)

Clinical manifestation
White or pale yellow, deep dermal or subcutaneous, medium-firm papule or nodule, often with a central pore; cheesy, foulsmelling material sometimes exuded with lateral pressure

Differential diagnosis
Lipoma; trichilemmoma; steatocystoma multiplex; granuloma annulare; sarcoidosis; lymphocytic infiltrates; insect bite reaction; acquired perforating disease; metastasis

Therapy

Simple excision by sharp dissection[*]; elliptical excision; marsupialization of large lesions; inflamed lesion: incision and drainage of purulent material; triamcinolone (3–5 mg per ml) injected intralesionally

References

Pariser RJ (1998) Benign neoplasms of the skin. Medical Clinics of North America 82(6):1285–1307

Epidermolysis bullosa

Synonym(s)

None

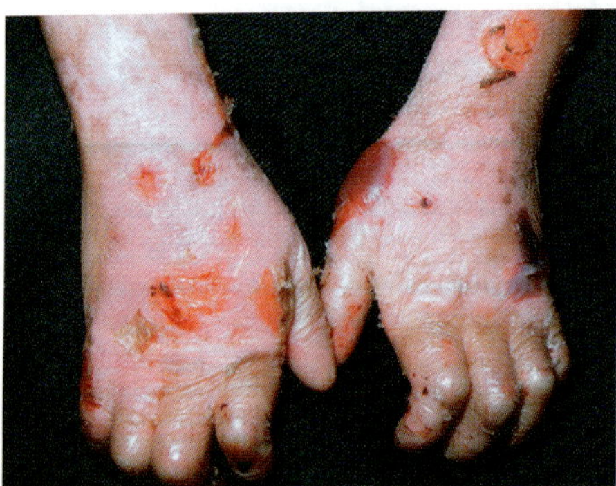

Epidermolysis bullosa. Bullae, erosions, and scarring of the hands

Definition

Group of inherited disorders characterized by blister formation in response to mechanical trauma

Pathogenesis

Epidermolysis bullosa simplex: associated with mutations of the genes coding for keratins 5 and 14; level of skin separation at the mid basal cell associated with variable intermediate filament clumping

Junctional epidermolysis bullosa: mutations in genes coding for laminin 5 subunits (α3 chain, laminin β3 chain, laminin γ2 chain), collagen XVII (BP180), α6 integrin, and β4 integrin

Dystrophic epidermolysis bullosa: mutations of the gene coding for type VII collagen (*COL7A1*); anchoring fibrils affected; degree of involvement ranging from subtle changes to complete absence

Clinical manifestation

Epidermolysis bullosa simplex:
• Weber-Cockayne variant: most common form; blisters usually precipitated by traumatic event; most frequently occurring on the palms and soles, often with hyperhidrosis
• Severe variant: generalized onset of blisters occurring at or shortly after birth; hands, feet, and extremities most common sites of involvement
• Koebner variant: sometimes has palmoplantar hyperkeratosis and erosions
• Dowling-Meara variant: involves oral mucosa with grouped herpetiform blisters.
Junctional epidermolysis bullosa:
• Letalis (Herlitz) variant: generalized blistering at birth; orificial erosions around the mouth, eyes, and nares; often accompanied by significant hypertrophic granulation tissue; involvement of the corneal, conjunctival, tracheobronchial, oral, pharyngeal, esophageal, rectal, and genitourinary mucosal surfaces; internal complications: hoarse cry, cough, and other respiratory difficulties; poor prognosis
• Nonlethal junctional variant (mitis form): usually survives infancy; generalized blistering; improves with age; scalp, nail, and tooth abnormalities; periorificial erosions and hypertrophic granulation tissue; mucous membranes erosions, resulting in strictures.
Dystrophic epidermolysis bullosa:
• Dominantly inherited variant; onset of disease usually at birth or during infancy; generalized blistering is common presentation; evolution to localized blistering with age

• Cockayne-Touraine variant: acral distribution and minimal oral or tooth involvement
• Pasini variant: more extensive blistering, scarlike papules on the trunk (albopapuloid lesions); involvement of the oral mucosa and teeth; dystrophic or absent nails common
• Mitis variant: involves acral areas and nails with little mucosal involvement; clinical manifestations similar to the dominantly inherited forms
• Severe recessive variant (Hallopeau-Siemens): generalized blistering at birth; subsequent extensive dystrophic scarring, most prominent on the acral surfaces, sometimes resulting in pseudosyndactyly (mitten-hand deformity) of the hands and feet; flexion contractures of the extremities increasingly common with age; dystrophy of nails and teeth; involvement of internal mucosa sometimes resulting in esophageal strictures and webs, urethral and anal stenosis, phimosis, and corneal scarring; intestinal malabsorption leading to a mixed anemia resulting from a lack of iron absorption and failure to thrive; significant risk of developing aggressive squamous cell carcinomas in areas of chronic erosions

Differential diagnosis
Linear IgA bullous disease; bullous pemphigoid; epidermolysis bullosa acquisita; friction blisters; pemphigus vulgaris; burn

Therapy
Avoidance of frictional trauma[*]; careful attention to skin and dental hygiene[*]; severe disease: soft diet to prevent esophageal trauma and blistering; skin equivalent dressings to promote epithelialization

References
Fine JD, Eady RA, Bauer EA, Briggaman RA, Bruckner-Tuderman L, et al. (2000) Revised classification system for inherited epidermolysis bullosa: report of the Second International Consensus Meeting on diagnosis and classification of epidermolysis bullosa. Journal of the American Academy of Dermatology 42(6):1051–1066

Epidermolysis bullosa acquisita

Synonym(s)
Acquired epidermolysis bullosa; dermolytic pemphigoid

Definition
Chronic autoimmune blistering disease, with lesions often occurring at sites of trauma

Pathogenesis
IgG autoantibodies specific for anchoring fibrils (type VII collagen) of the skin basement membrane causes an inflammatory process which is a contributing factor to blister formation; skin trauma a contributing factor; genetic factors possibly important, since HLA-DR2 is overrepresented in those with this condition

Clinical manifestation
Non-inflammatory bullae at sites of minor skin trauma, which heal with scars and/or milia; widespread inflammatory bullae not related to trauma; mucous membrane blisters and erosions, leading to scarring

Differential diagnosis
Epidermolysis bullosa; bullous pemphigoid; cicatricial pemphigoid; linear IgA bullous dermatosis; bullous lupus erythematosus; porphyria cutanea tarda; bullous disease of diabetes mellitus; erythema multiforme

Therapy
Prednisone 1 mg per kg PO daily[*]; corticosteroid sparing agents – azathioprine; methotrexate; mycophenolate mofteil; cyclophosphamide; dapsone

References
Kirtschig G, Murrell D, Wojnarowska F, et al. (2002) Interventions for mucous membrane pemphigoid/cicatricial pemphigoid and epidermolysis bullosa acquisita: A systematic lit-

erature review. Archives of Dermatology 138:380–384

Epidermolysis bullosa dystrophica

▶ Epidermolysis bullosa

Epidermolysis bullosa, Herlitz variant

▶ Epidermolysis bullosa

Epidermolysis bullosa herpetiformis

▶ Epidermolysis bullosa

Epidermolysis bullosa letalis

▶ Epidermolysis bullosa

Epidermolysis bullosa simplex

▶ Epidermolysis bullosa

Epidermolytic hyperkeratosis

Synonym(s)
Bullous congenital ichthyosiform erythroderma; bullous ichthyotic erythroderma; ichthyosis bullosa of Siemens; ichthyosis hystrix of Curth-Macklin

Definition
Congenital ichthyosis with characteristic histologic finding of epidermolytic hyperkeratosis

Pathogenesis
Autosomal dominant trait; defect in the genes for keratin 1 and keratin 10

Clinical manifestation
Presents at birth or shortly thereafter as erythema, blistering, and/or scaling; marked hyperkeratosis shortly after birth; scales are small, dark, with corrugated appearance; scales sometimes shedand, reaccumulate; keratotic skin in intertriginous areas which may become macerated and foul smelling; blisters occur in crops, rupturing, and leaving red, painful, denuded base; bullae tend to disappear before age 20; NPS subtype – lacks severe palmoplantar involvement; PS subtype – severe palmoplantar involvement; no ectropion

Differential diagnosis
Non-bullous ichthyosiform erythroderma; lamellar ichthyosis; X-linked ichthyosis; epidermolysis bullosa; incontinentia pigmenti; bullous impetigo; staphylococcal scalded skin syndrome

Therapy
Prednisone; beta carotene; acetretin; tretinoin; alpha-hydroxy acid

References
Bale SJ, Compton JG, DiGiovanna JJ (1993) Epidermolytic hyperkeratosis. Seminars in Dermatology 12(3):202–209

Epiloia

▶ Tuberous sclerosis

Epithelial nevus

▶ Epidermal nevus

Epithelioid angiomatosis

▶ Bacillary angiomatosis

Epithelioid hemangioma

▶ Angiolymphoid hyperplasia with eosinophilia

Epithelioma adenoides cysticum

▶ Trichoepithelioma

Epithelioma contagiosum

▶ Molluscum contagiosum

Epithelioma cuniculatum

▶ Verrucous carcinoma

Erosio interdigitalis blastomycetica

▶ Candidiasis

Erosive adenomatosis of the nipple

Synonym(s)
Benign papillomatosis of the nipple; florid papillomatosis of the nipple; papillary adenoma of the nipple; subareolar adenomatosis; papillomatosis of the subareolar ducts

Definition
Benign tumor of the nipple, with apocrine differentiation

Pathogenesis
Hamartomatous proliferation of the lactiferous ducts

Clinical manifestation
Asymptomatic-to-slightly-pruritic, unilateral, eroded, crusted plaque on the nipple; nipple discharge sometimes occurs premenstrually

Differential diagnosis
Paget's disease of the breast; contact dermatitis; basal cell carcinoma; apocrine gland tumors; hidradenitis suppurativa

Therapy
Excision of the nipple and subareolar tissue★

References
Montemarano AD, Sau P, James WD (1995) Superficial papillary adenomatosis of the nipple: a case report and review of the literature. Journal of the American Academy of Dermatology 33(5 Pt 2):871–875

Erysipelas

Synonym(s)
None

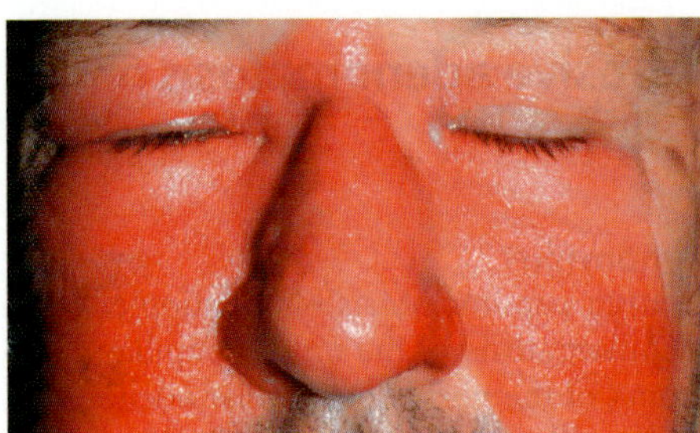

Erysipelas. Erythematous, edematous plaque on the central face

Definition
Skin infection involving the dermis and local lymphatics, usually caused by group A beta-hemolytic streptococci

Pathogenesis
Bacterial infection, typically caused by group A Streptococcus

Clinical manifestation
Abrupt onset of illness with fever and chills, muscle and joint pain, nausea, headache; skin change begins as small erythematous patch and progresses to red, indurated, shiny plaque; raised, sharply demarcated, advancing margins, with skin warmth, edema, and tenderness; lymphatic involvement with overlying skin streaking and regional lymphadenopathy

Differential diagnosis
Contact dermatitis; seborrheic dermatitis; lupus erythematosus; angioedema; herpes zoster; erysipeloid; necrotizing fasciitis

Therapy
Penicillin G procaine; Penicillin VK; dicolacillin if staphyloccocal infection present; cephalexin if patient is allergic to penicillin

References
Chartier C, Grosshans E (1996) Erysipelas: an update. International Journal of Dermatology 35(11):779–781

Erysipeloid

Synonym(s)
Erysipeloid of Rosenbach

Definition
Acute bacterial infection of traumatized skin caused by the microorganism Erysipelothrix rhusiopathiae (insidiosa)

Pathogenesis
Causative organism, E. rhusiopathiae, enters the skin through scratches or pricks; organism produces enzymes that help it dissect through the tissues; inflammation produced when immune system activated against foreign antigen

Clinical manifestation
Food handlers (home makers, farmers, fishermen, and butchers) at increased risk of acquiring the infection
Localized form: well demarcated, bright-red-to-purple, warm, tender plaques with a smooth, shiny surface, most commonly on the hands
Diffuse cutaneous form: multiple, well demarcated, violaceous plaques with an advancing border and central clearing
Systemic form: localized areas of swelling surrounding a necrotic center; sometimes presenting as follicular, erythematous papules; endocarditis as complication of septicemia

Differential diagnosis
Cellulitis; erysipelas; fixed medication reaction; erythema nodosum; leishmaniasis

Therapy
Penicillin*

References
Reboli AC, Farrar WE (1989) Erysipelothrix rhusiopathiae: an occupational pathogen. Clinical Microbiology Reviews 2(4):354–359

Erysipeloid of Rosenbach

▶ Erysipeloid

Erythema à calore

▶ Erythema ab igne

Erythema ab igne

Synonym(s)
Erythema ab igne elastosis; ephelis ab igne; erythema à calore; toasted skin syndrome

Definition
Changes in the skin caused by chronic and repeated exposure to infrared radiation

Pathogenesis
Unclear mechanism; repeated external heat exposure in the range of 43–47°C resulting in histopathologic changes similar to those seen in solar-damaged skin

Clinical manifestation
Reticulated violaceous and hyperpigmented plaques, most common on the legs of women; poikiloderma occurs with severe long-standing disease

Differential diagnosis
Livedo reticularis; poikiloderma of Civatte; poikiloderma atrophicans vasculare; morphea; livedo vasculitis

Therapy
Nd:YAG, ruby, or alexandrite laser

References
Page EH, Shear NH (1988) Temperature-dependent skin disorders. Journal of the American Academy of Dermatology 18(5 Pt 1):1003–1019

Erythema ab igne elastosis

▶ Erythema ab igne

Erythema annulare centrifugum

Synonym(s)
Erythema gyratum perstans; erythema exudativum perstans; erythema marginatum perstans; erythema perstans; erythema figuratum perstans; erythema microgyratum perstans; erythema simplex gyratum; erythema perstans

Definition
Figurate erythema with a characteristic advancing, scaly margin and central clearing

Pathogenesis
Probably represents hypersensitivity reaction to a variety of agents, including drugs, arthropod bites, infections (bacterial, mycobacterial, viral, fungal, filarial), ingestants (blue cheese penicillium), and malignancy

Clinical manifestation
Begins as asymptomatic, erythematous papules which spread peripherally while clearing centrally; often a trailing scale on the inner aspect of the advancing edge; appears on any skin surface other than the palms and soles; may be associated with an underlying disease (e.g., infection, malignancy, or other systemic illness)

Differential diagnosis
Erythema marginatum rheumaticum; erythema migrans; erythema gyratum repens; urticaria; granuloma annulare; sarcoidosis; tinea corporis; seborrheic dermatitis; lupus erythematosus; benign lymphocytic infiltrate; rheumatoid arthritis; psoriatic arthri-

tis; lupus erythematosus; Reiter syndrome; gonococcal arthritis

Therapy
Prednisone; high potency topical corticosteroids

References
Tyring SK (1993) Reactive erythemas: erythema annulare centrifugum and erythema gyratum repens. Clinics in Dermatology 11(1):135–139

Erythema areata migrans

▶ Benign migratory glossitis

Erythema chronicum figuratum melanodermicum

▶ Ashy dermatosis

Erythema circinata

▶ Benign migratory glossitis

Erythema contusiformis

▶ Erythema nodosum

Erythema craquelé

Definition
Manifestation of dry skin with large dry scales and fine fissures giving a cracked-pot appearance

References
Beacham BE (1993) Common dermatoses in the elderly. American Family Physician 47(6):1445–1450

Erythema dyschromicum perstans

▶ Ashy dermatosis

Erythema dyschronicum perstans

▶ Ashy dermatosis

Erythema dyspepsicum

▶ Erythema toxicum

Erythema elevatum diutinum

Synonym(s)
Extracellular cholesterosis

Definition
Leukocytoclastic vasculitis characterized by red, purple, brown, or yellow papules, plaques, or nodules

Pathogenesis
Possibly involves immune complex deposition with subsequent inflammatory cascade; associated with IgA monoclonal gammopathy, recurrent bacterial infections, (especially streptococcal), viral infections (including Hepatitis B or HIV), and rheumatologic disease

Clinical manifestation

Red, violaceous, smooth, brown or yellow papules, plaques, or nodules over extensor surfaces, especially over the joints; occasional crusting or bleeding

Differential diagnosis

Acute bebrile neutrophilic dermatosis; granuloma annulare; insect bite reaction; sarcoidosis; rheumatoid nodules; gouty tophi; multicentric reticulohistiocytosis; xanthomas; erythema multiforme

Therapy

Dapsone*

References

Gibson LE, el-Azhary RA (2000) Erythema elevatum diutinum. Clinics in Dermatology 18(3):295–299

Erythema exudativum

▶ Erythema multiforme

Erythema exudativum perstans

▶ Erythema annulare centrifugum

Erythema figuratum perstans

▶ Erythema annulare centrifugum

Erythema gyratum perstans

▶ Erythema annulare centrifugum

Erythema gyratum repens

Synonym(s)

None

Definition

Figurate erythema with a distinctive clinical appearance, which serves as a marker of internal malignancy

Pathogenesis

Possibly involves a cutaneous response to tumor antigens

Clinical manifestation

Eruption often precedes diagnosis of underlying malignancy; wood-grain appearance created by concentric, pruritic, mildly scaling bands of flat-to-slightly-palpable erythema, with rapid migration of the bands; course of eruption mirrors course of the underlying illness, with clearance of rash and relief of pruritus within 6 weeks of underlying illness resolution; sites of predilection trunk and extremities

Differential diagnosis

Erythema annulare centrifugum; granuloma annulare; tinea corporis; sarcoidosis; lupus erythematosus; glucagonoma syndrome; urticaria

Therapy

Treatment of underlying malignancy; prednisone; high potency topical corticosteroids

References

Eubanks LE, McBurney E, Reed R (2001) Erythema gyratum repens. American Journal of the Medical Sciences 321(5):302–305

Erythema induratum

▶ Nodular vasculitis

Erythema infectiosum

Synonym(s)
Fifth disease, slapped-cheek disease, academy rash, Sticker's disease, Sticker disease

Definition
Childhood exanthem caused by human Parvovirus B19, in which a 3-phased cutaneous eruption follows a mild prodrome

Pathogenesis
Parvovirus B19 viremia; production of specific immunoglobulin M (IgM) antibodies and subsequent formation of immune complexes; clinical findings probably result from the deposition of the immune complexes in the skin and joints

Clinical manifestation
4–14 day incubation period; virus spreads primarily via aerosolized respiratory droplets
Mild prodromal phase, including headache, coryza, low-grade fever, pharyngitis, and malaise
First stage: erythema of the cheeks, with nasal, perioral, and periorbital sparing (slapped-cheek appearance) and fades over 2–4 days
Second stage: within 1–4 days of the facial rash, erythematous macular-to-morbilliform eruption occurs primarily on the extremities
Third stage: after several days, most of the second stage eruption fades into a lacy pattern, particularly on the proximal extremities; lasts from 3 days to 3 weeks; after starting to fade, exanthem sometimes recurs over several weeks following exercise, sun exposure, friction, bathing in hot water, or stress; adults sometimes develop polyarthropathy

Differential diagnosis
Other viral exanthems; medication reaction; Lyme disease; lupus erythematosus; acute rheumatic fever; allergic hypersensitivity reaction

Therapy
Antihistamines, first generation, as sedative and mild anti-pruritic agent

References
Koch WC (2001) Fifth (human parvovirus) and sixth (herpesvirus 6) diseases. Current Opinion in Infectious Diseases 14(3):343–356

Erythema marginatum

Definition
Superficial, often asymptomatic, form of gyrate erythema, characterized by a transient eruption of macular to slightly palpable, non-scaling plaques on the trunk and extensor surfaces of the extremities; associated with rheumatic fever

References
Rullan E, Sigal LH (2001) Rheumatic fever. Current Rheumatology Reports 3(5):445–452

Erythema marginatum perstans

▶ Erythema annulare centrifugum

Erythema microgyratum perstans

▶ Erythema annulare centrifugum

Erythema migrans

▶ Lyme disease

Erythema multiforme

Synonym(s)
Erythema exudativum; Hebra's disease; erythema polymorphe

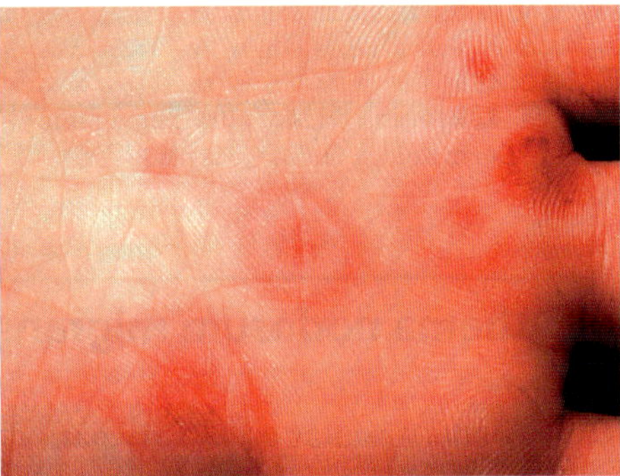

Erythema multiforme. Target-like papules on the palm

Definition
Acute inflammatory disorder related to numerous factors, characterized by distinctive clinical eruption, with hallmark of iris or target lesion

Pathogenesis
Unclear; herpes-associated disease appears to represent the result of a cell-mediated immune reaction associated with herpes simplex virus (HSV) antigen

Clinical manifestation
Most commonly associated with herpes simplex virus infection; also associated with other infections, drug ingestion, rheumatic diseases, vasculitides, non-Hodgkin's lymphoma, leukemia, multiple myeloma, myeloid metaplasia, polycythemia
Erythema multiforme minor variant: occasional mild flu-like prodrome; initial lesion dull red macule or urticarial plaque in the center, with small papule, vesicle, or bulla sometimes developing; raised, pale ring with edematous; periphery gradually becoming violaceous and forming concentric target lesion; lesions appear predominantly on the extensor surfaces of acral extremities and spread centripetally; mild erosions of one mucosal surface; palms, neck, and face frequently involved
Erythema multiforme major variant: prodrome of moderate fever, general discomfort, cough, sore throat, vomiting, chest pain, and diarrhea, usually for 1–14 days preceding the eruption; skin lesions same as with erythema multiforme minor; severe erosions of at least 2 mucosal surfaces; generalized lymphadenopathy

Differential diagnosis
Stevens-Johnson syndrome; toxic epidermal necrolysis; Henoch-Schönlein purpura; urticaria; viral exanthem; Kawasaki disease; figurate erythema; fixed drug eruption; lupus erythematosus; primary herpetic gingivostomatitis; Behçet's disease; aphthous stomatitis

Therapy
Antihistamines, first generation; prednisone; herpes simplex virus prophylaxis with valacyclovir, if more than 4–5 episodes per year

References
Salman SM, Kibbi AG (2002) Vascular reactions in children. Clinics in Dermatology 20(1):11–15

Erythema multiforme major

▶ Stevens-Johnson syndrome

Erythema neonatorum

▶ Erythema toxicum

Erythema neonatorum allergicum

▶ Erythema toxicum

Erythema nodosum

Synonym(s)
Dermatitis contusiformis; erythema contusiformis; focal septal panniculitis; nodose fever

Definition
Inflammatory vascular reaction pattern to multiple causes; characterized by tender subcutaneous nodules, usually on the anterior legs

Pathogenesis
Probably is delayed hypersensitivity reaction to a variety of antigens; most common associations with streptococcal infections in children and sarcoidosis in adults; other associations include tuberculosis, mycoplasma pneumonia, leprosy, coccidioidomycosis, North American blastomycosis, histoplasmosis, inflammatory bowel disease, pregnancy, and Behçet's disease; associated medications include oral contraceptives and sulfonamides

Clinical manifestation
Prodrome of flulike symptoms of fever and generalized aching; lesions begin as poorly-defined, red, tender nodules; become firm and painful during the second week; sometimes becoming fluctuant; not suppurating or ulcerating; individual lesions last approximately 2 weeks; associated leg edema and pain

Differential diagnosis
Nodular vasculitis; insect bite reaction; erysipelas; cellulitis; superficial thrombophlebitis; Weber-Christian disease; pancreatic panniculitis; lupus profundus; traumatic panniculitis; polyarteritis nodosa; rheumatoid nodules

Therapy
Non-steroidal anti-inflammatory agents; bed rest; leg elevation; prednisone

References
Requena L, Requena C (2002) Erythema nodosum. Dermatology Online Journal 8(1):4

Erythema nodosum migrans

▶ Subacute nodular migratory panniculitis

Erythema nuchae

▶ Salmon patch

Erythema papulosum

▶ Erythema toxicum

Erythema perstans

▶ Ashy dermatosis
▶ Erythema annulare centrifugum

Erythema polymorphe

▶ Erythema multiforme

Erythema simplex gyratum

▶ Erythema annulare centrifugum

Erythema solare

▶ Sunburn

Erythema toxicum

Synonym(s)
Erythema toxicum neonatorum; erythema neonatorum; toxic erythema; erythema neonatorum allergicum; erythema papulosum; urticaria neonatorum; erythema dyspepsicum

Definition
Benign, self-limited eruption occurring primarily in healthy newborns in the early neonatal period

Pathogenesis
Unknown

Clinical manifestation
Usual onset within the first 4 days of life in full-term infants, with peak onset occurring within the first 48 hours following birth; presents with a blotchy, evanescent, macular erythema, often on the face or trunk; sites of predilection include the forehead, face, trunk, and proximal extremities; mucous membranes usually spared

Differential diagnosis
Candidiasis; miliaria; pyoderma; insect bite reaction; varicella; herpes simplex virus infection; urticaria; folliculitis; transient neonatal pustular melanosis

Therapy
None

References
Wagner A (1997) Distinguishing vesicular and pustular disorders in the neonate. Current Opinion in Pediatrics 9(4):396–405

Erythema toxicum neonatorum

▶ Erythema toxicum

Erythemato-papulous acrodermatitis

▶ Gianotti-Crosti syndrome

Erythemato-vesiculo-papulous eruptive syndrome

▶ Gianotti-Crosti syndrome

Erythermalgia

▶ Erythromelalgia

Erythrasma

Synonym(s)
None

Definition
Chronic superficial infection of the intertriginous areas caused by Corynebacterium minutissimum

Pathogenesis
Under favorable conditions, such as heat and humidity, Corynebacteria organisms proliferate and cause clinical signs

Clinical manifestation
Well demarcated, brown-red, minimally scaly plaques, commonly occurring over inner thighs, crural region, scrotum, and toe webs; other intertriginous sites such as axillae, submammary area, periumbilical region, and intergluteal fold less commonly involved; toe web lesions appear macerated; predisposing factors: excessive sweating and hyperhidrosis, disrupted cutaneous barrier, obesity, diabetes mellitus, and immunocompromised state

Differential diagnosis
Tinea pedis; tinea corporis; tinea cruris; contact dermatitis; dyshidrotic eczema; intertrigo; contact dermatitis

Therapy
Erythromycin base; clarithromycin; drying powder applied twice daily

References
Holdiness MR (2002) Management of cutaneous erythrasma. Drugs 62(8):1131–41

Erythroderma

▶ Exfoliative dermatitis

Erythroderma exfoliativa recidivans faciei

▶ Riehl's melanosis

Erythrohepatic protoporphyria

▶ Erythropoietic protoporphyria

Erythrokeratoderma

▶ Erythrokeratodermia variabilis

Erythrokeratodermia figurata variabilis

▶ Erythrokeratodermia variabilis

Erythrokeratodermia papillaris et reticularis

▶ Confluent and reticulated papillomatosis

Erythrokeratodermia progressiva symmetrica

▶ Progressive symmetric keratoderma

Erythrokeratodermia variabilis

Synonym(s)
Erythrokeratoderma; keratosis rubra figurata; erythrokeratodermia figurata variabilis

Definition

Disorder of cornification associated with transient noninflammatory erythema and persistent, but changing, scaliness

Pathogenesis

Mutations identified in the connexin gene GJB3; possibly caused by impaired gap junctional intercellular communication due to a defect in gap junctions

Clinical manifestation

Transient, circumscribed, highly variable, figurate erythematous patches, sometimes surrounded by a hypomelanotic halo, involving any part of the skin; lesions most prevalent during childhood and sometimes becoming less frequent as the patient ages; burning sensation sometimes preceding or accompanying erythema; variably changing, brownish, hyperkeratotic plaques with geographic borders, symmetrically distributed over the limbs, buttocks, and trunk; flexures, face, and scalp usually spared

Differential diagnosis

Progressive symmetric erythrokeratodermia; Giroux-Barbeau erythrokeratodermia with ataxia; Greither disease; erythrokeratolysis hiemalis; ichthyosis linearis circumflexa; psoriasis; mycosis fungoides; lupus erythematosus; lamellar ichthyosis; gyrate erythema; atopic dermatitis

Therapy

Acitretin*; emollients and/or keratolytics, such as alpha hydroxy acids

References

Hendrix JD Jr, Greer KE (1995) Erythrokeratodermia variabilis present at birth: case report and review of the literature. Pediatric Dermatology 12(4):351–354

Erythrokeratolysis hiemalis

▶ **Keratolytic winter erythema**

Erythromelalgia

Synonym(s)

Erythermalgia

Definition

Disorder characterized by paroxysmal burning pain, warmth, and redness of the extremities

Pathogenesis

Unclear; arteriolar fibrosis and occlusion with platelet thrombi often present; prostaglandins and cyclooxygenase involved

Clinical manifestation

Most cases primary (idiopathic); secondary form sometimes precede myeloproliferative disorder with thrombocytosis; dramatic relief with aspirin typical of this type and useful in diagnosis; painful, warm extremities brought on by warming or dependency, lasting minutes to days, and relieved by cooling; lower extremities affected more often than upper extremities; symptoms worsening with warming of extremity or placing of extremity in a dependent position; symptoms sometimes decrease with cooling and elevation of extremity; no symptoms or signs between attacks

Differential diagnosis

Raynaud phenomenon; reflex sympathetic dystrophy; cellulitis; vasculitis; frostbite

Therapy

Cooling or elevating extremity to relieve symptoms of an attack*; aspirin 500 mg PO as needed; chemotherapy for myeloproliferative disorder

References

Cohen JS (2000) Erythromelalgia: new theories and new therapies. Journal of the American Academy of Dermatology 43(5 Pt 1):841–847

Erythromycin, systemic

Trade name(s)
Eryc; E-mycin; PCE; EES; Ilosone

Generic available
Yes

Drug class
Macrolide antibiotic

Mechanism of action
Inhibition of RNA-dependent protein synthesis by binding to the 50S subunit of the ribosome

Dosage form
250 mg, 333 mg, 400 mg, 500 mg tablet

Dermatologic indications and dosage
See table

Common side effects
Cutaneous: urticaria or other vascular reaction, stomatitis
Gastrointestinal: nausea and vomiting, diarrhea, abdominal cramps, jaundice
Laboratory: elevated liver enzymes; eosinophilia

Serious side effects
Bone marrow: suppression
Cardiovascular: arrhythmias, hypotension
Cutaneous: anaphylaxis, Stevens-Johnson syndrome

Drug interactions
Amiodarone; amitriptyline; budesonide; buspirone; carbamazepine; clozapine; oral contraceptives; cyclosporine; digoxin; ergot alkaloids; methadone; phenytoin; pimozide; protease inhibitors; quinidine; statins; tacrolimus; theophylline; valproic acid; vinca alkaloids; warfarin

Contraindications/precautions
Hypersensitivity to drug class or component; caution in patients with myasthenia gravis or impaired liver function

References
Alvarez-Elcoro S, Enzler MJ (1999) The macrolides: erythromycin, clarithromycin, and azithromycin. Mayo Clinic Proceedings 74(6):613–634

Erythromycin, topical

Trade name(s)
Emgel; Erycette; EryDerm; Erymax; Erythra-Derm; T-Stat; Theramycin; Staticin

Generic available
Yes

Drug class
Topical macrolide antibiotic; anti-inflammatory

Mechanism of action
Inhibition of RNA-dependent protein synthesis by binding to the 50S subunit of the ribosome

Dosage form
2% gel; 1.5, 2% solution

Dermatologic indications and dosage
See table

Common side effects
Cutaneous: burning sensation, dryness, peeling, pruritus, erythema

Serious side effects
None

Drug interactions
Topical clindamycin

Erythromycin, systemic. Dermatologic indications and dosage

Disease	Adult dosage	Child dosage
Acne vulgaris	250–1000 mg PO daily	250–500 mg PO daily
Acute necrotizing gingivitis	500 mg PO 4 times daily for 10 days	30–50 mg per kg daily divided into 4 doses for 10 days
Bacillary angiomatosis	500 mg PO 4 times daily for 3 weeks	30–50 mg per kg daily divided into 4 doses for 4 weeks
Bartonellosis	500 mg PO 4 times daily for 3 weeks	30–50 mg per kg daily divided into 4 doses for 10 days
Bejel	500 mg PO 4 times daily for 15 days	8 mg per kg daily divided into 4 doses for 15 days
Ecthyma	250–500 mg PO 4 times daily for 10 days	30–50 mg per kg daily divided into 4 doses for 10 days
Erythrasma	500 mg PO 4 times daily for 7–10 days	30–50 mg per kg daily divided into 4 doses for 7–10 days
Hidradenitis suppurativa	500 mg PO twice daily	30–50 mg per kg daily divided into 2 doses
Impetigo	250–500 mg PO 4 times daily for 10 days	30–50 mg per kg daily divided into 4 doses for 10 days
Leptospirosis	250–500 mg PO 4 times daily for 3 weeks	30–50 mg per kg daily divided into 4 doses for 3 weeks
Lyme disease	500 mg PO 4 times daily for 3 weeks	30–50 mg per kg daily divided into 4 doses for 10 days
Lymphogranuloma venereum	500 mg PO 4 times daily for 3 weeks	30–50 mg per kg daily divided into 4 doses for 3 weeks
Perioral dermatitis	250–500 mg PO twice daily for at least 30 days	125–250 mg PO 4 times daily for at least 30 days
Pinta	500 mg PO 4 times daily for 15 days	8 mg per kg daily divided into 4 doses for 15 days
Pitted keratolysis	250–500 mg PO 4 times daily for 10 days	30–50 mg per kg daily divided into 4 doses for 10 days
Pityriasis lichenoides	500 mg PO twice daily	30–50 mg per kg daily divided into 2 doses
Pityriasis rosea	500 mg PO 4 times daily for 2 weeks	30–50 mg per kg daily divided into 4 doses for 2 weeks
Relapsing fever (louse-borne)	500 mg PO for 1 dose	250 mg PO for 1 dose
Relapsing fever (tick-borne)	500 mg PO 4 times daily for 7 days	30–50 mg per kg daily divided into 4 doses for 7days
Rosacea	250–500 mg PO twice daily for at least 30 days	125–250 mg PO 4 times daily for at least 30 days
Scarlet fever	500 mg PO 4 times daily for 7–10 days	30–50 mg per kg daily divided into 4 doses for 10 days
Syphilis	500 mg PO 4 times daily for 2–4 weeks	30–50 mg per kg daily divided into 4 doses for 2–4 weeks

Erythromycin, systemic. Dermatologic indications and dosage (Continued)

Disease	Adult dosage	Child dosage
Trench fever	500 mg PO 4 times daily for 4 weeks	30–50 mg per kg daily divided into 3 doses for 15 days
Yaws	500 mg PO 4 times daily for 15 days	30–50 mg per kg daily divided into 4 doses for 15 days

Contraindications/precautions
Hypersensitivity to drug class or component; caution about resistant organisms when used without benzoyl peroxide

References
Greenwood R, Burke B, Cunliffe WJ (1986) Evaluation of a therapeutic strategy for the treatment of acne vulgaris with conventional therapy. British Journal of Dermatology 114(3):353–358

Erythroplasia of Queyrat

Synonym(s)
Carcinoma in situ of the penis

Definition
Precancerous epithelial proliferation of the penis, almost always occuring in uncircumcised men

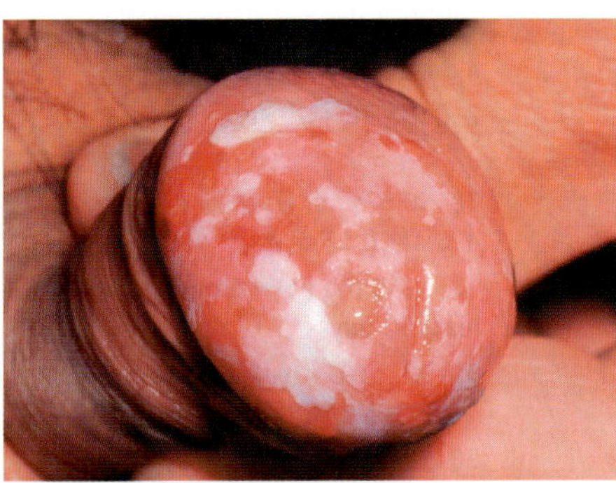

Erythroplasia of Queyrat. Ill-defined, scaly, eroded plaque of the glans penis

Pathogenesis
Arises from squamous epithelial cells of the glans penis or inner lining of prepuce; multiple contributing factors including chronic irritation (urine, smegma), inflammation (heat, friction, maceration) and infection (herpes simplex virus infection, human papillomavirus infection)

Clinical manifestation
Minimally raised, erythematous plaques, which may be smooth, velvety, scaly, crusted, or verrucous; ulceration or distinct papillomatous papules suggest progression to invasive squamous cell carcinoma

Differential diagnosis
Balanitis of Zoon; balanitis xerotica obliterans; candidiasis; contact dermatitis; squamous cell carcinoma; fixed drug reaction; psoriasis; lichen planus

Therapy
Fluorouracil, topical; destruction by liquid nitrogen cryotherapy or electrodesiccation and curettage

References
Fitzgerald DA (1998) Cancer precursors. Seminars in Cutaneous Medicine & Surgery 17(2):108–113

Erythroplasia of Zoon

▶ **Zoon balanitis**

Erythromycin, topical. Dermatologic indications and dosage

Disease	Adult dosage	Child dosage
Acne vulgaris	Apply twice daily	Apply twice daily
Familial benign chronic pemphigus	Apply twice daily	Apply twice daily
Perioral dermatitis	Apply twice daily	Apply twice daily
Pitted keratolysis	Apply twice daily for 2–4 weeks	Apply twice daily for 2–4 weeks
Rosacea	Apply twice daily	Apply twice daily

Erythropoietic porphyria

▶ Congenital erythropoietic porphyria

Erythropoietic protoporphyria

Synonym(s)
Erythrohepatic protoporphyria; congenital erythropoietic protoporphyria; protoporphyria

Definition
Inherited disorder of porphyrin-heme metabolism caused by mutations in the gene encoding ferrochelatase, resulting in accumulation of excess protoporphyrin that mediates a distinctive form of cutaneous photosensitivity

Pathogenesis
Mutations of the ferrochelatase gene, leading to excess protoporphyrin, a molecule capable of transformation to excited states by absorption of light energy; photoxidative damage to biomolecular targets in the skin, resulting in immediate phototoxic symptoms

Clinical manifestation
Immediate edema, erythema, and petechiae after sun exposure; occasional vesicles; chronic skin changes, including facial scars, perioral furrowing, and aged-appearing, thickened, or hyperkeratotic skin of the dorsal hands; with sustained, more intense, or frequent exposures, waxy scleroderma-like induration and/or weather-beaten or cobblestone textures of the face and dorsal aspects of hands; progressive liver failure in rare instances, with hepatosplenomegaly and jaundice

Differential diagnosis
Solar urticaria; acute tar photosensitivity; hereditary coproporphyria; porphyria cutanea tarda; pseudoporphyria; polymorphous light eruption; light-sensitive atopic dermatitis

Therapy
Beta-carotene 120–300 mg PO per day; sun avoidance★

References
Murphy GM (1999) The cutaneous porphyrias: a review. The British Photodermatology Group. British Journal of Dermatology 140(4):573–581

Erythropoietic uroporphyria

▶ Congenital erythropoietic porphyria

Essential lipoid histiocytosis

▶ Niemann-Pick disease

Essential melanotic pigmentation

▶ Laugier-Hunziger syndrome

Essential mixed cryoglobulinemia

▶ Cryoglobulinemia

Etat craquelé

▶ Asteatotic eczema

Eumycetoma

Synonym(s)
Madura foot; maduromycosis; fungal myce-toma; eumycotic mycetoma; melanoid myc-etoma; ochroid mycetoma

Definition
Chronic cutaneous and subcutaneous infec-tion caused by various genera of fungi and characterized by progressive destruction of soft tissue

Pathogen,esis
Infectious agents primarily saprophytic microorganisms found in the soil and on plant matter; inoculation occurrs as a result of traumatic implantation of thorns, splin-ters, and other plant matter; Pseudallesche-ria boydii most common etiologic agent of eumycetoma in the United States; Madurella mycetomatis most common causative organism worldwide

Clinical manifestation
Disease presents as a painless swelling or thickening of the skin and subcutaneous tissue, usually over the distal lower extrem-ity; with progression over months or years; lesion enlarges and eventually becomes tumorous; overlying skin sometimes smooth, dyspigmented, or shiny; abscesses and sinus tracts develops and sometimes contains a serosanguinous or seropurulent discharge, with white-to-yellow or black granules; predisposing factors: walking barefoot, agricultural work; poor personal hygiene; poor nutrition, and wounds or skin infections

Differential diagnosis
Tuberculosis; leprosy; leishmaniasis; squa-mous cell carcinoma; yaws; syphilis; actino-mycetoma; botryomycosis; chromoblasto-mycosis; sporotrichosis; blastomycosis; coc-cidioidomycosis; elephantiasis

Therapy
Ketoconazole; itraconazole; surgical exci-sion

References
Restrepo A (1994) Treatment of tropical mycoses. Journal of the American Academy of Dermatol-ogy 31(3 Pt 2):S91–102

Eumycotic mycetoma

▶ Eumycetoma

European blastomycosis

▶ Cryptococcosis

Exanthem subitum

▶ Roseola

Excoriated acne

▶ Acne excoriée

Exfoliative dermatitis

Definition
Eruption characterized by widespread erythema and scaling, often with pruritus, caused by multiple underlying conditions including generalization of pre-existing diseases such as psoriasis and atopic dermatitis; cutaneous T-cell lymphopma and reactions to medications

References
Rothe MJ, Bialy TL, Grant-Kels JM. (2000) Erythroderma. Dermatologic Clinics 18(3):405–415

External otitis

▶ Otitis externa

Extramammary Paget's disease

▶ Paget's disease

Exudative discoid and lichenoid dermatitis

▶ Sulzberger-Garbe syndrome

F

Fabry disease

▶ Angiokeratoma corporis diffusum

Fabry syndrome

▶ Angiokeratoma corporis diffusum

Fabry-Anderson disease

▶ Angiokeratoma corporis diffusum

Facial granuloma

▶ Granuloma faciale

Facial ringworm

▶ Tinea faciei

Factitial dermatitis

▶ Dermatitis artefacta

Factitious urticaria

▶ Dermatographism

Famciclovir

Trade name(s)
Famvir

Generic available
No

Drug class
Anti-viral

Mechanism of action
DNA polymerase inhibition

Dosage form
125 mg, 250 mg, 500 mg tablet

Dermatologic indications
See table

Common side effects
Gastrointestinal: nausea, vomiting
Neurologic: headache

Serious side effects
None

Drug interactions
Probenecid

Famciclovir. Dermatologic indications and dosage

Disease	Adult dosage	Child dosage
Herpes simplex virus infection, first epidose	250 mg PO 3 times daily for 7–10 days	Not established
Herpes simplex virus infection, prophylaxis	250 mg PO twice daily for up to 1 year	Not established
Herpes simplex virus infection, recurrent episode	125 mg PO twice daily for 5 days	Not established
Herpes zoster	500 mg PO 3 times daily for 7 days	Not established
Varicella	500 mg PO 3 times daily for 7 days	Not established

Contraindications/precautions

Hypersensitivity to drug class or component; elderly patients or those with renal failure may need lower dose

References

Brown TJ, Vander Straten M, Tyring S (2001) Antiviral agents. Dermatologic Clinics 19(1):23–34

Familial atypical mole-melanoma syndrome

▶ Atypical mole

Familial baldness

▶ Androgenetic alopecia

Familial benign chronic pemphigus

Synonym(s)

Hailey-Hailey disease; familial benign pemphigus

Definition

Inherited, intraepidermal, blistering disease, affecting the neck, axillae, and groin area

Pathogenesis

Autosomal dominant trait; overall defect in keratinocyte adhesion, apparently secondary to a primary defect in a calcium pump protein, ATP2C1; pump mutation in ATP2C1, a gene localized on chromosome 3

Clinical manifestation

Vesicles and erythematous plaques with overlying crusts, usually occurring in the genital area, the chest, neck, and axillary region; burning sensation and pruritus accompanying the eruption; malodorous drainage with secondary infection; factors known to exacerbate the disease: heat, friction, and infection

Differential diagnosis

Darier disease; impetigo; candidiasis; herpes simplex virus infection; pemphigus vulgaris; pemphigus foliaceus; atopic dermatitis; seborrheic dermatitis; extramammary Paget's disease

Therapy

Topical corticosteroids, mid potency; erythromycin, systemic; erythromycin, topical;

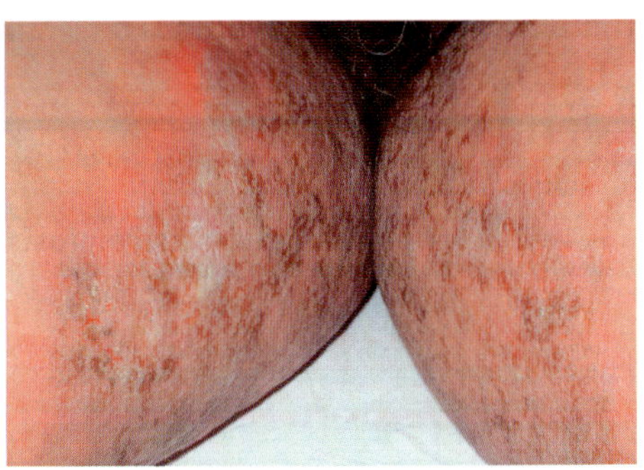

Familial benign chronic pemphigus. Eroded plaques on the thighs

clindamycin, topical; local CO_2 laser ablation; local dermabrasion

References

Gallagher TC (2000) Familial benign pemphigus. Dermatology Online Journal 6(1):7

Familial benign pemphigus

▶ Familial benign chronic pemphigus

Familial hemorrhagic angiomatosis

▶ Osler-Weber-Rendu syndrome

Familial Turner syndrome

▶ Noonan's syndrome

Familial white spotting

▶ Piebaldism

Fanconi-Prader syndrome

▶ Addison-Schilder disease

Farcy

▶ Glanders and melioidosis

Farmer's neck

▶ Actinic elastosis

Fatal cutaneointestinal syndrome

▶ Malignant atrophic papulosis

Fatal granulomatosis of childhood

▶ Chronic granulomatous disease

Fatty tumor

▶ Lipoma

Faun-tail nevus

▶ Nevoid hypertrichosis

Favre-Chaix disease

▶ Acroangiodermatitis

Favre-Racouchot syndrome

Synonym(s)
Syndrome of Favre-Racouchot; nodular cutaneous elastoidosis with cysts and comedones; senile comedones; solar comedones; smoker's comedones

Definition
Disorder characterized by multiple open and closed comedones in actinically damaged skin

Pathogenesis
Unknown; develops in individuals with a heavy smoking history and chronic exposure to ultraviolet light

Clinical manifestation
Multiple, bilaterally symmetrical, open and closed comedones in the periorbital and temporal areas; occasionally noted in the lateral neck, postauricular areas, and forearms; actinically damaged skin with yellowish discoloration, yellowish nodules, atrophy, wrinkles, and furrows

Differential diagnosis
Acne vulgaris; nevus comedonicus; colloid milia; milia; trichoepithelioma; syringoma; sebaceous hyperplasia; xanthoma

Therapy
Comedone extraction; surgical excision; tretinoin

References
Sharkey MJ, Keller RA, Grabski WJ, McCollough ML (1992) Favre-Racouchot syndrome. A combined therapeutic approach. Archives of Dermatology 128(5):615–616

Febrile neutrophilic dermatosis

▶ Acute febrile neutrophilic dermatosis

Female pattern baldness

▶ Androgenetic alopecia

Female pseudo Turner syndrome

▶ Noonan's syndrome

Fexofenadine

▶ Antihistamines, second generation

Fibroepithelial polyp

▶ Acrochordon

Fibroepithelioma of Pinkus

Synonym(s)
Pinkus tumor; premalignant fibroepithelial tumor

Definition
Premalignant epithelial tumor consisting of cells resembling those of basal cell carcinoma

Pathogenesis
Unknown

Clinical manifestation
Slowly enlarging, single or multiple, fleshy, pink or reddish, pedunculated papules with a broad base; occur exclusively on the trunk, particularly over the lumbosacral area

Differential diagnosis
Seborrheic keratosis; acrochordon; nevus sebaceus of Jadassohn; melanocytic nevus; amelanotic melanoma; neurofibroma

Therapy
Destruction by electrodesiccation and curettage; elliptical excision

References
Stern JB, Haupt HM, Smith RR (1994) Fibroepithelioma of Pinkus. Eccrine duct spread of basal cell carcinoma. American Journal of Dermatopathology 16(6):585–587

Fibroma

Synonym(s)
None

Definition
Benign fibrous tissue tumor

References
Weiss SW (1986) Proliferative fibroblastic lesions. From hyperplasia to neoplasia. American Journal of Surgical Pathology 10 Suppl 1:14–25

Fibroma durum

▶ Dermatofibroma

Fibroma simplex

▶ Dermatofibroma

Fibromatosis

Synonym(s)
None

Definition
Benign fibrous tissue proliferation, intermediate in biological behavior between benign fibroma and fibrosarcoma

References
Fisher C (1996) Fibromatosis and fibrosarcoma in infancy and childhood. European Journal of Cancer 32A(12):2094–2100

Fibrosarcoma of the skin

▶ Dermatofibrosarcoma protuberans

Fibrous dysplasia of bone

▶ McCune-Albright Syndrome

Fibrous dysplasia, polyostotic

▶ McCune-Albright syndrome

Fibrous papule

▶ Fibrous papule of nose/face

Fibrous papule of nose/face

Synonym(s)
Fibrous papule; fibrous papule of the nose

Definition
Small facial papule with a characteristic fibrovascular component on histological examination

Pathogenesis
Possibly remnant of a melanocytic nevus, or fibrohistiocytic lineage, or derived from dermal dendrocytes

Clinical manifestation
Solitary or multiple, dome-shaped, shiny, skin-colored or red-brown firm papules; usually located on the nose, but sometimes arising on the cheeks, chin, neck, lip, or the forehead

Differential diagnosis
Nevus; basal cell carcinoma; trichoepithelioma; syringoma; milium; seborrheic keratosis; pyogenic granuloma; angiofibroma

Therapy
Surgical excision for cosmesis

References
Shea CR, Salob S, Reed JA, Lugo J, McNutt NS 91996) CD34-reactive fibrous papule of the nose. Journal of the American Academy of Dermatology 35(2 Pt 2):342–345

Fibrous sclerosis of the penis

▶ Peyronie's disease

Fibroxanthoma, atypical

▶ Atypical fibroxanthoma

Fiessinger-Leroy syndrome

▶ Reiter syndrome

Fiessinger-Leroy-Reiter syndrome

▶ Reiter syndrome

Fifth disease

▶ Erythema infectiosum

Filariasis

Synonym(s)
Lymphatic filariasis; bancroftian filariasis; brugian filariasis; onchocerciasis; African river blindness; blinding filariasis; Robles' disease; loiasis; Loa loa

Definition
Disease group caused by nematode parasites of the order Filariidae, commonly called filariae

Pathogenesis
Lymphatic filariasis caused by Wuchereria bancrofti, Brugia malayi, and Brugia timori; cutaneous filariasis caused by Loa loa, Onchocerca volvulus, and Mansonella streptocerca; Microfilariae in insect host inoculated into vertebral host during feeding and completing their life cycle there

Clinical manifestation
Lymphatic filariasis – acute episode (adenolymphangitis): fever; inguinal or axillary lymphadenopathy;   testicular   and/or

Finasteride. Dermatologic indications and dosage

Disease	Adult dosage	Child dosage
Androgenetic alopecia in men	1 mg PO daily	Not indicated

inguinal pain; limb or genital swelling; skin exfoliation of the affected body part usually occurring with resolution of an episode; recurrent episodes of inflammation and lymphedema leading to lymphatic damage with chronic swelling and elephantiasis of the legs, arms, scrotum, vulva, and breasts
Onchocerciasis: skin nodules over bony prominences (i.e., onchocercomas); other skin lesions including edema, pruritus, erythema, papules, altered pigmentation, and lichenification
Loiasis: large transient area of localized nonerythematous subcutaneous edema (Calabar swelling), most common around joints

Differential diagnosis
Scrotal or testicular trauma; lymphoma; lymphogranuloma venereum; Milroy disease; bacterial or fungal lymphadenitis; leprosy; non-filarial elephantiasis; hydrocele

Therapy
Lymphatic filariasis: diethylcarbamazine 6 mg per kg PO per day for 12–21 days[*]
Oncocerciasis: ivermectin[*]
Loiasis: diethylcarbamazine 6 mg per kg PO per day for 12–21 days[*]; albendazole

References
Taylor MJ, Hoerauf A (2001) A new approach to the treatment of filariasis. Current Opinion in Infectious Diseases 14(6):727–731

Generic available
No

Drug class
Type II 5 α-reductase inhibitor

Mechanism of action
Inhibition of 5-α reductase causes reduced conversion of testosterone to dihydrotestosterone in hair follicles

Dosage form
1 mg tablet

Dermatologic indications and dosage
See table

Common side effects
Genitourinary: decreased libido, impotence, decreased ejaculate volume

Serious side effects
None

Drug interactions
None

Contraindications/precautions
Hypersensitivity to drug class or component

References
Messenger AG (2000) Medical management of male pattern hair loss. International Journal of Dermatology 39(8):585–586

Finasteride

Trade name(s)
Propecia

Finger infection

▶ **Paronychia**

Fingernail infection

▶ Paronychia

Finkelstein's disease

▶ Acute hemorrhagic edema of infancy

Fire ant bite

▶ Hymenoptera sting

Fish fancier's finger

▶ Mycobacterium marinum infection

Fish odor syndrome

Synonym(s)
None

Definition
Metabolic disorder causing the excretion of a compound in sweat with the odor of rotting fish

Pathogenesis
Autosomal dominant trait; trimethylamine derived from carnitine or choline by the action of bowel flora; defect in trimethylamine metabolism in the liver, resulting in compound with fish-like odor

Clinical manifestation
Foul body odor; no skin lesions

Differential diagnosis
Bromhidrosis from other causes

Therapy
Diet low in carnitine and choline (seafood, eggs, liver, peas, soy beans)*

References
Mitchell SC (1996) The fish-odor syndrome. Perspectives in Biology & Medicine 39(4):514–526

Fish skin ichthyosis

▶ Ichthyosis vulgaris

Fish tank granuloma

▶ Mycobacterium marinum infection

Fissured tongue

▶ Lingua plicata

Five-day fever

▶ Trench fever

Fixed drug eruption

Synonym(s)
Fixed medication reaction; fixed eruption

Definition
Eruption occurring at the same site or sites each time a given medication is administered

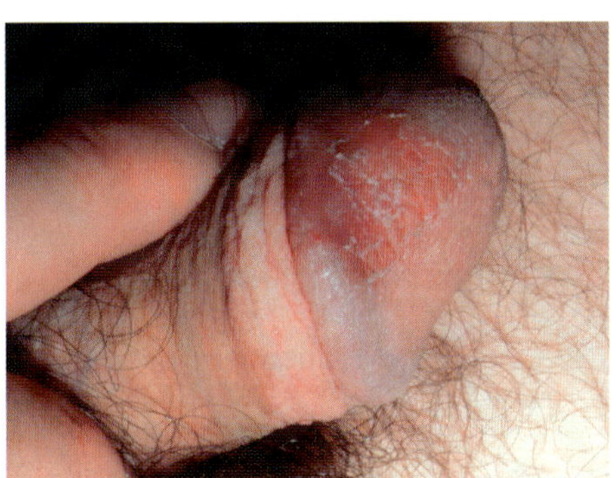

Fixed drug eruption. Scaly, red plaque on the glans penis

Pathogenesis
Probably results from an immunologically mediated inflammatory response to a given medication

Clinical manifestation
Develops 6–48 hours after administration of the causative drug; common etiologic agents: aspirin, barbiturates, co-trimoxazole, phenolphthalein, sulfonamides, and tetracycline; pruritus and burning, occasionally accompanied by fever; starts as a few sharply demarcated, erythematous macules that rapidly become erythematous plaques, usually on the lips, genitalia, and trunk; lesions heal hyperpigmentation; recurrence in the same site with readministration of the offending drug

Differential diagnosis
Contact dermatitis; herpes simplex virus infection; chemical burn; bullous pemphigoid; lupus erythematosus; psoriasis; porphyria cutanea tarda; erythema multiforme; erythema migrans; bullous disease of diabetes mellitus; post-inflammatory hyperpigmentation; factitial disease

Therapy
Withdrawal of offending drug★

References
Shiohara T, Mizukawa Y, Teraki Y (2002) Pathophysiology of fixed drug eruption: the role of skin-resident T cells. Current Opinion in Allergy & Clinical Immunology 2(4):317–323

Fixed eruption

▶ Fixed drug eruption

Fixed medication reaction

▶ Fixed drug eruption

Flegel disease

▶ Hyperkeratosis lenticularis perstans

Flegel's disease

▶ Hyperkeratosis lenticularis perstans

Florid cutaneous papillomatosis

Synonym(s)
None

Definition
Disorder characterized by the rapid onset of numerous warty papules on the trunk and extremities, often in association with malignant acanthosis nigricans and/or sign of Leser-Trelet and an internal malignancy

Pathogenesis
Unknown

Clinical manifestation
Multiple verrucous papules, beginning on the extremities, particularly on the dorsa of the hands and wrists; papules sometimes involve the entire body, including the face; usually associated with signs of internal cancer and malignant acanthosis nigricans and sign of Leser-Trélat

Differential diagnosis
Warts; acrokeratosis verruciformis of Hopf; seborrheic keratoses; epidermodysplasia verruciformis

Therapy
Treatment of underlying malignancy; topical therapies not effective

References
Schwartz RA (1993) Florid cutaneous papillomatosis. Clinics in Dermatology 11(1):89–91

Florid papillomatosis of nipple ducts

▶ Erosive adenomatosis of the nipple

Florid papillomatosis of the nipple

▶ Erosive adenomatosis of the nipple

Fluconazole

Trade name(s)
Diflucan

Generic available
No

Drug class
Tri-azole antifungal agent

Mechanism of action
Cell wall ergosterol inhibition by blocking 14α-demethlyation of lanosterol

Dosage form
50 mg, 100 mg, 150 mg, 200 mg tablet; 50 mg per ml, 200 mg/ml suspension

Dermatologic indications and dosage
See table

Common side effects
Cutaneous: skin eruption
Gastrointestinal: nausea and vomiting, diarrhea, abdominal pain, dyspepsia
Neurologic: headache, dizziness, taste changes

Serious side effects
Cutaneous: angioedema, Stevens-Johnson syndrome
Gastrointestinal: hepatotoxicity
Hematologic: agranulocytosis, leukocytosis
Neurologic: seizures

Drug interactions
Amitriptyline; barbiturates; buspirone; carbamazepine; celecoxib; cyclosporine; digoxin; ergot alkaloids; glyburide/metformin; phenytoin; pimozide; protease inhibitors; quinidine; rifampin; statins; sulfonylureas; tacrolimus; theophyllines; warfarin

Contraindications/precautions
Hypersensitivity to drug class or component; caution in patients with impaired renal or hepatic function

References
Meis JF, Verweij PE (2001) Current management of fungal infections. Drugs 61(Suppl 1):13–25

Fluocinolone acetonide

▶ Corticosteroids, topical, medium potency

Fluconazole. Dermatologic indications and dosage

Disease	Adult dosage	Child dosage
Angular cheilitis	150 mg PO once weekly for 2–4 weeks	3–6 mg per kg weekly for 2–4 weeks
Candidiasis associated with hyperimmuno-globulin E syndrome	150 mg PO daily for 1-3 weeks, depending on therapeutic response	3–6 mg per kg PO once weekly for 1-3 weeks, depending on therapeutic response
Candidiasis, cutaneous	150 mg PO once weekly for 2–4 weeks	3–6 mg per kg PO once weekly for 2–4 weeks
Candidiasis, oral (thrush)	150 mg PO once weekly for 2–4 weeks	3–6 mg per kg PO for 14–28 days
Candidiasis, vulvovaginal	150 mg PO for 1 dose	150 mg PO for 1 dose
Chronic paronychia	150 mg PO once weekly for 3–6 weeks	3–6 mg per kg PO once weekly for 3–6 weeks
Leishmaniasis	200 mg PO daily for 6 weeks	3–6 mg per kg PO once daily for 6 weeks
Onychomycosis	150 mg PO once weekly for 3–6 months	3–6 mg per kg PO once weekly for 3–6 months
Sporotrichosis	200-400 mg PO daily until infection clears	3–6 mg per kg PO once daily until infection clears
Tinea corporis	150 mg PO once weekly for 2–4 weeks	3–6 mg per kg PO once weekly for 2–4 weeks
Tinea cruris	150 mg PO once weekly for 2–4 weeks	3–6 mg per kg PO once weekly for 2–4 weeks
Tinea pedis	150 mg PO once weekly for 2–4 weeks	3–6 mg per kg PO once weekly for 2–4 weeks
Tinea versicolor	150 mg PO for 1–2 doses over 7-14 days	3–6 mg per kg PO for 1 dose; repeat in 7–14 days
White piedra	150 mg PO once weekly for 2–4 weeks	3–6 mg per kg PO once weekly for 2–4 weeks

Fluoroderma

▶ Halogenoderma

Fluorouracil, topical

Trade name(s)
Efudex; Fluoroplex; Carac; Adrucil

Generic available
No

Drug class
Antimetabolite

Mechanism of action
Inhibition of DNA synthesis by blocking thymidylate synthetase

Dosage form
0.5% cream; 1% cream; 5% cream; 1% solution; 2% solution; 5% solution; 50 mg/ml solution for intralesional injection

Fluorouracil, topical. Dermatologic indications and dosage

Disease	Adult dosage	Child dosage
Actinic keratosis	Apply 1–2 times daily for 3–6 weeks	Apply 1–2 times daily for 3–6 weeks
Basal cell carcinoma	Apply 1–2 times daily for 4–8 weeks	Not applicable
Basal cell nevus syndrome;	Apply 1–2 times daily for 4–8 weeks	Apply 1–2 times daily for 4–8 weeks
Bowenoid papulosis	Apply 1–2 times daily for 4–8 weeks	Not applicable
Carcinoma-in-situ (Bowen's disease)	Apply 1–2 times daily for 4–8 weeks	Not applicable
Disseminated superficial actinic porokeratosis	Apply twice daily for 4–8 weeks	Apply twice daily for 4–8 weeks
Hyperkeratosis lenticularis perstans	Apply 2 times daily for 2–4 months	Not applicable
Keratoacanthoma	50 mg per ml intralesional injection; repeat every 2 weeks for up to 5 times	Not applicable
Wart	Apply twice daily for 6 weeks	Apply twice daily for 6 weeks

Dermatologic indications and dosage
See table

Common side effects
Cutaneous: local pain, pruritus, burning, crusting, erosions, allergic contact dermatitis, photosensitivity, hypopigmentation, hyperpigmentation

Serious side effects
None

Drug interactions
None

Contraindications/precautions
Hypersensitivity to drug class or component; avoid excessive sun exposure while in use

References
Jeffes EW 3rd., Tang EH (2000) Actinic keratosis. Current treatment options. American Journal of Clinical Dermatology 1:167–179

Fluoxetine

▶ Selective serotonin reuptake inhibitor (SSRI)

Flurandrenolide

▶ Corticosteroids, topical, medium potency

Fluticasone propionate

▶ Corticosteroids, topical, medium potency

Focal acantholytic dyskeratosis

▶ **Warty dyskeratoma**

Focal dermal hypoplasia

Synonym(s)
Goltz's syndrome, Goltz syndrome

Definition
Genetic disorder characterized by distinctive skin abnormalities and a wide variety of defects affecting the eyes, teeth, and skeletal, urinary, gastrointestinal, cardiovascular, and central nervous system

Pathogenesis
X-linked dominant, typically lethal in males; mosaicism with random X-chromosome inactivation (lyonization) likely; profound dysplasia of ectodermal, neuroectodermal, endodermal, and mesodermal elements

Clinical manifestation
Present at birth, almost exclusively in females; skin findings – symmetric, linear, reticulated, frequently tender, pink or red, thin skin; involved areas angular, atrophic, slightly raised, or depressed macules, with telangiectasias; lesions follow the lines of Blaschko; prominent involvement on the lower extremities, forearms, and cheeks; hernia-like outpouchings of fatty tissue; multiple raspberry-like papillomas arising at junctions between the mucosa and the skin (i.e. perioral, perivulvar, perianal, periocular junctions); apocrine nevi; multiple hydrocystomas; hypohidrosis; scalp and body hair usually sparse; hair sometimes brittle; dysmorphic facial features; other abnormalities, include short stature, skeletal abnormalities, mental retardation, dysmorphic ears, and ocular abnormalities

Differential diagnosis
Aicardi syndrome; incontinentia pigmenti; proteus syndrome; MIDAS syndrome; aplasia cutis congenita; Adams-Oliver syndrome

Therapy
Flashlamp-pumped pulse dye laser for telangiectatic and erythematous skin lesions

References
Hardman CM, Garioch JJ, Eady RA, Fry L (1998) Focal dermal hypoplasia: report of a case with cutaneous and skeletal manifestations. Clinical & Experimental Dermatology 23(6):281–285

Focal facial dysplasia

▶ **Brauer's syndrome**

Focal septal panniculitis

▶ **Erythema nodosum**

Fogo selvagem

Synonym(s)
Endemic pemphigus foliaceus; Brazilian pemphigus; Brazilian pemphigus foliaceus; South American pemphigus

Definition
Variant of pemphigus foliaceus found in certain areas of Central America, South America, and Tunisia

Pathogenesis
Autoimmune disease, with autoantibodies specific for desmoglein, which results in acantholysis and linical blistering; black fly may be vector of spread

Clinical manifestation
Superficial vesicles that rupture easily and leave erosions; positive Nikolsky sign; occasional total body erythroderma; no mucous membrane involvement

Differential diagnosis
Impetigo; lupus erythematosus; pemphigus vulgaris; seborrheic dermatitis; atopic dermatitis; subcorneal pustular dermatosis; epidermolysis bullosa; glucagonoma syndrome; erythema multiforme
Other causes of erythroderma: drug reaction; cutaneous T-cell lymphoma; psoriasis; pityriasis rubra pilaris; contact dermatitis

Therapy
Severe disease: prednisone; steroid sparing agents: azathioprine; cyclophosphamide; mycophenolate mofetil
Mild-to-moderate disease: high potency topical corticosteroids

References
Sampaio SA, Rivitti EA, Aoki V, Diaz LA (1994) Brazilian pemphigus foliaceus, endemic pemphigus foliaceus, or fogo selvagem (wild fire). Dermatologic Clinics 12(4):765–776

Follicular mucinosis

Synonym(s)
Alopecia mucinosa

Definition
Degenerative mucinosis of pilosebaceous units

Pathogenesis
Primary idiopathic form; secondary form associated with benign diseases such as lupus erythematosus, lichen simplex chronicus, and angiolymphoid hyperplasia, and with malignant diseases such as mycosis fungoides, Kaposi's sarcoma, and Hodgkin's disease

Clinical manifestation
Pruritic, pink to yellow-white, follicular papules and plaques; may be solitary or multiple; face and scalp most common sites; non-scarring alopecia

Differential diagnosis
Alopecia areata; telogen effluvium; androgenetic alopecia; keratosis pilaris; lichen spinulosus; lichen planopilaris

Therapy
High potency topical corticosteroid; triamcinolone 3–5 mg per ml intralesional

References
Truhan AP, Roenigk HH Jr (1986) The cutaneous mucinoses. Journal of the American Academy of Dermatology 14(1):1–18

Folliculitis

Synonym(s)
None

Definition
Inflammation of the hair follicles caused by infection or physical or chemical irritation

Pathogenesis
Inflammatory process caused by obstruction or disruption of individual hair follicles and the associated pilosebaceous units

Clinical manifestation
Primary lesion a perifollicular papule or pustule; often appears as grid-like pattern of multiple red papules and/or pustules on hair-bearing areas, such as the face, scalp, thighs, axilla, and inguinal area; predisposing factors: friction; perspiration; occlusion; shaving; hyperhidrosis; diabetes mellitus or immunologic disorders; Staphylococcal nasal carriage; skin injuries; abrasions; surgical wounds; draining abscesses; skin occlusion for topical corticosteroid therapy

Clinical variants:
• Hot tub folliculitis: caused by psedomonas organisms in tub or pool water; pruritic, edematous, erythematous papules or pustules in areas of skin occluded by a bathing suit
• Pityrosporum folliculitis: pruritic acneform papules on the upper back, chest, upper arms, neck, chin, and sides of the face; caused by yeast forms of Pityrosporum ovale
• Fungal folliculitis: caused by candidal species and dermatophytes; principle etiologic agents: Trichophyton verrucosum and Trichophyton mentagrophytes; affects the coarse hairs in the mustache and beard area in men
• Staphylococcal folliculitis: follicular-based red papules and pustules, caused by Staphylococcal aureus

Differential diagnosis
Erythema toxicum; miliaria; insect bite reaction; scabies; acne; rosacea; perioral dermatitis; keratosis pilaris; acquired perforating disease; pemphigus foliaceus; Darier disease; Hailey-Hailey disease; pseudofolliculitis barbae

Therapy
Treatment of infection as per culture results; removal of inciting factors, such as tight-fitting clothing; anti-inflammatory therapy: tetracycline; doxycycline; minocycline; dapsone

References
Sadick NS (1997) Current aspects of bacterial infections of the skin. Dermatologic Clinics 15(2):341–349

Folliculitis decalvans

Synonym(s)
None

Definition
Final common pathway of various types of chronic folliculitis, producing progressive scarring

Pathogenesis
Inflammatory process caused by obstruction or disruption of individual hair follicles and the associated pilosebaceous units, leading to scarring alopecia because of destruction of the follicular units; role of staphylococcal follicular infection uncertain

Clinical manifestation
Occurs in women after age 30 and in men from adolescence onward; bogginess or induration of affected areas of the scalp or other hair-bearing sites; successive crops of pustules; late finding of scarring alopecia

Differential diagnosis
Dissecting folliculitis; lupus erythematosus; lichen planopilaris; kerion; pseudopelade of Brocq; follicular degeneration syndrome; pemphigus vulgaris; pemphigus foliaceus; Darier disease; Hailey-Hailey disease; pseudofolliculitis barbae

Therapy
Treatment of infection as per culture results

References
Brooke RC, Griffiths CE (2001) Folliculitis decalvans. Clinical & Experimental Dermatology 26(1):120–122

Folliculitis barbae traumatica

▶ Pseudofolliculitis barbae

Folliculitis, eosinophilic pustular

▶ Eosinophilic pustular folliculitis

Folliculitis keloidalis

▶ Acne keloidalis

Folliculitis keloidalis nuchae

▶ Acne keloidalis

Folliculitis, perforating

▶ Perforating folliculitis

Folliculitis, pityrosporom

▶ Folliculitis

Folliculitis ulerythema reticulata

▶ Ulerythema ophryogenes

Folliculoma

▶ Trichofolliculoma

Fong disease

▶ Nail-patella syndrome

Fordyce angiokeratoma

▶ Angiokeratoma of scrotum

Fordyce's disease

Synonym(s)
Fordyce's spots; Audry's glands; pseudocolloid lip mucous membrane sebacous milia; pseudocolloid of the buccal mucosa; pseudocolloid of the lips; mucosal sebaceous cysts

Definition
Developmental anomaly characterized by enlarged ectopic sebacous glands on the mucosa of the mouth and genitals

Pathogenesis
Unknown

Clinical manifestation
Asymptomatic, 1–2 mm yellow papules on the mucosal surfaces of the mouth and genitalia; papules sometimes coalesce into plaques

Differential diagnosis
Warts; lichen planus; white sponge nevus

Therapy
None indicated

References
Massmanian A, Sorni Valls G, Vera Sempere FJ (1995) Fordyce spots on the glans penis. British Journal of Dermatology 133(3):498–500

Fordyce's spots

▶ Fordyce's disease

Foreign body granuloma

Synonym(s)
Foreign body reaction

Definition
Inflammatory response with granuloma formation as a reaction to exogenous material, usually an inanimate object

Pathogenesis
Reaction to inert foreign materials too large to be ingested by either neutrophils or macrophages

Clinical manifestation
Firm, red papule or nodule, clearly distinguishable from the surrounding normal tissue

Differential diagnosis
Sarcoidosis; granuloma annulare; granuloma faciale; kerion; epidermoid cyst; zirconium or beryllium granuloma; Wegener's granulomatosis; lymphoma; tuberculosis; leprosy; lymphogranuloma venereum; sporotrichosis

Therapy
Surgical removal of foreign body*

References
Yoshitatsu S, Takagi T (2000) A case of giant pencil-core granuloma. Journal of Dermatology 27(5):329–332

Foreign body reaction

▶ Foreign body granuloma

Fort Bragg fever

▶ Leptospirosis

Fox impetigo

▶ Impetigo

Fox-Fordyce disease

Synonym(s)
Fox-Fordyce syndrome; apocrine miliaria

Definition
Chronic, pruritic, papular eruption localize to areas where apocrine glands are found, such as the axilla

Pathogenesis
Unknown; keratin plug in the hair follicle infundibulum obstructs the apocrine acrosyringium and produces apocrine anhidrosis; extravasation of sweat and inflammation possible causes of the intense itching

Clinical manifestation
Pruritic, flesh-colored-to-reddish, smooth, dome-shaped, discrete, follicular or perifollicular papules, most commonly in the axilla, but sometimes also affecting the periareolar, inframammary, and pubic areas; appear under conditions of heat, humidity, and friction; anhidrosis in the affected area; more common in women

Differential diagnosis
Folliculitis; pseudofolliculitis of the axilla; miliaria; milia; follicular hamartomas; hidradenitis suppurativa

Therapy
Tretinoin; surgical excision of the axilla; liposuction-assisted curettage

References
Chae KM, Marschall MA, Marschall SF (2002) Axillary Fox-Fordyce disease treated with liposuction-assisted curettage. Archives of Dermatology 138(4):452–454

Fox-Fordyce syndrome

▶ Fox-Fordyce disease

Foxhole foot

▶ Immersion foot

Frambesia tropica

▶ Yaws

Francois dyscephaly syndrome

▶ Hallermann-Streiff syndrome

Freckles

▶ Ephelides

Freezing of tissue

▶ Frostbite

Frey's syndrome

▶ Auriculotemporal syndrome
▶ Gustatory sweating

Frostbite

Synonym(s)
Freezing of tissue

Definition
Damage to the skin and underlying tissues caused by extreme cold

Pathogenesis
Extreme cold temperatures cause ice crystals to form in and around cells; red blood cells and platelets congeal, causing clots and ischemic damage; with skin warming, damage also caused by reperfusion

Clinical manifestation
Frostnip: mildest and completely reversible form of cold injury; blanching and numbness of the exposed area
Superficial frostbite: early signs and symptoms: sticking or pricking sensation, followed by development of pale, waxy skin; involved area becomes anesthetic; deeper tissues remain soft
Deep frostbite: same signs and symptoms as superficial variant, but deep tissues become hard and solid, and mottled bluish-gray discoloration develops; after warming, skin turns erythematous, edematous, with throbbing pain; within 6 hours, bullae appear, sometimes filled with clear fluid or with blood; wet or dry gangrene sometimes occurs after severe tissue injury

Differential diagnosis
Chilblains; Raynaud phenomenon; subcutaneous fat necrosis; acrocyanosis; trench foot

Therapy
Rapid rewarming in warm water bath at 37°-44° but avoidance of rewarming if danger of refreezing is present[*]; aloe vera gel applied 4 times daily; avoidance of thawing of frostbitten area if it cannot be kept thawed; no direct dry heat, such as a radiator, campfire, heating pad, or hair dryer, to thaw the frostbitten areas; no rubbing or

massaging of affected area; no disturbance of blisters on frostbitten skin; avoidance of smoking or drinking alcoholic beverages while recovering*

References
Murphy JV, Banwell PE, Roberts AH, McGrouther DA (2000) Frostbite: pathogenesis and treatment. Journal of Trauma-Injury Infection & Critical Care 48(1):171–178000

Frostnip

▶ Frostbite

Fuchs' syndrome III

▶ Ascher's syndrome

Fujimoto's disease

▶ Kikuchi's syndrome

Fuller-Albright syndrome

▶ McCune-Albright syndrome

Fungal mycetoma

▶ Eumycetoma

Fungal nail infection

▶ Onychomycosis

Furrowed tongue

▶ Lingua plicata

Furuncle

Synonym(s)
Boil; carbuncle (aggregation of several furuncles); abscess; furunculosis (multiple or recurrent furuncles)

Definition
Acute infection of the hair follicle and perifollicular tissue, usually caused by a Staphlococcal pathogen

Pathogenesis
S. aureus usual infective organism; host factors: follicular abnormality; maceration; ingrown hair; friction; minor skin trauma; colonization in the nares; diabetes mellitus; immunosuppression; poor nutrition or hygiene; exposure to harsh irritants; carbuncles with predisposition to thicker areas of skin, such as nape of neck and thigh

Clinical manifestation
Occurs only in hair-bearing areas; most common on neck, face, axillae, buttocks, thighs; presents as red, painful papule or nodule, enlarging over a few days; spontaneous rupture yields pus and necrotic debris; resolution with post-inflammatory hyperpigmentation

Differential diagnosis
Hidradenitis suppurativa; folliculitis; acne; inflamed epidermoid cyst; myiasis; foreign body reaction; factitial disease

Therapy
Medical therapy: dicloxacillin; cephalexin; azithromycin.
Surgical therapy: incision and drainage if fluctuance.

General therapy: warm compresses applied
3–4 times per day

References

Stulberg DL, Penrod MA, Blatny RA (2002) Common bacterial skin infections. American Family Physician 66(1):119–124

Furunculosis

▶ Furuncle

G

Gamasid rickettsiosis

▶ Rickettsialpox

Gangrene

Synonym(s)
Mortification

Definition
Term used to describe the decay or death of an organ or tissue caused by a lack of blood supply; a complication of infectious or inflammatory processes, injury, or degenerative changes associated with chronic diseases

References
Cha JY, Releford BJ Jr, Marcarelli P (1994) Necrotizing fasciitis: a classification of necrotizing soft tissue infections. Journal of Foot & Ankle Surgery 33(2):148–155

Gardner syndrome

Synonym(s)
Gardner's syndrome; familial adenomatous polyposis; familial polyposis of the colon

Definition
Disorder characterized by gastrointestinal polyps, multiple osteomas, and skin and soft tissue tumors

Pathogenesis
Autosomal dominant trait; mutations in the adenomatous polyposis coli gene on chromosome 5q21-22, which is a tumor suppressor gene

Clinical manifestation
Multiple epidermoid cysts; desmoid tumors; fibrous tumors; osteomas, often on the maxilla or mandible; congenital hypertrophy of retinal pigment epithelium; miscellaneous findings: tyroid carcinoma; adrenal adenoma; urinary bladder carcinoma; hepatoblastoma

Differential diagnosis
Peutz-Jeghers syndrome; Cowden disease; juvenile polyposis syndrome

Therapy
Early prophylactic colectomy[*]; genetic counseling; surgical excision of cysts and desmoids only for symptomatic relief

References
Tsao H (2000) Update on familial cancer syndromes and the skin. Journal of the American Academy of Dermatology 42(6):939-969

Garlic glove fibroma

▶ **Acquired digital fibrokeratoma**

Gas gangrene

Synonym(s)
Clostridial myonecrosis

Definition
Infection of muscle tissue by toxin-producing clostridia organisms

Pathogenesis
Anaerobic, gram-positive, spore-forming bacillus of the genus *Clostridium*, of which *C perfringens* is the most common species; organism produces multiple exotoxins injurious to tissue

Clinical manifestation
Posttraumatic gas gangrene: recent serious injury to the skin or soft tissues or open fractures
Postoperative gas gangrene: history of recent surgery of the gastrointestinal tract or the biliary tract
Occult malignancy-associated spontaneous gas gangrene: no obvious preceding event; gas gangrene presents with sudden onset of pain, with low-grade fever and apathetic mental status; local swelling and serosanguineous exudate appear soon after onset of pain; skin turns to a bronze color, then progresses to a blue-black color with hemorrhagic bullae; entire region sometimes becomes markedly edematous within hours; wound may be nonodorous or have a sweet mousy odor; crepitus following gas production; pain and tenderness to palpation disproportionate to wound appearance; late signs: hypotension, renal failure, and a paradoxical heightening of mental acuity

Differential diagnosis
Cellulitis; necrotizing fasciitis; abortion; bacterial sepsis; abdominal abscess

Therapy
Combination of penicillin G and intravenous clindamycin⋆; combination of clindamycin and metronidazole in penicillin-allergic patients; fasciotomy for compartment syndrome⋆; surgical debridement of necrotic tissue; hyperbaric oxygen

References
Chapnick EK, Abter EI (1996) Necrotizing soft-tissue infections. Infectious Disease Clinics of North America 10(4):835–855

Gastrointestinal polyposis syndrome, generalized, associated with hyperpigmentation, alopecia, and nail atrophy

▶ **Cronkhite-Canada syndrome**

Gaucher's disease

Synonym(s)
Glucosyl cerebroside lipidosis; glucosylceramide lipidosis

Definition
Group of diseases resulting from an inborn error of glycosphingolipid metabolism caused by the deficient activity of the lysosomal hydrolase, acid beta-glucosidase, and resulting in progressive accumulation of undegraded glycolipid substrates, particularly glucosylceramide, in the bone marrow, liver, and spleen

Pathogenesis
Autosomal recessive disorder; inborn error of glycosphingolipid metabolism caused by

the deficient activity of the lysosomal hydrolase, acid beta-glucosidase

Clinical manifestation
Presenting symptom in all types: excessive fatigue associated with a hypochromic anemia and splenomegaly
Type 1 (adult nonneuronopathic form): onset of the manifestations from early childhood to late adulthood; generalized yellowish bronze hyperpigmentation; bleeding, secondary to thrombocytopenia, manifested as epistaxis and ecchymoses; sequlae of monoclonal gammopathy or multiple myeloma
Type 2 (infantile or acute neuronopathic type): collodion-type skin changes or ichthyosis; hepatosplenomegaly; rapid neurologic deterioration, leading to death within the first year of life
Type 3 (juvenile, Norrbotten, or subacute neuronopathic form): neurologic signs such as deficits in eye movements, cerebellar abnormalities, tonic-clonic seizures, or myoclonus; hypersplenism and skeletal changes similar to those in the chronic nonneuronopathic form

Differential diagnosis
Addison's disease; phytophotodermatitis; traumatic ecchymosis

Therapy
Human placental and recombinant glucocerebrosidase; bone marow transplantation

References
Schiffmann R, Brady RO (2002) New prospects for the treatment of lysosomal storage diseases. Drugs 62(5):733–742

Generalized lentiginosis

▶ LEOPARD syndrome

Generalized lipodystrophy

▶ Berardinelli-Seip syndrome

Genetic hemochromatosis

▶ Hemochromatosis

Genital wart

▶ Condyloma acuminatum

Geographic tongue

▶ Benign migratory glossitis

German measles

▶ Rubella

Gianotti-Crosti syndrome

Synonym(s)
Papular acrodermatitis of childhood; papulovesicular acrolocated syndrome; acropapulo-vesicular syndrome; infantile papular acrodermatitis; infantile lichenoid acrodermatitis; erythemato-papulous acrodermatitis; erythemato-vesiculo-papulous eruptive syndrome; acrodermatitis papulosa eruptiva infantilis; papular infantile acrodermatitis; acrodermatitis papulosa

infantum; infantile eruptive papulous dermatitis

Definition
Self-limited, childhood exanthem occurring in characteristic distribution and associated with multiple infectious agents

Pathogenesis
Associated with mostly viral agents, including hepatitis B, Epstein-Barr virus (EBV), respiratory syncytial virus (RSV), coxsackievirus and other enteroviruses, parainfluenza virus, parvovirus B19, poxvirus, cytomegalovirus (CMV), human herpesvirus 6 (HHV-6); some occurrences follow immunization with measles-mumps-rubella, poliovirus, and influenza virus vaccines

Clinical manifestation
Pale, pink-to-flesh-colored papules localized symmetrically over the extremities, the buttocks, and the face; papules sometimes have a smooth-topped, polished, or lichenoid appearance; occasional pruritus; occasional lymphadenopathy and mild constitutional symptoms, such as low-grade fever and malaise; complete resolution after at least 2 months

Differential diagnosis
Pityriasis rosea; pityriasis lichenoides; atopic dermatitis; lichen planus; lichen nitidus; drug eruption; Langerhans cell histiocytosis; flat warts; polymorphous light eruption; sarcoidosis; granuloma annulare; scabies

Therapy
None

References
Nelson JS, Stone MS (2000) Update on selected viral exanthems. Current Opinion in Pediatrics 12(4):359–364

Giant cell arteritis

▸ Temporal arteritis

Giant cell reticulohistiocytosis

▸ Multicentric reticulohistiocytosis

Giant condyloma of Buschke and Löwenstein

Synonym(s)
Giant condylomata acuminata of Buschke and Löwenstein; anogenital verrucous carcinoma; Buschke-Löwenstein tumor; giant malignant condyloma

Definition
Slow-growing, locally destructive, verrucous carcinoma, typically appearing on the penis but sometimes occurring elsewhere in the anogenital region

Pathogenesis
Unclear; possibly a human papilloma virus-induced neoplasm; other possible etiologic factors: chronic phimosis and poor penile hygiene

Clinical manifestation
Presents on the prepuce as a keratotic plaque, slowly expanding into a cauliflower-like mass; sometimes ulcerate or forms a penile horn; associated with a foul odor; expansion to the corpus cavernosum and urethra may occur with subsequent fistulation; regional lymphadenopathy common, primarily due to secondary infection

Differential diagnosis
Condyloma acuminata; squamous cell carcinoma

Therapy
Surgical excision*; interferon

References
Kanik AB, Lee J, Wax F, Bhawan J (1997) Penile verrucous carcinoma in a 37-year-old circumcised man. Journal of the American Academy of Dermatology 37(2 Pt 2):329–331

Giant condylomata acuminata of Buschke and Löwenstein

► Giant condyloma of Buschke and Löwenstein

Giant follicle

► Dilated pore

Giant hemangioma syndrome

► Kasabach-Merritt syndrome

Giant malignant condyloma

► Giant condyloma of Buschke and Löwenstein

Gingivitis, desquamative

► Desquamative gingivitis

Glanders and melioidosis

Synonym(s)
Farcy; morve; malleus (glanders); Whitmore disease (melioidosis)

Definition
Related diseases produced by bacteria of the *Burkholderia* species, which are gram-negative rods

Pathogenesis
Causative agent of Glanders: Burkholderia mallei; primarily a disease of animals such as horses, mules, and donkeys; once in the host, synthesis and release of certain toxins occur; melioidosis: caused by the bacterium Burkholderia pseudomallei; organism distributed widely in the soil and water of the tropics and spread to humans through direct contact with a contaminated source

Clinical manifestation
Similar clinical syndrome in both diseases.
Localized form: bacteria enter the skin through a laceration or abrasion; local infection with ulceration and regional lymphadenopathy; incubation period 1–5 days; bacteria that enter the host through mucous membranes sometimes cause increased mucus production in the affected areas
Pulmonary form: occurs when bacteria are aerosolized and enter respiratory tract via inhalation or hematogenous spread; with inhalational melioidosis, cutaneous abscesses may develop; septicemia: when bacteria disseminated in the bloodstream in glanders, usually fatal within 7–10 days
Chronic form: multiple abscesses affecting the liver, spleen, skin, or muscles

Differential diagnosis
Anthrax; plague; tuberculosis; atypical mycobacterial infection; brucellosis; North American blastomycosis; coccidioidomycosis; nocardia infection

Therapy
Amoxicillin; tetracycline

References
Rosenbloom M, Leikin JB, Vogel SN, Chaudry ZA (2002) Biological and chemical agents: a brief synopsis. American Journal of Therapeutics 9(1):5–14

Glomangioma

▶ Glomus tumor

Glomus tumor

Synonym(s)
Glomangioma

Definition
Benign neoplasm of modified smooth muscle cells (glomus cells)

Pathogenesis
Unknown cause for solitary lesion; multiple glomus tumors, especially those of the disseminated form, inherited as autosomal-dominant trait with incomplete penetrance; tumors arise from the arterial portion of the glomus body

Clinical manifestation
Solitary glomus tumor: paroxysmal pain, which can be severe and exacerbated by pressure or temperature changes, especially cold; blanchable blue or purple papule, located most commonly in acral areas, especially subungual areas of fingers and toes
Multiple glomus tumors: pain relatively uncommon
• Regional variant: blue-to-purple, compressible papules or nodules that are grouped and limited to a specific area, most commonly an extremity
• Disseminated variant: multiple lesions distributed over the body with no specific grouping; congenital plaquelike glomus tumors: grouped papules coalescing into indurated plaques or clusters of discrete nodules

Differential diagnosis
Angioleiomyoma; angiolipoma; arteriovenous malformation; blue nevus; hemangioma; melanoma; spiradenoma; tufted angioma; Kaposi's sarcoma; blue rubber bleb nevus; neurilemmoma

Therapy
Solitary glomus tumor: surgical excision[★]; multiple glomus tumors: surgical removal for cosmetic reasons only

References
Alam M, Scher RK (1999) Current topics in nail surgery. Journal of Cutaneous Medicine & Surgery 3(6):324–335
Parsons ME, Russo G, Fucich L, Millikan LE, Kim R (1997) Multiple glomus tumors. International Journal of Dermatology 36(12):894–900

Glossodynia

Definition
Painful sensation in the tongue

References
Marbach JJ (1999) Medically unexplained chronic orofacial pain. Temporomandibular pain and dysfunction syndrome, orofacial phantom pain, burning mouth syndrome, and trigeminal neuralgia. Medical Clinics of North America 83(3):691–710

Glucagonoma syndrome

Synonym(s)
Necrolytic migratory erythema

Definition
Glucagon-secreting tumor associated with hyperglucagonemia, necrolytic migratory

erythema, and diabetes mellitus; hypoaminoacidemia; cheilosis; normochromic, normocytic anemia; venous thrombosis; weight loss; neuropsychiatric signs and symptoms; pseudoglucagonoma syndrome: necrolytic migratory erythema without a glucogon-secreting tumor, but with another underlying cause such as cirrhosis, celiac sprue, or pancreatitis

Pathogenesis
Unclear relation between glucagonoma and skin findings; levels of glucagon not well correlated with the episodic course of the skin manifestations; possible role of relative zinc deficiency; theories of causation: related to glucagon-induced hypoalbuminemia; zinc-dependent delta-6 desaturation of linoleic acid; poor hepatic breakdown of glucagon contributing to an excessive prostaglandin-mediated inflammatory response

Clinical manifestation
Presents with nonspecific complaints, such as weight loss, diabetes mellitus, diarrhea, and stomatitis; necrolytic migratory erythema: found anywhere on the body, but most common in the perineum, buttocks, groin, lower abdomen, and lower extremities; eruption starts as a pruritic or painful, erythematous patch that blisters centrally, erodes, crusts over, and heals with hyperpigmentation; annular lesions with confluence into plaques; confluence in severely affected areas; associated mucocutaneous findings, including atrophic glossitis, cheilosis, dystrophic nails, and buccal mucosal inflammation

Differential diagnosis
Acrodermatitis enteropathica; candidiasis; paraneoplastic pemphigus; Hailey-Hailey disease; Darier disease; pellagra; kwashiorkor

Therapy
Surgical resection of the tumor, if localized[*]; in the absence of tumor, treat underlying cause[*]

References
Chastain MA (2001) The glucagonoma syndrome: a review of its features and discussion of new perspectives. American Journal of the Medical Sciences 321(5):306–320

Glucosyl cerebroside lipidosis

▶ Gaucher's disease

Glucosylceramide lipidosis

▶ Gaucher's disease

Glycolic acid

▶ Alpha hydroxy acid

Glyderm plus

▶ Alpha hydroxy acids

Goltz syndrome

▶ Focal dermal hypoplasia

Goltz-Gorlin syndrome

▶ Focal dermal hypoplasia

Goltz's syndrome

▶ **Focal dermal hypoplasia**

Gonadal dysgenesis

▶ **Turner syndrome**

Gonococcal dermatitis-arthritis syndrome

▶ **Gonococcemia**

Gonococcemia

Synonym(s)
Gonococcal dermatitis-arthritis syndrome; disseminated gonococcal infection

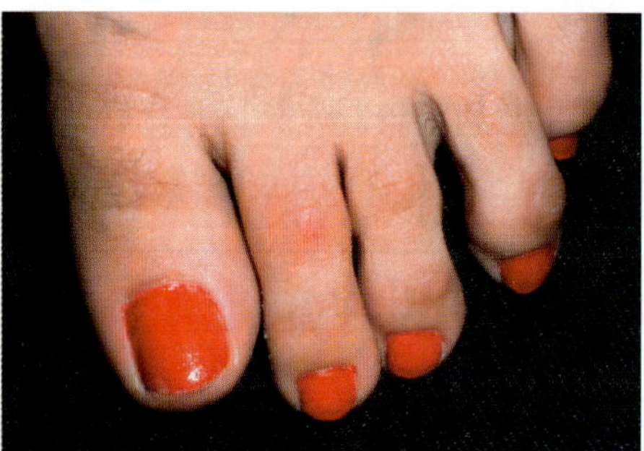

Gonococcemia. Violaceous papule on the toe

Definition
Sexually transmitted disease caused by the bacterium Neisseria gonorrhoeae, which spreads from the initial site of infection through the bloodstream to other parts of the body

Pathogenesis
Neisseria gonorrhoeae transmitted through vaginal, oral, and anal intercourse; infection also transmitted by a woman to her newborn during childbirth; dissemination often occurs during menses

Clinical manifestation
More common in women, often with asymptomatic infection; disseminated disease generally follows the primary genital infection by several days to 2 weeks; fever; myalgias; tenosynovitis; monoarticular septic arthritis, affecting large, weight-bearing joints; acral palpable purpuric papules and pustules, usually relatively few in number

Differential diagnosis
Meningococcemia or other infectious causes of septic vasculitis; lupus erythematosus; cryoglobulinemia; Reiter syndrome; infective endocarditis

Therapy
Ceftriaxone 1 gm intramuscularly or intravenously every 24 hours for 3 days or until 24 hours after symptomatic improvement; complete 7-day course with ciprofloxacin 500 mg PO twice daily or cefixime 400 mg PO twice daily or azithromycin 500 mg PO per day*; concurrent therapy for presumed chlamydia with doxycycline 100 mg PO twice daily for 7 days

References
Brown TJ, Yen-Moore A, Tyring SK (1999) An overview of sexually transmitted diseases. Part I. Journal of the American Academy of Dermatology 41(4):511–532

Gorlin syndrome

▶ **Basal cell nevus syndrome**

Gorlin-Goltz syndrome

▶ Basal cell nevus syndrome

Gottron's syndrome

▶ Acrogeria

Gougerot and Blum, lichenoid pigmented purpura

▶ Benign pigmented purpura

Gougerot-Carteaud papillomatosis

▶ Confluent and reticulated papillomatosis

Gougerot-Houwer-Sjögren syndrome

▶ Sjögren syndrome

Gowers' local panatrophy

▶ Panatrophy of Gowers

Gowers' panatrophy

▶ Panatrophy of Gowers

Graft versus host disease

Synonym(s)

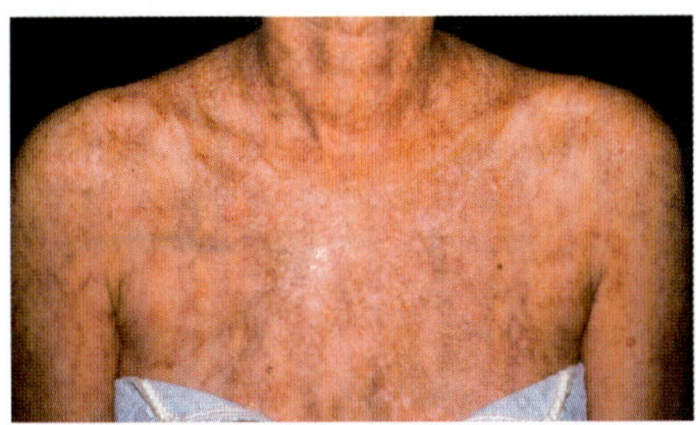

Graft versus host disease. Sclerotic, hyperpigmented and hypopigmented plaques on the upper trunk

Definition
Immunologic assault and its consequences when immunologically competent cells are introduced into an immunoincompetent host

Pathogenesis
Three criteria for development – (1) graft containing immunologically competent cells, (2) host appearing foreign to the graft, (3) host incapable of reacting sufficiently against the graft; recognition of epithelial target tissues as foreign by the immunocompetent cells, with subsequent induction of an inflammatory response and eventual apoptotic death of the target tissue; reaction against the host's keratinocytes, resulting in the clinical syndrome

Clinical manifestation
Incidence higher in recipients of allogeneic hematopoietic cells than in patients receiving syngeneic or autologous hematopoietic

cells; greatest incidence in patients in whom bone marrow is used as the source of hematopoietic cells

Acute graft versus host disease: observed 10–30 days posttransplant; eruptions usually begin as faint, tender, erythematous macules, often centered around hair follicles; as disease progresses, macules sometimes coalesce to form confluent plaques or papules; subepidermal bullae may occur

Chronic graft versus host disease: evolves from acute form in 70–90% of patients; risk increases with the severity of acute reaction; violaceous lichenified papules, often on the ventral skin surfaces, very similar to those of lichen planus; lacy white plaques on the buccal mucosa; scattered sclerodermatous plaques; widespread disease resulting in ulcerations, joint contractures, and esophageal dysmotility

Differential diagnosis

Acute graft versus host disease: erythema multiforme; drug eruption; Stevens-Johnson syndrome/toxic epidermal necrolysis; eruption of lymphocyte recovery

Chronic graft versus host disease: scleroderma; lichen planus; lichenoid drug eruption; lupus erythematosus

Therapy

Acute graft versus host disease: prednisone; extracorporeal photochemotherapy

Chronic graft versus host disease: photochemotherapy; methotrexate; extracorporeal photochemotherapy; hydroxychloroquine; etretinate

References

Jacobsohn DA, Vogelsang GB (2002) Novel pharmacotherapeutic approaches to prevention and treatment of GVHD. Drugs 62(6):879–889

Granular bacteriosis

▶ **Botryomycosis**

Granular cell myoblastoma

▶ Granular cell tumor

Granular cell neurofibroma

▶ Granular cell tumor

Granular cell neuroma

▶ Granular cell tumor

Granular cell schwannoma

▶ Granular cell tumor

Granular cell tumor

Synonym(s)

Granular cell myoblastoma; granular cell schwannoma; granular cell neuroma; granular cell neurofibroma; Abrikossof's tumor

Definition

Acquired tumor of neural crest origin, characterized by cells with eosinophilic cytoplasmic granules

Pathogenesis

Possible tumor derivation from Schwann cells

Clinical manifestation

Discrete, asymptomatic, firm, flesh-colored nodule, located within or beneath the dermis, occurring in the tongue, head, and neck region or dorsal aspect of the forearms

Differential diagnosis
Fibroma; squamous cell carcinoma; wart; dermatofibroma; neurofibroma; epidermoid cyst

Therapy
Surgical excision*

References
Becelli R, Perugini M, Gasparini G, Cassoni A, Fabiani F (2001) Abrikossoff's tumor. Journal of Craniofacial Surgery 12(1):78–81

Granuloma, actinic

▶ Actinic granuloma

Granuloma annulare

Synonym(s)
None

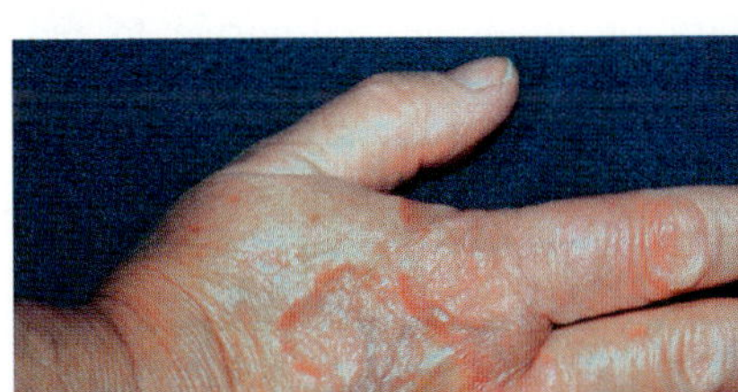

Granuloma annulare. Annular red-brown plaques on the dorsal aspect of the hand

Definition
Inflammatory skin disease characterized by annular plaques consisting of small papules

Pathogenesis
May involve immune mechanisms

Clinical manifestation
Localized variant: flesh-colored to dull red papules, often in an annular arrangement, over distal extremities; often occur over dorsal surfaces of feet, hands and fingers, and the extensor aspects of arms and legs
Generalized variant: few to thousands of flesh-colored to dull red papules involving multiple body regions, often in symmetrical distribution; papules may coalesce into annular or arcuate plaques; may have large red patches (vascular granuloma annulare)
Subcutaneous variant: firm, nontender, flesh-colored-to-pinkish papules or nodules without overlying epidermal alteration, often over the lower extremity

Differential diagnosis
Erythema annulare centrifugum; tinea corporis; lichen planus; lupus erythematosus; insect bite reaction; sarcoidosis; Lyme disease; necrobiosis lipoidica; rheumatoid nodules; acquired perforating disease; lichen myxedematosus; cutaneous T-cell lymphoma; erythema multiforme

Therapy
Localized disease: intralesional triamcinolone; corticosteroids, topical, superpotent
Generalized disease: photochemotherapy

References
Smith MD, Downie JB, DiCostanzo D (1997) Granuloma annulare. International Journal of Dermatology 36(5):326–333

Granuloma faciale

Synonym(s)
Facial granuloma; granuloma faciale eosinophilicum, granuloma faciale with eosinophilia

Definition
Benign chronic skin disease of unknown origin, characterized by single or multiple cutaneous nodules, usually occurring over the face

Pathogenesis
Sun exposure possible factor in development

Clinical manifestation
Solitary or multiple, sharply marginated, red or violaceous papules or nodules; surface sometimes has telangiectasias and/or enlarged follicular orifices; usually occurs on the face, but also on the upper extremities or trunk

Differential diagnosis
Sarcoidosis, granuloma annulare; discoid lupus erythematosus; mycosis fungoides; fixed drug eruption; Jessner's lymphocytic infiltrate; lymphoma; leprosy; lupus vulgaris; foreign body granuloma

Therapy
Triamcinolone 3–4 mg per ml intralesional; dapsone

References
Inanir I, Alvur Y (2001) Granuloma faciale with extrafacial lesions. British Journal of Dermatology 145(2):360–362

Granuloma faciale eosinophilicum

► Granuloma faciale

Granuloma faciale with eosinophilia

► Granuloma faciale

Granuloma fissuratum

► Acanthoma fissuratum

Granuloma gluteale infantum

Synonym(s)
Kaposi's sarcoma-like granuloma; granuloma intertriginosum infantum; infantile vegetating halogenosis; vegetating potassium bromide toxic dermatitis; vegetating bromidism

Definition
Disease characterized by oval, granulomatous nodules on the gluteal surfaces and groin areas of infants

Pathogenesis
Unclear; unusual cutaneous response to local inflammation, maceration, and secondary infection; contact occlusion probably predisposing factor

Clinical manifestation
Solitary or mulptiple, red-purple to red-brown, firm-to-hard, discrete dermal nodules with smooth or slightly lichenified surfaces; aligned with the long axis parallel to the skin folds; located on the gluteal surfaces, in the groin area, upper thighs, lower abdomen, or rarely the neck and face

Differential diagnosis
Langerhans cell histiocytosis; candidiasis; contact dermatitis; lymphoma; mastocytosis; scabies; syphilis; juvenile xanthogranuloma; pyogenic granuloma; sarcoma; foreign body granuloma

Therapy
Spontaneous resolution; no therapy indicated

References

Bluestein J, Furner BB, Phillips D (1990) Granuloma gluteale infantum: case report and review of the literature. Pediatric Dermatology 7(3):196–198

References

Brown TJ, Yen-Moore A, Tyring SK (1999) An overview of sexually transmitted diseases. Part 1. Journal of the American Academy of Dermatology 41(4):511–532

Granuloma inguinale

Synonym(s)
Donovanosis

Definition
Sexually transmitted disease characterized by genital lesions presenting as indolent, progressive ulcerations with a granulomatous appearance

Pathogenesis
Infection caused by a gram-negative pleomorphic bacillus, Calymmatobacterium granulomatis; mode of transmission primarily through sexual contact; mildly contagious

Clinical manifestation
Occurs on glans penis and scrotum in men, and labia minora, mons veneris, and fourchette in women; rare cervical involvement; soft, red papules or nodules arising at the site of inoculation; lesions eventually ulcerate and produce red, friable, granulomatous plaques and nodules; ulcers with clean, friable bases and distinct, raised, rolled margins; autoinoculation results in lesions on adjacent skin; occasional hypertrophic or verrucous plaques, with formation of large, vegetating masses resembling genital warts; swelling of the external genitalia in later-stage lesions

Differential diagnosis
Syphilis; lymphogranuloma venereum; chronic herpes simplex virus infection; squamous cell carcinoma; lichen sclerosus

Therapy
Trimethoprim/sulfamethoxazole; doxycycline

Granuloma intertriginosum infantum

▶ Granuloma gluteale infantum

Granuloma pyogenicum

▶ Pyogenic granuloma

Granuloma telangiectaticum

▶ Pyogenic granuloma

Granuloma trichophyticum

▶ Majocchi granuloma

Granuloma tricofitico

▶ Majocchi granuloma

Granulomatosis disciformis chronica et progressiva

▶ Actinic granuloma

Granulomatosis, lymphomatoid

▶ Lymphomatoid granulomatosis

Granulomatosis, Miescher's

▶ Miescher's granulomatosis

Granulomatous arteritis

▶ Temporal arteritis

Granulomatous cheilitis

▶ Cheilitis granulomatosa

Granulomatous disease of childhood

▶ Chronic granulomatous disease

Granulomatous perioral dermatitis

▶ Perioral dermatitis

Granulomatous rosacea

▶ Rosacea

Granulomatous vasculitis

▶ Wegener's granulomatosis

Granulomatous vasculitis with asthma

▶ Churg-Strauss syndrome

Griscelli syndrome

Synonym(s)
Partial albinism with immunodeficiency

Definition
Disease characterized by partial pigmentary dilution with silvery gray hair, frequent infections, cellular immune deficiency, neurologic abnormalities, and fatal outcome from an uncontrolled T lymphocyte and macrophage activation syndrome

Pathogenesis
Caused by two genes: MYA5 and RAB27A; gene MYA5 produces severe neurological problems; gene RAB27A causes accelerated phase sometimes lethal within a short period of time

Clinical manifestation
Silvery blond hair; occasional subtle pigmentary dilution of the skin and iris and hyperpigmentation in sun-exposed areas; accelerated phase of the disease with fever, jaundice, hepatosplenomegaly, lymphadenopathy, pancytopenia and generalized lymphohistiocytic infiltrates of various organs including the central nervous system; neurologic manifestations: hyperreflexia, seizures, signs of intracranial hypertension, regression of developmental milestones,

Griseofulvin. Dermatologic indications and dosage

Disease	Adult dosage	Child dosage
Onychomycosis	500 mg PO twice daily for 6–12 months	5–10 mg per kg PO daily for 6–12 months
Tinea capitis	250–500 mg PO twice daily for 6–8 weeks	25 mg per kg PO daily for 6–8 weeks
Tinea corporis	250–500 mg PO twice daily for 2–6 weeks	5–10 mg per kg PO daily for 2–4 weeks
Tinea cruris	250–500 mg PO twice daily for 2–6 weeks	5–10 mg per kg PO daily for 2–4 weeks
Tinea faciei	250–500 mg PO twice daily for 2–6 weeks	25 mg per kg PO daily for 6–8 weeks

hypertonia, nystagmus, and ataxia; variety of immunological abnormalities, restricted to the patients with RAB27A defect

Differential diagnosis
Hematophagic lymphohistiocytosis; familial lymphohistiocytosis; Chediak-Higashi syndrome; X-linked lymphoproliferative syndrome

Therapy
Bone marrow transplantation*; chemotherapy for accelerated phase

References
Klein C, Philippe N, Le Deist F, Fraitag S, Prost C, Durandy A, Fischer A, Griscelli C (1994). Partial albinism with immunodeficiency (Griscelli syndrome). Journal of Pediatrics 125(6):886–895

Griseofulvin

Trade name(s)
Fulvicin P/G; Gris-PEG; Grifulvin V

Generic available
Yes

Drug class
Oral anti-fungal agent

Mechanism of action
Inhibition of fungal cell wall synthesis

Dosage form
125 mg, 165 mg, 250 mg, 330 mg tablet; 125 mg per 5 ml suspension

Dermatologic indications and dosage
See table

Common side effects
Cutaneous: photosensitivity, vascular reaction
Gastrointestinal: nausea, vomiting, diarrhea, flatulence
Neurologic: dizziness, paresthesias, confusion

Serious side effects
Bone marrow: granulocytopenia
Gastrointestinal: hepatotoxicity

Drug interactions
Amiodarone; barbiturates; carbamazepine; clarithromycin; oral contraceptives; cyclosporine; erythromycin; itraconazole; ketoconazole; protease inhibitors; tacrolimus; warfarin

Other interactions
Ethanol

Contraindications/precautions
Hypersensitivity to drug class or component; acute intermittent porphyria; pregnancy; caution in patients with penicillin allergy or impaired liver function

References
Bennett ML, Fleischer AB. Loveless JW, Feldman SR (2000) Oral griseofulvin remains the treatment of choice for tinea capitis in children. Pediatric Dermatology 17(4):304–309

Groin dermatophytosis

▶ Tinea cruris

Grönblad-Strandberg syndrome

▶ Pseudoxanthoma elasticum

Groove sign

Definition
Enlargement of the nodes above and below the inguinal ligament in patients with lymphogranuloma venereum

References
Brown TJ, Yen-Moore A, Tyring SK (1999) An overview of sexually transmitted diseases. Part I. Journal of the American Academy of Dermatology 41(4):511–532

Grover disease

▶ Transient acantholytic dermatosis

Grover's disease

▶ Transient acantholytic dermatosis

Gumma

Definition
Soft, tumor-like granulomatous growth caused by syphilis, appearing during the late stage, tertiary syphilis, most frequently in the liver but also occurring in the brain, testis, heart, skin, and bone

References
Quinn P, Weisberg L (1997) Cerebral syphilitic gumma. New England Journal of Medicine. 336(14):1027–1028

Günther's disease

▶ Erythropoietic porphyria
▶ Congenital erythropoietic porphyria

Gustatory hyperhidrosis

▶ Auriculotemporal syndrome

Gustatory sweating

▶ Auriculotemporal syndrome

Guttate parapsoriasis

▶ Pityriasis lichenoides
▶ Small plaque parapsoriasis

Guttate psoriasis

▶ Psoriasis

Gym itch

▶ Tinea cruris

H

Haber's syndrome

Synonym(s)
None

Definition
Rosacea-like eruption with keratotic papules and pitted scars

Pathogenesis
Unknown; familial incidence

Clinical manifestation
Permanent flushing of the cheeks, nose, forehead and chin, with erythema and telangiectasia; keratotic papules; atrophic, pitted papules; prominent follicles; comedones

Differential diagnosis
Rosacea; polymorphous light eruption; seborrheic dermatitis; lupus erythematosus; tinea faciei; Dowling Degos disease

Therapy
Light hyfrecation or cryotherapy of keratotic papules; no effective therapy for erythema

References
McCormack CJ, Cowen P (1997) Haber's syndrome. Australasian Journal of Dermatology 38(2):82–84

Hailey-Hailey disease

▶ Familial benign chronic pemphigus

Hair follicle nevus

▶ Trichofolliculoma

Hairy leukoplakia

Synonym(s)
Oral hairy leukoplakia

Definition
Oral infection caused by the Epstein-Barr virus, appearing as white, mildly verrucous lesions on the lateral surfaces of the tongue

Pathogenesis
Caused by Epstein-Barr virus; unclear whether a development following superinfection with EBV or activation of latent infection due to reduced immune surveillance

Clinical manifestation
Asymptomatic, white plaque along the lateral tongue borders, with accentuation of vertical folds; occasionally spreads to the

mouth floor, tonsillar pillars, ventral tongue, and pharynx; occurs almost exclusively in immunocompromised patients, particularly those infected with HIV

Differential diagnosis
Wart; syphilis; premalignant leukoplakia ("smoker's leukoplakia"); traumatic leukoplakia; squamous cell carcinoma; candidiasis; geographic tongue; lichen planus

Therapy
None

References
Itin PH, Lautenschlager S, Fluckiger R, Rufli T (1993) Oral manifestations in HIV-infected patients: diagnosis and management. Journal of the American Academy of Dermatology 29(5 Pt 1):749–760

Hairy tongue

Synonym(s)
Black hairy tongue; lingua nigra; lingua villosa; lingua villosa nigra

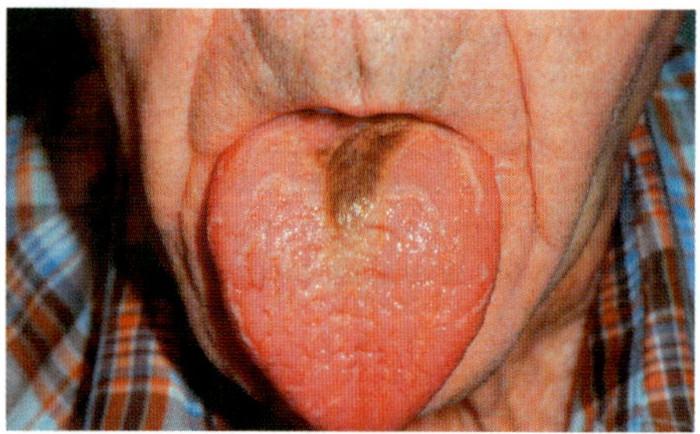

Hairy tongue. Brown, hypertrophic plaque on the tongue

Definition
Condition of defective desquamation of the filiform papillae of the tongue that results in an irregular, discolored plaque, with elongation of filiform papillae and a lack of normal desquamation

Pathogenesis
Inadequate hygiene or microbial overgrowth stimulates elongation of filiform papillae; lack of mechanical stimulation and debridement

Clinical manifestation
Elongation of the filiform papillae on the dorsal surface of the tongue, which retain pigments from food, beverages, and tobacco, resulting in brown, black or reddish discoloration

Differential diagnosis
Candidiasis; lichen planus; oral hairy leukoplakia

Therapy
Mechanical removal of elongated papillae by brushing the tongue with a toothbrush or using a tongue scraper; destruction by electrodesiccation and curettage or CO_2 laser vaporization; tretinoin; acitretin

References
Sarti GM, Haddy RI, Schaffer D, Kihm J (1990) Black hairy tongue. American Family Physician 41(6):1751–1755

Halcinonide

▶ **Corticosteroids, topical, high potency**

Half-and-half nails

Definition
Distal portion of the nail plate assuming a reddish-brown color while more proximal portion remaining white; seen in patients with renal disease and in many normal people

References
Mazuryk HA, Brodkin RH (1991) Cutaneous clues to renal disease. Cutis 47(4):241–248

Hallermann-Streiff syndrome

Synonym(s)
Francois dyscephaly syndrome; Hallermann-Streiff-Francois syndrome; oculomandibulodyscephaly with hypotrichosis; oculomandibulofacial syndrome

Definition
Genetic disorder characterized by malformations of the skull and facial region, sparse hair, ocular abnormalities, dental defects, degenerative skin changes, and short stature

Pathogenesis
Unknown

Clinical manifestation
Skin findings: sparse hair; atrophy, particularly in the scalp and nasal regions
Craniofacial features: brachycephaly with frontal and/or parietal bossing; small, underdeveloped lower jaw; narrow, highly arched palate; thin, pinched, tapering nose
Ocular findings: congenital cataracts; microphthalmia; other ocular abnormalities
Dental defects: presence of natal teeth; hypodontia or partial adontia malformation; and/or improper alignment of teeth
Skeletal findings: short stature

Differential diagnosis
Progeria; Werner's syndrome

Therapy
None

References
Cohen MM Jr (1991) Hallermann-Streiff syndrome: a review. American Journal of Medical Genetics 41(4):488–499

Hallermann-Streiff-Francois syndrome

▶ Hallermann-Streiff syndrome

Hallopeau, acrodermatitis continua

▶ Acrodermatitis continua of Hallopeau

Halo nevus

Synonym(s)
Sutton's nevus; nevus of Sutton; leukoderma acquisita centrifugum

Definition
Benign skin lesion representing melanocytic nevus in which an inflammatory response produces zone of depigmentation surrounding the lesion

Pathogenesis
Unclear; apparently an immunologic reaction against melanocyte; cells predominantly T lymphocytes; precipitating cause and exact role of lymphocytes unknown

Clinical manifestation
One or more, uniformly colored, evenly shaped, round or oval pigmented papules or macule, with regular peripheral hypopigmentation; seen most frequently on the trunk; repigmentation may take place over months or years, but lesion sometimes remains white indefinitely

Differential diagnosis
Vitiligo; atypical mole; melanoma; tinea versicolor; lichen sclerosus; morphea; post-traumatic hypopigmentation

Therapy
None indicated for childhood lesions; surgical excision for adult-onset lesions, although considered controversial

References
Zeff RA, Freitag A, Grin CM, Grant-Kels JM (1997) The immune response in halo nevi. Journal of the American Academy of Dermatology 37(4):620–624

Halobetasol propionate

▶ Corticosteroids, topical, super potency

Halodermia

▶ Knuckle pads

Halogenoderma

Synonym(s)
Bromoderma; iododerma; fluoroderma

Definition
Skin eruption resulting from exposure to bromide-containing drugs or substances such as potassium bromide (bromoderma), iodide-containing drugs or substances such as water-soluble contrast media (iododerma), or fluoride-containing drugs or substances such as fluoride teeth gels (fluoroderma)

Pathogenesis
May represent a delayed hypersensitivity allergic response

Clinical manifestation
Bromoderma: multiple, vegetative, ulcerating and pustular plaques with elevated papillomatous borders, located mainly on the legs, but also on the face
Iododerma: vesicular, pustular, hemorrhagic, suppurative, and/or ulcerative papules and plaques occurring on the areas of skin with the highest concentration of sebaceous glands, such as the face
Fluoroderma: resembles iododerma, with numerous and scattered papules and nodules

Differential diagnosis
Tuberculosis; sarcoidosis; North American blastomycosis; rosacea; pyoderma gangrenosum; acute febrile neutrophilic dermatosis; syphilitic gumma; pemphigus vegetans

Therapy
Discontinuation of causative agent[*]

References
Alagheband M, Engineer L (2000) Lithium and halogenoderma. Archives of Dermatology 136(1):126–127

Hanhart-Richner syndrome

▶ Tyrosinemia II

Hansen disease

▶ Leprosy

Hansen's disease

▶ Leprosy

Harada syndrome

▶ Vogt-Koyanagi-Harada syndrome

Harlequin baby

▶ Ichthyosis fetalis

Harlequin fetus

▶ Ichthyosis fetalis

Harlequin ichthyosis

▶ Ichthyosis fetalis

Hartnup aminoaciduria

▶ Hartnup disease

Hartnup disease

Synonym(s)
Hartnup disorder, Hartnup aminoaciduria, Hartnup syndrome

Definition
Disorder caused by defective transport of neutral amino acids in the small intestine and kidney, resulting in a pellagra-like skin eruption, cerebellar ataxia, and aminoaciduria

Pathogenesis
Failure of the transport of tryptophan and other neutral alpha-amino acids in the small intestine and renal tubules; abnormality in tryptophan transport, leading to niacin deficiency that is responsible for pellagra-like eruption and photosensitivity

Clinical manifestation
Gingivitis, stomatitis, glossitis; photosensitivity; multiple sun exposures leading to dry, scaly, well-marginated plaques, resembling chronic eczema, affecting preferentially the forehead, cheeks, periorbital regions, dorsal surface of the hands, and other light-exposed areas; vesiculobullous eruption with exudation sometimes occurs; hypopigmentation and/or hyperpigmentation that is intensified with further sunlight exposure; intermittent cerebellar ataxia with wide-based gait, spasticity, delayed motor development, and tremulousness, all reversible with niacin therapy; diarrhea; attacks sometimes provoked by a febrile illness, poor nutrition, sulfonamides, and possibly emotional stress

Differential diagnosis
Polymorphous light eruption; lupus erythematosus; atopic dermatitis; seborrheic dermatitis; nutritional pellagra; Cockayne syndrome; carcinoid syndrome; ataxia telangiectasia; xeroderma pigmentosum

Therapy
Niacin 50–100 mg PO 3 times per day[*]; avoidance of sun exposure; high protein diet

References
Kahn G (1986) Photosensitivity and photodermatitis in childhood. Dermatologic Clinics 4(1):107–116

Hartnup disorder

▶ Hartnup disease

Hartnup syndrome

▶ Hartnup disease

Hashimoto-Pritzker disease

▶ Congenital self-healing Langerhans cell histiocytosis

HAT

▶ African trypanosomiasis

Haverhill fever

▶ Rat-bite fever

Haxthausen's disease

▶ Cold panniculitis

Heat rash

▶ Miliaria

Hebra's disease

▶ Erythema multiforme

Hecht-Beals syndrome

▶ Beals-Hecht syndrome

Heloma

▶ Clavus

Hemangiectasia hypertrophicans

▶ Klippel-Trenaunay-Weber syndrome

Hemangioendothelioma

Synonym(s)
None

Definition
Varied group of proliferative and neoplastic vascular lesions, with a biological behavior falling somewhere between the benign hemangioma and malignant angiosarcoma

Pathogenesis
Unknown

Clinical manifestation
Epithelioid hemangioendothelioma: soliatary, sometimes painful, soft tissue mass, sometimes ulcerating, most commonly on the lower extremities
Spindle cell hemangioendothelioma: firm blue papules or nodules, often multifocal within given anatomic sites, occurring over the distal extremities
Kaposiform hemangioendothelioma: usually in retroperitoneum, but sometimes

occurring in the skin; bluish papule or nodule; associated with consumption coagulopathy and lymphangiomatosis

Retiform hemangioendothelioma: slow-growing plaque with ill-defined borders, usually on the distal extremities

Differential diagnosis
Angiosarcoma; Dabska tumor; Kaposi's sarcoma; hemangioma

Therapy
Wide local excision*

References
Grezard P, Balme B, Ceruse P, Bailly C, Dujardin T, Perrot H (1999) Ulcerated cutaneous epithelioid hemangioendothelioma. European Journal of Dermatology 9(6):487–490

Hemangioma

Synonym(s)
Angioma

Definition
Dense collections of dilated vessels occurring in the skin or internal organs

References
Dinehart SM, Kincannon J, Geronemus R (2001) Hemangiomas: evaluation and treatment. Dermatologic Surgery 27(5):475–485

Hemangioma, capillary

▶ Capillary hemangioma

Hemangioma, cavernous

▶ Capillary hemangioma

Hemangioma, cherry

▶ Cherry hemangioma

Hemangiopericytoma

Synonym(s)
None

Definition
Vascular sarcoma derived from pericytes, with distinctive histologic features and a variable course depending on the degree of cellular atypia

Pathogenesis
Unknown

Clinical manifestation
Rapidly enlarging, asymptomatic, well demarcated, soft or rubbery, red or bluish tumor; sessile or somewhat pedunculated; sometimes has surface lobularity or telangiectasis; located at one of many sites, including orbit, neck, mediastinum, epicardium, retroperitoneum, and upper and lower extremity; occurs in all age groups, but rare prior to the second decade or after the seventh decade

Differential diagnosis
Fibrous histiocytoma; malignant fibrous histiocytoma; synovial sarcoma; juxtaglomerular tumor; vascular leiomyoma; juvenile hemangioma; myxoid lipoma; myxoid liposarcoma; mesenchymal chondrosarcoma

Therapy
Bland lesions with minimal mitotic activity: wide local excision*; active and dysplastic lesions: radical surgical excision, with or without adjunctive radiotherapy*

References

Pandey M, Kothari KC, Patel DD (1997) Haemangiopericytoma: current status, diagnosis and management. European Journal of Surgical Oncology 23(4):282–285

Hematoma

Synonym(s)
None

Definition
Collection of blood within soft tissue that results in swelling

References

McGillis ST, Ratner D, Clark R, Madani S, et al. (1998) Atlas of excision and repair. Dermatologic Clinics 16(1):181–194

Hemochromatosis

Synonym(s)
Bronze diabetes, iron deposition disease, hereditary hemochromatosis; genetic hemochromatosis; primary hemochromatosis

Definition
Abnormal accumulation of iron in parenchymal organs, leading to organ toxicity

Pathogenesis
Autosomal recessive trait; associated with two mutations in the *HFE* gene; error of iron metabolism characterized by excess dietary iron absorption and iron deposition in tissues; presence of free iron in biological systems leads to rapid formation of damaging reactive oxygen metabolites, which can produce DNA cleavage, impaired protein synthesis, and impairment of cell integrity and cell proliferation, resulting in cell injury and fibrosis

Clinical manifestation
Generalized hyperpigmentation; ichthyosis; skin atrophy; koilonychia; partial alopecia; diabetes mellitus; cirrhosis; congestive heart failure; hepatomegaly; splenomegaly; arthritis; amenorrhea; loss of libido; impotence; symptoms of hypothyroidism

Differential diagnosis
Addison's disease; polymorphous light eruption; post-inflammatory hyperpigmentation; sun-induced tanning; drug-induced hyperpigmentation; actinic reticuloid; poikiloderma of Civatte; argyria; iron overload associated with chronic anemia; multiple blood transfusions; hyperplastic erythroid marrow from diseases such as hereditary sideroblastic anemias, severe alpha and beta thalassemia; myelodysplastic syndrome variants

Therapy
Phlebotomy[*]; limiting of alcohol consumption; avoidance of iron supplements and raw oysters

References

Powell LW (2002) Hereditary hemochromatosis and iron overload diseases. Journal of Gastroenterology & Hepatology 17 Suppl:S191–195

Hemorrhagic jaundice

▶ **Leptospirosis**

Henoch-Schönlein purpura

Synonym(s)
Anaphylactoid purpura; Schönlein-Henoch purpura

Definition
Immunoglobulin (Ig)A-mediated small-vessel vasculitis with involvement of the skin,

gastrointestinal tract, joints, and kidneys, occurring primarily in children

Pathogenesis
Vascular deposition of IgA immune complexes, which activate complement components, which mediate tissue injury

Clinical manifestation
Prodrome of fever, anorexia, and headache; erythematous macules and papules on buttocks and extremities, which become purpuric; colic, vomiting, and diarrhea; polyarthralgia; proteinuria and hematuria

Differential diagnosis
Urticaria; lupus erythematosus; Churg-Strauss syndrome; essential mixed cryoglobulinemia; polyarteritis nodosa; rheumatoid arthritis; benign pigmented purpura; child abuse; bacterial endocarditis; meningococcemia; Rocky Mountain spotted fever

Therapy
Prednisone; dapsone; azathioprine; intravenous immunoglobulin (IVIG)

References
Saulsbury FT (2001) Henoch-Schonlein purpura. Current Opinion in Rheumatology 13(1):35–40

Heparin necrosis

Synonym(s)
None

Definition
Necrotic areas of skin, usually at the site of heparin injection, characterizing a localized hypersensitivity reaction

Pathogenesis
Possible immunologic basis

Clinical manifestation
Begins as localized erythema, typically at heparin injection sites, usually in women;

burning pain; progression to bulla formation and necrosis over a few days; more common in obese or diabetic patients

Differential diagnosis
Pyoderma gangrenosum; calciphylaxis; spider bite reaction; factitial disease; bacterial pyoderma; herpes simplex virus infection; fixed drug eruption

Therapy
Discontinuance of heparin therapy[*]; hydrocolloid dressings to ulcerated area; ulcer excision and skin grafting if ulceration persists

References
Levine LE, Bernstein JE, Soltani K, Medenica MM, Yung CW (1983) Heparin-induced cutaneous necrosis unrelated to injection sites. Archives of Dermatology 119(5):400–403

Hepatic porphyria

▶ Porphyria cutanea tarda

Hepatolenticular degeneration

▶ Wilson disease

Hereditary angioedema

Synonym(s)
None

Definition
Hereditary disorder characterized by painless, nonpruritic swelling of the skin

Pathogenesis
Mutations in the C1-INH gene, transmitted as an autosomal dominant trait; two vari-

ants: type I – low antigenic and functional plasma levels of C1-INH protein; type II – presence of normal or elevated antigenic levels of a dysfunctional mutant protein together with reduced levels of the functional protein; C1-INH deficiency permits autoactivation of the first component of complement (C1) with consumption of C4 and C2

Clinical manifestation

Recurrent, noninflammatory swelling of the skin and mucous membranes; erythema or mild urticarial eruption occasionally preceding edema; sometimes precipitated by trauma, anxiety, or stress; associated with lupus erythematosus and other autoimmune diseases

Differential diagnosis

Chronic urticaria; pressure-induced urticaria; acquired angioedema; ACE inhibitor-induced angioedema

Therapy

Acute episodes: replacement with C1-INH concentrates[*]; fresh-frozen plasma; prophylaxis: danazol 400–600 mg PO per day

References

Nzeako UC, Frigas E, Tremaine WJ (2001) Hereditary angioedema: a broad review for clinicians. Archives of Internal Medicine 161(20):2417–2429

Hereditary baldness

▶ Androgenetic alopecia

Hereditary coproporphyria

Synonym(s)

None

Definition

One of the porphyrias, characterized by abdominal pain, neuropsychiatric problems, constipation, and skin changes

Pathogenesis

Autosomal dominant disease, resulting from defects in coproporphyrinogen oxidase; related to deposition of formed porphyrins in the skin which become photoactive after sunlight exposure

Clinical manifestation

Skin changes: blisters forming in sun-exposed areas; skin fragility; scarring; hypertrichosis in sun-exposed areas
Neurologic changes: central nervous system signs, including seizures, mental status changes, cortical blindness, and coma; peripheral neuropathies predominantly motor neuropathies; diffuse pain, especially in the upper body; autonomic neuropathies, including hypertension and tachycardia; psychiatric abnormalities

Differential diagnosis

Porphyria cutanea tarda; acute intermittent porphyria; adrenal crisis; biliary disease; fibromyalgia; Addison's disease; acute abdomen from diverse causes; psychosis; lead intoxication

Therapy

Glucose 400 mg IV per day for mild attacks; hematin 4 mg per kg per day for 4 days for acute attacks[*]

References

Lim HW, Cohen JL (1999) The cutaneous porphyrias. Seminars in Cutaneous Medicine & Surgery 18(4):285–292

Hereditary hemochromatosis

▶ Hemochromatosis

Hereditary hemorrhagic telangiectasia

▶ Osler-Weber-Rendu syndrome

Hereditary hidrotic ectodermal dysplasia

▶ Hidrotic ectodermal dysplasia

Hereditary ichthyosis vulgaris

▶ Ichthyosis vulgaris

Hereditary leukokeratosis

▶ White sponge nevus

Hereditary osteo-onychodysplasia

▶ Nail-patella syndrome

Hereditary palmo-plantar keratoderma

▶ Unna-Thost palmoplantar kerato-derma

Hereditary papulotranslucent acrokeratoderma

▶ Acrokeratoelastoidosis

Hereditary symmetrical aplastic nevi of the temples

▶ Brauer's syndrome

Heredofamilial angiomatosis

▶ Osler-Weber-Rendu syndrome

Heredopathia atactica polyneuritiformis

▶ Refsum disease

Herlitz syndrome

▶ Epidermolysis bullosa

Hermansky-Pudlak syndrome

Synonym(s)
None

Definition
Oculocutaneous albinism associated with a mild hemorrhagic diathesis

Pathogenesis
Autosomal recessive inheritance, many with a mutation of the HPS1 gene; storage pool platelet defect with poor platelet aggregation; accumulation of a ceroid lipofuscin in the lysosomes of a variety of tissues

Clinical manifestation
Variable degrees of hypopigmentation; pigmented nevi and freckles common; mild bleeding disorder with epistaxis, easy bruising, hemoptysis, gingival bleeding, and postpartum bleeding; interstitial lung fibrosis; restrictive lung disease; granulomatous colitis

Differential diagnosis
Albinism; Chediak-Higashi syndrome

Therapy
Avoidance of aspirin; low vision evaluation and rehabilitation; sun avoidance

References
Toro J, Turner M, Gahl, WA (1999) Dermatologic manifestations of Hermansky-Pudlak syndrome in patients with and without a 16-base pair duplication in the HPS1 gene. Archives of Dermatology 135(7)774–780

Herpes gestationis

Synonym(s)
Pemphigoid gestationis; autoimmune dermatosis of pregnancy; pregnancy-associated autoimmune disease

Definition
Autoimmune bullous eruption developing in association with pregnancy

Pathogenesis
Immunoglobulin G (IgG) autoantibodies produced against bullous pemphigoid (BP)

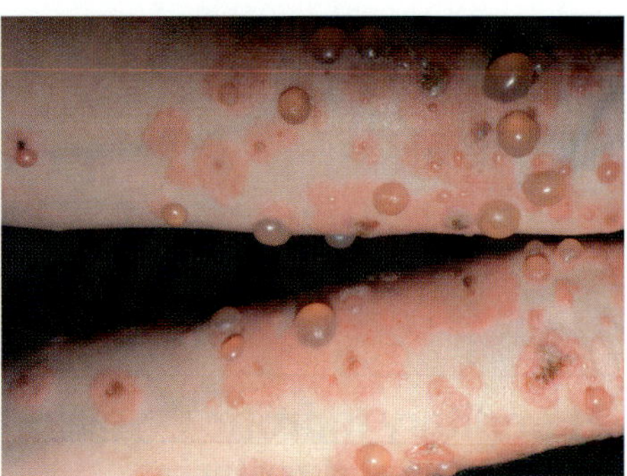

Herpes gestationis. Multiple vesicles and bullae on the upper extremities in a pregnant woman

antigen 2 (BPAG2) (also known as BP 180), which is component of the hemidesmosome; trigger for autoantibody production unknown

Clinical manifestation
Eruption develops during the second and third trimesters; in 25% of patients, lesions appear immediately after delivery, begin as intensely pruritic erythematous urticarial patches and plaques, often periumbilical; lesions progress to tense vesicles and bullae, spreading peripherally, often sparing the face, palms, soles, and mucous membranes; disease activity usually remits within days after parturition; some patients have persistent disease activity that lasts months or years; sometimes recurs with the resumption of menses, use of oral contraceptives, and with subsequent pregnancies

Differential diagnosis
Bullous pemphigoid; linear IgA bullous dermatosis; dermatitis herpetiformis; herpes simplex virus infection; drug-induced bullous disorder; papular dermatitis of pregnancy; prurigo gestationis of Besnier; pruritic urticarial papules and plaques of pregnancy (PUPPP)

Therapy
Mild disease: corticosteroids, topical, high potency.
Severe disease: prednisone*

References

Scott JE, Ahmed AR (1998) The blistering diseases. Medical Clinics of North America 82(6):1239–1283

Herpes gladiatorum

▶ Herpes simplex virus infection

Herpes simplex virus infection

Synonym(s)
None

Definition
Viral infection caused by Herpesvirus hominis (herpes simplex virus)

Pathogenesis
Transmitted through close personal contact; two viral subtypes: HSV-1 transmitted primarily by contact with infected saliva; HSV-2 mainly transmitted sexually; after direct exposure to infectious material (i.e., saliva, genital secretions), initial viral replication occurs at either the skin or mucous membrane entry site; after retrograde axonal flow from neurons at viral point of entry and local replication, viral genome becomes latent and no viral particles are produced; stimulus (e.g., physical or emotional stress, fever, ultraviolet light) causes reactivation of the virus

Clinical manifestation
Neonatal infection: onset of illness within 24 hours of birth; most often, symptoms of illness within the first week of life; rash noted after symptoms begin; manifestations of illness representative of the organ systems involved (i.e., CNS, lungs, gastrointestinal tract, heart, kidneys); skin vesicles develops on an erythematous base, which may coalesce into playues; localized eye infection with conjunctival injection and a watery discharge; dendritic lesions on fluorescein staining of the cornea; acute gingivostomatitis: most frequent clinical presentation of first-episode, primary HSV infection, although most patients have asymptomatic first infection; fever (102–104°F); listlessness or irritability; inability to eat and/or drink; gingivitis with markedly swollen, erythematous, bleeding gums; occasional increased drooling noted in infants; vesicular lesions develop on the tongue, buccal mucosa, and palate, with extension to lips and face; tender submandibular or cervical adenopathy; disease lasting from 3–7 days; recurrent orolabial herpetic infection (herpes labialis): heralded by a prodrome of pain, tingling, burning, or itching, usually lasts up to 6 hours; vesicular rash in crops of 3–5 vesicles, frequently arising near the vermillion border; recurrences often associated with febrile illnesses, local trauma, sun exposure, or menstruation; primary genital infections: most infections asymptomatic; severe constitutional symptoms: fever, malaise, myalgias, and occasional headache; vesicular rash; lesions sometimes persist for up to 3 weeks; painful inguinal lymphadenopathy; dysuria; vaginal discharge; recurrent genital infections: vulvar irritation and/or ulcerating or vesicular lesions; symptoms more severe in females; recurrent infections in males sometimes present with vesicular lesions on the shaft of the penis; local symptoms of recurrence: pain, itching, and dysuria; CNS infection: encephalitis possible manifestation of primary or recurrent infection; other sequelae: aseptic meningitis, transverse myelitis; herpetic whitlow (infection of a digit): presents with acute onset of edema, erythema, and localized pain and tenderness in the finger; associated fever and enlarged regional adenopathy; herpes gladiatorum: begins with painful vesicular lesions, frequently over the shoulders and neck in wrestlers (sites of skin-to-skin contact); Kaposi's varicelliform eruption (eczema herpeticum): clusters of umbilicated vesiculopustules in areas of a pre-existent derma-

titis; transmission occurs through contact with an infected person or by dissemination of primary or recurrent herpes; recurrent episodes sometimes occur, but milder and not usually associated with systemic symptoms; severe cases sometimes cause scarring

Differential diagnosis
Impetigo; candidiasis; varicella; herpes zoster; vesicular dermatophytosis; bullous pemphigoid; pemphigus vulgaris; aphthous stomatitis; Behçet's disease; contact dermatitis

Therapy
Neonatal infection, CNS infection: acyclovir[*]; first episode mucocutaneous infection, recurrent mucocutaneous infection, herpetic whitlow, herpes gladiatorum: valacyclovir, famciclovir; chronic suppression: valacyclovir[*]; famciclovir

References
Simmons A (2002) Clinical manifestations and treatment considerations of herpes simplex virus infection. Journal of Infectious Diseases 186 Suppl 1:S71–77

Herpes zoster

Synonym(s)
Shingles; zoster

Definition
Neurocutaneous infection caused by the varicella-zoster virus, which occurs in people who have had chickenpox; represents a reactivation of the dormant varicella-zoster virus

Pathogenesis
Reactivation of dormant varicella-zoster virus (VZV); results most often from a failure of the immune system to contain latent VZV replication; most commonly occurs in one or more posterior spinal ganglia or cranial sensory ganglia; trigger of reactivation unclear, but some cases possibly related to external re-exposure to the virus, acute or chronic disease processes such as malignancies and other infections, medications, and emotional stress

Clinical manifestation
May begin with non-specific constitutional symptoms and signs; prodromal pain or parathesias along one or more dermatomes, lasting 1–10 days, followed by patchy erythema in the dermatomal area of involvement and regional lymphadenopathy; unilateral, grouped vesicles on erythematous base, with severe local pain; vesicles initially clear, but eventually becoming pustular, rupturing, crusting, and involuting; scarring ensues if deeper epidermal and dermal layers compromised by scratching, secondary infection, or other complications

Zoster oticus (geniculate zoster, zoster auris, Ramsay-Hunt syndrome, Hunt syndrome): Ménière disease, Bell palsy, cerbrovascular accident or abscess of the ear; beginning with otalgia and herpetiform vesicles on the external ear canal, with or without features of facial paralysis, resulting from facial nerve involvement, auditory symptoms (e.g., deafness), and vestibular symptoms

Disseminated zoster: generalized eruption of more than 15–25 extradermatomal vesicles, occurring 7–14 days after the onset of dermatomal disease; occurs rarely in the general population, but commonly in elderly, hospitalized, or immunocompromised patients; often an indication of depressed cell-mediated immunity caused by various underlying clinical situations, including malignancies, radiation therapy, cancer chemotherapy, organ transplants, and chronic use of systemic corticosteroids; dissemination sometimes includes involvement of the lungs and central nervous system

Differential diagnosis
Varicella; herpes simplex virus infection; impetigo; candidiasis; erysipelas; cellulitis; bullous pemphigoid; pemphigus; contact

dermatitis; urticaria; photoallergic reaction; folliculitis; insect bite reaction; brachioradial pruritus

Therapy
Famciclovir; valacyclovir; post-herpetic neuralgia prophylaxis: prednisone; post-herpetic neuralgia: capsaicin; tricyclic antidepressants, such as amitriptyline: 25–100 mg PO daily; gabapentin: 300–2400 mg PO daily

References
Chen TM, George S, Woodruff CA, Hsu S (2002) Clinical manifestations of varicella-zoster virus infection. Dermatologic Clinics 20(2):267–282

Herpetic whitlow

▶ Herpes simplex virus infection

Hidradenitis suppurativa

Synonym(s)
Suppurative hidradenitis; apocrine acne; apocrinitis

Definition
Disorder of the terminal follicular epithelium in the apocrine gland–bearing skin, characterized by comedone-like follicular occlusion, chronic relapsing inflammation, mucopurulent discharge, and progressive scarring

Pathogenesis
Unknown disorder of follicular occlusion; earliest change: follicular plugging which obstructs apocrine gland ducts; earliest inflammatory event: rupture of the follicular epithelium: friction in intertriginous locations considered possible contributing factor; rupture followed by spillage of foreign-body material into the dermis, initiating an inflammatory response resulting in foreign-body granuloma; bacterial infection a risk factor for destructive scarring, but not a primary cause of the disease; genetic factors may be operative

Clinical manifestation
Hirsutism and obesity common findings among affected women; early symptoms of pruritus, erythema, and local hyperhidrosis; lesions occur in the axillae, groin area, nipples, and buttocks; painful and/or tender red papules and nodules; lesion heal with fibrosis and eventual recurrence in the adjacent area; painful or tender abscesses and inflamed, discharging papules or nodules; nodules coalesce and sometimes become infected, resulting in acute abscesses; dermal contractures and rope-like elevation of the skin; multiple abscesses and sinus tracts form a subcutaneous honeycomb; double-ended comedones; associated arthropathy sometimes presenting with asymmetric pauciarticular arthritis, symmetric polyarthritis, or polyarthralgia syndrome

Differential diagnosis
Granuloma inguinale; lymphogranuloma venereum; actinomycosis; staphylococcal abscesses; Bartholin cyst; carbuncle; Crohn disease; infected or inflamed epidermoid cyst; tuberculosis; tularemia; ulcerative colitis

Therapy
Wide surgical excision, preferably taking as much apocrine gland-bearing skin as possible*; localized disease: surgical techniques including incision and drainage; exteriorization; curettage; electrocoagulation of the sinus tracts; simple excision; triamcinolone 3–5 mg per kg intralesionally to inflamed nodules; tetracycline; erythromycin; isotretinoin; acitretin; dapsone

References
Brown TJ, Rosen T, Orengo IF (1998) Hidradenitis suppurativa. Southern Medical Association Journal 91(12):1107–1114

Hidradenoma, clear cell

► Eccrine hidradenoma

Hidradenoma papilliferum

Synonym(s)
Papillary hidradenoma; hidradenoma vulvae; apocrine adenoma; adenoma hidradenoides

Definition
Benign tumor with apocrine differentiation, most commonly seen in the genital area of women

Pathogenesis
Unknown

Clinical manifestation
Solitary, well-circumscribed, firm-to-cystic, bluish papule or nodule, with occasional ulceration, usually noted in the vulvar area of middle-aged women

Differential diagnosis
Leiomyoma; epidermoid cyst; squamous cell carcinoma; hemangioma; pyogenic granuloma; melanoma; Bartholin cyst

Therapy
Surgical excision*

References
Vang R, Cohen PR (1999) Ectopic hidradenoma papilliferum: a case report and review of the literature. Journal of the American Academy of Dermatology 41(1):115–118

Hidradenoma vulvae

► Hidradenoma papilliferum

Hidroacanthoma simplex

► Poroma

Hidrocystoma, apocrine

► Apocrine hidrocystoma

Hidrocystoma, eccrine

► Eccrine hidrocystoma

Hidrotic ectodermal dysplasia

Synonym(s)
Hereditary hidrotic ectodermal dysplasia; Clouston's disease

Definition
Genodermatosis characterized by nail dystrophy, alopecia, and hyperkeratosis of the palms and soles

Pathogenesis
Autosomal dominant trait; abnormal α-proteins in hair and nails

Clinical manifestation
Dystrophic nails; sparse, thin, fragile hair; thickening of the palms and soles; normal sweat function; skin dryness

Differential diagnosis
Anhidrotic ectodermal dysplasia; pachonychia congenita; Basan syndrome; chondroectodermal dysplasia; dyskeratosis congenita

Therapy
None

References
Chitty LS, Dennis N, Baraitser M (1996) Hidrotic ectodermal dysplasia of hair, teeth, and nails: case reports and review. Journal of Medical Genetics 33(8):707–710

Hirsutism

Definition
Development of androgen-dependent terminal body hair in a woman at sites where terminal hair not normally found

References
Marshburn PB, Carr BR (1995) Hirsutism and virilization. A systematic approach to benign and potentially serious causes. Postgraduate Medicine 97(1):99–102, 105–106

His-Werner disease

▶ Trench fever

Histiocytic

▶ Kikuchi's syndrome

Histiocytoid hemangioma

▶ Angiolymphoid hyperplasia with eosinophilia

Histiocytoma

▶ Dermatofibroma

Histiocytoma cutis

▶ Dermatofibroma

Histiocytosis, Langerhans cell

▶ Langerhans cell histiocytosis

Histiocytosis, regressing atypical

▶ Cutaneous CD30+ (Ki-1) anaplastic large-cell lymphoma

Histiocytosis X

▶ Langerhans cell histiocytosis

Histoplasmosis

Synonym(s)
Darling's disease

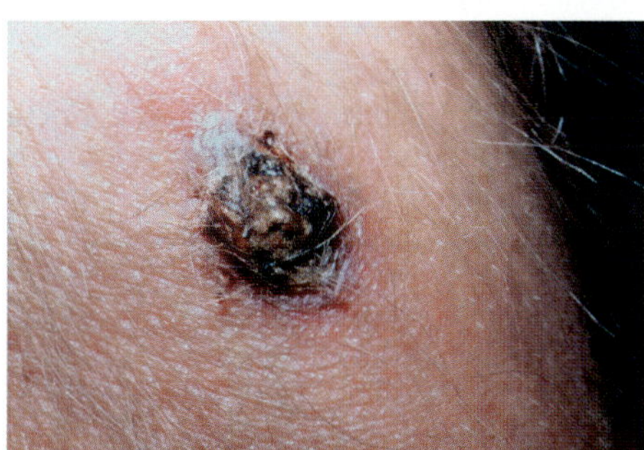

Histoplasmosis. Crusted, infiltrated nodule on the leg

Definition
Pulmonary and systemic infection caused by the fungus Histoplasma capsulatum

Pathogenesis
Alveolar deposition caused by aerosolization of conidia and mycelial fragments from contaminated soil; susceptibility to dissemination increased with impaired cellular host defenses; intracellular conversion from mycelial to pathogenic yeast form after macrophage phagocytosis; clinical manifestations occur with continued exposure to large inocula; pulmonary infection may disseminate, with hematogenous spread

Clinical manifestation
Acute pulmonary infection usually asymptomatic; with symptomatic disease, fever, headache, malaise, myalgia, abdominal pain, and chills; with exposure to large inoculum, severe dyspnea may occur; nonspecific signs of infection: erythema nodosum and erythema multiforme; occsional joint pain and infiltrated papules in the skin

Chronic pulmonary disease mostly in patients with underlying pulmonary disease; associated with cough, weight loss, fevers, and malaise; if cavitations present, hemoptysis, sputum production, and increasing dyspnea.

Progressive disseminated disease occurs mostly in immunocompromised patients; skin lesions begins as small papules and ulcerations; oropharyngeal ulcers sometimes involve buccal mucosa, tongue, gingiva, and larynx

Differential diagnosis
Bacterial or mycoplasma pneumonia; North American blastomycosis; coccidioidomycosis; tuberculosis; sarcoidosis; aspergillosis; squamous cell carcinoma; lymphoma

Therapy
None for asymptomatic disease or for cutaneous disease as sole sign of dissemination; progressive disease, particularly with meningitis – amphotericin B – 0.7–1 mg per kg per day IV to a total dose of 35 mg per kg★; mildly symptomatic or prolonged acute pulmonary disease – ketoconazole; itraconazole

References
Mocherla S, Wheat LJ (2001) Treatment of histoplasmosis. Seminars in Respiratory Infections 16(2):141–148

HIV-associated eosinophilic folliculitis

▶ Eosinophilic pustular folliculitis

HIV-related eosinophilic folliculitis

▶ Eosinophilic pustular folliculitis

Hives

▶ Urticaria

Hoffman's disease

▶ Dissecting cellulitis of scalp

Homocystinuria

Synonym(s)
None

Definition
Inherited disorder of methionine metabolism

Pathogenesis
Three main causes: (1) deficiency of cystathionine synthase; gene for this deficiency located on chromosomal band 21q22.3; (2) insufficient vitamin B-12 synthesis resulting from a defect in the remethylation of homocysteine to methionine; (3) deficiency in methylenetetrahydrofolate reductase; high concentrations of amino acids that are competitive inhibitors of tyrosinase results in pigment dilution, regardless of the cause of increased homocystine levels

Clinical manifestation
Cutaneous findings: red macules on buccal mucosa; enlarged pores on the face; livedo-like pattern of blood vessels; atrophic scars on the arms and hands; multiple small angiomas; hypopigmentation, which is reversible in patients with pyridoxine-responsive disease; coarse hair texture; hyperhidrosis; xerosis; acrocyanosis; Marfan's-like habitus; generalized osteoporosis; arterial and venous thrombosis; mental retardation; visual impairment

Differential diagnosis
Marfan syndrome; thrombophlebitis

Therapy
Pyridoxine 300–600 mg PO per day; betaine 3 g PO twice daily in adults, 100 mg per kg PO per day in children less than 3 years old as initial dose.
Cyanocobalamin: 25–250 mcg PO per day; low methionine diet

References
Kabra M (2002) Dietary management of inborn errors of metabolism. Indian Journal of Pediatrics 69(5):421–426

Homogentisic acid oxidase deficiency

► Alcaptonuria
► Ochronosis

Honeycomb atrophy

► Keratosis pilaris atrophicans
► Ulerythema ophryogenes

Hori nevus

► Nevus of Ota and Ito

Hori's nevus

► Nevus of Ota and Ito

Hornet sting

► Hymenoptera sting

Horse-collar neck

► Benign symmetric lipomatosis

Horton disease

► Temporal arteritis

Hospital gangrene

► Necrotizing fasciitis

Hot tub dermatitis

▶ Hot tub folliculitis

Hot tub folliculitis

Synonym(s)
Hot tub dermatitis; splash rash; pseudomonas folliculitis; whirlpool folliculitis

Definition
Community-acquired pseudomonas skin infection, resulting from bacterial colonization of hair follicles after exposure to contained, contaminated water

Pathogenesis
Bacterial organism, Pseudomonas aeruginosa, found in soil and fresh water, gains entry through hair follicles or via breaks in the skin; predisposing factors: hot water, high pH (>7.8), and low chlorine level (<0.5 mg/L); predisposing environmental conditions: prolonged water exposure, excessive numbers of bathers, inadequate pool care; risk factors: crowding, wearing of snug bathing suits, and frequency and duration of exposure

Clinical manifestation
Onset usually about 48 hours after contaminated water exposure; follicular papules, vesicles, and pustules, which may be crusted, on exposed skin, but usually sparing the face, neck, palms and soles; lesions progress to erythematous papules and pustules; clear spontaneously in 2–10 days; rarely recur; heal without scarring, but sometimes cause desquamation or hyperpigmented macules; occasional mild accompanying constitutional symptoms and signs

Differential diagnosis
Insect bite reaction; inflammatory folliculitis; staphylococcal folliculitis; Grover's disease; pityriasis lichenoides et varioliformis acuta; scabies

Therapy
No effective therapy, including systemic or topical antibiotics

References
Bhatia A, Brodell RT (1999) "Hot tub folliculitis". Test the waters – and the patient – for Pseudomonas. Postgraduate Medicine 106(4):43–46

Howell-Evans syndrome

▶ Tylosis

Human African trypanosomiasis

▶ African trypanosomiasis

Human threadworm infection

▶ Strongyloidosis

Hunter syndrome

Synonym(s)
Mucopolysaccharidosis type II

Definition
Inherited metabolic storage disease arising from a deficiency of L-sulfoiduronate sulfatase

Pathogenesis
X-linked trait; deficiency of L-sulfoiduro-nate sulfatase, which results in accumulation of mucopolysaccharides in the lysosomes of the cells in the connective tissue and increase in their excretion in the urine

Clinical manifestation
Mild and severe form of disease; organs most involved: bone, the various viscera, the connective tissue, and the brain; onset by age 3 years; hirsutism; skin thickening, particularly over the fingers; multiple, ivory-white, pebbly papules or nodules overlying the scapula and near posterior axillary fold; progressive deafness; hepatosplenomegaly, joint stiffness; coarse facial features; cardiovascular involvement

Differential diagnosis
Hurler syndrome; Sanfilippo syndrome; Scheie syndrome; Gaucher's disease; osteogenesis imperfecta; vitamin D-resistant rickets; Niemann-Pick disease

Therapy
Bone marrow transplantation; investigational enzyme replacement therapy with iduronate-2-sulfatase

References
Peters C, Krivit W (2000) Hematopoietic cell transplantation for mucopolysaccharidosis IIB (Hunter syndrome). Bone Marrow Transplantation 25(10):1097–1099

Hurler syndrome

Synonym(s)
Mucopolysaccharidosis type I-H

Definition
Inherited metabolic storage disease arising from a deficiency of alpha-L-iduronidase

Pathogenesis
Autosomal recessive trait; deficiency of alpha-L-iduronidase, which results in accumulation of mucopolysaccharides in the lysosomes of the cells in the connective tissue

Clinical manifestation
Onset in early childhood; organs most involved: the bone, the viscera, the connective tissue, and the brain; lichenified, dry, thick skin with diminished elasticity; increased pigmentation on the dorsum of the hands; sclerodermalike changes; hypertrichosis of the extremities; pale colored hair; neurologic symptoms: hypertensive hydrocephalus syndrome, changes in the tonus of the musculature and the tendon reflex, and damage of the cranial nerves; myxedema in patients with associated hypothyroidism; dwarfism; hepatosplenomegaly; cardiovascular involvement; progressive deterioration of intellect after a period of apparently normal development; speech disturbances; ocular symptoms: progressive clouding of the cornea, megalocornea, hereditary glaucoma, and congestion and atrophy of the optic disc; death often occurs before age 10 years from progressive neurologic and cardiovascular deterioration

Differential diagnosis
Hunter syndrome; Sanfilippo syndrome; Scheie syndrome; Gaucher's disease; osteogenesis imperfecta; vitamin D-resistant rickets; Niemann-Pick disease

Therapy
Bone marrow transplantation; investigational enzyme replacement therapy with alronidase

References
Wraith JE (2001) Enzyme replacement therapy in mucopolysaccharidosis type I: progress and emerging difficulties. Journal of Inherited Metabolic Disease 24(2):245–250

Hurler-Scheie syndrome

▶ Scheie syndrome

Hutchinson melanotic freckle

▶ Lentigo maligna

Hutchinson's melanotic freckle

▶ Lentigo maligna

Hyalinosis cutis et mucosae

▶ Lipoid proteinosis

Hydroa herpetiformis

▶ Dermatitis herpetiformis

Hydrocortisone

▶ Corticosteroids, topical, low potency

Hydroquinone

Trade name(s)
Solaquin Forte; Eldoquin; Eldopaque; Nuquin; Lustra; Melanex; Esoterica; Porcelana Fade Cream; Esoterica; Tri-Luma

Generic available
Yes

Drug class
Depigmenting agent

Mechanism of action
Inhibits enzymatic oxidation of tyrosine; suppresses other melanocytic metabolic processes

Dosage form
1.5% cream (Eldopaque; Esoterica; Porcelana); 2% cream (Nuquin); 3% lotion (Melanex); 4% cream (Solaquin Forte, Lustra); 4% gel (Solaquin Forte); 4% cream with tretinoin and fluocinolone (Tri-Luma)

Dermatologic indications and dosage
See table

Hydroquinone. Dermatologic indications and dosage

Disease	Adult dosage	Child dosage
Berloque dermatitis	Apply 1–2 times daily	Apply 1–2 times daily
Lentigo	Apply 1–2 times daily	Apply 1–2 times daily
Melasma	Apply 1–2 times daily	Apply 1–2 times daily
Postinflammatory hyperpigmentation	Apply 1–2 times daily	Apply 1–2 times daily

Common side effects
Cutaneous: contact dermatitis, burning sensation, erythema

Serious side effects
Cutaneous: ochronosis-like pigmentation

Drug interactions
None

Contraindications/precautions
Hypersensitivity to drug class or component

References
Glaser DA, Rogers C (2001) Topical and systemic therapies for the aging face. Facial Plastic Surgery Clinics of North America 9(2):189–196

Hydroxychloroquine

Trade name(s)
Plaquenil

Generic available
Yes

Drug class
Antimalarial

Mechanism of action
Not completely elucidated; may work by immunosuppressive effects, DNA binding, photo-protective effects, and/or anti-inflammatory mechanisms

Dosage form
200 mg tablet

Dermatologic indications and dosage
See table

Common side effects
Cutaneous: exacerbation of psoriasis, blue-gray skin discoloration, transverse nail bands; skin eruptions

Gastrointestinal: nausea and vomiting, diarrhea
Laboratory: elevated liver enzymes
Neurologic: headache, nervousness, mood swings, vertigo
Ocular: halos, blurred vision

Serious side effects
Hematologic: agranulocytosis, aplastic anemia
Neurologic: seizures
Ocular: visual changes from retinopathy

Drug interactions
None

Contraindications/precautions
Hypersensitivity to drug class or component; porphyria cutanea tarda; history of retinal field changes

References
Van Beek MJ, Piette WW (2001) Antimalarials. Dermatologic Clinics 19(1): 147–160

Hydroxyurea

Trade name(s)
Hydrea

Generic available
Yes

Drug class
Cytotoxic agent

Mechanism of action
Ribonucleotide reductase inhibition, which is the rate-limiting enzyme in DNA synthesis

Dosage form
500 mg tablets

Dermatologic indications and dosage
See table

Hydroxychloroquine. Dermatologic indications and dosage

Disease	Adult dosage	Child dosage
Chronic actinic dermatitis	Start at 200 mg PO twice daily; titrate downward after a favorable response has occurred	Start at 3–5 mg per kg PO daily; titrate downward after a favorable response has occurred
Chronic graft versus host disease	Start at 200 mg PO twice daily; titrate downward after a favorable response has occurred	12 mg per kg daily PO, divided into 2 doses
Dermatomyositis	Start at 200 mg PO twice daily; titrate downward after a favorable response has occurred	Start at 3–5 mg per kg PO daily; titrate downward after a favorable response has occurred
Granuloma annulare	Start at 200 mg PO twice daily; titrate downward after a favorable response has occurred	Start at 3–5 mg per kg PO daily; titrate downward after a favorable response has occurred
Lupus erythematosus, discoid	Start at 200 mg PO twice daily; titrate downward after a favorable response has occurred	Start at 3–5 mg per kg PO daily; titrate downward after a favorable response has occurred
Lupus erythematosus, subacute cutaneous	Start at 200 mg PO twice daily; titrate downward after a favorable response has occurred	Start at 3–5 mg per kg PO daily; titrate downward after a favorable response has occurred
Lymphocytic infiltration of the skin	Start at 200 mg PO twice daily; titrate downward after a favorable response has occurred	Start at 3–5 mg per kg PO daily; titrate downward after a favorable response has occurred
Pemphigus foliaceus	Start at 200 mg PO twice daily; titrate downward after a favorable response has occurred	Start at 3–5 mg per kg PO daily; titrate downward after a favorable response has occurred
Polymorphous light eruption	Start at 200 mg PO twice daily; titrate downward after a favorable response has occurred	Start at 3–5 mg per kg PO daily; titrate downward after a favorable response has occurred
Porphyria cutanea tarda	200 mg twice weekly for first month; gradually titrate dose upward over 3–6 months to 200 mg daily	3 mg per kg PO weekly for first month; gradually titrate dose upward over 3–6 months to 3 mg per kg PO daily
Reticular erythematous mucinosis	Start at 200 mg PO twice daily; titrate downward after a favorable response has occurred	Start at 3–5 mg per kg PO daily; titrate downward after a favorable response has occurred
Sarcoidosis	Start at 200 mg PO twice daily; titrate downward after a favorable response has occurred	Start at 3–5 mg per kg PO daily; titrate downward after a favorable response has occurred
Solar urticaria	Start at 200 mg PO twice daily; titrate downward after a favorable response has occurred	Start at 3–5 mg per kg PO daily; titrate downward after a favorable response has occurred
Weber-Christian disease	Start at 200 mg PO twice daily; titrate downward after a favorable response has occurred	Start at 3–5 mg per kg PO daily; titrate downward after a favorable response has occurred

Hydroxyurea. Dermatologic indications and dosage

Disease	Adult dosage	Child dosage
Hypereosinophilic syndrome	20–30 mg per kg PO daily	15–30 mg per kg PO daily
Psoriasis	20–30 mg per kg PO daily	15–30 mg per kg PO daily
Reiter syndrome	20–30 mg per kg PO daily	15–30 mg per kg PO daily

Common side effects
Cutaneous: stomatitis, alopecia, erythema, skin eruption, leg ulcers
Gastrointestinal: hepatitis, anorexia, nausea and vomiting, diarrhea, dyspepsia
Neurologic: headache, dizziness, hallucinations, seizures
Renal: renal insufficiency

Serious side effects
Bone marrow: anemia, thrombocytopenia, leukopenia
Neoplastic: possible increased risk of leukemia
Pulmonary: pulmonary fibrosis

Drug interactions
Bone marrow suppressants

Contraindications/precautions
Hypersensitivity to drug class or component; bone marrow depression; pregnancy; caution in patients with impaired renal function or with other myelosuppressive agents

References
Kumar B, Saraswat A, Kaur I (2001) Rediscovering hydroxyurea: its role in recalcitrant psoriasis. International Journal of Dermatology 40(8):530–534

Hydroxyzine

▶ **Antihistamines, first generation**

Hymenoptera sting

Synonym(s)
Bee sting, hornet sting, wasp sting, yellow jacket sting, fire ant bite

Definition
Reaction to a sting or bite from an insect of order Hymenoptera, which includes bees, hornets, wasps, yellow jackets, and ants

Pathogenesis
Over 30 individual compounds contained in venom of winged Hymenoptera, including biogenic amines, polypeptides, protein toxins and enzymes; small amounts of low molecular weight protein contained in venom of fire or stinging ants; reactions to envenomation either directly toxic (either local or systemic) or allergic (either localized or anaphylactic)

Clinical manifestation
Simple sting: results in a local reaction with swelling and pain initially and itching a few hours later; swelling sometimes increases over several days and usually resolves within one week
Immediate hypersensitivity reaction: local swelling or urticaria with pain and itching; sometimes spreads to become more generalized, with urticaria, which may progress to involve the upper or lower airway in an anaphylactic reaction
Delayed hypersensitivity reaction: either immune-complex mediated (either immunoglobulin M or immunoglobulin G)

or systemic (serum sickness type) or local (Arthus type); occurs within 1 week of envenomation; symptoms: fever, arthralgias and myalgias, headache, and general malaise; signs: eruption of either red macules and papules or palpable purpura; joint swelling and tenderness with or without effusions; lymphadenopathy; glomerulitis or nephrotic syndrome
Fire ant bite: usually multiple; presents as swelling and pain with early vesicle formation, followed by ulceration and possible secondary infection

Differential diagnosis

Anaphylaxis from other causes; allergic cutaneous vasculitis; foreign body reaction; spider bite

Therapy

Simple envenomations: ice water soaks; pain control with ibuprofen or acetaminophen
Generalized reactions: epinephrine: 0.15–0.3 mg SC or 0.2–1 mg IV, repeated every 20–30 minutes if indicated★; diphenhydramine – 25-75 mg PO or IM or IV, repeated every 6 hours as needed★

References

Metry DW, Hebert AA (2000) Insect and arachnid stings, bites, infestations, and repellents. Pediatric Annals 29(1):39–48

Hyper-IgE syndrome

▶ Hyperimmunoglobulin E syndrome

Hypercare Certain-Dri

▶ Aluminium chloride

Hypercorticalism

▶ Cushing syndrome

Hypereosinophilic syndrome

Synonym(s)
Idiopathic hypereosinophilic syndrome

Definition
Group of leukoproliferative disorders characterized by an overproduction of eosinophils, resulting in organ damage

Pathogenesis
Underlying cause of eosinophil overproduction not well understood; cytokine-mediated eosinophils survive in the tissues for longer periods of time than normal, thus increasing the amount of tissue damage; cells contain granules that store toxic cationic proteins, the primary mediators of tissue injury; toxins: major basic protein, eosinophil peroxidase, eosinophil-derived neurotoxin, and eosinophil cationic protein; eosinophils also release specific cytokines that recruit additional eosinophils

Clinical manifestation
Cutaneous findings: pruritius; angioedema, urticaria, often with dermatographism; erythematous, pruritic papules, plaques and nodules, with or without ulceration
Cardiac findings: chest pain, dyspnea, or orthopnea
Hematologic changes: splenomegaly; thrombotic episodes
Neurologic findings: encephalopathy; cerebrovascular accidents or transient ischemic episodes

Pulmonary changes: chronic, persistent cough, usually nonproductive; dyspnea from congestive heart failure or pleural effusions; pulmonary fibrosis
Rheumatologic findings: arthralgias and myalgias; occasional Raynaud phenomenon
Gastrointestinal findings: abdominal pain; nausea; diarrhea; hepatomegaly

Differential diagnosis
Angiolymphoid hyperplasia with eosinophilia; atopic dermatitis; lupus erythematosus; drug reaction; parasitic infection; malignancy with secondary eosinophilia; Churg-Strauss syndrome; eosinophilia-myalgia syndrome; eosinophilic fasciitis

Therapy
Prednisone*; aggressive disease unresponsive to corticosteroids: hydroxyurea; vincristine: 1–2 mg IV every 2 weeks; chlorambucil: pulse of 4–10 mg/m²/d PO for 4 days every other month; interferon; photochemotherapy for symptomatic control of skin eruption and pruritus; bone marrow transplantation for life-threatening disease

References
Assa'ad AH, Spicer RL, Nelson DP, Zimmermann N, Rothenberg ME (2000) Hypereosinophilic syndromes. Chemical Immunology 76:208–229

Hyperhidrosis

Definition
Excessive sweating of certain body areas, particularly axillae, palms, and soles

References
Togel B, Greve B, Raulin C (2002) Current therapeutic strategies for hyperhidrosis: a review. European Journal of Dermatology 12(3):219–223

Hyperimmunoglobulin E syndrome

Synonym(s)
Job syndrome; hyper-IgE syndrome, Job's syndrome

Definition
Heritable disorder characterized by the production of high levels of the antibody immunoglobulin E (IgE), causing serious skin and lung infections and atopic eczema-like eruption

Pathogenesis
Autosomal dominant trait; no clearly defined defect of either T or B cell function; chemotactic defect in neutrophils; activation of Th2 lymphocytes producing cytokines responsible for activation and differentiation of eosinophils

Clinical manifestation
Characteristic coarse facies; early non-specific papular or pustular eruption, favoring the scalp, proximal flexures, and buttocks; eczematous eruption; recurrent staphylococcal abscesses, often described as cold abscesses because of lack of pain, heat, or redness; cellulitis; recurrent bronchitis, caused by S. aureus or Haemophilus influenzae; other systemic bacterial infections; chronic mucocutaneous candidiasis and onychomycosis; skeletal abnormalities: frequent painless bone fractures; scoliosis; hyperextensible joints

Differential diagnosis
Atopic dermatitis; chronic mucocutaneous candidiasis; recurrent folliculitis; staphylococcal carriage state with recurrent skin infections; DiGeorge syndrome; Wiskott-Aldrich syndrome; chronic granulomatous disease; common variable immunodeficiency; X-linked hypogammaglobulinemia; leukocyte adhesion deficiency

Therapy

Active bacterial infection: nafcillin 500–2000 mg IV every 6 hours for 1–5 days, depending on therapeutic response; then dicloxacillin 500 mg PO 4 times daily for 10–21 days, depending on therapeutic response; pediatric patient: 100–200 mg per kg IV per day in 4 divided doses for 1–5 days, depending on therapeutic response; then dicloxacillin 250 mg PO 4 times daily for 10–21 days, depending on therapeutic response; incision and drainage of fluctuant abscesses; fluconazole for active candidiasis; cyclosporine; prophylaxis: cimetidine: 20–40 mg per kg PO 3–4 times per day; ascorbic acid: 500 mg PO per day; antibacterial soaps used 1–2 times per day

References

Shemer A, Weiss G, Confino Y, Trau H (2001) The hyper-IgE syndrome. Two cases and review of the literature. International Journal of Dermatology 40(10):622–628

Hyperkeratosis eccentrica

▶ **Porokeratosis**

Hyperkeratosis figurata centrifuga atrophicans

▶ **Porokeratosis**

Hyperkeratosis follicularis et parafollicularis in cutem penetrans

▶ **Kyrle's disease**

Hyperkeratosis haemorrhagica

▶ **Black heel**

Hyperkeratosis lenticularis perstans

Synonym(s)

Flegel disease; Flegel's disease

Definition

Disease of localized abnormal keratinization, characterized by inflammatory keratotic papules

Pathogenesis

Ultraviolet light possibly a factor

Clinical manifestation

Asymptomatic, small, red-brown, hyperkeratotic papules on the lower extremities, sparing the trunk; removal of the scale reveals bright red base, with pinpoint bleeding

Differential diagnosis

Disseminated superficial actinic porokeratosis; porokeratosis of Mibelli; stucco keratosis; actinic keratosis; flat warts; acrokeratosis verruciformis of Hopf; Kyrle's disease

Therapy

Fluorouracil; acitretin; dermabrasion

References

Fathy S, Azadeh B (1988) Hyperkeratosis lenticularis perstans. International Journal of Dermatology 27(2):120–121

Hyperkeratosis palmaris et plantaris

▶ Unna-Thost palmoplantar keratoderma

Hypermelanotic macule

▶ Café au lait macule

Hyperpituitarism

▶ Acromegaly

Hypertrichosis

Definition
Abnormally increased growth of hair, regardless of location

References
Vashi RA, Mancini AJ, Paller AS (2001) Primary generalized and localized hypertrichosis in children. Archives of Dermatology 137(7):877–884

Hypertrichosis lanuginosa acquisita

▶ Hypertrichosis lanuginosa

Hypertrichosis universalis congenita, Ambras type

▶ Ambras syndrome

Hypertrichotic osteochondrodysplasia

▶ Cantu syndrome

Hypertrophic morphea

▶ Dermatofibrosarcoma protuberans

Hypoadrenalism

▶ Addison's disease

Hypocorticism

▶ Addison's disease

Hypohidrotic ectodermal dysplasia

▶ Anhidrotic ectodermal dysplasia

Hypomelanosis guttata ideopathica

▶ Idiopathic guttate hypomelanosis

Hypomelanosis of Cummins and Cottel

▶ Idiopathic guttate hypomelanosis

Hypomelanosis of Ito

Synonym(s)
Incontinentia pigmenti achromians

Definition
Syndrome characterized by hypopigmented whorls of skin along the Blaschko lines

Pathogenesis
Chromosomal mosaicism and sporadic mutations; identity of a specific gene not confirmed

Clinical manifestation
Asymmetric, hypopigmented or white macules coalescing to form reticulated patches along the lines of Blaschko; macules covering more than 2 dermatomes and often on both sides of the body, present at birth; occasional associations with neurologic, skeletal, and other congenital abnormalities

Differential diagnosis
Incontinentia pigmenti; nevoid hypermelanosis; nevus depigmentosus; congenital nevocellular nevus; post-inflammatory hyperpigmentation

Therapy
None for pigmentary abnormality

References
Pinto FJ, Bolognia JL (1991) Disorders of hypopigmentation in children. Pediatric Clinics of North America 38(4):991–1017

I

Iatrogenic acrodermatitis enteropathica

▶ Acrodermatitis enteropathica

IBIDS

▶ Tay syndrome

Ichthyosiform erythroderma with vacuolation

▶ Chanarin-Dorfman syndrome

Ichthyosiform nevus

▶ CHILD syndrome

Ichthyosis

Synonym(s)
None

Definition
Groups of diseases represented by thick, scaly skin

References
Shwayder T (1999) Ichthyosis in a nutshell. Pediatrics in Review 20(1):5–12

Ichthyosis bullosa of Siemens

▶ Epidermolytic hyperkeratosis

Ichthyosis congenita

▶ Ichthyosis fetalis

Ichthyosis congenita larva

▶ Lamellar ichthyosis

Ichthyosis fetalis

Synonym(s)
Harlequin ichthyosis; harlequin baby; ichthyosis congenita; keratosis diffusa fetalis; harlequin fetus

Definition
Severe form of congenital ichthyosis, characterized by profound thickening of the keratin layer in fetal skin, producing a horny shell of platelike scale and contraction abnormalities of the eyes, ears, mouth, and appendages

Pathogenesis
Probable autosomal recessive trait; abnormal lamellar granule structure and function; abnormal conversion of profilaggrin to filaggrin

Clinical manifestation
Condition present at birth; skin severely thickened with large, shiny plates of hyperkeratotic scale; deep fissures separate the scales; severe ectropion, leaving the conjunctiva at risk for desiccation and trauma; pinnae sometimes small and rudimentary, or absent; severe traction on lips causes eclabium and fixed open mouth; nasal hypoplasia and eroded nasal alae; limbs encased in the thick membrane, causing flexion contractures of the arms, legs, and digits; limb motility poor or absent; hypoplasia of the fingers, toes, and fingernails; temperature dysregulation; heat intolerance; occasional hyperthermia; restriction of chest-wall expansion sometimes results in respiratory distress, hypoventilation, and respiratory failure; dehydration from excess water loss

Differential diagnosis
Trichorrhexis invaginata; congenital ichthyosiform erythroderma; lamellar ichthyosis; Conradi's disease; trichothiodystrophy; Sjogren-Larsson syndrome; X-linked ichthyosis; lamellar ichthyosis; Netherton's syndrome

Therapy
Acitretin

References
Singh S, Bhura M, Maheshwari A, Kumar A, Singh CP, Pandey SS (2001) Successful treatment of harlequin ichthyosis with acitretin. International Journal of Dermatology 40(7):472–473

Ichthyosis hystrix

▶ Epidermolytic hyperkeratosis

Ichthyosis hystrix of Curth-Macklin

▶ Epidermolytic hyperkeratosis

Ichthyosis, lamellar

▶ Lamellar ichthyosis

Ichthyosis linearis circumflexa

▶ Netherton syndrome

Ichthyosis nacrée

▶ Ichthyosis vulgaris

Ichthyosis nigricans

▶ X-linked ichthyosis

Ichthyosis nitida

▶ Ichthyosis vulgaris

Ichthyosis palmaris et plantaris

▶ Unna-Thost palmoplantar keratoderma

Ichthyosis sebacea

▶ Lamellar ichthyosis

Ichthyosis simplex

▶ Ichthyosis vulgaris

Ichthyosis vulgaris

Synonym(s)
Common ichthyosis; autosomal dominant ichthyosis; hereditary ichthyosis vulgaris; ichthyosis simplex; xeroderma; pityriasis vulgaris; ichthyosis nacrée; ichthyosis nitida; fish skin ichthyosis

Definition
Hereditary retention hyperkeratosis characterized by large, plate-like, scaly plaques

Pathogenesis
Autosomal dominant trait; altered profilaggrin expression leading to retained scale; chemical abnormality correlated with decreased numbers of keratohyalin granules

Clinical manifestation
Symmetrical, variable scaling; small, fine, irregular, and polygonal scales, often curling at the edges to give the skin a rough feel; color ranging from white to dirty gray to brown; most scaling occurring on extensor surfaces of extremities, with sharp demarcation between normal flexural folds and surrounding affected areas; lower extremities generally more affected than upper extremities; on trunk, scaling often more pronounced on back than abdomen; sparing of flexural folds; palmoplantar thickening and hyperlinearity; relative sparing of face; improvement in summer or in warm climate

Differential diagnosis
X-linked ichthyosis; asteatosis; atopic dermatitis; lamellar ichthyosis; sarcoidosis; dermatophytosis; acquired ichthyosis

Therapy
Alpha hydroxy acids; emollients; keratolytics such as salicylic acid; urea

References
Rabinowitz LG, Esterly NB (1994) Atopic dermatitis and ichthyosis vulgaris. Pediatrics in Review 15(6):220–226

Ichthyosis, X-linked

▶ X-linked ichthyosis

Ichthyotic neutral lipid storage disease

▶ Chanarin-Dorfman syndrome

Id reaction

Synonym(s)
Autoeczematization, autosensitization

Definition
Acute, generalized reaction to a variety of stimuli, including infections and inflammatory skin diseases

Pathogenesis
Unknown; theories of causation: (1) abnormal immune recognition of autologous skin antigens; (2) increased stimulation of normal T cells by altered skin constituents; (3) dissemination of infectious antigen with a secondary response; and (4) dissemination of cytokines from a primary site

Clinical manifestation
Acute onset of a pruritic, symmetrial, erythematous, papular or papulovesicular eruption, usually preceded by acute flare of underlying dermatitis or infection, at a site distant from the primary infection or dermatitis; vesicles sometimes present on the hands or feet; underlying conditions: dermatophytes, mycobacteria, viruses, bacteria, parasites, contact dermatitis, stasis dermatitis, or other eczematous processes

Differential diagnosis
Atopic dermatitis; stasis dermatitis; seborrheic dermatitis; contact dermatitis; dyshidrotic eczema; dermatophytosis; scabies; Gianotti-Crosti syndrome; pityriasis lichenoides et varioliformis acuta; drug eruption; folliculitis

Therapy
Prednisone*; corticosteroids, topical, medium-potency

References
Gianni C, Betti R, Crosti C (1996) Psoriasiform id reaction in tinea corporis. Mycoses 39(7-8):307–308

Idiopathic anetoderma of Schweninger and Buzzi

▶ **Anetoderma**

Idiopathic atrophoderma of Pasini and Pierini

▶ **Atrophoderma of Pasini and Pierini**

Idiopathic guttate hypomelanosis

Synonym(s)
Hypomelanosis of Cummins and Cottel; hypomelanosis guttata ideopathica; leukodermia lenticular disseminata; leukopathia guttata et reticularis symmetrica; senile depigmented spots; symmetric progressive leukopathy of extremities

Definition
Acquired, benign leukoderma, most commonly seen in light-skinned women with a history of significant chronic sun exposure

Pathogenesis
Possibly related to sun exposure and its effect on melanocytes; defect of the epidermal melanin unit, resulting in hypopigmentation

Clinical manifestation
Most commonly seen on the legs of fair-skinned, women, but also occurring on the dorsal aspect of the forearms; multiple, confetti-like, hypopigmented macules

Differential diagnosis
Post-inflammatory hypopigmentation; scars; lichen sclerosus; vitiligo; tinea versicolor; flat warts; pinta

Therapy
Corticosteroids, topical, medium potency; tretinoin; cryosurgery; sun avoidance

References
Falabella R (1988) Idiopathic guttate hypomelanosis. Dermatologic Clinics 6(2):241–247

Imiquimod. Dermatologic indications and dosage

Disease	Adult dosage	Child dosage
Basal cell carcinoma	Apply 3 times weekly	Not indicated
Extramammary Paget's disease	Apply every other day for 16 weeks	Not indicated
Genital warts	Apply 3 times weekly	Not indicated
Keloid, post-excision	Apply daily to excision site for 8 weeks	Not indicated

Idiopathic hypereosinophilic syndrome

▶ Hypereosinophilic syndrome

Idiopathic hypertrophic osteoarthropathy

▶ Pachydermoperiostosis

Idiopathic inflammatory myopathy

▶ Dermatomyositis

Idiopathic lenticular mucocutaneous pigmentatio

▶ Laugier-Hunziger syndrome

Idiopathic lobular panniculitis

▶ Weber-Christian disease

Imiquimod

Trade name(s)
Aldara

Generic available
No

Drug class
Immunomodulator

Mechanism of action
Induction of cytokines, including tumor necrosis factor-α, interferon-α, interferon-γ, IL-1 and IL-6

Dosage form
5% cream

Dermatologic indications and dosage
See table

Common side effects
Cutaneous: burning sensation, irritant dermatitis, pruritus, local pain, hypopigmentation

Serious side effects
None

Drug interactions
None

Contraindications/precautions
Hypersensitivity to drug class or component

References
Dahl M (2002) Imiquimod: a cytokine inducer. Journal of the American Academy of Dermatology 47(9 suppl):205–208

Immersion foot

Synonym(s)
Trench foot; sea boot foot; paddy-field foot; tropical jungle foot; foxhole foot

Definition
Condition produced by prolonged exposure of the feet to non-freezing, moist, occlusive microenvironment

Pathogenesis
Hyperhydration causes maceration of the stratum corneum; aggravating factors: tight shoes, foot dependency, immobility, dehydration, trauma, history of peripheral vascular disease; cold exposure causes increased blood viscosity, thrombosis, ischemia and cell injury

Clinical manifestation
Cold water immersion foot: pre-hyperemic stage with cyanotic, absent pulses, and cold, waxy feet; hyperemic stage with painful feet, bounding pulses, brawny edema; occur several hours after removing footwear; post-hyperemic stage with cold sensitivity and hyperhidrosis that lasts from weeks to years; warm water immersion foot: severely painful and/or pruritic, edematous, white wrinkled feet, with sharp demarcation between involved and uninvolved skin

Differential diagnosis
Chilblains; Raynaud phenomenon; frostbite; sweaty sock dermatitis; pitted keratolysis

Therapy
Bed rest, leg elevation, and drying of feet[*]

References
Wrenn K (1991) Immersion foot. A problem of the homeless in the 1990s. Archives of Internal Medicine 151(4):785-788

Immune complex urticaria

▶ Urticarial vasculitis

Impetigo

Synonym(s)
Impetigo contagiosa, Fox impetigo, impetigo bullosa, impetigo contagiosa bullosa

Definition
Bacterial infection of the superficial layers of the epidermis caused by gram-positive bacterial pathogens

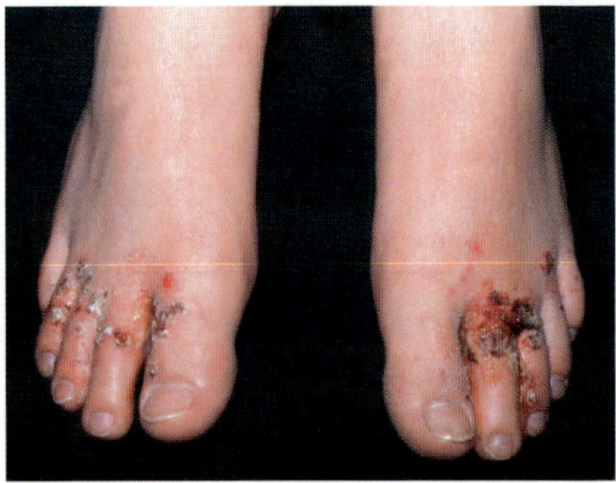

Impetigo. Exudative, eroded plaques with honey-colored crusts on the feet

Pathogenesis

Bullous variant: gram-positive, coagulase-positive, group II Staphylococcus aureus, most often phage type 71; organisms often spread from nasal carriage site

Non-bullous variant: in the United States, group A beta hemolytic streptococcal infection and Staphylococcus aureus occur with equal frequency; in other parts of the world, group A beta hemolytic streptococcal infection is most common cause; organism often transmitted through hand contact, entering through abraded or otherwise traumatized skin

Clinical manifestation

Bullous variant: acute onset of vesicles that enlarge and quickly rupture, often leaving a peripheral collarette ofk scale; occurs in milieu of hot and humid environments with crowded living conditions and poor hygiene

Non-bullous variant: fragile vesicle or pustule that readily ruptures and becomes a honey-yellow, adherent, crusted papule or plaque; located around the nose, mouth, and exposed parts of the body, sparing the palms and soles; regional, tender lymphadenopathy

Differential diagnosis

Herpes simplex virus infection; varicella; dermatophytosis; pediculosis; thermal or chemical burn; erythema multiforme; fixed drug reaction; arthropod bite reaction; incontinentia pigmenti; scabies; contact dermatitis; cutaneous candidiasis

Therapy

Bullous variant: dicloxacillin; cephalexin; mupirocin; bacitracin

Non-bullous variant: dicloxacillin; cephalexin; erythromycin; mupirocin; bacitracin

References

Sadick NS (1997) Current aspects of bacterial infections of the skin. Dermatologic Clinics 15(2):341–349

Impetigo bullosa

▶ Impetigo

Impetigo contagiosa

▶ Impetigo

Impetigo contagiosa bullosa

▶ Impetigo

Incontinentia pigmenti

Synonym(s)

Bloch-Sulzberger syndrome, Bloch-Siemens syndrome

Definition

Hereditary disorder characterized by neurologic, ophthalmologic, dental, and cutaneous abnormalities

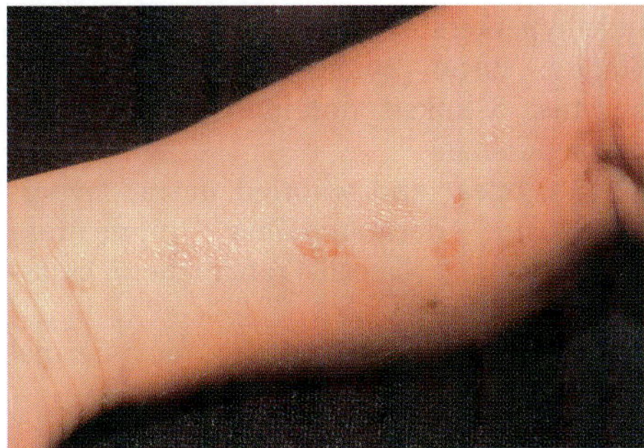

Incontinentia pigmenti. Linear, hyperpigmented, verrucous plaques on the leg

Pathogenesis

X-linked dominant, single gene disorder; mutations in NEMO/IKK-g, which encodes a critical component of the nuclear factor-B (NF-B) signaling pathway; patchy distribution of skin lesions resulting from tissue mosaicism due to random X-inactivation

Clinical manifestation

Cutaneous changes:

Stage 1: linear, red papules and vesicles grouped on an erythematous base, mainly on the extremities

Stage 2: linear, verrucous plaques on an erythematous base

Stage 3: streaks and whorls of brown or slate-gray pigmentation along the lines of Blaschko, particularly on the trunk

Stage 4: hypopigmented, atrophic, reticulated patches, mostly on the lower extremities; lusterless, thin hair; nail dystrophy, ranging from mild pitting or ridging to severely thickened, abnormally ridged nails; dental abnormalities

• Ocular findings: retinal detachment; proliferative retinopathy; fibrovascular retrolental membrane; cataracts; atrophy of the ciliary body

• Neurologic findings: seizures; developmental delay; mental retardation; ataxia, spasticity; microcephaly; cerebral atrophy; hypoplasia of the corpus callosum; periventricular cerebral edema

Differential diagnosis

Stage 1: bullous impetigo; herpes simplex virus infection; varicella; epidermolysis bullosa; bullous mastocytosis; epidermolytic hyperkeratosis; erythema toxicum

Stage 2: linear epidermal nevus; lichen striatus; X-linked dominant chondrodysplasia punctata

Stage 3: linear and whorled nevoid hypermelanosis; dermatopathia pigmentosa reticularis; Naegeli-Franceschetti-Jadassohn syndrome

Stage 4: hypomelanosis of Ito; focal dermal hypoplasia syndrome

Therapy

None for skin abnormalities

References

Tomaraei SN, Bajwa RP, Dhiman P, Marwaha RK (1995) Incontinentia pigmenti (Bloch-Sulzberger syndrome): report of a case and review of the Indian literature. Indian Journal of Pediatrics 62(1):118–122

Incontinentia pigmenti achromians

▶ **Hypomelanosis of Ito**

Indian tick typhus

▶ **Boutonneuse fever**

Infantile acropustulosis

▶ **Acropustulosis of infancy**

Infantile digital fibromatosis

Synonym(s)

Digital fibrous tumor of childhood; Reye tumor; recurring digital fibroma of childhood

Definition

Benign, nodular proliferation of fibrous tissue occurring almost exclusively on the dorsal and lateral aspects of the fingers or toes in infants and small children

Pathogenesis

Unknown

Clinical manifestation

Single or multiple, firm, erythematous, smooth, dome-shaped papules on the dorsal-lateral aspect of distal phalanges of the fingers and toes; sparing of the thumbs and great toes; occasional spontaneous regression

Differential diagnosis
Acquired digital fibrokeratoma; wart; knuckle pad; dermatofibroma; granuloma annulare; angiofibroma; fibrosarcoma; xanthoma; neurilemmoma; sarcoidosis

Therapy
Surgery only if impairment or deformity of the digits; triamcinolone 3–5 mg per ml intralesional

References
Kawaguchi M, Mitsuhashi Y, Hozumi Y, Kondo S (1998) A case of infantile digital fibromatosis with spontaneous regression. Journal of Dermatology 25(8):523–526

Infantile eczema

▶ Atopic dermatitis

Infantile eruptive papulous dermatitis

▶ Gianotti-Crosti syndrome

Infantile fibromatosis

▶ Juvenile fibromatosis

Infantile hemangioma

▶ Capillary hemangioma

Infantile lichenoid acrodermatitis

▶ Gianotti-Crosti syndrome

Infantile myofibromatosis

▶ Juvenile fibromatosis

Infantile papular acrodermatitis

▶ Gianotti-Crosti syndrome

Infantile scurvy

▶ Barlow's disease

Infantile vegetating halogenosis

▶ Granuloma gluteale infantum

Infantile/childhood eosinophilic pustulosis of the scalp

▶ Eosinophilic pustular folliculitis

Infection by achlorophillic algae

▶ Protothecosis, cutaneous

Inflammatory angiomatous nodules

▶ Angiolymphoid hyperplasia with eosinophilia

Inflammatory linear verrucous epidermal nevus

▶ Epidermal nevus

Insect bite reaction

▶ Papular urticaria

Interface parapsoriasis

▶ Large plaque parapsoriasis

Interferon-α

Trade name(s)
Roferon A; Intron A

Generic available
No

Drug class
Immune modulator

Mechanism of action
Anti-viral; anti-proliferative; immunoregulatory

Dosage form
Powder for reconstitution for subcutaneous or intramuscular injection

Dermatologic indications and dosage
See table

Common side effects
General: flu-like symptoms
Laboratory: decreased white blood cell count, elevated liver enzymes

Serious side effects
Bone marrow: suppression
Immunologic: autoimmune thyroiditis
Neurologic: spastic hemiplegia, mood disorders, seizures; peripheral neuropathy
Pulmonary: toxic effects

Drug interactions
Bone marrow suppressants; vinca alkaloids; zidovudine; aminophylline; interleukin-2

Contraindications/precautions
Hypersensitivity to drug class or component; pregnancy; autoimmune hepatitis

References
Edwards L (2001) The interferons. Dermatologic Clinics 19:139–146

Intertriginous inflammation

▶ Intertrigo

Intertrigo

Synonym(s)
Intertriginous inflammation

Interferon-α. Dermatologic indications and dosage

Disease	Adult dosage	Child dosage
AIDS-associated Kaposi's sarcoma	30 million IU/m^2 subcutaneously or intramuscularly 3 times weekly	Not applicable
Basal cell carcinoma	500,000 IU subcutaneously 3 times weekly for 3 weeks	Not applicable
Behçet's disease	2 million IU subcutaneously weekly, escalating to 12 million IU over 2 months	Not indicated
Cutaneous T cell lymphoma	1 million IU intralesional weekly for 4 weeks	Not indicated
Genital warts	250,000 IU intralesional twice weekly for 8 weeks	Not indicated
Giant condyloma of Buschke and Löwenstein	250,000 IU intralesional twice weekly for 8 weeks	Not applicable
High risk melanoma adjuvant therapy	20 million IU per m^2 IV 5 days weekly for 4 weeks, followed by 10 million IU per m^2 subcutaneously 3 times weekly for 48 weeks	20 million IU per m^2 IV 5 days weekly for 4 weeks, followed by 10 million IU per m^2 subcutaneously 3 times weekly for 48 weeks
Infantile hemangioma	Not applicable	3 million IU subcutaneously daily for up to 18 months
Keloid, post-excision	1.5 million IU intralesional twice over 4 days	1.5 million IU intralesional twice over 4 days
Squamous cell carcinoma	500,000 IU subcutaneously 3 times weekly for 3 weeks	Not applicable

Definition

Superficial inflammation of skin caused by moisture, bacteria, or fungi in the skin folds

References

Guitart J, Woodley DT (1994) Intertrigo: a practical approach. Comprehensive Therapy 20(7):402–409

Intestinal amebiasis

▶ Amebiasis

Intra-oral fistula

▶ Oral cutaneous fistula

Intraepidermal adenocarcinoma

▶ Paget's disease

Intravascular endothelioma

▶ Angioendotheliomatosis

Intravascular lymphomatosis

▶ Angioendotheliomatosis

Inverted follicular keratosis

Synonym(s)
None

Definition
Benign proliferation characterized by endophytic growth and histologic follicular differentiation

Pathogenesis
Unknown

Clinical manifestation
Solitary, skin-colored papule or nodule with a smooth or minimally keratotic surface, most commonly on the face of middle-aged patients

Differential diagnosis
Seborrheic keratosis; wart; squamous cell carcinoma; keratoacanthoma; basal cell carcinoma

Therapy
Simple excision[*]

References
Soylu L, Akcali C, Aydogan LB, Ozsahinoglu C, Tuncer I (1993) Inverted follicular keratosis. American Journal of Otolaryngology 14(4):247–248

Iododerma

▶ Halogenoderma

Iron deposition disease

▶ Hemochromatosis

Ischemic ulcer

▶ Decubitus ulcer

Isotretinoin

Trade name(s)
Accutane; Amnesteem; Sotret

Generic available
No

Drug class
Retinoid

Mechanism of action
Inhibition of sebaceous gland differentiation and proliferation; reduction in sebaceous gland activity; normalization of follicular epithelial differentiation

Dosage form
10 mg, 20 mg, 40 mg capsule

Dermatologic indications and dosage
See table

Common side effects
Dermatologic: peeling on hands and feet, cheilitis, skin fragility, alopecia, dry skin, pruritus, paronychia
Eyes: dry eyes, with contact lens intolerance; dry mucous membranes
Musculoskeletal: myalgias, arthralgias
Laboratory: hyperlipidemia

Serious side effects
Eye: decreased night vision
Neurologic: spinal hyperostosis, pseudotumor cerebri, mood disorder
Gastrointestinal: hepatotoxicity, pancreatitis

Isotretinoin. Dermatologic indications and dosage

Disease	Adult dosage	Child dosage
Acne conglobata	0.5 mg/kg PO daily for 1 month followed by 1 mg/kg daily for 4 months	0.5 mg/kg PO daily for 1 month followed by 1 mg/kg daily for 4 months
Acne necrotica	0.5 mg/kg PO daily for 1 month followed by 1 mg/kg daily for 4 months	0.5 mg/kg PO daily for 1 month followed by 1 mg/kg daily for 4 months
Acne vulgaris	0.5 mg/kg PO daily for 1 month followed by 1 mg/kg daily for 4 months	0.5 mg/kg PO daily for 1 month followed by 1 mg/kg daily for 4 months
Basal cell nevus syndrome	0.5 mg/kg PO daily for 1 month followed by 1 mg/kg daily for 4–6 months	0.5 mg/kg PO daily for 1 month followed by 1 mg/kg daily for 4–6 months
Chloracne	0.5 mg/kg PO daily for 1 month followed by 1 mg/kg daily for 4 months	0.5 mg/kg PO daily for 1 month followed by 1 mg/kg daily for 4 months
Darier disease	0.2–0.3 mg/kg PO daily for 1 month, followed by 0.5–1.0 mg/kg daily indefinitely	0.2–0.3 mg/kg PO daily for 1 month, followed by 0.5–1.0 mg/kg daily indefinitely
Dissecting cellulitis of the scalp	0.5 mg/kg PO daily for 1 month followed by 1 mg/kg daily for 4 months	0.5 mg/kg PO daily for 1 month followed by 1 mg/kg daily for 4 months
Eosinophilic pustular folliculitis	0.5 mg/kg PO daily for 1 month followed by 1 mg/kg daily for 4 months	0.5 mg/kg PO daily for 1 month followed by 1 mg/kg daily for 4 months
Gram negative folliculitis	0.5 mg/kg PO daily for 1 month followed by 1 mg/kg daily for 4 months	0.5 mg/kg PO daily for 1 month followed by 1 mg/kg daily for 4 months
Hidradenitis suppurativa	0.5 mg/kg PO daily for 1 month followed by 1 mg/kg daily for 4 months	0.5 mg/kg PO daily for 1 month followed by 1 mg/kg daily for 4 months
Keratosis pilaris atrophicans	0.5 mg/kg PO daily for 1 month followed by 1 mg/kg daily for 4 months	0.5 mg/kg PO daily for 1 month followed by 1 mg/kg daily for 4 months
Lamellar ichthyosis	0.2–0.3 mg/kg PO daily for 1 month, followed by 0.5–1.0 mg/kg daily indefinitely	0.2–0.3 mg/kg PO daily for 1 month, followed by 0.5–1.0 mg/kg daily indefinitely
Lichen sclerosus	0.5 mg/kg PO daily for 1 month followed by 1 mg/kg daily for 4 months	0.5 mg/kg PO daily for 1 month followed by 1 mg/kg daily for 4 months
Lupus erythematosus, discoid	0.5 mg/kg PO daily for 1 month followed by 1 mg/kg daily for 4 months	0.5 mg/kg PO daily for 1 month followed by 1 mg/kg daily for 4 months
Muir-Torre syndrome	0.5–1.0 mg per kg PO indefinitely	0.5–1.0 mg per kg PO indefinitely

Isotretinoin. Dermatologic indications and dosage (Continued)

Disease	Adult dosage	Child dosage
Pityriasis rubra pilaris	0.5 mg/kg PO daily for 1 month followed by 1 mg/kg daily for 4 months	0.5 mg/kg PO daily for 1 month followed by 1 mg/kg daily for 4 months
Reactive perforating collagenosis	0.5 mg/kg PO daily for 1 month followed by 1 mg/kg daily for 4 months	0.5 mg/kg PO daily for 1 month followed by 1 mg/kg daily for 4 months
Rosacea	10–20 mg PO daily for 4–6 months	Not indicated
Sebaceous gland hyperplasia	10–20 mg PO daily or every other day indefinitely	Not indicated
Steatocystoma mutiplex	0.5 mg/kg PO daily for 1 month followed by 1 mg/kg daily for 4–6 months	0.5 mg/kg PO daily for 1 month followed by 1 mg/kg daily for 4–6 months
T-cell lymphoma, cutaneous	1 mg per kg PO daily for 4–6 months	1 mg per kg PO daily for 4–6 months
Transient acantholytic dermatosis	0.5–1.0 mg per kg PO daily for 4–5 months	Not applicable

Genitourinary: major birth defects; pseudotumor cerebri

Drug interactions
Tretinoin; benzoyl peroxide; carbamazepine; tetracyclines

Contraindications/precautions
Hypersensitivity to drug class or component; pregnancy; caution in patients with renal or hepatic dysfunction, history of pancreatitis or diabetes mellitus; children may be more sensitive to effects on bones, which may prevent normal bone growth during puberty

References
Hirsch RJ, Shalita AR (2001) Isotretinoin dosing: past, present, and future trends. Seminars in Cutaneous Medicine & Surgery 20(3):162–165

Itching purpura of Loewenthal

▶ Benign pigmented purpura

Ito, nevus of

▶ Nevus of Ota and Ito

Itraconazole

Trade name(s)
Sporanox

Generic available
No

Drug class
Azole antifungal agent

Mechanism of action
Cell wall ergosterol inhibition secondary to blockade of 14α-demethlyation of lanosterol

Dosage form
100 mg tablet; 10 mg per ml oral solution

Itraconazole. Dermatologic indications and dosage

Disease	Adult dosage	Child dosage
Aspergillosis	200 mg PO daily until clearing	Not indicated
Chromoblastomycosis	200 mg twice daily one week per month for 7 months	Not established
Eumycetoma	300 mg PO daily for months to years	Not established
Histoplasmosis	200–400 mg PO daily for 6–12 months	3–5 mg per kg PO once daily for 6–12 months
Majocchi granuloma	200 mg PO daily for 4–6 weeks	5 mg per kg PO once daily for 4–6 weeks
North American blastomycosis	200–400 mg PO daily for a minimum of 6 months	5–7 mg per kg PO daily for a minimum of 6 months
Onychomycosis	200 mg PO twice daily one week per month for 3 months	5 mg per kg once daily for 7 consecutive days each month for 3 months
Oropharyngeal candidiasis	200 mg PO daily for 1–2 weeks	5 mg per kg PO once daily for 1–2 weeks
Prototothecosis	200 mg PO daily for 2–6 weeks	Not established
South American blastomycosis	100 mg PO daily for 6 months	5–7 mg per kg PO daily or divided into 2 doses for 6 months
Sporotrichosis, disseminated	200 mg PO twice daily indefinitely	5 mg per kg PO daily indefinitely
Sporotrichosis, lymphocutaneous variant	100 mg PO twice daily for 4–8 weeks; if no obvious improvement or if evidence of progressive fungal disease occurs, increase dose in 100 mg increments	100 mg PO daily; contintue for at least 1 week following clinical resolution
Tinea capitis	200 mg PO daily for 1–3 weeks	5 mg per kg PO daily for 2–4 weeks
Tinea corporis	200 mg PO daily for 1–3 weeks	5 mg per kg PO once daily for 1–3 weeks
Tinea cruris	200 mg PO daily for 1–3 weeks	5 mg per kg PO once daily for 1–3 weeks
Tinea faciei	200 mg PO daily for 1–3 weeks	5 mg per kg PO once daily for 1–3 weeks
Tinea pedis	200 mg PO daily for 1–3 weeks	5 mg per kg PO once daily for 1–3 weeks
White piedra	100 mg daily until culture-negative	Not established

Dermatologic indications and dosage
See table

Common side effects
Cutaneous: skin eruption, vasculitis
Gastrointestinal: nausea and vomiting, diarrhea, dyspepsia

Laboratory: elevated liver enzymes, hypertriglyceridemia

Serious side effects
Cutaneous: anaphylaxis, Stevens-Johnson syndrome reaction
Gastrointestinal: hepatotoxicity

Ivermectin. Dermatologic indications and dosage

Disease	Adult dosage	Child dosage
Cutaneous larva migrans	200 mcg per kg PO for 1 dose, repeat in 10 days	200 mcg per kg PO for 1 dose, repeat in 10 days
Onchocerciasis	150 mcg per kg PO for 1 dose	150 mcg per kg PO for 1 dose
Scabies	200 mcg per kg PO for 1 dose, repeat in 10 days	200 mcg per kg PO for 1 dose, repeat in 10 days
Strongyloidosis	200 mcg per kg PO for 1 dose, repeat in 10 days	200 mcg per kg PO for 1 dose, repeat in 10 days

Drug interactions
Amiodarone; amitriptyline; antacids; barbiturates; buspirone; carbamazepine; cyclosporine; digoxin; glyburide/metformin; protease inhibitors; phenytoin; pimozide; quinidine; rifampin; statins; sulfonylureas; tacrolimus; theophylline; vinca alkaloids; warfarin

Contraindications/precautions
Hypersensitivity to drug class or component; use of the following medications – cisapride, midazolam, triazolam, pimozide, quinidine, dofetilide, lovastatin, simvastatin; history of congestive heart failure; caution in patients with cardiovascular or pulmonary disease or impaired liver or renal function

References
Moosavi M, Bagheri B, Scher R (2001) Systemic antifungal therapy. Dermatologic Clinics 19(1):35–52

Ivermectin

Trade name(s)
Stromectol

Generic available
Yes

Drug class
Anti-helminthic

Mechanism of action
Increases nerve and muscle cell permeability of targetpathogens

Dosage form
3 mg, 6 mg tablet

Dermatologic indications and dosage
See table

Common side effects
Cutaneous: pruritus, skin eruption, edema
Lymph nodes: lymphadenopathy
Neurologic: dizziness

Serious side effects
None

Drug interactions
None

Contraindications/precautions
Hypersensitivity to drug class or component

References
del Giudice P (2002) Ivermectin in scabies. Current Opinion in Infectious Diseases 15(2):123–126

Jacob's ulcer

▶ Basal cell carcinoma

Jadassohn-Lewandowsky syndrome

▶ Pachyonychia congenita

Jessner's lymphocytic infiltrate

▶ Jessner lymphocytic infiltration of skin

Jessner's lymphocytic infiltration of skin

Synonym(s)
Jessner's lymphocytic infiltrate, lymphocytic infiltrate of Jessner; benign chronic T-cell infiltrative disorder

Definition
Chronic benign T-cell infiltrative process of the skin

Pathogenesis
Possibly a photosensitivity disorder

Clinical manifestation
One or a few asymptomatic, erythematous papules, which expand peripherally to form well demarcated, infiltrated, red plaques, usually on sun-exposed skin; occasional-spontaneous resolution after several months

Differential diagnosis
Lupus erythematosus; polymorphous light eruption; granuloma faciale; lymphoma; cutaneous metastasis; granuloma annulare; sarcoidosis; fixed drug eruption

Therapy
Triamcinolone 3–4 mg per ml intralesional; corticosteroids, topical, high potency; hydroxychloroquine; prednisone; thalido-mide; surgical excision of individual lesions; superficial orthovoltage radiation; cryotherapy

References
Guillaume JC, Moulin G, Dieng MT, Poli F, Morel P, et al. (1995) Crossover study of thalidomide vs placebo in Jessner's lymphocytic infiltration of the skin. Archives of Dermatology 131(9):1032–1035

Jeunes filles, des

▶ Acne excoriée

Job syndrome

▶ **Hyperimmunoglobulin E syndrome**

Job's syndrome

▶ **Hyperimmunoglobulin E syndrome**

Jock itch

▶ **Tinea cruris**

Jogger's nipples

Synonym(s)
None

Definition
Irritation of the nipples secondary to frictional trauma from clothing worn by runners

Pathogenesis
Frictional trauma on sensitive skin from hard shirt fabrics

Clinical manifestation
Soreness, dryness, erythema, erosions, and bleeding of the nipples, worse in those with erect nipples; occurs in women who do not wear bras when running or in men who wear shirts made of hard, synthetic fibers

Differential diagnosis
Contact dermatitis; atopic dermatitis; xerotic eczema; Paget's disease of the nipple

Therapy
Protective bras in women*; soft-fiber outer garments, made of materials such as silk; protective tape over nipples before running; emollient creams

References
Ramsey ML (1997) Skin care for active people. Physician and Sportsmedicine 25(3):131–132

Junctional epidermolysis simplex

▶ **Epidermolysis bullosa**

Juvenile fibromatosis

Synonym(s)
Infantile fibromatosis

Definition
Group of disorders of infancy and childhood, characterized by proliferation of fibroblasts

Pathogenesis
Unknown; juvenile hyaline fibromatosis variant a disorder of glycosaminoglycan synthesis

Clinical manifestation
Infantile myofibromatosis: one or multiple, rubbery or hard, skin-colored papules, either superficial or deep to the muscle, most commonly occurring on the head, neck, and trunk; usually present at birth or within the first few months of life; regression by age 2 years; viscera rarely involved, but if so, prognosis is poor
Fibrous hamartoma of infancy: usually present at birth, often in the axillary area, shoulder or groin region; presents as enlarging subcutaneous nodule; occasional spontaneous resolution
Juvenile hyaline fibromatosis (systemic hyalinosis): onset in early infancy with multiple, hard or soft, fixed or mobile, translucent papules and nodules of the scalp, face,

gingivae, neck and trunk; osteolytic lesions of skull, long bones, or phalanges; poor muscle development; joint contractures in adult life
Infantile digital fibromatosis: multiple, firm, smooth, pink or flesh-colored papules of the fingers or toes, at birth or early childhood, often with spontaneous regression after 2–3 years

Differential diagnosis
Acquired digital fibrokeratoma; granuloma annulare; angiofibroma; fibrosarcoma; leiomyoma; leiomyosarcoma; juvenile xanthogranuloma; sarcoidosis; multicentric reticulohistiocytosis; knuckle pads

Therapy
Infantile myofibromatosis: none indicated if limited to superficial structures; chemotherapy if visceral involvement
Fibrous hamartoma of infancy: surgical excision
Juvenile hyaline fibromatosis: no effective therapy
Infantile digital fibromatosis: excisional surgery only if impairment or deformity of the digits

References
Campbell RJ, Garrity JA (1991) Juvenile fibromatosis of the orbit: a case report with review of the literature. British Journal of Ophthalmology 75(5):313–316

Juvenile giant cell granuloma

▸ Juvenile xanthogranuloma

Juvenile hyaline fibromatosis

▸ Juvenile fibromatosis

Juvenile xanthogranuloma

Synonym(s)
Nevoxanthoendothelioma; xanthoma multiplex; juvenile xanthoma; congenital xanthoma tuberosum; xanthoma naviforme; juvenile giant cell granuloma

Definition
Benign papules and nodules, composed of histiocytic cells, that predominantly occur in infancy and childhood

Pathogenesis
Possibly a granulomatous reaction of histiocytes to an unknown stimulus

Clinical manifestation
Occurs in infancy or early childhood, with asymptomatic, smooth, firm papules that initially are red-brown, then quickly change color to yellow, usually on the trunk or upper extremities; lesions resolve spontaneously in months to years, leaving small, atrophic scars

Differential diagnosis
Xanthoma; mastocytoma; insect bite reaction; granuloma annulare; sarcoidosis; Spitz nevus; Langerhans cell histiocytosis; non-Langerhans cell histiocytosis; benign cephalic histiocytosis; generalized eruptive histiocytoma; self-healing reticulohistiocytoma; xanthoma disseminatum

Therapy
Excision for cosmetic reasons only

References
Chang MW (1999) Update on juvenile xanthogranuloma: unusual cutaneous and systemic variants. Seminars in Cutaneous Medicine & Surgery 18(3):195–205

Juvenile xanthoma

▸ Juvenile xanthogranuloma

Juxtaepidermal poroma

▶ Poroma

K

K-M syndrome

▸ Kasabach-Merritt syndrome

Kaltostat

▸ Alginates

Kaposi sarcoma

▸ Kaposi's sarcoma

Kaposi varicelliform eruption

▸ Eczema herpeticum

Kaposi's dermatosis

▸ Xeroderma pigmentosum

Kaposi's sarcoma

Synonym(s)
Kaposi sarcoma; multiple idiopathic hemorrhagic sarcoma

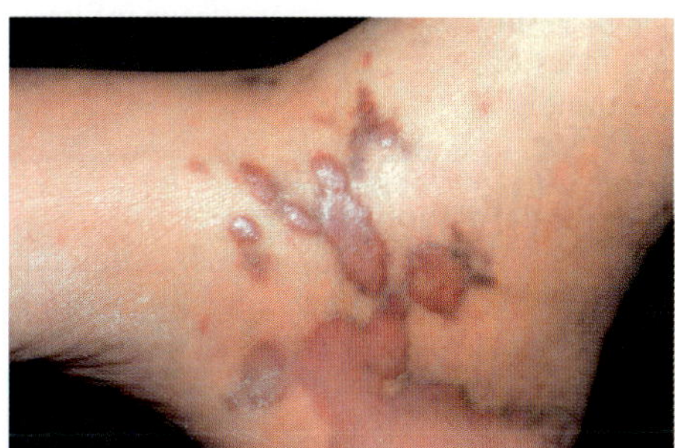

Kaposi's sarcoma. Violaceous papules and plaques on the lower extremity

Definition
Neoplasm of endothelial origin, involving the skin, mucosal surfaces, and internal organs

Pathogenesis
Unclear whether a hyperplastic disease or a true neoplasm; Herpes hominis virus-8 (HHV-8) linked to all subtypes; co-factors: immunosuppression, genetics, country of residence, and male sex

Clinical manifestation
Classic subtype: usually affects older men of Mediterranean or eastern European

backgrounds; sometimes arises in chronically edematous extremities; violaceous patches, plaques, or nodules on the lower extremities, which can be painful and can ulcerate

African endemic subtype: primarily affects boys and men; appears same as classic subtype or in a more deadly form involving bones and lymph system

Iatrogenic subtype: seen in kidney and liver transplant patients on immunosuppressive drugs; usually regresses after immunosuppressive drug stopped

AIDS-related subtype: lesions often appear on the upper body, including the oral cavity, head, neck, back, and in viscera; begin as discrete, red or purple patches that are bilaterally symmetric and initially tend to involve the lower extremities; patches become elevated, evolving into nodules and plaques; sometimes arise as a large infiltrating mass or as multiple, cone-shaped, friable tumors

Differential diagnosis
Pyogenic granuloma; tufted angioma; melanocytic nevus; melanoma; cavernous hemangioma; angiokeratoma; metastasis; myofibromatoma; arteriovenous malformations

Therapy
None indicated for indolent skin tumors in elderly patients; localized disease: cryotherapy; radiation therapy; surgical excision or laser ablation; intralesional vinblastine chemotherapy; disseminated disease: vinblastine 3.5–10 mg IV weekly, or chemotherapy combinations, with vinblastine, bleomycin, and doxorubicin; AIDS-associated disease: antiviral therapy

References
Geraminejad P, Memar O, Aronson I, Rady PL, Hengge U, Tyring SK (2002) Kaposi's sarcoma and other manifestations of human herpesvirus 8. Journal of the American Academy of Dermatology 47(5):641–655

Kaposi's sarcoma-like granuloma

▶ Granuloma gluteale infantum

Kaposi's varicelliform eruption

▶ Herpes simplex virus infection

Kasabach-Merritt syndrome

Synonym(s)
K-M syndrome; consumptive thrombocytopenia; giant hemangioma syndrome

Definition
Thrombocytopenia caused by sequestration and destruction of platelets in a large vascular lesion, usually a cavernous hemangioma

Pathogenesis
Vascular lesion cause platelet trapping and activation, with consumption of coagulation factors

Clinical manifestation
Presents as a reddish-brown skin plaque or nodule that progresses to a large violaceous mass; petechiae, bruising, and bleeding; high-output cardiac failure; may occur in cavernous hemangioma, Kaposi hemangioendothelioma, or tufted angioma

Differential diagnosis
Coagulation abnormality of other cause; angiosarcoma; port-wine stain; congenital hemangiopericytoma; kaposiform heman-

gioendothelioma of infancy and childhood; teratoma; lymphatic malformation; venous malformation; infantile fibrosarcoma; infantile myofibromatosis; congenital hemangiopericytoma; epithelioid hemangioendothelioma

Therapy
Prednisone; interferon; hematologic agents such as epsilon aminocaproic acid, aspirin, and dipyridamole, pentoxifylline, and cryoprecipitate

References
Hall GW (2001) Kasabach-Merritt syndrome: pathogenesis and management. British Journal of Haematology 112(4):851–862

Kawasaki disease

Synonym(s)
Mucocutaneous lymph node syndrome; Kawasaki syndrome; acute febrile mucocutaneous lymph node syndrome

Definition
Acute systemic vasculitis associated with a febrile illness; skin and mucous membrane involvement

Pathogenesis
May be caused by a ubiquitous infectious agent in certain genetically predisposed individuals

Clinical manifestation
Prolonged fever; polymorphous exanthem; swelling and induration of the hands and feet, with subsequent desquamation; non-exudative conjunctival injection; hemorrhagic, dry, fissured lips; "strawberry tongue"; non-suppurative cervical lymphadenopathy; myocarditis and pancarditis; coronary artery abnormalities; arthralgias and arthritis; urethritis with sterile pyuria; aseptic meningitis; diarrhea, vomiting, abdominal pain; hydrops of the gallbladder; auditory abnormalities; testicular swelling, pneumonitis

Differential diagnosis
Viral exanthem; erythema multiforme; scarlet fever; rubeola; staphylococcal scalded skin syndrome; Stevens-Johnson syndrome/toxic epidermal necrolysis; leptospirosis; Rocky Mountain spotted fever; acrodynia; juvenile rheumatoid arthritis; polyarteritis nodosa

Therapy
Intravenous immunoglobulin (IVIG), 2 g per kg, as a single infusion over 10–12 hours[*]; aspirin 80–100 mg per kg per day PO in 4 divided doses until the fever has abated for several days

References
Rowley AH, Shulman ST (1999) Kawasaki syndrome. Pediatric Clinics of North America 46(2):313–329

Kawasaki syndrome

▶ Kawasaki disease

Kelley-Seegmiller syndrome

▶ Lesch-Nyhan syndrome

Keloid

Synonym(s)
Cheloid

Definition
Overgrowth of fibrous tissue that usually develops at the site of a skin injury, where

the tissue extends beyond borders of the original wound, usually does not regress spontaneously, and tends to recur after excision

Pathogenesis

Probable genetic factors; imbalance between the anabolic and catabolic phases of healing process; more collagen produced than degraded

Clinical manifestation

Rubbery or hard, reddish-brown papule or nodule, with regular margins; some with clawlike pseudopods extending beyond the areas of trauma, projecting above the level of the surrounding skin; no spontaneous regression; lesion become less red over many months or years; most common locations: earlobes, face, neck, lower extremities, breast, chest, back, and abdomen

Differential diagnosis

Hypertrophic scar; squamous cell carcinoma; dermatofibroma; dermatofibrosarcoma protuberans; fibromatosis; North American blastomycosis

Therapy

Triamcinolone 10–20 mg per ml intralesional; cryotherapy; silicone gel sheet; compression dressing; superficial orthovoltage radiation therapy; surgical excision with postoperative interferon or imiquimod

References

Shaffer JJ, Taylor SC, Cook-Bolden F (2002) Keloidal scars: a review with a critical look at therapeutic options. Journal of the American Academy of Dermatology 46(2):S63–97

Keratinous cyst

▶ Pilar cyst

Keratoacanthoma

Synonym(s)

Self-healing squamous cell carcinoma; self-healing epithelioma

Definition

Low-grade malignancy of the pilosebaceous epithelium, characterized by rapid growth over a few weeks to months, followed by spontaneous resolution over several months

Pathogenesis

Possible etiologic factors: sun exposure, trauma, human papilloma virus, genetic factors, and immunosuppression

Clinical manifestation

Solitary, firm, round, skin-colored or reddish papule rapidly progressing to dome-shaped nodule, with a smooth shiny surface and a central keratinous plug; occurs on sun-exposed areas of face, neck, and dorsum of the upper extremities; spontaneous involution after many months

Differential diagnosis

Squamous cell carcinoma; basal cell carcinoma; wart; seborrheic keratosis; inverted follicular keratosis; atypical fibroxanthoma; Merkel cell carcinoma; metastasis; sporotrichosis; coccidioidomycosis; North American blastomycosis; prurigo nodularis

Therapy

Surgical excision[*]; radiation therapy; methotrexate 25 mg per ml intralesional, repeated every 2–3 weeks for up to 5 treatments; fluorouracil 50 mg per ml intralesional, repeated every 2–3 weeks for up to 5 treatments

References

Schwartz RA (1994) Keratoacanthoma. Journal of the American Academy of Dermatology 30(1):1–19

Keratoconjunctivitis sicca

▶ Sjögren syndrome

Keratoderma

Synonym(s)
Keratodermia

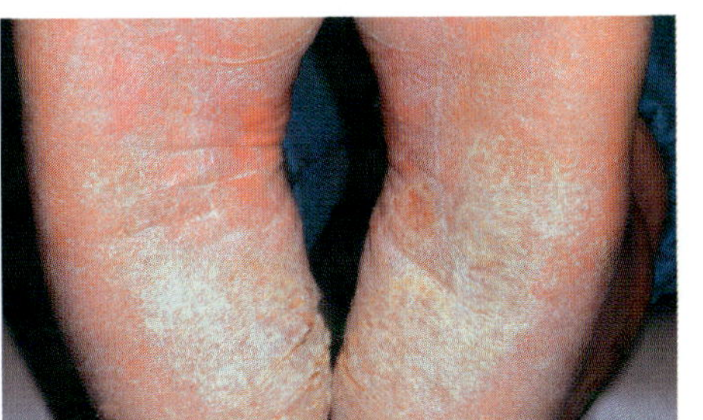

Keratoderma. Scaly plaques on the plantar aspects of the feet

Definition
Skin disorder consisting of a surface that appears horny or scaly

References
Ratnavel RC, Griffiths WA (1997) The inherited palmoplantar keratodermas. British Journal of Dermatology 137(4):485–490

Keratoderma blennorrhagica

Definition
Hyperkeratotic and pustular condition of the palms and soles associated with Reiter disease

References
Shupack JL, Stiller MJ, Haber RS (1991) Psoriasis and Reiter's syndrome. Clinics in Dermatology 9(1):53–58

Keratoderma hereditaria mutilans

▶ Vohwinkel syndrome

Keratoderma palmoplangtaris diffusa with periodontosis

▶ Papillon-Lefèvre syndrome

Keratoderma palmoplantaris striata

▶ Striate keratoderma

Keratoderma palmoplantaris transgradiens

▶ Mal de Meleda

Keratodermia

▶ Keratoderma

Keratoelastoidosis

▶ Acrokeratoelastoidosis

Keratolysis plantaris sulcatum

▶ Pitted keratolysis

Keratolytic winter erythema

Synonym(s)
Winter erythrokeratolysis; erythrokeratolysis hiemalis; Oudtshoorn skin

Definition
Form of ichthyosis characterized by cyclical erythema, hyperkeratosis, and recurrent and intermittent peeling of the palms and soles, particularly during winter

Pathogenesis
Unknown; autosomal dominant trait

Clinical manifestation
Palmoplantar erythema with skin scaling; more pronounced in winter months

Differential diagnosis
Erythrokeratodermia variabilis; progressive symmetric erythrokeratodermia; Giroux-Barbeau erythrokeratodermia with ataxia; Greither disease; ichthyosis linearis circumflexa; psoriasis; mycosis fungoides; lupus erythematosus; lamellar ichthyosis; gyrate erythema; atopic dermatitis

Therapy
Emollients

References
Danielsen AG, Weismann K, Thomsen HK (2001) Erythrokeratolysis hiemalis (keratolytic winter erythema): a case report from Denmark. Journal of the European Academy of Dermatology & Venereology 15(3):255–256

Keratoma plantarum sulcatum

▶ Pitted keratolysis

Keratomycosis nigricans palmaris

▶ Tinea nigra

Keratosis diffusa fetalis

▶ Ichthyosis fetalis

Keratosis follicularis

▶ Darier disease

Keratosis follicularis et parafollicularis serpiginosa

▶ Elastosis perforans serpiginosa

Keratosis follicularis serpiginosa

▶ Elastosis perforans serpiginosa

Keratosis follicularis spinosa of Unna

▶ Lichen spinulosus

Keratosis follicularis spinulosa

▶ Lichen spinulosus

Keratosis, inverted follicular

▶ Inverted follicular keratosis

Keratosis, lichenoid

▶ Lichenoid keratosis

Keratosis palmaris et plantaris

Synonym(s)
Palmoplantar keratosis; palmoplantar keratoderma

Definition
Heterogeneous group of disorders characterized by scaling and thickening of palms and soles

References
Ratnavel RC, Griffiths WA (1997) The inherited palmoplantar keratodermas. British Journal of Dermatology 137(4):485–490

Keratosis palmaris et plantaris with carcinoma of the esophagus

▶ Tylosis

Keratosis palmo-plantaris circumscripta

▶ Tyrosinemia II

Keratosis pilaris

Synonym(s)
Lichen pilaris; keratosis suprafollicularis; pityriasis pilaris

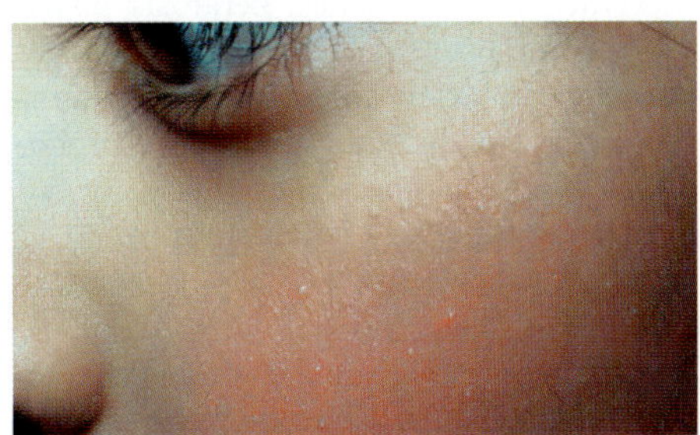

Keratosis pilaris. Acuminate, follicular papules on the cheek

Definition
Disorder of follicular keratinization, characterized by follicular keratotic papules

Pathogenesis
Autosomal dominant trait; arises from excessive accumulation of keratin at the follicular orifice

Clinical manifestation
Multiple accuminate follicular keratotic papules, sometimes with surounding erythema, most common on lateral arms, thighs and cheeks; association with ichthyosis vulgaris and atopic dermatitis; worse in dry climates and in the winter months; tends to improve with age

Differential diagnosis
Lichen spinulosus; folliculitis; milia; phrynoderma; ichthyosis; pityriasis rubra pilaris; Darier disease; lichen planus

Therapy
Emollients; tretinoin; alpha hydroxy acids; corticosteroids, topical, medium potency

References
Lateef A, Schwartz RA (1999) Keratosis pilaris. Cutis 63(4):205–207

Keratosis pilaris atrophicans

Synonym(s)
Ulerythema ophryogenes; keratosis pilaris rubra atrophicans faciei; keratosis pilaris atrophicans faciei; folliculitis ulerythema reticulata; honeycomb atrophy; atrophoderma vermiculatum; ulerythema acneiforme; atrophoderma reticulatum

Definition
Group of clinically related disorders characterized by follicular keratotic papules, variable perifollicular inflammation, and end-stage atrophy

Pathogenesis
Unknown; hereditary component

Clinical manifestation
Keratosis pilaris rubra atrophicans faciei (ulerythema ophryogenes) variant: follicular papules with erythematous halo, located over the lateral eyebrows; beginning shortly after birth and diminishing with age
Atrophoderma vermiculatum variant: onset between age 5 and 12 years; follicular keratotic papules with surrounding erythema; evolving into atrophic pits in a reticulate honeycomb pattern

Differential diagnosis
Keratosis pilaris; folliculitis; acne vulgaris; milia; pityriasis rubra pilaris

Therapy
Keratolytics such as lactic acid 5% cream, urea 10% cream, or salicylic acid 2–5% cream or gel applied twice daily; alpha hydroxy acids; isotretinoin

▶ **Ulerythema ophryogenes**

References
Frosch PJ, Brumage MR, Schuster-Pavlovic C, Bersch A (1988) Atrophoderma vermiculatum. Case reports and review. Journal of the American Academy of Dermatology 18(3):538–542

Keratosis pilaris atrophicans faciei folliculitis ulerythema reticulata

▶ **Keratosis pilaris atrophicans**

Keratosis pilaris rubra atrophicans faciei

▶ **Keratosis pilaris atrophicans**
▶ **Ulerythema ophryogenes**

Keratosis rubra congenita

▶ Lamellar ichthyosis

Keratosis rubra figurata

▶ Erythrokeratodermia variabilis

Keratosis supracapitularis

▶ Knuckle pads

Keratosis suprafollicularis

▶ Keratosis pilaris

Keratosis-ichthyosis-deafness syndrome

▶ KID syndrome

Ketoconazole

Trade name(s)
Nizoral

Generic available
Yes

Drug class
Azole antifungal agent

Mechanism of action
Inhibition of fungal cell membrane ergosterol synthesis

Dosage form
200 mg tablet

Dermatologic indications and dosage
See table

Common side effects
Dermatologic: skin eruption, pruritus
Gastrointestinal: nausea and vomiting, diarrhea, abdominal pain
Neurologic: somnolence, dizziness, lethargy, headache, nervousness
Laboratory: elevated liver enzymes

Serious side effects
Dermatologic: anaphylaxis
Gastrointestinal: hepatic failure

Ketoconazole. Dermatologic indications and dosage

Disease	Adult dosage	Child dosage
Eumycetoma	400 mg PO daily for months to years	Not established
Histoplasmosis	200–400 mg PO daily for 6–12 months	5–10 mg per kg PO daily for 6–12 months
North American blastomycosis	400–800 mg PO daily for a minimum of 6 months	5–7 mg per kg PO daily for 6 months
Protothecosis	200–400 mg PO daily for 2–6 weeks	Not established
South American blastomycosis	200–400 mg PO dailyfor 6–12 months	5–10 mg per kg PO daily for 6–12 months
Tinea versicolor	400 mg PO for 1 dose; repeat in 7 days	6.6 mg per kg PO for 1 dose; repeat in 7 days

Endocrine: adrenal insufficiency
Laboratory: leukopenia, hemolytic anemia

Drug interactions
Amiodarone; amitriptyline; antacids; barbiturates; buspirone; carbamazepine; cyclosporine; digoxin; glyburide/metformin; H-2 blockers; protease inhibitors; phenytoin; pimozide; quinidine; rifampin; statins; sulfonylureas; tacrolimus; theophylline; vinca alkaloids; warfarin

Contraindications/precautions
Hypersensitivity to drug class or component; achlorhydria; fungal meningitis; caution in patients with hepatic insufficiency or with use of other potentially hepatotoxic medications

References
Rheney CC, Saddler CM (1998) Oral ketoconazole in cutaneous fungal infections. Annals of Pharmacotherapy 32(6):709–711

KID syndrome

Synonym(s)
Keratosis-ichthyosis-deafness syndrome

Definition
Disorder characterized by keratitis, ichthyosis-like keratoderma, and deafness

Pathogenesis
Unknown

Clinical manifestation
Vascularizing keratitis, with recurrent corneal ulcerations; congenital erythrokeratoderma; reticulated hyperkeratosis of the palms and soles; sensorineural deafness; may develop chronic infections, scarring alopecia, squamous cell carcinoma, and neuromuscular disease

Differential diagnosis
Congenital ichthyosiform erythroderma; lamellar ichthyosis; epidermolytic hyperkeratosis; Netherton's syndrome

Therapy
Emollients; cyclosporine 2% ophthalmic solution for keratitis

References
Langer K, Konrad K, Wolff K (1990) Keratitis, ichthyosis and deafness (KID)-syndrome: report of three cases and a review of the literature. British Journal of Dermatology 122(5):689–697

Kikuchi's disease

▶ Kikuchi's syndrome

Kikuchi's syndrome

Synonym(s)
Kikuchi's disease; Fujimoto's disease; Kikuchi-Fujimoto disease; histiocytic necrotizing lymphadenitis

Definition
Benign, self-limited disorder characterized by fever, chills, weight loss, and lymphadenopathy

Pathogenesis
Possibly hypersensitivity reaction to infectious agent

Clinical manifestation
Painless lymphadenopathy; mainly of the cervical lymph nodes; constitutional signs and symptoms: fever, chills, sore throat, myalgias; skin lesions including red plaques, facial erythema, crusted papules and nodules, ulcerated papules; spontaneous resolution in 1–4 months, with recurrences

Differential diagnosis
Viral exanthem; bacterial skin infection; mononucleosis; lupus erythematosus; lymphoma; metastatic disease; sarcoidosis

Therapy
None

References
Yasukawa K, Matsumura T, Sato-Matsumura KC, Takahashi T, Fujioka Y, Kobayashi H, Shimizu H (2001) Kikuchi's disease and the skin: case report and review of the literature. British Journal of Dermatology 144(4):885–889

Kikuchi-Fujimoto disease

▶ Kikuchi's syndrome

Kimura disease

▶ Kimura's disease

Kimura's disease

Synonym(s)
Kimura disease; eosinophilic granuloma of soft tissue; eosinophilic hyperplastic lymphogranuloma; eosinophilic lymphofolliculosis; eosinophilic lymphofollicular granuloma; eosinophilic lymphoid granuloma

Definition
Benign, self-limited process, characterized by subcutaneous tumors with a characteristic histologic appearance and lymphadenopathy, and peripheral eosinophilia

Pathogenesis
Abnormal proliferation of lymphoid follicles and vascular endothelium; may represent hypersensitivity reaction, perhaps to arthropod bites, parasitic or candidal infections

Clinical manifestation
Solitary or multiple, firm, subcutaneous nodules, which usually are located on the head or neck; lymphadonopathy; peripheral eosinophilia

Differential diagnosis
Angiolymphoid hyperplasia with eosinophilia; pyogenic granuloma; Kaposi's sarcoma; eccrine cylindroma; Langerhans cell histiocytosis; metastatic disease; Mikulicz disease; parotid tumor

Therapy
Surgical excision*; triamcinolone 3–5 mg per ml intralesional; prednisone; radiation therapy

References
Gumbs MA, Pai NB, Saraiya RJ, Rubinstein J, Vythilingam L, Choi YJ (1999) Kimura's disease: a case report and literature review. Journal of Surgical Oncology 70(3):190–193

Kindler syndrome

Synonym(s)
Kindler's syndrome; poikiloderma of Kindler

Definition
Disorder characterized by signs and symptoms of both epidermolysis bullosa and poikiloderma

Pathogenesis
Unknown

Clinical manifestation
Congenital acral bullae; poikiloderma, beginning on sun-exposed skin and spreading to other areas over time; atrophy over the hands and feet; gingivostomatitis

Differential diagnosis

Rothmund-Thomson syndrome; hereditary acrokeratotic poikiloderma of Weary; epidermolysis bullosa; Werner syndrome; Bloom's syndrome

Therapy
None

References

Patrizi A, Pauluzzi P, Neri I, Trevisan G, De Giorgi LB, Pasquinelli G (1996) Kindler syndrome: report of a case with ultrastructural study and review of the literature. Pediatric Dermatology 13(5):397–402

Kindler's syndrome

▶ Kindler syndrome

Kinky hair syndrome

▶ Menke's kinky hair syndrome

Kitamura's acropigmentatio reticularis

▶ Reticulate acropigmentation of Kitamura

Kitamura's reticulate acropigmentation

▶ Reticulate Acropigmentation of Kitamura

Klein-Waardenburg syndrome

▶ Waardenburg syndrome

Klippel-Trenaunay syndrome

▶ Klippel-Trenaunay-Weber syndrome

Klippel-Trenaunay-Weber syndrome

Synonym(s)

Klippel-Trenaunay syndrome; Angio-osteohypertrophy; nevus verrucosus osteohypertrophicus syndrome; hemangiectasia hypertrophicans; nevus verucosus hypertrophicans

Definition

Disorder characterized by triad of port-wine stain, varicose veins, and bony and soft tissue hypertrophy of an extremity

Pathogenesis
Unknown

Clinical manifestation

Multiple port wine stains or other vascular nevi; hypertrophy of bones and soft tissue in the area of increased vascularity, most commonly in the lower limbs, the face and head, or internal organs; occasional arteriovenous fistulas; varicose veins; occasional syndactyly and polydactyly, mental retardation, and seizures

Differential diagnosis

Parkes-Weber syndrome; Mafucci syndrome; proteus syndrome

Therapy
Compression garments; surgical removal of varicosities; flashlamp-pumped pulse dye laser for port wine stain

References
Blei F (2002) Vacular anomalies: From bedside to bench and back again. Current Problems in Pediatric & Adolescent Health Care 32(3):72–93

Knuckle pads

Synonym(s)
Halodermia; subcutaneous fibroma; keratosis supracapitularis; discrete keratoderma

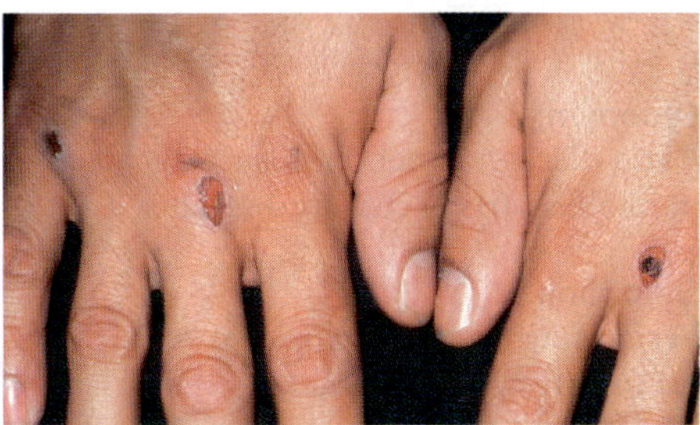

Knuckle pads. Thickened skin over the knuckles, with erosions

Definition
Asymptomatic papules or nodules over the knuckles of the hands, often occurring after repetitive trauma to the area

Pathogenesis
Often of unknown cause; some cases associated with trauma, such as boxing or biting of the knuckles in children; occasional familial disorder

Clinical manifestation
Well-circumscribed, flesh-colored papules or nodules over the knuckles of the hands, most commonly over the proximal interphalangeal joint; may have erosion with frictional trauma

Differential diagnosis
Acanthosis nigricans; wart; granuloma annulare; callus; foreign body reaction; gouty tophus; osteoarthritis with Heberden nodules; rheumatoid nodule

Therapy
Protective gloves or other form of padding over the knuckles

References
Won YH, Seo JJ, Kim SJ, Lee SC, Chun IK (1998) Knuckle pad-like keratoderma: a new cutaneous side reaction induced by tegafur. International Journal of Dermatology 37(4):315–317

Koebner phenomenon

Definition
Appearance of skin lesions of lichen planus, warts, molluscum contagiosum, psoriasis, or lichen nitidus along a site of injury

References
Weiss G, Shemer A, Trau H (2002) The Koebner phenomenon: review of the literature. Journal of the European Academy of Dermatology & Venereology 16(3):241–248

Kohlmeier-Degos syndrome

▶ **Malignant atrophic papulosis**

Koilonychia

Definition
Abnormal shape of the fingernail where the nail plate has raised ridges and is thin and concave

References
Gao XH, Li X, Zhao Y, Wang Y, Chen HD (2001) Familial koilonychia. International Journal of Dermatology 40(4):290–291

Koplik's spots

Definition
Punctate, white papules, often on an erythematous base, occurring on the buccal mucosa early in the course of rubeola

References
Rosa C (1998) Rubella and rubeola. Seminars in Perinatology 22(4):318–322

Kraurosis vulvae

▶ Lichen sclerosus

Kunze riehm syndrome

▶ Michelin tire baby syndrome

Kwashiorkor

Synonym(s)
None

Definition
Nutritional syndrome due to severe protein malnutrition with relative carbohydrate excess

Pathogenesis
Caused by lack of essential amino acids, trace elements such as zinc, and vitamins in the diet

Clinical manifestation
Failure to thrive; edema; muscle wasting; retarded mental development; red, violaceous, and brown exfoliating plaques, giving skin a "flaky paint" appearance; hair dry, lusterless, and light brown to gray in color; dyschromia with hypopigmentation and hyperpigmentation; mucosal cheilosis

Differential diagnosis
Marasmus; pellagra

Therapy
Increase in dietary animal protein

References
Latham MC (1991) The dermatosis of kwashiorkor in young children. Seminars in Dermatology 10(4):270–272

Kyrle disease

▶ Kyrle's disease

Kyrle's disease

Synonym(s)
Kyrle disease; hyperkeratosis follicularis et parafollicularis in cutem penetrans

Definition
Perforating disease associated with diabetes mellitus and renal failure, characterized by formation of large papules with central keratin plugs

Pathogenesis
Possible contributing factors: metabolic derangements, mechanical trauma (e.g., rubbing and scratching), or coiled-up hairs within hyperkeratotic follicular lumina

Clinical manifestation
Small, scaly papule which enlarges to form red-brown papule or nodule with a central keratin plug; some follicular lesions; papules sometimes coalesce to form larger keratotic plaques

Differential diagnosis
Reactive perforating collagenosis; perforating folliculitis; elastosis perforans serpiginosa; prurigo nodularis; scabies; keratoacanthoma; Darier disease; keratosis pilaris

Therapy

Tretinoin; isotretinoin; acitretin; vitamin A 100,000 units PO daily for 30 days, repeated after a 1-month rest period

References

Harman M, Aytekin S, Akdeniz S, Derici M (1998) Kyrle's disease in diabetes mellitus and chronic renal failure. Journal of the European Academy of Dermatology & Venereology 11(1):87–88

L

L-tryptophan-induced eosinophilia-myalgia syndrome

▶ Eosinophilia-myalgia syndrome

Labial lentigo

▶ Lentigo

Lactic acid

▶ Alpha hydroxy acid

Laffer-Ascher syndrome

▶ Ascher's syndrome

Lamellar ichthyosis

Synonym(s)
Nonbullous congenital ichthyosiform erythroderma; ichthyosis sebacea; ichthyosis congenita larva; keratosis rubra

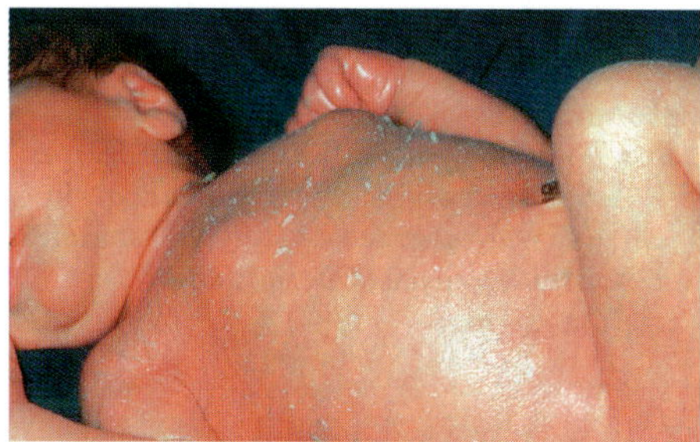

Lamellar ichthyosis. Generalized erythema and scale in a neonate

Definition
Hereditary disorder of cornification, characterized by large, dark, plate-like scales and underlying erythroderma

Pathogenesis
Autosomal recessive trait; mutation in the gene for transglutaminase 1(TGM1), enzyme involved in cornified cell envelope formation

Clinical manifestation
Neonate presents with tough, film-like membrane that fissures when stretched (collodion membrane); membrane shed in 10–14 days, leaving redness and scale, ranging from fine and white to thick, dark, and plate-like, arranged in a pattern resembling fish skin; generalized pattern with accentuation in flexural areas such as the axilla, groin, antecubital fossa, and neck, while sparing mucous membranes; scarring alopecia; nail dystrophy; ectropion; eclabium;

conjunctivitis; small, deformed ears; inflexible digits due to taut skin

Differential diagnosis
X-linked ichthyosis; congenital ichthyosiform erythroderma; Conradi disease; Netherton syndrome; trichothiodystrophy; erythrodermic psoriasis; generalized seborrheic dermatitis; Rud syndrome; Sjögren-Larsson syndrome

Therapy
Emollients; alpha hydroxy acids; tretinoin; acitretin

References
Lacour M, Mehta-Nikhar B, Atherton DJ, Harper JI (1996) An appraisal of acitretin therapy in children with inherited disorders of keratinization. British Journal of Dermatology 134(6):1023–1029

Langerhans cell histiocytosis

Synonym(s)
Histiocytosis X; Langerhans cell granulomatosis; type II histiocytosis

Definition
Group of disorders characterized by proliferation of bone-marrow-derived Langerhans cells and mature eosinophils

Pathogenesis
Unclear whether disorders are neoplastic or inflammatory

Clinical manifestation
Unifocal disease (eosinophilic granuloma): solitary bony lesion, usually asymptomatic
Multifocal disease (Hand-Schuler-Christian variant): diabetes insipidus; bony defects; exophthalmos; other features: liver, spleen, lymph node infiltration; skin lesions, including noduloulcerative lesions in the oral, perineal, perivulvar, or retroauricular regions

Acute disseminated disease (Letterer-Siwe): skin findings, including petechiae; scaly or crusted yellow-brown papules, sometimes coalescing to form plaques, often in seborrheic distribution; exudative intertriginous lesions sometimes ulcerating; fever; anemia; thrombocytopenia; pulmonary infiltrates; lymphadenopathy; hepatosplenomegaly; neurologic involvement

Differential diagnosis
Seborrheic dermatitis; dermatomyositis; mastocytosis; Wiskott-Aldrich syndrome; acrodermatitis enteropathica; Rosai-Dorfman disease; xanthoma disseminatum; candidiasis; listeriosis; herpes simplex virus infection; varicella; infantile acropustulosis; leukemia; lymphoma; myeloma

Therapy
Localized skin involvement: high potency topical corticosteroids
Extensive skin involvement: topical nitrogen mustard; photochemotherapy
Multisystem disease: chemotherapy

References
Zelger B, Burgdorf WH (2001) The cutaneous histiocytoses. Advances in Dermatology 17:77–114

Langerhans cell granulomatosis

▶ Langerhans cell histiocytosis

Large plaque parapsoriasis

Synonym(s)
Interface parapsoriasis; atrophic parapsoriasis; variegate dermatitis; poikiloderma atrophicans vasculare; poikiloderma vasculare atrophicans; lichenoid mycosis fungoides

Definition
Chronic, inflammatory skin disorder characterized by large scaly plaques

Pathogenesis
Unclear; may represent exaggerated host response to chronic antigenic stimulation

Clinical manifestation
Faint, salmon-colored plaques with arcuate geographic borders, often greater than 5 cm in diameter; may have an atrophic, cigarette, or tissue paper surface quality; lesions appear on proximal extremities and trunk in a bathing trunk distribution; rare spontaneous remission; sometimes progresses to cutaneous T-cell lymphoma

Differential diagnosis
Small plaque parapsoriasis; psoriasis; seborrheic dermatitis; dermatophytosis; lupus erythematosus; lichen planus; pityriasis rosea; syphilis; mycosis fungoides; xerosis; nummular eczema

Therapy
Corticosteroids, topical, super potency; UVB phototherapy; photochemotherapy

References
Lambert WC, Everett MA (1981) The nosology of parapsoriasis. Journal of the American Academy of Dermatology 5(4):373–395

Larva currens

▶ Strongyloidosis

Larva migrans

▶ Cutaneous larva migrans

Late-onset prurigo of pregnancy

▶ **Pruritic urticarial papules and plaques of pregnancy**

Lateral cervical cyst

▶ **Branchial cleft cyst**

Latrodectism

▶ **Brown recluse spider bite**

Laugier disease

▶ **Laugier-Hunziger syndrome**

Laugier-Hunziger syndrome

Synonym(s)
Laugier disease; essential melanotic pigmentation; idiopathic lenticular mucocutaneous pigmentation

Definition
Acquired, benign, macular hyperpigmentation of the lips and buccal mucosa, associated with longitudinal melanonychia and pigmentation elsewhere

Pathogenesis
Unknown

Clinical manifestation
Solitary or confluent macular hyperpigmentation of buccal mucosa, lips, gingiva, tongue, soft palate, and hard palate; pigmentation also noted on neck, thorax, abdomen, dorsal and lateral aspects of fingers, soles, genitalia, perineum, perianal skin, and anal mucosa; nail pigmentation without dystrophy of fingers and toes; one or two longitudinal bands per nail, which tend to occur along the lateral aspects of the nail plate; half nail pigmentation or complete nail pigmentation

Differential diagnosis
Nevus; melanoma; Addison's disease; hemochromatosis; lichen planus; lupus erythematosus; amalgam tattoo; contact mucositis; drug-induced or chemical-induced hyperpigmentation; traumatic melanonychia of the toenails; Peutz-Jeghers syndrome; physiologic melanoplakia and melanonychia

Therapy
Frequency-doubled Q-switched Nd:YAG laser, or HGM K1 krypton laser, or 532-nm diode-pumped vanadate laser

References
Veraldi S, Cavicchini S, Benelli C, Gasparini G (1001) Laugier-Hunziker syndrome: a clinical, histopathologic, and ultrastructural study of four cases and review of the literature. Journal of the American Academy of Dermatology 25(4): 632–636

Launois-Bensaude syndrome

▶ Benign symmetric lipomatosis

Lawrence syndrome

▶ Berardinelli-Seip syndrome

Ledderhose disease

▶ Plantar fibromatosis

Leiomyoma

Synonym(s)
None

Definition
Benign soft-tissue neoplasm that arises from smooth muscle

Pathogenesis
Unknown; three subtypes:
Piloleiomyoma: arising from the arrector pili muscle of the pilosebaceous unit.
Angioleiomyoma: arising from smooth muscle (i.e., tunica media) within the walls of arteries and veins.
Genital leiomyoma: derived from the dartos muscle of the scrotum or labia majora, or from the erectile muscle of the nipple

Clinical manifestation
Piloleiomyoma: smooth, firm, tender, reddish-brown papule or nodule; multiple piloleiomyomas sometimes occur on face, trunk, or extremities; grouped, dermatomal, or linear pattern; solitary piloleiomyoma usually found on lower extremity; angioleiomyoma: well defined, deep dermal papule or nodule which may be painful; genital leiomyoma: found on vulva, scrotum, or nipple

Differential diagnosis
Neurilemmoma; mastocytoma; dermatofibroma; glomus tumor; neuroma; angiofibroma; eccrine spiradenoma; breast carcinoma; plasmacytoma; leiomyosarcoma; neurofibroma

Therapy
Pain relief: nifedipine SR: 30–60 mg PO per day; phenoxybenzamine: 20–40 mg PO 2–

3 times per day; surgical excision of solitary tumor

References

Fearfield LA, Smith JR, Bunker CB, Staughton RC (2000) Association of multiple familial cutaneous leiomyoma with a uterine symplastic leiomyoma. Clinical & Experimental Dermatology 25(1):44–47

Leishmaniasis, cutaneous

Synonym(s)

Aleppo boil; Delhi boil; Baghdad boil; Biskra button; oriental sore

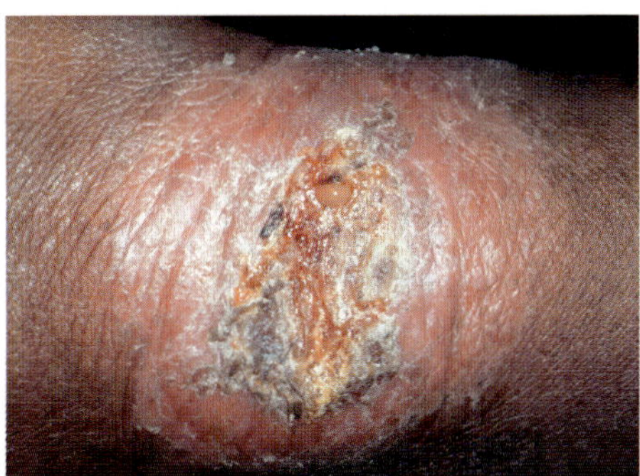

Leishmaniasis, cutaneous. Infiltrated, exudative, scaly, and crusted nodule on the knee

Definition

Protozoal parasitic disease spread by the bite of the sandfly

Pathogenesis

Protozoal promastigotes inoculated into the host during the sandfly's blood meal; promastigotes enter macrophages, transform back into amastigotes, multiply, and spread throughout the reticuloendothelial system; helper T-cell subtype 1 (Th1) immune response which induces disease resolution

Clinical manifestation

Asymptomatic red papule which ulcerates; occurs at site of sandfly bite; heals over weeks to many months

Differential diagnosis

Cutaneous tuberculosis; syphilis; leprosy; basal cell carcinoma; squamous cell carcinoma; deep fungal infection; pyoderma gangrenosum

Therapy

Sodium antimony gluconate 20 mg per kg per day IV or IM for 20 days; ketoconazole 600 mg PO daily for 4 weeks; hyperthermia

References

Hepburn NC (2001) Management of cutaneous leishmaniasis. Current Opinion in Infectious Diseases 14(2):151–154

Lentiginosis-deafness-cardiopathy syndrome

▶ LEOPARD syndrome

Lentiginosis profusa syndrome

▶ LEOPARD syndrome

Lentiginous hyperpigmentation

▶ Nevoid hypermelanosis

Lentigo

Synonym(s)

Sun spot; liver spot

Definition

Small, sharply circumscribed, non-inflammatory pigmented macule

Pathogenesis
Unknown; solar lentigo and ink-spot lentigo associated with sun exposure in fair-skinned people; PUVA lentigo associated with photochemotherapy (PUVA); radiation lentigo caused by local high-dose irradiation

Clinical manifestation
Lentigo simplex: asymptomatic, round or oval, uniformly tan-brown to black macule, with jagged or smooth margins; lesions few in number and occurring anywhere on skin or mucous membranes

Solar lentigo: most commonly appearing on the face, arms, dorsa of the hands, and upper part of the trunk; stellate-shaped, round or oval, uniformly tan-brown to black macule; slowly increasing in number and in size; lesions sometimes coalesce to form larger patches

Ink spot lentigo: reticulated pattern, resembling spot of ink; limited to sun-exposed areas; single ink-spot lentigo among an extensive number of solar lentigines; PUVA lentigo: persistent, pale brown macule appearing 6 months or longer after the start of PUVA therapy for psoriasis; resembling solar lentigo, but often with more irregular borders which may mimic ephelides; occurrence closely associated with greater cumulative doses of PUVA

Radiation lentigo: resembles sun-induced lentigo, but often has other histopathologic signs of long-term cutaneous radiation damage; considered an indicator of a prior exposure to a large single dose of ionizing radiation

Tanning-bed lentigo: usually occurs in women with history of tanning-bed use; similar to PUVA lentigo

Mucosal melanotic macule (labial lentigo; vulvar lentigo; penile lentigo):
Labial lentigo almost always on the vermilion of the lower lip and usually solitary and asymptomatic; color ranges from brown to blue to blue-black

Oral lentigo: appears on the gingiva, buccal mucosa, palate, and tongue

Penile lentigo: most common sites: glans penis, corona, coronal sulcus, and penile shaft; varies in color from tan to brown to dark brown, with irregular borders and skip areas

Vulvar lentigo: occurs anywhere on the genital mucosa as a mottled, pigmented patch with skip areas

Differential diagnosis
Melanocytic nevus; lentigo maligna; melanoma; ephelides; actinic keratosis; seborrheic keratosis; traumatic tattoo; phyto-photodermatitis

Therapy
Frequency-doubled Q-switched Nd:YAG laser, or HGM K1 krypton laser, or 532-nm diode-pumped vanadate laser; hydroquinone, with or without tretinoin

References
Schaffer JV, Bolognia JL (2000) The clinical spectrum of pigmented lesions. Clinics in Plastic Surgery 27(3):391–408

Lentigo maligna

Synonym(s)
Hutchinson's melanotic freckle; Hutchinson melanotic freckle

Definition
Intraepidermal melanocytic neoplasm, characterized by slow growth, on the face or other sun-exposed areas in fair-skinned, elderly individuals

Pathogenesis
Related to chronic, cumulative sun exposure

Clinical manifestation
Most commonly affects the sun-exposed skin of the head and neck, with a predilection for the nose and cheek; less common sites: arm, leg, and trunk; conjunctivae and oral mucosa sometimes may be involved by contiguous spread from cutaneous lesion; irregular mottling or flecking as lesion

enlarges, with areas of dark brown or black in some parts and lightening in others; lesion may be present for many years before dermal invasion occurs

Differential diagnosis
Melanocytic nevus, including atypical mole; lentigo; seborrheic keratosis; pyogenic granuloma; basal cell carcinoma; squamous cell carcinoma

Therapy
Surgical excision with 0.5 cm margin*; cryotherapy; radiation therapy

References
Kaufmann R (2000) Surgical management of primary melanoma. Clinical & Experimental Dermatology 25(6):476–481

Lentigo maligna melanoma

▶ Melanoma

Lentigo senilis

▶ Lentigo

Lentigo simplex

▶ Lentigo

LEOPARD syndrome

Synonym(s)
Cardiocutaneous lentiginosis syndrome; multiple lentigines syndrome; generalized lentiginosis; centrofacial lentiginosis; lentiginosis profusa syndrome; lentiginosis-deafness-cardiopathy syndrome; cardiocutaneous syndrome; progressive cardiomyopathic lentiginosis

Definition
Acronym depicting the main findings of a syndrome characterized by lentigines, electrocardiographic conduction abnormalities, ocular hypertelorism, pulmonary stenosis, abnormalities of genitalia, retardation of growth, and deafness

Pathogenesis
Possible mutation in the stem cell pool of the neural crest in embryonic life

Clinical manifestation
Many affected patients lack one or more components of the defined syndrome; small, dark brown, polygonal, irregularly shaped macules, often present on the face, neck, and upper part of the trunk, but also on palms, soles, and sclerae; axillary freckling; café au lait spots; localized hypopigmentation; mild mental retardation; sensorineural hearing loss; short stature; mostly asymptomatic cardiac defects; dysmorphic face and/or skull; skeletal abnormalities

Differential diagnosis
Albright syndrome; Carney's syndrome; neurofibromatosis; Noonan syndrome; Peutz-Jeghers syndrome; nevi-atrial myxoma-myxoid neurofibromata-ephelides (NAME or LAMB) syndrome

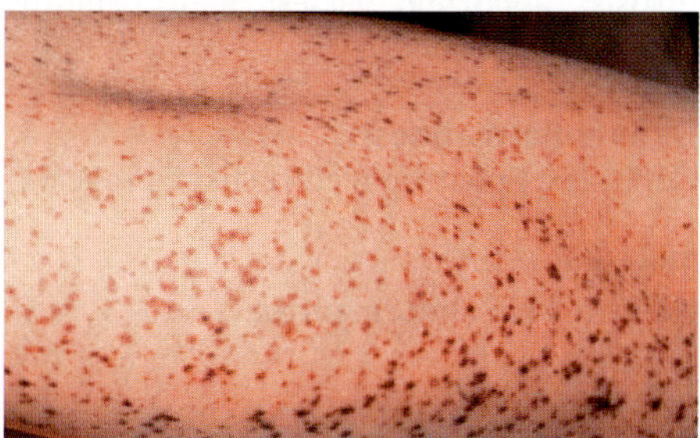

LEOPARD syndrome. Multiple brown macules on the forearm

Therapy

Cosmetically disfiguring lentigines – frequency-doubled Q-switched Nd:YAG laser, or HGM K1 krypton laser, or 532-nm diode-pumped vanadate laser; hydroquinone, with or without tretinoin

References

Jozwiak S, Schwartz RA; Janniger CK (1996) LEOPARD syndrome (cardiocutaneous lentiginosis syndrome). Cutis 57(4):208–214

Leprechaunism

Synonym(s)
Donohue syndrome

Definition
Hereditary disorder characterized by insulin resistance resulting in growth delays, abnormalities affecting the endocrine system, distinctive characteristics of the head and face, low birth weight, skin abnormalities, and enlargement of the breast and clitoris in females and the penis in males

Pathogenesis
Autosomal recessive disorder; exact genetic defect unknown

Clinical manifestation
Insulin resistance; acanthosis nigricans; diffuse, increased skin pigmentation; decreased subcutaneous tissue; skin atrophy; hirsutism; gingival hypertrophy; ichthyosis; abnormal facies; short stature; abnormal genitalia

Differential diagnosis
Cutis laxa; lipoatrophy; dwarfism; progeria

Therapy
None for skin abnormalities

References

Kosztolanyi G (1997) Leprechaunism/Donohue syndrome/insulin receptor gene mutations: a syndrome delineation story from clinicopathological description to molecular understanding. European Journal of Pediatrics 156(4):253–255

Lepromatous leprosy

▶ Leprosy

Leprosy

Synonym(s)
Hansen's disease; Hansen disease

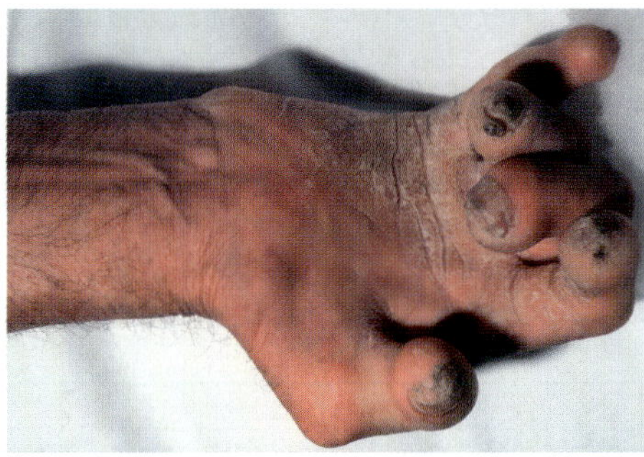

Leprosy. Scaly plaques, digital tip erosions, and sclerosis of the hand

Definition
Chronic granulomatous disease, caused by Mycobacterium leprae, which principally affects the skin and peripheral nervous system

Pathogenesis
Causative organism, M. leprae, an obligate intracellular acid-fast bacillus with ability to enter nerves which are in cooler parts of the body; tissue damage depends on degree to which cell-mediated immunity expressed, the extent of bacillary spread and multiplication, appearance of tissue-damaging immunologic complications (i.e., lepra reactions), and the development of nerve damage and its sequelae

Clinical manifestation
Indeterminate leprosy: one to a few hypopigmented or erythematous macules, with intact sensation

Tuberculoid leprosy: skin lesions few in number; well-defined, erythematous large plaques, with elevated borders with atrophic center; arciform or annular plaques; found on the face, limbs, or elsewhere, but sparing intertriginous areas and the scalp; alternate presentation: large, asymmetric, hypopigmented macule; both types of lesions anesthetic, have localized alopecia, and sometimes spontaneously resolve in a few years, leaving pigmentary disturbances or scars; neural involvement causes tender, thickened nerves with subsequent loss of function; great auricular nerve and superficial peroneal nerves often prominent

Borderline tuberculoid leprosy: similar to tuberculoid form, but lesions smaller and more numerous, nerves less enlarged, and less alopecia

Borderline leprosy: numerous, asymmetric, moderately anesthetic, red, irregularly shaped plaques less well defined than those in the tuberculoid type; regional adenopathy sometimes present

Lepromatous leprosy: only infectious stage; early cutaneous lesions consisting mainly of pale, small, diffuse, symmetric macules, which become infiltrated later, with little loss of sensation; nerves not thickened and sweating normal; alopecia of lateral eyebrows, eyelashes, and trunk, but scalp hair intact; lepromatous infiltrations either diffuse nodules (lepromas) or plaques, which result in appearance of leonine facies; brawny lower extremity edema; neuritic lesions symmetric and slow to develop; eye involvement causes pain; photophobia, decreased visual acuity, glaucoma, and blindness; testicular atrophy produces sterility and gynecomastia; lymphadenopathy and hepatomegaly result from organ infiltration; stridor and hoarseness from laryngeal involvement; nasal infiltration sometimes produces a saddle-nose deformity; aseptic necrosis and osteomyelitis

Reactional state: lepra type I reaction: usually affects patients with borderline disease; downgrading reaction represents shift toward the lepromatous pole before the initiation of therapy; reversal reaction disease shift toward tuberculoid pole after the initiation of therapy; lepra type II reactions (erythema nodosum leprosum): immune complex–mediated reaction occurring in patients with borderline lepromatous or polar lepromatous disease; crops of painful red papules, usually manifesting after a few years of therapy and resolving spontaneously after about 5 years; associated fever, malaise, joint pain, nerve pain, iridocyclitis, dactylitis, and orchitis; Lucio phenomenon: common in Mexico and Central America; cutaneous hemorrhagic infarcts in patients with diffuse lepromatous leprosy

Differential diagnosis
Vitiligo; post-inflammatory hypopigmentation; lupus erythematosus; syphilis; sarcoidosis; tuberculosis; leishmaniasis; granuloma annulare; psoriasis

Therapy
Paucibacillary disease: dapsone and rifampin[*]; multibacillary disease: dapsone indefinitely, rifampin and clofazimine 50 mg PO per day for 3 years[*]; reactional states: prednisone; thalidomide

References
Ramos-e-Silva M, Rebello PF (2001) Leprosy. Recognition and treatment. American Journal of Clinical Dermatology 2(4):203–211001

Leptospirosis

Synonym(s)
Autumnal fever; seven-day fever; swineherd's disease; swamp fever; mud fever; Fort Bragg fever; Weil disease; canicola fever; rice-field fever; cane-cutter fever; hemorrhagic jaundice; Stuttgart disease

Definition
Bacterial infection caused by one of several species of spirochete of genus Leptospira, which can be found in fresh water contaminated by animal urine

Pathogenesis
Caused by pathogenic spirochetes of the genus Leptospira; organisms enter host through abrasions in healthy skin, through sodden and waterlogged skin, directly through intact mucus membranes or conjunctiva, through the nasal mucosa and cribriform plate, or through the lungs; during acute infection, organisms multiply in the small blood vessel endothelium, resulting in damage and vasculitis, the direct cause of the various clinical manifestations

Clinical manifestation
Anicteric leptospirosis: self-limited disease similar to a mild flu-like illness; icteric leptospirosis (Weil disease): severe illness with multiple organ system involvement; skin changes: warm and flushed; transient petechial eruption that can involve the palate; in severe disease, jaundice and purpura; conjunctival suffusion; myalgia; signs of meningitis, including neck stiffness and rigidity, delirium, and photophobia; liver enlargement and tenderness from hepatitis

Differential diagnosis
Enteric fever; viral hepatitis; hantavirus infection; rickettsial disease; encephalitis; typhoid fever; dengue fever; viral meningitis; malaria

Therapy
Mild disease: doxycycline; amoxicillin; erythromycin; severe disease: penicillin G 20–24 million units IV per day, divided into 4 doses for 5–10 days*

References
Vinetz JM (2001) Leptospirosis. Current Opinion in Infectious Diseases 14(5):527–538

Lesch-Nyhan disease

▶ Lesch-Nyhan syndrome

Lesch-Nyhan syndrome

Synonym(s)
Kelley-Seegmiller syndrome; Lesch-Nyhan disease

Definition
Genetic disorder associated with overproduction of uric acid, neurological disability, and behavioral problems

Pathogenesis
Mutations in the HPRT gene on the X chromosome lead to deficiency of hypoxanthine-guanine phosphoribosyl transferase (HPRT), which plays a key role in the recycling of the purine bases, hypoxanthine and guanine, into the purine nucleotide pools; with absence of HPRT, purine bases not salvaged, but degraded and excreted as uric acid; synthetic rate for purines accelerated markedly, to compensate for purines lost by the failure of the salvage process, resulting in overproduction of uric acid; pathogenesis of neurological and behavioral features unclear

Clinical manifestation
Growth retardation; impaired cognitive function; behavioral problems with attempts at self-injury, such as self-amputations of the fingers, biting of the lips, tongue, or oral mucosa; marked hyperuricemia leading to nephrolithiasis

Differential diagnosis
Mental retardation; sociopathic behavior; cerebral palsy

Therapy
Control of hyperuricemia: allopurinol 300 mg PO per day*; behavior modification therapy

References

Jinnah HA, De Gregorio L, Harris JC, Nyhan WL, O'Neill JP (2000) The spectrum of inherited mutations causing HPRT deficiency: 75 new cases and a review of 196 previously reported cases. Mutation Research 463(3):309–326

Lethal cutaneous and gastrointestinal arterial thrombosis

▶ Malignant atrophic papulosis

Lethal midline granuloma

▶ Lymphomatoid granulomatosis

Letterer-Siwe disease

▶ Langerhans cell histiocytosis

Leukocytoclastic vasculitis

Synonym(s)

Allergic angiitis; small vessel vasculitis; allergic cutaneous vasculitis

Definition

Histopathologic term used to denote a small vessel vasculitis, occurring in a heterogeneous group of disorders

Pathogenesis

Exact mechanism unclear; possibly involves immune complexes, other autoantibodies such as antineutrophil cytoplasmic antibody (ANCA), other inflammatory mediators, and local factors that affect endothelial cells and other adhesion molecules; associated with medications, infections, foods and food additives, rheumatic diseases such as lupus erythematosus, and, rarely, malignant processes

Clinical manifestation

Asymptomatic, pruritic or painful, palpable purpuric papules, sometimes coalescing into plaques and/or ulcerating; most frequently observed on the legs, but any site possible; some lesions begin as urticarial papules; systemic manifestations of lung, gastrointestinal, renal, or rheumatologic involvement reflected in signs and symptoms referable to those organs

Differential diagnosis

Septic vasculitis (e.g., meningococcemia, gonococcemia); Wegener's granulomatosis; polyarteritis nodosa; erythema multiforme; Churg-Strauss syndrome; cholesterol emboli; benign pigmented purpura; amyloidosis; Buerger disease; infective endocarditis; Rocky Mountain spotted fever; thrombotic thrombocytopenic purpura; urticaria; Waldenström hypergammaglobulinemia; idiopathic thrombocytopenia purpura; or other causes of decreased platelets

Therapy

Colchicine; dapsone; prednisone

References

Stone JH, Calabrese LH, Hoffman GS, Pusey CD, Hunder GG, Hellmann DB (2001) Vasculitis. A collection of pearls and myths. Rheumatic Diseases Clinics of North America 27(4):677–728

Leukoderma acquisita centrifugum

▶ Halo nevus

Leukodermia lenticular disseminata

▶ Idiopathic guttate hypomelanosis

Leukopathia guttata et reticularis symmetrica

▶ Idiopathic guttate hypomelanosis

Lice

▶ Pediculosis

Lichen amyloidosis

Synonym(s)
Primary localized cutaneous amyloidosis

Definition
Disorder characterized by deposition of amyloid fibrils in the skin, without evidence of deposition in internal organs

Pathogenesis
Fibrils arise from degenerating keratinocytes, probably secondary to chronic itching and scratching

Clinical manifestation
Intensely pruritic, flesh-colored or red-brown, hyperkeratotic papules, most commonly seen on the pretibial surfaces but also on the feet and thighs; macular variant: irregular hyperpigmented patches over the back or chest

Differential diagnosis
Post-inflammatory hyperpigmentation; lichen simplex chronicus; mycosis fungoides; contact dermatitis; prurigo nodularis; lichen planus; lichenoid drug eruption; pretibial myxedema; necrobiosis lipoidica; acanthosis nigricans; ashy dermatosis

Therapy
Corticosteroids, topical, super potent; UVB phototherapy; severe underlying atopic dermatitis: cyclosporine

References
Behr FD, Levine N, Bangert J (2001) Lichen amyloidosis associated with atopic dermatitis: clinical resolution with cyclosporine. Archives of Dermatology 137(5):553–555

Lichen aureus

▶ Benign pigmented purpura

Lichen myxedematosus

▶ Papular mucinosis

Lichen nitidus

Synonym(s)
None

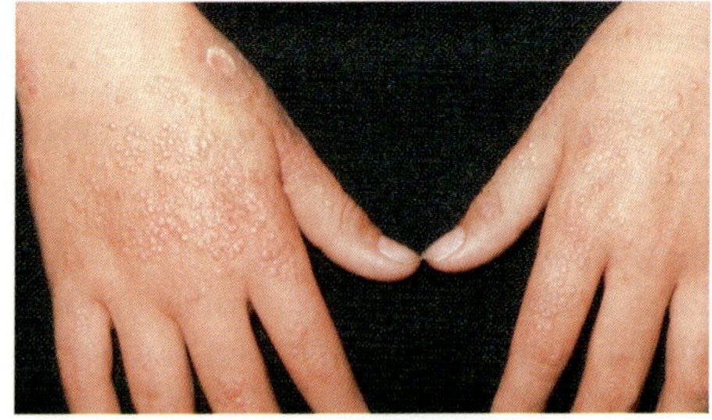

Lichen nitidus. Flat-topped, flesh-colored papules, coalescing into plaques on the hands

Definition
Chronic skin eruption characterized by asymptomatic, small, flat-topped, skin-colored papules

Pathogenesis
Unknown

Clinical manifestation
Multiple 1–3 mm, sharply demarcated, clustered, round or polygonal, flat-topped, skin-colored shiny papules, most commonly on trunk, thighs, forearms, and genitalia; Koebner phenomenon sometimes occurs

Differential diagnosis
Lichen planus; flat warts; lichen spinulosus; lichen amyloidosis; keratosis pilaris; lichen striatus; id reaction; sarcoidosis

Therapy
Corticosteroids, topical, super potent; photochemotherapy

References
Arizaga AT, Gaughan MD, Bang RH (2002) Generalized lichen nitidus. Clinical & Experimental Dermatology 27(2):115–117

Lichen pigmentosus

▶ Ashy dermatosis

Lichen pilaris

▶ Keratosis pilaris

Lichen pilaris seu spinulosus of Crocker

▶ Lichen spinulosus

Lichen planopilaris

▶ Lichen planus

Lichen planus

Synonym(s)
Lichen rubor

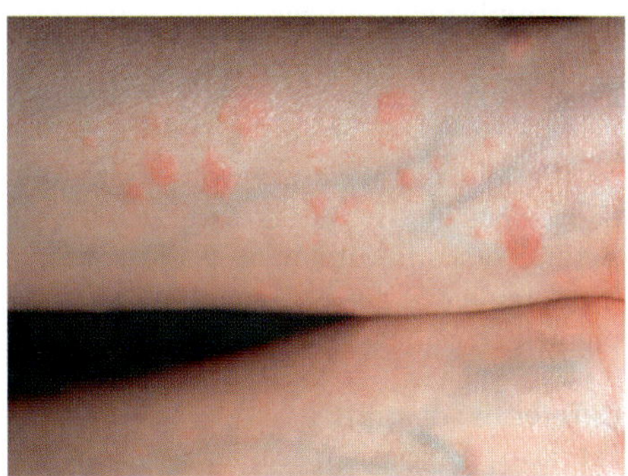

Lichen planus. Violaceous, polygonal, flat-topped papules over the wrist

Definition
Pruritic eruption characterized by violaceous, polygonal papules, with fine reticulated scale

Pathogenesis
Unknown; cell-mediated immune response to unknown stimuli; associated with hepatitis C infection, chronic active hepatitis, and primary biliary cirrhosis

Clinical manifestation
Pruritic, discrete or confluent, polygonal violaceous papules, with fine white scale (Wickham's stria); mucous membrane involvement with white or gray streaks forming a linear or reticular pattern on a violaceous background, most commonly on the buccal mucosa and tongue; genital involvement with annular papules on the

glans penis; vulvar involvement with reticulate papules or erosions, with dyspareunia, burning sensation, pruritus and vulvar and urethral stenosis; nail plate thinning with longitudinal grooving and ridging and occasional destruction of nail plate with ptyrigium formation; follicular and perifollicular, violaceous, scaly, pruritic papules on the scalp, sometimes progressing to atrophic cicatricial alopecia (lichen planopilaris)

Hypertrophic variant: pruritic, thick, scaly, violaceous plaques, usually on the anterior leg; atrophic variant: few lesions, often representing the resolution of annular or hypertrophic lesions

Erosive variant: chronic, painful erosions on the mucosal surfaces; evolve from sites of previous non-erosive disease

Actinic variant: nummular plaques with a hypopigmented zone surrounding a hyperpigmented center

Differential diagnosis

Psoriasis; pityriasis rosea; lupus erythematosus; lichenoid drug eruption; scabies; graft versus host disease; lichen simplex chronicus; lichen nitidus; syphilis; pemphigus foliaceus; squamous cell carcinoma of the oral mucosa

Therapy

Corticosteroids, topical, super potent;[*]; severe, generalized disease – prednisone; acitretin; isotretinoin; photochemotherapy

References

Capella GL, Finzi AF (2000) Psoriasis, lichen planus, and disorders of keratinization: unapproved treatments or indications. Clinics in Dermatology 18(2):159–169

Lichen ruber planus cum pigmentatione

▶ **Riehl's melanosis**

Lichen rubor

▶ **Lichen planus**

Lichen sclerosus

Synonym(s)

Lichen sclerosus et atrophicus; kraurosis vulvae; balanitis xerotica obliterans

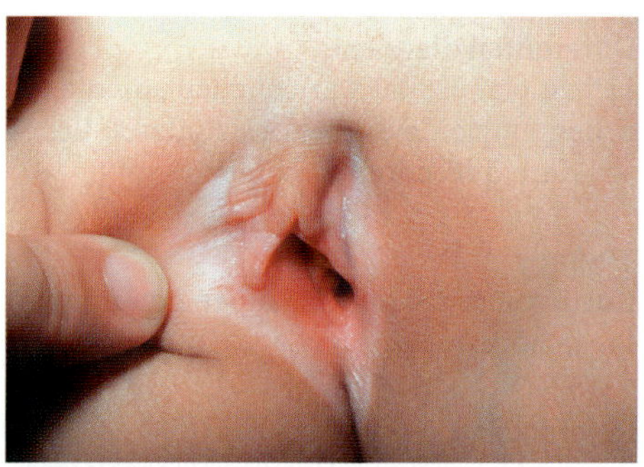

Lichen sclerosus. Hypopigmented, sclerotic plaques, with effacement of the labia minora

Definition

Chronic inflammatory dermatosis resulting in white plaques with epidermal atrophy

Pathogenesis

Unknown; inflammation and abnormal fibroblast function in the upper dermis causing fibrosis of the upper dermis

Clinical manifestation

Asymptomatic or slightly pruritic, white, polygonal papules coalescing into shiny plaques, often with follicular prominence and occasional isomophic response (Koebner phenomenon); vulvar variant (kraurosis vulvae): often intense pruritus; gradual obliteration of the labia minora and stenosis of the introitus; occasional vesicles or hemorrhagic bullae; hourglass, butterfly pattern involving perivaginal and perianal areas; male genital variant (balanitis xerotica obliterans): usually confined to glans penis and prepuce or foreskin remnants; sometimes causes phimosis after extensive sclerosis of prepuce

Differential diagnosis
Morphea; scleroderma; child abuse; lichen planus; psoriasis; tinea versicolor; vitiligo; idiopathic guttate hypomelanosis; post-inflammatory hypopigmentation; anetoderma; Bowen's disease

Therapy
Genital disease: corticosteroids, topical, super potent[*]; tretinoin; acitretin; isotretinoin; extragenital disease: no effective therapy

References
Neill SM, Ridley CM (2001) Management of anogenital lichen sclerosus. Clinical & Experimental Dermatology 26(8):637–643

Lichen sclerosus et atrophicus

▶ Lichen sclerosus

Lichen sclerosus et atrophicus of the penis

▶ Balanitis xerotica obliterans

Lichen sclerosus of the penis

▶ Balanitis xerotica obliterans

Lichen scrofulosorum

▶ Cutaneous tuberculosis

Lichen simplex chronicus

Synonym(s)
Neurodermatitis circumscripta; circumscribed neurodermatitis; lichen simplex chronicus of Vidal

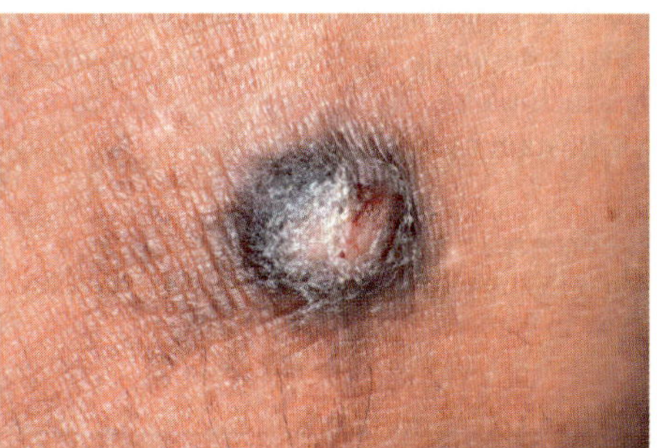

Lichen simplex chronicus. Irregular eroded nodule with surrounding lichenification

Definition
Lichenification of the skin with variable scale, due to repetitive scratching or rubbing

Pathogenesis
Unknown; occurs more frequently in those with atopic diathesis; psychological factors operative in some cases; caused by chronic rubbing or scratching

Clinical manifestation
One or more slightly erythematous, scaly, well-demarcated, lichenified, firm plaques, often with hyperpigmentation; most common locations: posterior neck, scalp, extensor aspect of extremities, vulva in women, and scrotum in men

L

Prurigo nodularis variant: discrete, firm, purpuric nodules or papules, often with overlying erosion; occurs on extensor surfaces of arms and legs, posterior neck, upper back and trunk

Differential diagnosis
Acanthosis nigricans; lichen amyloidosis; insect bite reaction; psoriasis; contact dermatitis; lupus erythematosus; dermatophytosis; stasis dermatitis; nummular eczema; lichen planus; acne keloidalis; atopic dermatitis

Therapy
Corticosteroids, topical, high potency, or corticosteroids, topical, super potency★; triamcinolone 3–5 mg per ml intralesional; antihistamines, first generation

References
Jones RO (1996) Lichen simplex chronicus. Clinics in Podiatric Medicine & Surgery 13(1):47–54

Lichen simplex chronicus of Vidal

▶ Lichen simplex chronicus

Lichen spinulosus

Synonym(s)
Keratosis follicularis spinulosa; lichen pilaris seu spinulosus of Crocker; keratosis follicularis spinosa of Unna

Definition
Disorder characterized by plaques consisting of follicular keratotic papules

Pathogenesis
Unknown

Clinical manifestation
Symmetrical, accuminate, keratotic papules, affecting the neck, buttocks, abdomen, trochanters, knees, and extensor surfaces of the arms; may coalesce into plaques

Differential diagnosis
Lichen nitidus; lichen simplex chronicus; keratosis pilaris; phrynoderma; flat warts; lichen planopilaris; pityriasis rubra pilaris; Darier disease

Therapy
Alpha hydroxy acids

References
Strickling WA, Norton SA (2000) Spiny eruption on the neck. Diagnosis: Lichen spinulosus (LS). Archives of Dermatology 136(9):1165–1170

Lichen striatus

Synonym(s)
Linear lichenoid dermatosis; linear neurodermatitis; blaschkitis; Blaschko linear acquired inflammatory skin eruption; zonal dermatosis; linear dermatosis; systematized lichenification; linear eczema

Definition
Inflammatory papular eruption with a distinctive linear distribution, often following Blaschko's lines

Pathogenesis
Unknown

Clinical manifestation
Most common on extremities, trunk, and neck; flat- topped, erythematous or skin-colored, lichenoid, scaly papules, coalescing into small plaques in a continuous or interrupted linear band; spontaneous resolution in months to 1 year, often in the same proximal to distal fashion in which they appeared, leaving variable dyspigmentation

Differential diagnosis
Inflammatory linear verrucous epidermal nevus; lichen planus; atopic dermatitis; lichen simplex chronicus; Darier disease; wart; porokeratosis

Therapy
Corticosteroids, topical, high potency; emollients

References
Hauber K, Rose C, Brocker EB, Hamm H (2000) Lichen striatus: clinical features and follow-up in 12 patients. European Journal of Dermatology 10(7):536–539

Lichen tropicus

▶ Miliaria

Lichenoid benign keratosis

▶ Lichenoid keratosis

Lichenoid chronic dermatosis

▶ Sulzberger-Garbe syndrome

Lichenoid keratosis

Synonym(s)
Benign lichenoid keratosis; solitary lichen planus; solitary lichen planus-like keratosis; lichenoid benign keratosis

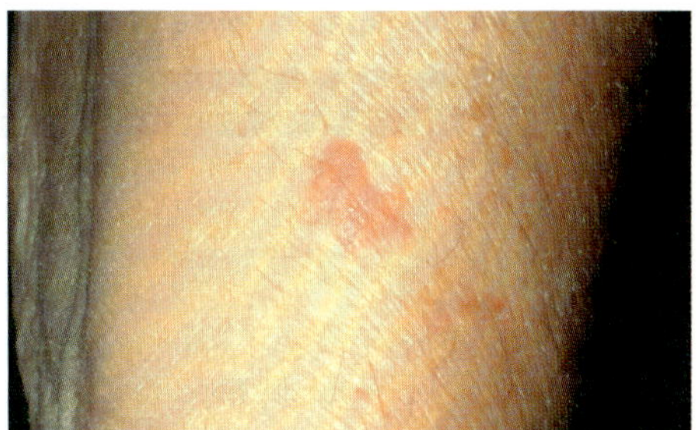

Lichenoid keratosis. Sharply demarcated, reddish-brown verrucous papule on the leg

Definition
Solitary, benign skin lesion with the histologic features of a lichenoid reaction

Pathogenesis
Unclear; may be inflammatory stage of lentigo or seborrheic keratosis

Clinical manifestation
Sharply demarcated, scaly, red-brown, almost flat papule, often on sun-exposed skin of the extremities

Differential diagnosis
Lentigo; seborrheic keratosis; lichen planus; lichenoid drug eruption; lupus erythematosus; wart; Bowen's disease; superficial basal cell carcinoma

Therapy
Destruction by liquid nitrogen cryotherapy or electrodesiccation and curettage

References
Jang KA, Kim SH, Choi JH, Sung KJ, Moon KC, Koh JK (2000) Lichenoid keratosis: a clinicopathologic study of 17 patients. Journal of the American Academy of Dermatology 43(3):511–516

Lichenoid mycosis fungoides

▶ Large plaque parapsoriasis

Lindane. Dermatologic indications and dosage

Disease	Adult dosage	Child dosage
Pediculosis capitis	Apply shampoo for 30 minutes	> 2 years old – apply shampoo for 30 minutes
Pediculosis pubis	Apply shampoo for 30 minutes	> 2 years old – apply shampoo for 30 minutes
Scabies	Apply lotion to whole body except for the head; reapply in 7 days	> 2 years old – apply lotion to whole body except for the head; reapply in 7 days

Lichenoid pigmented purpura of Gougerot and Blum

▶ **Benign pigmented purpura**

Light-sensitive seborrheid

▶ **Perioral dermatitis**

Lindane

Trade name(s)
None

Generic available
Yes

Drug class
Organochloride anti-parasitic agent

Mechanism of action
Blocks neural transmission

Dosage form
1% lotion; 1% shamopoo

Dermatologic indications and dosage
See table

Common side effects
Cutaneous: irritant dermatitis
Neurologic: dizziness, anxiety, CNS stimulation

Serious side effects
Neurologic: neurotoxicity; seizures

Drug interactions
None

Contraindications/precautions
Hypersensitivity to drug class or component; pregnancy; lactating mother

References
Wendel K, Rompalo A (2002) Scabies and pediculosis pubis: an update of treatment regimens and general review. Clinical Infectious Diseases 35(Suppl 2):S146–51

Linea alba (bite line)

Definition
Thin, white line running from angle of mouth to pterygomandibular raphae, caused by pressure of cheek into line of occlusion

References
Laude TA (1995) Approach to dermatologic disorders in black children. Seminars in Dermatology 14(1):15–20

Linear and whorled nevoid hypermelanosis

▶ Nevoid hypermelanosis

Linear dermatosis

▶ Lichen striatus

Linear eczema

▶ Lichen striatus

Linear IgA bullous dermatosis

▶ Linear IgA dermatosis

Linear IgA bullous disease

▶ Linear IgA dermatosis

Linear IgA dermatosis

Synonym(s)
Linear IgA bullous dermatosis; linear IgA bullous disease; chronic bullous disease of childhood

Definition
Autoimmune, subepidermal, vesiculobullous disease with IgA immunoreactants deposited in the skin

Pathogenesis
Antibody to 97 kDa protein in the basement membrane zone causes complement activation and neutrophil chemotaxis; loss of adhesion at the dermal-epidermal junction produces blisters; 97 kDa protein may represent a portion of the extracellular domain of the 180 kDa bullous pemphigoid antigen

Clinical manifestation
Clear and/or hemorrhagic vesicles or bullae on normal, erythematous, or urticarial skin; may also have erythematous plaques, blanching macules and papules, or erythema multiforme-like lesions; oral mucous membrane lesions, including red patches, vesicles, ulcerations, erosions, desquamative gingivitis, or cheilitis; possibly medication related in some cases, most commonly with vancomycin

Differential diagnosis
Bullous pemphigoid; erythema multiforme; epidermolysis bullosa; epidermolysis bullosa acquisita; dermatitis herpetiformis; impetigo; pemphigus foliaceus; pemphigus vulgaris; herpes simplex virus infection; herpes zoster

Therapy
Dapsone; prednisone; tetracycline; niacinamide

References
Rabinowitz LG, Esterly NB (1993) Inflammatory bullous diseases in children. Dermatologic Clinics 11(3):565–581

Linear lichenoid dermatosis

▶ Lichen striatus

Linear neurodermatitis

▶ Lichen striatus

Linear porokeratosis

▶ Porokeratosis

Lingua nigra

▶ Hairy tongue

Lingua plicata

Synonym(s)
Fissured tongue; scrotal tongue; furrowed tongue

Definition
Condition characterized by grooves varying in depth and noted along the dorsal and lateral aspects of the tongue

Pathogenesis
Possibly polygenic or autosomal inheritance pattern

Clinical manifestation
Asymptomatic fissured tongue, affecting the dorsum and often extending to the lateral borders; fissures or grooves sometimes interconnected, artificially separating the dorsum of the tongue into lobules

Differential diagnosis
Geographic tongue; cheilitis granulomatosa

Therapy
No therapy if asymptomatic; brushing of tongue with toothbrush to remove embedded debris

References
Fisher BK. Linzon CD (1997) Scrotal glans penis (glans penis plicatum) associated with scrotal tongue (lingua plicata). International Journal of Dermatology 36(10):762–763997

Lingua villosa

▶ Hairy tongue

Lingua villosa nigra

▶ Hairy tongue

Lipid histiocytosis

▶ Niemann-Pick disease

Lipoatrophy

▶ Progressive lipodystrophy

Lipodermoid

▶ Dermoid cyst

Lipoglycoproteinosis

▶ Lipoid proteinosis

Lipogranulomatosis subcutanea

▶ Rothman-Makai syndrome

Lipoid dermatoarthritis

▶ Multicentric reticulohistiocytosis

Lipoid proteinosis

Synonym(s)

Hyalinosis cutis et mucosae, Urbach-Wiethe disease; lipoproteinosis; lipoglycoproteinosis; lipoidosis cutis et mucosae

Definition

Hereditary disease characterized by deposition of eosinophilic hyaline-like material in the skin, larynx, mucous membranes, brain, and other internal organs

Pathogenesis

Autosomal recessive trait; unclear whether deposit of eosinophilic material in organs is primary or secondary phenomenon; possibly an abnormality of collagen metabolism or a lysosomal disease

Clinical manifestation

Hoarseness in infancy; presents early in life with recurrent vesicles, bullae, and hemorrhagic crusts, particularly on the face, on mucous membranes, and on distal extremities, which heal with ice-pick scarring; later in life, skin becomes waxy, thickened, and yellow; papules, plaques, and nodules on the face, axillae, and scrotum; verrucous lesions on the elbows, knees, and sites of trauma; beaded papules along the eyelid margins (moniliform blepharitis); patchy alopecia where hyaline deposits are present; cobblestone appearance with multiple papules on the tongue, lips, and gingiva; tongue may have woody induration and ulceration; transient swelling of the lips and tongue; abnormal dentition; involvement of larynx and vocal cords sometimes causes respiratory distress; bilateral temporal lobe calcifications sometimes lead to seizures

Differential diagnosis

Amyloidosis; papular mucinosis; xanthomas; colloid milia; myxedema; erythropoetic protoporphyria

Therapy

Acitretin; dermabrasion; surgical resection of vocal cord papules

References

Touart DM, Sau P (1998) Cutaneous deposition diseases. Part I. Journal of the American Academy of Dermatology 39(2 Pt 1):149–171

Lipoid rheumatism

▶ Multicentric reticulohistiocytosis

Lipoidosis cutis et mucosae

▶ Lipoid proteinosis

Lipoma

Synonym(s)

Fatty tumor

Definition

Benign tumor of fat cells, presenting as subcutaneous nodules

Pathogenesis

Unknown; differs biochemically from normal fat by increased lipoprotein lipase levels and larger number of precursor cells

Clinical manifestation

Asymptomatic, slow-growing, soft, subcutaneous nodule, most commonly over the back, neck, shoulders, and proximal upper extremities

Differential diagnosis
Epidermoid cyst; liposarcoma; panniculitis; neurofibroma; leiomyoma; blue rubber bleb nevus syndrome; glomus tumor

Therapy
Surgical excision; liposuction

References
Salam GA (2002) Lipoma excision. American Family Physician. 65(5):901–904

Lipomatosis

▶ Lipoma

Lipophagic panniculitis of childhood

▶ Rothman-Makai syndrome

Lipoproteinosis

▶ Lipoid proteinosis

Liposarcoma

Synonym(s)
Atypical lipoma; atypical lipomatous tumors; malignancy of fat cells

Definition
Malignancy of fat cells

Pathogenesis
Trauma possibly a co-factor in some cases

Clinical manifestation
Asymptomatic, exophytic, slow-growing, dome-shaped or polypoid tumor

Differential diagnosis
Lipoma; neurofibroma; dermatofibrosarcoma; angiofibroma; rhabdomyosarcoma; leiomyosarcoma; fibrous histiocytoma lipoblastoma in infants and children

Therapy
Wide local excision[*]

References
Wong CK, Edwards AT, Rees BI (1997) Liposarcoma: a review of current diagnosis and management. British Journal of Hospital Medicine 58(11):589–591

Livedo reticularis

Definition
Mottling of the skin, usually on the legs

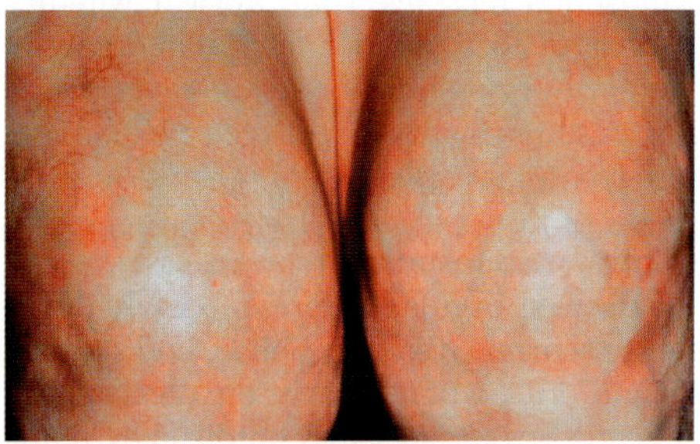

Livedo reticularis. Reticulated red-brown patches on the lower extremities

References
Piette WW (1994) The differential diagnosis of purpura from a morphologic perspective. Advances in Dermatology 9:3–23

Livedo reticularis with summer/winter ulcerations

▶ Livedoid vasculitis

Livedo vasculitis

▶ Livedoid vasculitis

Livedoid vasculitis

Synonym(s)
Livedo vasculitis; livedo reticularis with summer/winter ulcerations; segmental hyalinizing vasculitis

Definition
Chronic vasculopathy characterized by recurrent lower extremity ulcerations that heal with stellate white scars

Pathogenesis
Unknown; deposition of fibrinoid material in dermal vessels causes overlying ischemic change, suggesting occlusive or thrombotic mechanism

Clinical manifestation
Small, painful, purpuric macules and papules that ulcerate and heal with stellate white atrophic scars, with surrounding telangiectasias and hyperpigmentation; seasonal course, with outbreaks in the summer and winter; occurs more often in women

Differential diagnosis
Livedo reticularis (retiform purpura); hypersensitivity vasculitis; stasis ulceration; cholesterol emboli; septic emboli; anti-phospholipid antibody syndrome; lupus erythematosus

Therapy
Antiplatelet therapy, such as aspirin and dipyridamole; fibrinolytic agents, such as tissue plasminogen activator or danazol; anticoagulants, such as warfarin; anti-inflammatory agents, such as prednisone or non-steroidal anti-inflammatory agents; pentoxifylline

References
Fogelman JP (2001) Livedoid vasculitis. Dermatology Online Journal 7(1):19

Liver spot

▶ Lentigo

Loa loa

▶ Filariasis

Lobular capillary hemangioma

▶ Pyogenic granuloma

Localized scleroderma

▶ Morphea

Loiasis

▶ Filariasis

Loose anagen hair of childhood

▶ Loose anagen hair syndrome

Loose anagen hair syndrome

Synonym(s)
Loose anagen syndrome; short anagen syndrome; loose anagen hair of childhood

Definition
Disorder characterized by anagen hairs with abnormal morphology, easily and painlessly pulled or plucked from the scalp, leading to short, abnormal-appearing hair

Pathogenesis
Unknown; abnormal keratinization of the inner root sheath may be part of the pathological process

Clinical manifestation
Sparse growth of thin, fine hair and diffuse or patchy alopecia without inflammation or scarring; hair easily pulled out and unmanageable, lusterless, dry, dull, or matted; hair grows only to relatively short length

Differential diagnosis
Alopecia areata; tinea capitis; traction alopecia; trichotillomania; telogen effluvium; lichen planopilaris; thyroid disease; iron deficiency anemia; anagen effluvium

Therapy
None

References
Li VW, Baden HP, Kvedar JC (1996) Loose anagen syndrome and loose anagen hair. Dermatologic Clinics 14(4):745–751

Loose anagen syndrome

▶ Loose anagen hair syndrome

Loratadine

▶ Antihistamines, second generation

Loss of hair, partial or complete

▶ Alopecia

Louis-Bar syndrome

▶ Ataxia-telangiectasia

Louse-borne relapsing fever

▶ Relapsing fever

Louse borne typhus

▶ Epidemic typhus

Loxoscelism

▶ Brown recluse spider bite

Lues

▶ Syphilis

Lupus anticoagulant syndrome

▶ Antiphospholipid syndrome

Lupus erythematosus, acute

Synonym(s)
Acute lupus erythematosus

Definition
Heterogeneous connective tissue disease associated with polyclonal B-cell activation and multisystem involvement

Pathogenesis
Unclear; interplay of genetic, environmental, and hormonal factors; association with human leukocyte antigen DR2 and human leukocyte antigen DR3; ultraviolet light acts as trigger; certain viruses may be co-factors

Clinical manifestation
Confluent erythema and edema, most commonly over malar eminence and nasal bridge (butterfly eruption); vesicles and bullae, often over lower extremities; morbilliform eruption in a sunlight distribution; other sites of involvement: forehead, periorbital area, and sides of the neck; superficial ulceration, primarily involving the posterior surface of the hard palate

Differential diagnosis
Rosacea; tinea faciei; seborrheic dermatitis; polymorphous light eruption; erythema multiforme; phototoxic drug eruption; solar urticaria; dermatomyositis

Therapy
Prednisone*; azathioprine; cyclophosphamide; thalidomide; hydroxychloroquine; intravenous IgG (IVIG): 0.5–1 g per kg per day for 4 days

References
Callen JP (2002) Management of skin disease in patients with lupus erythematosus. Best Practice & Research in Clinical Rheumatology 16(2):245–264

Lupus erythematosus, discoid

Synonym(s)
Chronic cutaneous lupus erythematosus; discoid lupus erythematosus

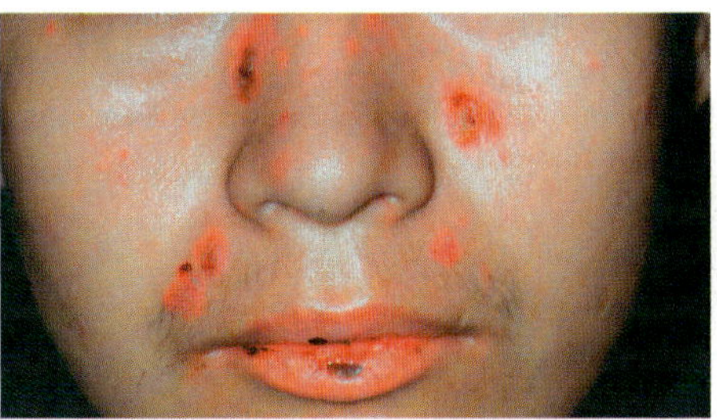

Lupus erythematosus, discoid. Multiple, red eroded papules on the face and lip

Definition
Chronic, scarring, atrophy-producing, photosensitive dermatosis, sometimes occurring in patients with systemic lupus erythematosus

Pathogenesis
Possible genetic predisposition; triggered by ultraviolet light

Clinical manifestation
Minimally scaly, erythematous papule or plaque, evolving with hypopigmentation in the central area and hyperpigmentation at the active border, often starting after sun exposure; as lesion evolves, dilation of follicular openings occurs with keratinous plug (follicular plugging; patulous follicles); resolution with atrophy and scarring; localized variant: head and neck affected; usually only a few lesions; widespread vari-

ant: areas other than head and neck affected; more likely to develop systemic lupus erythematosus

Differential diagnosis
Lichen planus; actinic keratosis; granuloma faciale; Jessner lymphocytic infiltration of the skin; granuloma annulare; sarcoidosis; dermatomyositis; rosacea; tinea faciei; squamous cell carcinoma

Therapy
Corticosteroids, topical, super potent; triamcinolone 3–4 mg per ml intralesional; hydroxychloroquine; prednisone; thalidomide

References
Callen JP (1994) Treatment of cutaneous lesions in patients with lupus erythematosus. Dermatologic Clinics 12(1):201–206

Lupus erythematosus panniculitis

▶ Lupus panniculitis

Lupus erythematosus, subacute cutaneous

Synonym(s)
Subacute cutaneous lupus erythematosus

Definition
Nonscarring, photosensitive dermatosis that may occur in patients with systemic lupus erythematosus, Sjögren syndrome, deficiency of the second component of complement, or after exposure to certain medications

Pathogenesis
Genetic predisposition; strong association with anti-Ro (SS-A) autoantibodies; ultraviolet light modulation of autoantigens, epidermal cytokines, and adhesion molecules, with keratinocyte injury and apoptosis

Clinical manifestation
Begins as a minimally scaly, erythematous papule or a small plaque, in sun-exposed distribution
Papulosquamous variant: mimics psoriasis or lichen planus
Annular variant: similar to erythema annulare centrifugum
Neonatal variant: transient infiltrated red papules and plaques on the face; usually resolves by age 4–6 months; some patients with congenital heart block requires pacemaker
Systemic signs and symptoms: Sjögren syndrome, fatigue, arthritis, pleuritis or pericarditis; several drugs capable of producing this syndrome, most commonly thiazide diuretics

Differential diagnosis
Psoriasis; erythema annulare centrifugum; erythema multiforme; tinea corporis; lichen planus; sarcoidosis; granuloma annulare; Lyme disease; dermatomyositis; hypersensitivity vasculitis; polymorphous light eruption

Therapy
Hydroxychloroquine★; corticosteroids, topical, super potent; prednisone; thalidomide

References
McCauliffe DP (2001) Cutaneous lupus erythematosus. Seminars in Cutaneous Medicine & Surgery 20(1):14–26

Lupus miliaris disseminatus faciei

▶ Rosacea

Lupus panniculitis

Synonym(s)
Lupus profundus; lupus erythematosus panniculitis

Definition
Variant of chronic cutaneous lupus erythematosus, characterized by subcutaneous nodules and atrophy

Pathogenesis
Unknown

Clinical manifestation
Multiple, discrete, firm, subcutaneous nodules, with evolution into atrophic papules or nodules; sometimes associated with lesions of discoid lupus erythematosus; occasionally occurs in patients with systemic lupus erythematosus

Differential diagnosis
Erythema nodosum; erythema induratum (nodular vasculitis); superficial thrombophlebitis; Weber-Christian disease; pancreatic panniculitis; inflamed epidermoid cyst; atrophoderma of Pasini and Pierini; morphea

Therapy
Hydroxychloroquine★; surgical excision

References
Peters MS, Su WP (1989) Lupus erythematosus panniculitis. Medical Clinics of North America 73(5):1113–1126

Lupus profundus

▶ Lupus panniculitis

Lupus vulgaris

▶ Cutaneous tuberculosis

Lutz mycosis

▶ South American blastomycosis

Lyell syndrome

▶ Toxic epidermal necrolysis

Lyme borreliosis

▶ Lyme disease

Lyme borreliosis, late phase

▶ Acrodermatitis chronica atrophicans

Lyme disease

Synonym(s)
Lyme borreliosis

Definition
Systemic infection caused by the spirochete Borrelia burgdorferi, after inoculation into the skin by a tick bite

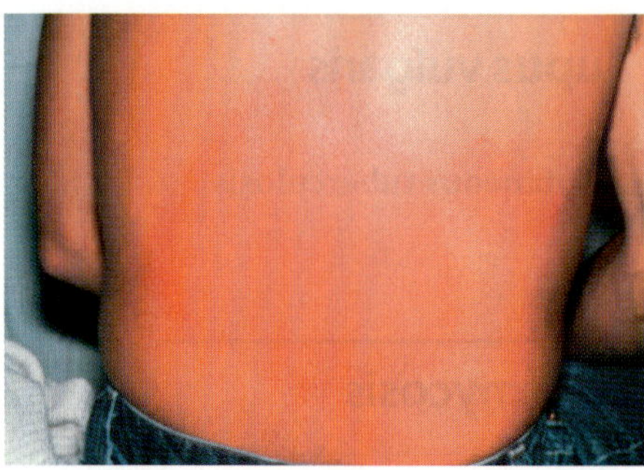

Lyme disease. Large, red plaque with an active advancing margin

Pathogenesis
Spriochetes introduced into the skin by a bite from an infected Ixodes tick; three tick species: B burgdorferi sensu stricto strain constituting all North American isolates; B garinii found exclusively in Europe; B afzelii most common organism causing acrodermatitis chronica atrophicans

Clinical manifestation
Early Lyme disease: sometimes presents with flulike illness; erythema migrans: begins as an erythematous macule or papule at the site of tick bite, often with central punctum at the site of the bite; eruption gradually expands with central clearing over days to weeks; multiple lesions may occur; borrelial lymphocytoma: bluish red nodules, usually on earlobe or nipple; acrodermatitis chronica atrophicans: begins as an inflammatory phase marked with edema and erythema, usually on the distal extremities; lesions on posterior heels and dorsal surfaces of the hands, feet, elbows, and knees; gradual central progression over months to years; systemic involvement, including Bell's palsy, arthritis; chronic fatigue syndrome; meningoradiculoneuritis (Bannwarth syndrome); carditis; and chronic meningoencephalitis

Differential diagnosis
Erythema marginatum rheumaticum; erythema gyratum repens; urticaria; granuloma annulare; sarcoidosis; tinea corporis; seborrheic dermatitis; lupus erythematosus; benign lymphocytic infiltrate; rheumatoid arthritis; psoriatic arthritis; lupus erythematosus; Reiter syndrome; gonococcal arthritis

Therapy
Doxycycline; amoxicillin; erythromycin

References
Ravishankar J, Lutwick LI (2001) Current and future treatment of Lyme disease. Expert Opinion on Pharmacotherapy 2(2):241–251

Lymphadenosis benigna cutis

▶ **Pseudolymphoma**

Lymphangioma

Synonym(s)
Cutaneous lymphangioma; lymphangioma circumscriptum; cavernous lymphangioma; cystic hygroma

Definition
Congenital hamartomatous malformation of the lymphatic system, involving the skin and subcutaneous tissues

Pathogenesis
Cisterns arising from primitive lymph sac failing to connect with the rest of the lymphatic system during embryonic development; contractions increase the intramural pressure, causing dilated channels to protrude from the walls of the cisterns toward the skin; vesicles seen in lymphangioma circumscriptum represent outpouchings of these dilated vessels

Clinical manifestation
Lymphangioma circumscriptum: small clusters of vesicles, varying in color from pink to red to black (secondary to hemorrhage); sometimes have verrucous surface
Cavernous lymphangioma: rubbery, multi-lobulated subcutaneous nodules
Cystic hygroma: large, soft, and translucent cystic lesion, occurring in the neck, axilla, and parotid area

Differential diagnosis
Herpes simplex virus infection; herpes zoster; wart; epidermoid cyst; lipoma; hemangioma; neurofibroma; epidermal nevus; melanoma; lymphangiectasia; branchiogenic cyst; thyroglossal duct cyst

Therapy
Complete surgical excision*; laser ablation; cryotherapy, sclerotherapy; electrocautery

References
Mulliken JB, Fishman SJ, Burrows PE (2000) Vascular anomalies. Current Problems in Surgery 37(8):517–584

Lymphangioma circumscriptum

▶ Lymphangioma

Lymphangiosarcoma of Stewart-Treves

▶ Stewart-Treves syndrome

Lymphatic filariasis

▶ Filariasis

Lymphocytic infiltrate of Jessner

▶ Jessner lymphocytic infiltration of skin

Lymphocytic infiltration of skin

▶ Jessner's lymphocytic infiltration of skin

Lymphocytoma cutis

▶ Pseudolymphoma

Lymphogranuloma inguinale

▶ Lymphogranuloma venereum

Lymphogranuloma venereum

Synonym(s)
Lymphogranuloma inguinale; climatic bubo; Nicholas-Favre disease

Definition
Sexually transmitted chlamydial disease, characterized by genital ulceration and marked regional lymphadenopathy

Pathogenesis
Caused by Chlamydia trachomatis, an obligate intracellular organism which travels

through the lymphatics to multiply within macrophages in regional lymph nodes; risk factors: anal intercourse, unprotected sexual intercourse; multiple sex partners, sex with partners in endemic areas

Clinical manifestation

Primary stage: small, painless papule or herpetiform ulcer, usually on glans penis or vaginal wall, which heals within a few days; unilateral painful inguinal lymphadenopathy; horizontal group of inguinal nodes most commonly involved; enlargement of the nodes above and below the inguinal ligament (groove sign)

Tertiary stage: proctocolitis; perirectal abscess; fistulas; anal strictures; hyperplasia of intestinal and perirectal lymphatics; end result sometimes elephantiasis of the female genitalia, characterized by fibrotic labial thickening, or elephantiasis and deformation of the penis in men

Differential diagnosis

Chancroid; syphilis; granuloma inguinale; cat-scratch disease; infectious mononucleosis; tuberculosis; tularemia; brucellosis; bubonic plague; lymphoma; metastasis; Crohn disease

Therapy

Doxycycline; erythromycin, systemic

References

Mabey D, Peeling RW (2002) Lymphogranuloma venereum. Sexually Transmitted Infections 78(2):90–92

Lymphomatoid granulomatosis

Synonym(s)

Angiocentric lymphoproliferative lesion; polymorphic reticulosis

Definition

Systemic angiodestructive lymphoproliferative disease, characterized by prominent pulmonary involvement

Pathogenesis

Probably distinctive type of B-cell lymphoma associated with exuberant, benign, T-cell reaction

Clinical manifestation

Skin: patchy, occasionally painful, erythematous macules, papules, and plaques involving gluteal regions and extremities; subcutaneous nodules which may ulcerate

Pulmonary involvement: cough; dyspnea; hemoptysis; sputum production possibly reflecting associated pneumonia

Neurological manifestations: lymphocytic infiltration of the meninges, cerebral vessels, and peripheral nerves; mass lesions; mental status changes, ataxia, hemiparesis, seizures, distal sensory neuropathy, mononeuritis multiplex; associated with Sjögren syndrome, chronic viral hepatitis, rheumatoid arthritis, renal transplantation, and human immune deficiency virus (HIV) infection

Lethal midline granuloma variant: destructive lesions of midface, nasal cavity, nasal sinuses

Differential diagnosis

Bronchocentric granulomatosis; Churg-Strauss disease; sarcoidosis; Wegener's granulomatosis; non-Hodgkin's lymphoma

Therapy

Systemic corticosteroids with or without chemotherapy

References

Jaffe ES, Wilson WH (1997) Lymphomatoid granulomatosis: pathogenesis, pathology and clinical implications. Cancer Surveys 30:233–248

Lymphomatoid papulosis

Synonym(s)
Macaulay disease; Macaulay's disease

Definition
Chronic lymphoproliferative disease of the skin, characterized by recurrent crops of papules that may ulcerate and heal with scarring

Pathogenesis
Unknown; CD30 (Ki-1) positive lymphoproliferative disorder; possibly either benign chronic disorder of activated T cells responding to external or internal stimuli or low-grade T-cell lymphoma localized to skin

Clinical manifestation
Crops of mildly pruritic red papules evolving into red-brown, often hemorrhagic, vesicles or pustules with necrotic crust; healing with depressed scars; most common distribution on trunk and extremities; associated systemic lymphoma in some patients

Differential diagnosis
Pityriasis lichenoides et varioliformis acuta; leukemia cutis; drug eruption; pityriasis lichenoides et varioliformis acuta (Mucha-Habermann disease); cutaneous B-cell lymphoma; Hodgkin's disease; scabies; insect bite reaction; pseudolymphoma; Langerhans cell histiocytosis; miliaria; folliculitis

Therapy
Methotrexate[*]; photochemotherapy

References
Karp DL, Horn TD (1994) Lymphomatoid papulosis. Journal of the American Academy of Dermatology 30(3):379–395

M

Macaulay disease

▶ Lymphomatoid papulosis

Macaulay's disease

▶ Lymphomatoid papulosis

Macroglobulinemia

▶ Waldenström macroglobulinemia

Macular atrophy of the skin

▶ Malignant atrophic papulosis

Madelung's disease

▶ Benign symmetric lipomatosis

Madura foot

▶ Eumycetoma
▶ Mycetoma

Maduromycosis

▶ Eumycetoma
▶ Mycetoma

Maffucci syndrome

Synonym(s)
Enchondromatosis; dyschondrodysplasia with hemangiomas; enchondromatosis with multiple cavernous hemangiomas

Definition
Disorder characterized by benign cartilaginous tumors (enchondromas), bone deformities, and hemangiomas

Pathogenesis
Unknown

Clinical manifestation
Hemangiomas in various areas of the body, including leptomeninges, eyes, pharynx, tongue, trachea, and intestines; enchondromas, usually on the hands

Differential diagnosis
Kaposi's sarcoma; Klippel-Trenaunay-Weber syndrome; dyschondrodysplasia with hemangiomas; enchondromatosis with multiple cavernous hemangiomas;

Gorham syndrome; Ollier disease; proteus syndrome

Therapy
None for asymptomatic lesions; surgical repair for bone fractures, as needed

References
Kuwahara RT, Skinner RB Jr (2002) Maffucci syndrome: a case report. Cutis 69(1):21–22

Majocchi granuloma

Synonym(s)
Majocchi's granuloma; granuloma trichophyticum; granuloma tricofitico

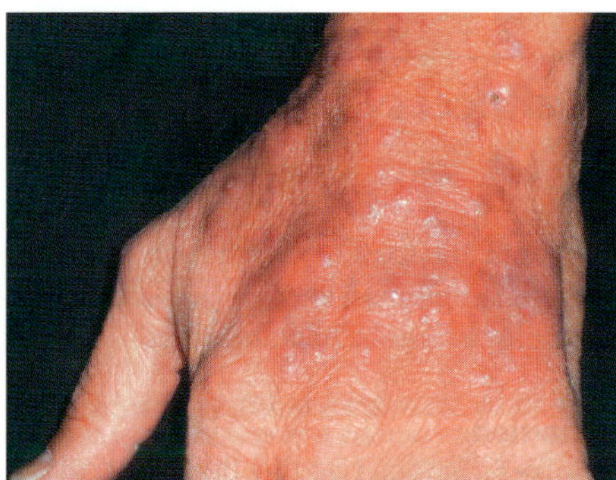

Majocchi granuloma. Red-brown plaque on the hand, studded with follicular papules and pustules

Definition
Nodular perifolliculitis secondary to a dermatophyte infection

Pathogenesis
Type IV hypersensitivity reaction, most commonly due to Trichophyton rubrum infection; possibly a response to the organism itself or non-specific inflammatory response to follicular contents

Clinical manifestation
Develops on any hair-bearing area, but most often on the scalp, face, forearms, dorsal aspect of hands, and legs; solitary or multiple, well-circumscribed, oval, scaly plaques with perifollicular papules and pustules

Differential diagnosis
Folliculitis; pseudofolliculitis barbae; scabies; acne keloidalis; psoriasis; lupus erythematosus; acquired perforating disease; contact dermatitis; coccidioidomycosis; rosacea; herpes simplex virus infection; ecthyma

Therapy
Terbinafine; itraconazole; azole antifungal agents

References
Elgart ML (1996) Tinea incognito: an update on Majocchi granuloma. Dermatologic Clinics 14(1):51–55

Majocchi's disease

▶ Majocchi granuloma

Majocchi's granuloma

▶ Majocchi granuloma

Mal de Meleda

Synonym(s)
Acroerythrokeratoderma; keratoderma palmoplantaris transgradiens

Definition
Keratoderma of the palms and soles occuring as a genetic disease, mainly in residents of the island of Meleda

Pathogenesis
Recessive or variable dominant mode of transmission; exact genetic defect unknown

Clinical manifestation
Keratoderma of the palms and soles, with extension onto the dorsa of the affected limbs; extension to the elbows and knees; associated eczema in many patients; hyperhidrosis; nail thickening and koilonychia

Differential diagnosis
Olmsted syndrome; keratosis lichenoides chronica striata; mutilating keratoderma (Vohwinkel's syndrome); progressive palmoplantar keratoderma; tylosis (Unna-Thost syndrome)

Therapy
Keratolytic therapy, such as 6% salicylic acid in 70% propylene glycol; acetretin

References
Ratnavel RC, Griffiths WA (1997) The inherited palmoplantar keratodermas. British Journal of Dermatology 137(4):485–90

Mal de pinto

▶ Pinta

Malacoplakia

▶ Malakoplakia, cutaneous

Malakoplakia, cutaneous

Synonym(s)
Malacoplakia

Definition
Immunodeficiency disease characterized by variable and non-specific skin lesions and associated with macrophage dysfunction

Pathogenesis
Caused by inadequate bacterial killing by macrophages or monocytes that exhibit defective phagolysosomal activity; risk factors: chronic corticosteroid use, rheumatoid arthritis, diabetes mellitus, and organ transplantation

Clinical manifestation
Yellow-to-pink papules, nodules, or ulcers, most commonly in perianal or inguinal areas, the buttocks and abdominal wall, or in mucous membranes; occasional secondary infection, most commonly Escherichia coli; chronic, benign, self-limited course

Differential diagnosis
Squamous cell carcinoma; sarcoidosis; Langerhans cell histiocytosis; lymphoma histiocytoma; granular cell tumor; furuncle; actinomycosis; botryomycosis

Therapy
Surgical excision[★]; ciprofloxacin; trimethoprim-sulfamethoxazole: 160 mg TMP/ 800 mg SMZ PO twice daily for 7–14 days

References
Remond B, Dompmartin A, Moreau A, Esnault P, Thomas A, Mandard JC, Leroy D (1994) Cutaneous malacoplakia. International Journal of Dermatology 33(8):538–542

Male genital lichen sclerosus

▶ Balanitis xerotica obliterans

Male pattern baldness

▶ Androgenetic alopecia

Male Turner syndrome

▶ Noonan's syndrome

Malherbe, calcifying epithelioma of

▶ Pilomatricoma

Mali's disease

▶ Acroangiodermatitis

Malignancy of fat cells

▶ Liposarcoma

Malignant angioendotheliomatosis

▶ Angioendotheliomatosis

Malignant angioma

▶ Angiosarcoma

Malignant atrophic papulosis

Synonym(s)
Degos' disease; Degos' syndrome; Kohlmeier-Degos syndrome; papulosis atrophicans maligna; macular atrophy of the skin; fatal cutaneointestinal syndrome; lethal cutaneous and gastrointestinal arterial thrombosis

Definition
Multisystem disorder involving small-caliber blood vessels, characterized by narrowing and occlusion of the lumen by intimal proliferation and thrombosis, leading to ischemia and infarction in the involved organs

Pathogenesis
Unknown

Clinical manifestation
Skin findings: multiple, small, asymptomatic papules appearing in crops and primarily involving the trunk and limbs while sparing the palms, soles, face, and scalp; pinkish papules become umbilicated, with depressed centers, and turn porcelain-white
Gastrointestinal manifestations: nonspecific; including abdominal pain, abdominal distention, nausea, vomiting, diarrhea or constipation, weakness, fatigue, weight loss, or symptoms of malabsorption; in late stage, gastrointestinal hemorrhage, bowel infarction, and perforation
Neurological findings: involvement of both central and peripheral nervous systems; paresthesias of the face and extremities, headaches, dizziness, seizures, hemiplegia, aphasia, paraplegia, and gaze palsy

Differential diagnosis
Pyoderma gangrenosum; lupus erythematosus; Crohn disease; polyarteritis nodosa; thromboangiitis obliterans; lichen planus; morphea; lichen sclerosus; burn or other skin trauma

Therapy
No effective therapy, including anticoagulants, antiplatelet drugs such as aspirin and dipyridamole, corticosteroids, immunosuppressants, sulfonamide, tetracycline, and penicillin

References

Demitsu T, Nakajima K, Okuyama R, Tadaki T (1992) Malignant atrophic papulosis (Degos' syndrome). International Journal of Dermatology 31(2):99–102

Malignant carcinoid syndrome

Synonym(s)
Carcinoid syndrome

Definition
Constellation of symptoms seen in patients with metastases from carcinoid tumors

Pathogenesis
Primary tumors arise from neuroendocrine cells secreting serotonin; variety of vasoactive peptides produced, causing clinical symptoms

Clinical manifestation
Flushing of the face and neck, sometimes brief (e.g., 2–5 min) or lasting for several hours; fixed telangiectasia and/or violaceous hue, primarily on the face and neck, most marked in the malar area; tachycardia without significant change in blood pressure

Differential diagnosis
Urticaria; anaphylaxis; angioedema; pheochromocytoma; mastocytosis; pellagra

Therapy
Antihistamines, first generation; octreotide 100 mcg subcutaneously 3–4 times per day; various cancer chemotherapy regimens

References
Bax ND, Woods HF, Batchelor A, Jennings M (1996) Clinical manifestations of carcinoid disease. World Journal of Surgery 20(2):142–146

Malignant down

▶ Hypertrichosis lanuginosa

Malignant endothelioma

▶ Angiosarcoma

Malignant endovascular papillary angioendothelioma

▶ Endovascular papillary angioendothelioma of childhood

Malignant melanoma

▶ Melanoma

Malignant mole

▶ Melanoma

Malignant nonchromaffin paraganglioma

▶ Alveolar soft part sarcoma

Malignant organoid granular cell myoblastoma

▶ Alveolar soft part sarcoma

Malignant papillary dermatosis

▶ Paget's disease

Malignant pustule

▶ Anthrax, cutaneous

Malignant rhabdomyoma

▶ Rhabdomyosarcoma

Malignant tumors with eccrine differentiation

▶ Eccrine carcinoma

Malleus

▶ Glanders and melioidosis

Mallorca acne

▶ Acne aestivalis

Marasmus

Synonym(s)
Protein energy malnutrition

Definition
Type of malnutrition resulting from chronic inadequate consumption of protein and energy, characterized by wasting of muscle, fat, and other body tissue

Pathogenesis
Negative energy balance from decreased energy intake, increased energy expenditure, or both

Clinical manifestation
Occurs mostly in young children; shrunken wasted appearance, with withdrawn behavior; loss of muscle and subcutaneous fat mass

Differential diagnosis
Kwashiorkor; underlying systemic malignancy

Therapy
Nutritional supplementation[*]

References
Akner G, Cederholm T (2001) Treatment of protein-energy malnutrition in chronic nonmalignant disorders. American Journal of Clinical Nutrition 74(1):6–24

Marchiafava-Micheli syndrome

▶ Paroxysmal nocturnal hemoglobinuria

Marfan disease

▶ Marfan syndrome

Marfan syndrome

Synonym(s)
Marfan's syndrome, Marfan disease, Marfan's disease

Definition
Inherited connective tissue disorder characterized by abnormalities in skeletal system, cardiovascular system, eyes, and skin

Pathogenesis
Autsomal dominant trait; mutations in the fibrillin-1 (FBN1) gene located on chromosome 15q21.1; production of abnormal fibrillin-1 monomers from the mutated gene disrupt multimerization of fibrillin-1 and prevent microfibril formation, leading to abnormal connective tissue structure

Clinical manifestation
Skin findings: striae; hyperextensible skin; elastosis perforans serpiginosa; high, arched palate; poor wound healing
Skeletal findings: joint hypermobility; pectus excavatum; scoliosis; long arms and legs
Ocular findings: ectopic lens; early cataracts
Cardiopulmonary findings: aortic root dilatation and dissection; aortic valve prolapse; spontaneous pneumothorax
Neurologic findings: dura ectasia

Differential diagnosis
Ehlers-Danlos syndrome; Klinefelter's syndrome; fragile X syndrome

Therapy
None for skin changes

References
Aburawi EH, O'Sullivan J, Hasan A (2001) Marfan's syndrome: a review. Hospital Medicine (London) 62(3):153–157

Marfan's disease

▶ Marfan syndrome

Marfan's syndrome

▶ Marfan syndrome

Marjolin ulcer

Synonym(s)
Marjolin's ulcer

Definition
Malignant tumor that arises in chronic burn wounds or other skin ulcerations

References
Phillips TJ, Salman SM, Bhawan J, Rogers GS (1998) Burn scar carcinoma. Diagnosis and management. Dermatologic Surgery 24(5):561–565

Marjolin's ulcer

▶ Marjolin ulcer

Market men's disease

▶ Tularemia

Mask of pregnancy

▶ Melasma

Massage alopecia

▶ Traction alopecia

Mastocytosis

Synonym(s)
Urticaria pigmentosa; mastocytosis syndrome

Definition
Disorder characterized by mast cell proliferation and accumulation within various organs, including the skin

Pathogenesis
May be abnormal mast cell response to unknown stimuli; increased local concentrations of mast cell growth factors stimulate mast cell proliferation; systemic manifestations reflect the release of mast cell-derived mediators, such as histamine, prostaglandins, heparin, neutral proteases, and acid hydrolases

Clinical manifestation
Most common in children, who have 25–100 red-brown macules or barely elevated papules, usually over the trunk; lesion becomes a wheal when rubbed (Darier's sign); solitary mastocytoma: usually appears within first month of life; rubbery, yellow to brown, plaques, urticate with or without vesiculation after rubbing (bullous urticaria pigmentosa); telangiectasia macularis eruptiva perstans: brown macules and telangiectasias with erythema, often over upper trunk; associated with peptic ulcer disease; diffuse mastocytosis: bullae in infancy, replaced by doughy skin, with generalized pruritus; dermatographism, bullae after minor skin trauma; mast cell infiltration of liver, spleen, skeleton, and gastrointestinal tract; flushing syndrome, most common in early life

Differential diagnosis
Spitz nevus; juvenile xanthogranuloma; amyloidosis; sarcoidosis; granuloma annulare; melanocytic nevus; fixed drug eruption; insect bite reaction; lymphoma; Jessner lymphocytic infiltrate; lentigo; berloque dermatitis; Langerhans cell histiocytosis

Therapy
Antihistamines, second generation*; photochemotherapy; corticosteroids, topical, super potency

References
Hartmann K, Bruns SB, Henz BM (2001) Mastocytosis: review of clinical and experimental aspects. Journal of Investigative Dermatology Symposium Proceedings 6(2):143–147

Mastocytosis syndrome

▶ **Mastocytosis**

McCune-Albright Syndrome

Synonym(s)
Albright syndrome; Albright's syndrome; osteitis fibrosa disseminata; fibrous dysplasia of bone; polyostotic dysplasia; polyostotic fibrous dysplasia; osteitis fibrosa cystica; Fuller-Albright syndrome; Albright-Sternberg-McCune syndrome; brown spot syndrome

Definition
Fibrous dysplasia of bone; sexual precocity; hyperpigmentation

Pathogenesis
Mutation in the GNAS1 gene coding for guanine nucleotide-binding protein G alpha subunit (protein Gs); mosaic pattern of autonomously functioning clones of cells in the affected organs

Clinical manifestation
Hyperpigmented patches, often following Blaschko's lines; precocious puberty; other endocrine dysfunction: thyroid storm (particularly during general anesthesia), tachyarrhythmia, and fever; cushingoid habi-

tus; acromegaly; hirsutism; galactorrhea; skeletal deformities

Differential diagnosis
Hyperpigmented skin lesions: neurofibromatosis; tuberous sclerosis; Bloom syndrome; ataxia-telangiectasia; Russell-Silver syndrome; Fanconi anemia; precocious puberty; ovarian/testicular tumors; adrenal tumors; congenital adrenal hyperplasia; exogenous estrogens/androgen intake

Therapy
Surgical excision of hyperfunctional endocrine tissue if severe endocrine imbalance present

References
de Sanctis C, Lala R, Matarazzo P, Balsamo A, et al. (1999) McCune-Albright syndrome: A longitudinal clinical study of 32 patients. Journal of Pediatric Endocrinology 12(6):817–826

MD Forte facial cream

▶ Alpha hydroxy acids

Measles

▶ Rubella
▶ Rubeola

Median canal dystrophy

▶ Median nail dystrophy

Median nail dystrophy

Synonym(s)
Median canal dystrophy

Definition
Acquired nail plate disorder characterized by longitudinal split in the center of the nail plate

Pathogenesis
Sometimes related to trauma of the proximal nail fold area from habitual picking, etc.

Clinical manifestation
Longitudinal split appears in center of nail plate; several fine cracks project from the line laterally, giving the appearance of fir tree; thumb most often affected; spontaneous remission after months to years, with recurrences possible

Differential diagnosis
Underlying anatomic defects, including mucous cyst, squamous cell carcinoma; melanoma; wart; exostosis; onychomycosis; psoriasis; lichen planus

Therapy
None

References
Griego RD, Orengo IF, Scher RK (1995) Median nail dystrophy and habit tic deformity: are they different forms of the same disorder? International Journal of Dermatology 34(11):799–800

Median rhomboid glossitis

Synonym(s)
Central papillary atrophy; posterior lingual papillary atrophy

Definition
Defective embryonic posterior dorsal tongue point of fusion, leaving a rhomboid-shaped, smooth, erythematous mucosa lacking in papillae or taste buds

Pathogenesis
Onset occurring during embryonic tongue development

Clinical manifestation

Smooth, flat, or slightly lobulated plaque on posterior midline of the dorsum of the tongue, just anterior to the V-shaped grouping of the circumvalate papillae; secondary chronic candida infection

Differential diagnosis

Squamous cell carcinoma; black hairy tongue; lingual thyroid; tertiary syphilis; tuberculosis; granular cell tumor

Therapy

Azole antifungal troches for candida superinfection

References

Carter LC (1990) Median rhomboid glossitis: review of a puzzling entity. Compendium 11(7):446, 448–451

Mediterranean spotted fever

▶ Boutonneuse fever

Meibomian cyst

▶ Chalazion

Melandodermic leukodystrophy

▶ Addison-Schilder disease

Melanoacanthoma

Synonym(s)

Benign mixed tumor of melanocytes and malpighian cells; melanoepithelioma; melanoacanthosis

Definition

Benign mixed tumor of keratinocytes and melanocytes

Pathogenesis

Trauma a possible factor in this reactive process; may be a seborrheic keratosis variant

Clinical manifestation

Solitary, hyperpigmented or verrucous, round or oval papule, plaque, cutaneous horn, or nodule, usually on trunk, lip, or eyelid; also occur in oral mucosa

Differential diagnosis

Melanocytic nevus; melanoma; seborrheic keratosis; wart; actinic keratosis; pigmented basal cell carcinoma; mucosal melanosis

Therapy

Cryotherapy; destruction by electrodessication and curettage; simple excision

References

Tomich CE, Zunt SL (1990) Melanoacanthosis (melanoacanthoma) of the oral mucosa. Journal of Dermatologic Surgery & Oncology 16(3):231–236

Melanoacanthosis

▶ Melanoacanthoma

Melanoepithelioma

▶ Melanoacanthoma

Melanoid mycetoma

▶ Eumycetoma

Melanoma

Synonym(s)
Malignant melanoma; malignant mole

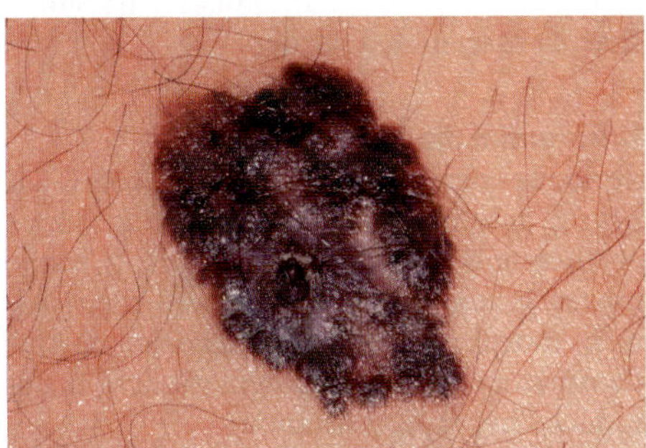

Melanoma. Irregular pigmented plaque, with shades of red, white, and blue

Definition
Malignant tumor of melanocytes

Pathogenesis
Multiple contributing factors: (1) fair complexion; (2) excessive childhood sun exposure and blistering childhood sunburns; (3) increased number of common acquired and atypical moles; (4) family history of melanoma; (5) xeroderma pigmentosum; (6) familial atypical mole melanoma syndrome

Clinical manifestation
Occurs most commonly on the trunk in white males and the lower legs and back in white females, in pigmented races; most common sites are plantar foot, subungual, palmar, and mucosal sites
Superficial spreading subtype: most common, occurring in approximately 70% of patients; a flat or slightly elevated papule or plaque, with variegate pigmentation (black, brown, blue, or pink discoloration), usually greater than 6 mm in diameter; irregular asymmetric borders
Nodular subtype: most commonly seen on the legs and trunk; rapid growth of a dark brown-to-black papule or dome-shaped nodule, which may be friable and ulcerate; lentigo maligna melanoma: arises in intraepithelial precursor lesion, lentigo maligna; slow growing, irregular, pigmented patch, located on the sun-damaged skin of head, neck, and arms of fair-skinned older individuals; over time, dark brown-to-black macular pigmentation or raised blue-black nodules evolves
Acral lentiginous subtype: least common variety, but most common type in dark-skinned individuals; occurs on the palms, soles, or beneath the nail plate; subungual lesion presents as diffuse nail discoloration or longitudinal pigmented band within the nail plate, with pigment spreading to the proximal or lateral nail folds (Hutchinson sign)

Differential diagnosis
Melanocytic nevus, including atypical mole; lentigo; seborrheic keratosis; pyogenic granuloma; basal cell carcinoma; squamous cell carcinoma; dermatofibroma; cherry hemangioma; metastasis; keratoacanthoma; chronic paronychia; subungual hematoma; melanonychia striata

Therapy
Wide local excision★; sentinel node biopsy and node dissection as needed for 1-4 mm deep primary tumors; adjuvant interferon (IFN) alfa-2b for high risk primary tumors or regional micrometastatic disease

References
Lang PG (2002) Current concepts in the management of patients with melanoma. American Journal of Clinical Dermatology 3(6):401–426

Melanosis faciei feminae

▶ Riehl's melanosis

Melanosis lenticularis progressiva

▶ Xeroderma pigmentosum

Melanotic hyperpigmentation

▶ Postinflammatory hyperpigmentation

Melasma

Synonym(s)
Chloasma; mask of pregnancy; pregnancy mask

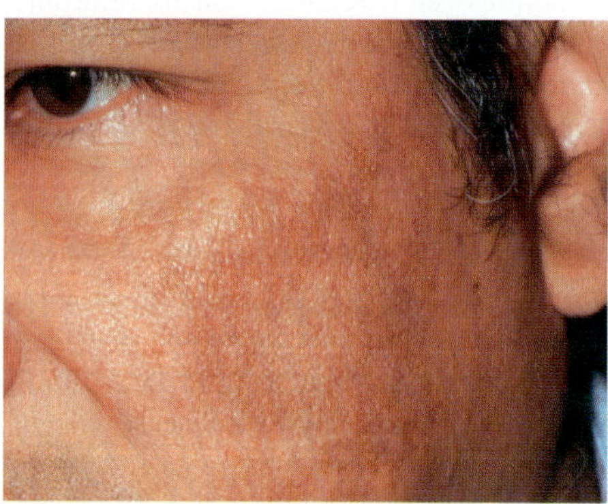

Melasma. Reticulated, brown plaque on the face

Definition
Acquired, chronic hypermelanosis, characterized by macular hyperpigmentation, mainly in sun-exposed skin

Pathogenesis
Multiple contributing factors, including genetic predispsition, sun exposure, hormonal stimulation; racial predisposition (e.g., common in Hispanics)

Clinical manifestation
Symmetric, tan-brown, macular hyperpigmentation; occurs in 1 of 3 patterns: central facial, malar, or mandibular; irregular, sharply marginated borders

Differential diagnosis
Berloque dermatitis; lentigo; nevocellular nevus; polymorphous light reaction; lupus erythematosus; poikiloderma of Civatte; mastocytosis; Addison disease; lichen planus; morphea; Riehl's melanosis; postinflammatory hyperpigmentation; drug-induced hyperpigmentation

Therapy
Hydroquinone; azelaic acid; tretinoin; sunscreen protection; chemical peel; laser therapy

References
Pandya AG, Guevara IL (2000) Disorders of hyperpigmentation. Dermatologic Clinics. 18(1):91–98

Melioidosis

▶ Glanders and melioidosis

Melkersson-Rosenthal syndrome

▶ Cheilitis granulomatosa

MEN IIB syndrome

▶ Mucosal neuroma syndrome

MEN III syndrome

▶ Mucosal neuroma syndrome

Meningococcal sepsis

▶ Meningococcemia

Meningococcemia

Synonym(s)
Meningococcal sepsis

Definition
Acute infection of the bloodstream and subsequent vasculitis with the bacteria Neisseria meningitidis

Pathogenesis
Caused by Neisseria meningitidis, an obligate, non-motile, aerobic, encapsulated gram-negative diplococcus; host factors: deficiencies of terminal complement components C_5 through C_9 or properdin, immunoglobulin deficiency, asplenia, and HIV infection; vascular injury the result of direct toxic effects of organism and immunologic reaction

Clinical manifestation
May follow upper respiratory infection; associated with headache, nausea, vomiting, myalgias, and arthralgias; fulminant disease: hemorrhagic eruption, hypotension, and cardiac depression occur within hours of initial presentation; skin findings of petechiae on the extremities and trunk, sometimes generalizing; progression: pustules, bullae, and hemorrhagic plaques with central necrosis and stellate purpura with a central "gun-metal" gray hue; neurologic findings: headache; altered mental status; neck stiffness; irritability; seizures; nerve palsies; gait disturbance; gastrointestinal findings: nausea and vomiting

Differential diagnosis
Bacterial sepsis other than that caused by Neisseria meningitidis, such as gonococcemia, Haemophilus influenzae, and Streptococcus pneumoniae; Rocky Mountain spotted fever; viral illnesses, especially enteroviruses; toxic shock syndrome; leptospirosis; hypersensitivity vasculitis; Henoch-Schönlein purpura; polyarteritis nodosa; dermatomyositis; lupus erythematosus; coagulopathies; idiopathic purpura fulminans

Therapy
Penicillin G in sensitive strains[*]: 300,000 U per kg per day, up to 24 million U per day IV in 4–6 divided doses until 5–7 days after temperature has returned to normal; ceftriaxone: 2 g IV or IM every 12 hours until 5–7 days after temperature has returned to normal; cefotaxime for adults: 1–2 g IV or IM every 6–12 hours; for children <50 kg: 50 mg/kg IV or IM every 8 hours

References
Levine N, Kunkel M, Nguyen T, Ackerman L (2002) Emergency Department Dermatology. Current Problems in Dermatology 14(6):183–220

Menke's kinky hair syndrome

Synonym(s)
Menkes kinky hair disease; kinky hair syndrome; steely hair syndrome; trichopoliodystrophy

Definition
Multisystem disorder of copper metabolism, characterized by fine silvery wiry hair,

doughy skin, connective tissue abnormalities, and progressive neurologic deterioration

Pathogenesis
X-linked recessive trait with gene locus in band Xq13.3; defect in intestinal copper transport with associated low serum copper and ceruloplasmin levels, resulting in a deficiency in copper-dependent enzyme activity; copper-dependent metalloenzymes relevant to the clinical phenotype: tyrosinase (pigmentation of skin and hair), lysyl oxidase (elastin and collagen cross-linking), ascorbate oxidase (skeletal development), monoamine oxidase (possibly responsible for pili torti), superoxide dismutase (free-radical detoxification), dopamine beta-hydroxylase (catecholamine production), peptidyl-glycine alpha-amidating mono-oxygenase (bioactivation of peptide hormones), and cytochrome c oxidase (electron transport and possibly responsible for hypothermia)

Clinical manifestation
Skin – hypopigmented, pale, cutis marmorata; lax doughy skin of cheeks; cupid's bow upper lip
Hair – pili torti; trichorrhexis nodosa; light-colored, sparse, short, brittle, kinky, steel wool-like hair; sparse, broken eyebrows and eyelashes
Abnormal facies; musculoskeletal abnormalities; progressive neurologic deterioration

Differential diagnosis
Ectodermal dysplasia; argininosuccinic aciduria; Björnstad syndrome; Crandall syndrome; Salti-Salem syndrome; Tay syndrome; Conradi-Hünermann chondrodysplasia punctata; Bazex syndrome; citrullinemia; hypohidrotic ectodermal dysplasia; Salamon syndrome; tricho-odontonychial dysplasia with pili torti; pili torti and enamel hypoplasia

Therapy
None for skin and hair problems

References
Kodama H, Murata Y, Kobayashi M (1999) Clinical manifestations and treatment of Menkes disease and its variants. Pediatrics International 41(4):423–429

Merkel cell carcinoma

Synonym(s)
Trabecular carcinoma; small cell carcinoma of the skin; primary cutaneous neuroendocrine carcinoma

Definition
Aggressive primary cutaneous neoplasm with neuroendocrine differentiation

Pathogenesis
Cell of origin may be epidermal Merkel Cell, a dermal Merkel Cell equivalent, a neural-crest-derived cell of the APUD (amine precursor uptake and decarboxylation) system, or a residual epidermal stem cell; chronic exposure to solar ultraviolet radiation possibly a co-factor

Clinical manifestation
Single, painless, firm, shiny, red or violaceous papule, with predilection for individuals with fair skin; most common in seventh decade and older; occurs most commonly in the head and neck region and extremities; regional nodal metastases first site of dissemination; increased incidence in immunocompromised patients

Differential diagnosis
Squamous cell carcinoma; basal cell carcinoma; melanoma; metastasis; Kaposi's sarcoma; hemangioma; dermatofibroma; lymphoma

Therapy
Wide local excision[*]; Mohs micrographic surgery; regional lymph node dissection; radiation therapy for local palliation

References

Goessling W, McKee PH, Mayer RJ (2002) Merkel cell carcinoma. Journal of Clinical Oncology 20(2):588–598

Methotrexate

Trade name(s)
Rheumatrex

Generic available
Yes

Drug class
Anti-metabolite

Mechanism of action
Immunosuppressive: inhibits dihydrofolate reductase; inhibits lymphocyte proliferation

Dosage form
2.5 mg tablet; 25 mg per ml solution for intramuscular injection

Dermatologic indications and dosage
See table

Common side effects
Cutaneous: stomatitis, photosensitivity, skin eruption, alopecia
Gastrointestinal: nausea, vomiting
Laboratory: elevated liver function enzymes

Serious side effects
Bone marrow: marrow suppression
Cutaneous: Stevens-Johnson syndrome, toxic epidermal necrolysis, exfoliative dermatitis, radiation recall reactions
Pulmonary: pulmonary fibrosis

Drug interactions
Acitretin; COX-2 inhibitors; salicylates; non-steroidal anti-inflammatory agents; penicillins; sulfonamides; trimethoprim

Contraindications/precautions
Hypersensitivity to drug class or component; pregnancy; alcohol abuse; severe liver dysfunction; immunodeficiency syndromes; caution in patients with impaired renal function or ulcerative colitis

References

Silvis NG (2001) Antimetabolites and cytotoxic drugs. Dermatologic Clinics 19(1):105–118

Methoxsalen

Trade name(s)
Oxsoralen Ultra; Oxsoralen lotion

Generic available
No

Drug class
Psoralen

Mechanism of action
Suppression of DNA synthesis; photo-immunologic effects; selective cytotoxicity; melanocyte stimulation

Dosage form
10 mg capsules; 1% solution for dilution

Dermatologic indications and dosage
See table

Common side effects
Cutaneous: phototoxic reaction, exanthem, herpes simplex virus infection recurrence, photo-aging after chronic use
Gastrointestinal: nausea, vomiting, hepatic toxicity

Serious side effects
Cutaneous: carcinogenesis
Ocular: cataract formation

Drug interactions
Doxycycline; fluoroquinolones; carbamazepine; phenytoin

Methotrexate. Dermatologic indications and dosage

Disease	Adult dosage	Child dosage
Bullous pemphigoid	7.5–25 mg PO as a single dose weekly	5–15 mg PO as a single weekly dose
Chronic graft versus host disease	7.5–25 mg PO as a single dose weekly	5–15 mg PO as a single weekly dose
Dermatomyositis	7.5–25 mg PO as a single dose weekly	5–15 mg PO as a single weekly dose
Epidermolysis bullosa acquisita	7.5–25 mg PO as a single dose weekly	5–15 mg PO as a single weekly dose
Lupus erythematosus	7.5–25 mg PO as a single dose weekly	5–15 mg PO as a single weekly dose
Lymphomatoid papulosis	5–7.5 mg PO as a single weekly dose	2.5–5 mg PO as a single weekly dose
Mycosis fungoides	7.5–25 mg PO as a single dose weekly	5–15 mg PO as a single weekly dose
Pemphigus vulgaris	7.5–25 mg PO as a single dose weekly	5–15 mg PO as a single weekly dose
Pityriasis lichenoides	5–7.5 mg PO as a single weekly dose	2.5–5 mg PO as a single weekly dose
Pityriasis rubra pilaris	7.5–25 mg PO as a single dose weekly	5–15 mg PO as a single weekly dose
Progressive systemic sclerosis	7.5–25 mg PO as a single dose weekly	5–15 mg PO as a single weekly dose
Psoriasis	7.5–25 mg PO as a single dose weekly	5–15 mg PO as a single weekly dose
Pyoderma gangrenosum	7.5–25 mg PO as a single dose weekly	5–15 mg PO as a single weekly dose
Reiter syndrome	7.5–25 mg PO as a single dose weekly	5–15 mg PO as a single weekly dose
Relapsing polychondritis	7.5–25 mg PO as a single dose weekly	5–15 mg PO as a single weekly dose
Sarcoidosis	7.5–25 mg PO as a single dose weekly	5–15 mg PO as a single weekly dose
Sézary syndrome	7.5–25 mg PO as a single dose weekly	5–15 mg PO as a single weekly dose
Vasculitis, including polyarteritis nodosa	7.5–25 mg PO as a single dose weekly	5–15 mg PO as a single weekly dose

Methoxsalen. Dermatologic indications and dosage

Disease	Adult dose	Child dose
Component of photochemotherapy – psoriasis; Reiter syndrome; cutaneous T cell lymphoma (mycosis fungoides; Sézary syndrome; vitiligo; polymorphous light eruption; solar urticaria; chronic actinic dermatitis; morphea; linear scleroderma; graft versus host disease; lymphomatoid papulosis	Systemic photochemotherapy – 0.4–0.6 mg per kg PO 1.5 hours before exposure to ultraviolet A light, either via light box, outdoor sunlight, or photopheresis; topical therapy – 0.1% lotion applied 30 minutes before exposure to ultraviolet A light	Systemic photochemotherapy – 0.4–0.6 mg per kg PO 1.5 hours before exposure to ultraviolet A light, either via light box, outdoor sunlight, or photopheresis; topical therapy – 0.1% lotion applied 30 minutes before exposure to ultraviolet A light
Component of photopheresis – T-cell lymphoma (mycosis fungoides; Sézary syndrome)	0.4–0.6 mg per kg PO 1.5 hours before exposure to ultraviolet A light	0.4–0.6 mg per kg PO 1.5 hours before exposure to ultraviolet A light

M

Contraindications/precautions
Hypersensitivity to drug class or component

References
Laube S, George SA (2001) Adverse effects with PUVA and UVB phototherapy. Journal of Dermatological Treatment 12(2):101–105
Lim HW, Edelson RL (1995) Photopheresis for the treatment of cutaneous T-cell lymphoma. Hematology – Oncology Clinics of North America 9(5):1117–1126

Metronidazole, topical

Trade name(s)
MetroGel; MetroCream; MetroLotion; Noritate

Generic available
Yes

Drug class
Nitroimidazole antibiotic

Mechanism of action
DNA disruption and inhibition of nucleic acid synthesis (may not be mechanism in skin disease treatment)

Dosage form
0.75% cream, gel; 1% cream

Dermatologic indications and dosage
See table

Common side effects
Cutaneous: burning sensation, erythema, skin eruption

Serious side effects
None

Drug interactions
None

Metronidazole, topical. Dermatologic indications and dosage

Disease	Adult dosage	Child dosage
Rosacea	Apply once daily	Apply once daily

Contraindications/precautions
Hypersensitivity to drug class or component

References
Cohen AF, Tiemstra JD (2002) Diagnosis and treatment of rosacea. Journal of the American Board of Family Practice 15(3):214–217

Michelin tire baby syndrome

Synonym(s)
Michelin tire syndrome; Kunze Riehm syndrome

Definition
Heterogeneous group of disorders characterized by ringed creases of the extremities

Pathogenesis
Autosomal dominant trait; at least two distinct chromosomal abnormalities

Clinical manifestation
Deep, gyrus-like skin folds on the back; circumferential, deep skin folds of limbs, with spontaneous resolution of skin creases in childhood; loose, thick skin; xanthomas and/or lipomas; hypertrichosis with underlying smooth muscle hamartoma; cleft palate; neuroblastoma; congenital heart defects

Differential diagnosis
Nevus lipomatosis

Therapy
None

References
Glover MT, Malone M, Atherton DJ (1989) Michelin-tire baby syndrome resulting from diffuse smooth muscle hamartoma. Pediatric Dermatology 6(4):329–331

Michelin tire syndrome

► Michelin tire baby syndrome

Miescher syndrome 2

► Berardinelli-Seip syndrome

Miescher-Melkersson-Rosenthal syndrome

► Cheilitis granulomatosa

Miescher's cheilitis granulomatosa

► Cheilitis granulomatosa

Miescher's granulomatosis

► Actinic granuloma
► Cheilitis granulomatosa

Migratory necrolytic erythema

Definition
Migratory eruption on face, abdomen, perineum, buttocks, or lower extremities, usually associated with underlying glucagonoma

▶ Glucogonoma

References
Schwartz RA (1997) Glucagonoma and pseudoglucagonoma syndromes. International Journal of Dermatology 36(2):81–89

Mikulicz disease

▶ Rhinoscleroma

Miliaria

Synonym(s)
Prickly heat; sudamina; heat rash; lichen tropicus; tropical anhidrosis

Definition
Disorder of the eccrine sweat glands often occurring in conditions of increased heat and humidity, caused by blockage of the sweat ducts that results in the leakage of eccrine sweat into skin

Pathogenesis
Occlusion of the skin, due to clothing or bandages, resulting in pooling of sweat on the skin surface and overhydration of the stratum corneum; in susceptible persons, including infants, with relatively immature eccrine glands, stratum corneum overhydration causes transient blockage of the acrosyringium, resulting in leakage of sweat; other contributing factors: immaturity of the sweat ducts in neonates, lack of acclimitization, occlusive clothing, hot and humid conditions, vigorous exerciose, and bacterial overgrowth

Clinical manifestation
Miliaria crystallina: usually affects neonates and adults who are febrile or who recently moved to a tropical climate; asymptomatic, clear, superficial vesicles appear in crops, often confluent, and without surrounding erythema; rupture easily and resolve with superficial, branny desquamation; occur within days to weeks of exposure to hot weather and disappear within hours to days; in infants, lesions occur on the head, neck, and upper part of the trunk; in adults, lesions appear on the trunk

Miliaria rubra: occurs in hot, humid environments; pruritic or painful, small, discrete, non-follicular, erythematous papules and vesicles; lesions on the neck and in the groin and axillae; lesions on covered skin subject to friction, such as the neck, scalp, upper part of the trunk, and flexures in adults

Miliaria profunda: occurs in those in a tropical climate who have had repeated episodes of miliaria rubra; asymptomatic, firm, flesh-colored papules, usually on the trunk, developing within minutes or hours after the stimulation of sweating and resolves quickly after removal of stimulus that caused sweating; increased sweating in unaffected skin; lymphadenopathy; hyperpyrexia and symptoms of heat exhaustion, including dizziness, nausea, dyspnea, and palpitations

Differential diagnosis
Folliculitis; milia; viral exanthem; cutaneous candidiasis; erythema toxicum; insect bite reaction; scabies; foreign body reaction; drug eruption; cholinergic urticaria

Therapy
Miliaria crystallina: no therapy indicated
Miliaria rubra: removal of occlusive clothing; limiting of activity; air conditioning
Miliaria profunda: removal of occlusive clothing; limited activity; air conditioning;

anhydrous lanolin lotion applied 2–3 times daily and before activity that may produce excess sweating

References
Wenzel FG, Horn TD (1998) Nonneoplastic disorders of the eccrine glands. Journal of the American Academy of Dermatology 38(1):1–17

Miliaria cystallina

▶ Miliaria

Miliaria profunda

▶ Miliaria

Miliaria pustulosa

▶ Miliaria

Miliary tuberculosis of the skin

▶ Cutaneous tuberculosis

Milium

Synonym(s)
None

Definition
Small, benign, keratin-filled cyst

Pathogenesis
Derived from the pilosebaceous follicle; primary lesions arise from vellus hair follicles; secondary milia result from damage to pilosebaceous unit after skin trauma

Clinical manifestation
Uniform, pearly-white to yellowish, small, domed papules, often in groups; primary milia: usually on the face of newborns; seen around the eye in children and adults; secondary lesions: arise after blistering or trauma, including bullous pemphigoid, inherited and acquired epidermolysis bullosa, bullous lichen planus, porphyria cutanea tarda, and burns

Differential diagnosis
Acne vulgaris; flat wart; syringoma; trichoepithelioma; xanthoma

Therapy
Incision and drainage; light hyfrecation

References
Touart DM, Sau P (1998) Cutaneous deposition diseases. Part I. Journal of the American Academy of Dermatology. 39(2 Pt 1):149–171

Minocycline

Trade name(s)
Minocin; Dynacin; Vectrin

Generic available
Yes

Drug class
Tetracycline

Mechanism of action
Antibiotic activity: protein synthesis inhibition by binding to the 30S ribosomal subunit; anti-inflammatory activity: unclear mechanism

Dosage form
50 mg, 75 mg, 100 mg tablets

Dermatologic indications and dosage
See table

Minocycline. Dermatologic indications and dosage

Disease	Adult dosage	Child dosage
Acne vulgaris	50–100 mg PO twice daily	> 8 years old – 50–100 mg PO twice daily
Atrophoderma of Pasini-Pierini	50–100 mg PO twice daily	> 8 years old – 50–100 mg PO twice daily
Bullous pemphigoid	50–100 mg PO twice daily	> 8 years old – 50–100 mg PO twice daily
Confluent and reticulate papillomatosis of Gougerot and Carteaud	50–100 mg PO twice daily	> 8 years old – 50–100 mg PO twice daily
Dermatitis herpetiformis	50–100 mg PO twice daily	> 8 years old – 50–100 mg PO twice daily
Folliculitis	50–100 mg PO twice daily	> 8 years old – 50–100 mg PO twice daily
Linear IgA bullous dermatosis	50–100 mg PO twice daily	> 8 years old – 50–100 mg PO twice daily
Mycobacterium marinum infection	100 mg PO twice daily for 4–6 weeks after clinical resolution	> 8 years old – 50–100 mg PO twice daily for 4–6 weeks after clincial resolution
Nocardiosis	100-200 mg PO daily for 2–4 weeks	> 8 years old – 100-200 mg PO daily for 2–4 weeks
Pemphigus foliaceus	50–100 mg PO twice daily	> 8 years old – 50–100 mg PO twice daily
Perioral dermatitis	50–100 mg PO twice daily for at least 30 days	> 8 years old – 50–100 mg PO twice daily for at least 30 days
Rosacea	50–100 mg PO twice daily for at least 30 days	> 8 years old – 50–100 mg PO twice daily for at least 30 days
Rosacea	50–100 mg PO twice daily	> 8 years old – 50–100 mg PO twice daily

Common side effects
Cutaneous: photosensitivity, stomatitis, oral candidiasis, urticaria or other vascular reaction
Gastrointestinal: nausea and vomiting, diarrhea, esophagitis
Neurologic: tinnitus, dizziness, drowsiness, headache, ataxia

Serious side effects
Gastrointestinal: pseudomembranous colitis, hepatotoxicity

Hematologic: neutropenia, thrombocytopenia
Neurologic: pseudotumor cerebri

Drug interactions
Antacids; calcium salts; oral contraceptives; digoxin; iron salts; isotretinoin; magnesium salts; warfarin

Contraindications/precautions
Hypersensitivity to drug class or component; pregnancy; patient < 8 years old; cau-

tion in patients with impaired renal or liver function

References

Sadick N (2000) Systemic antibiotic agents. Dermatologic Clinics 19(1):1–22

Minoxidil, topical

Trade name(s)
Rogaine

Generic available
Yes

Drug class
Peripheral vasodilator

Mechanism of action
Unclear; may involve vasodilatation and/or anti-androgen mechanisms

Dosage form
2%, 5% solution

Dermatologic indications and dosage
See table

Common side effects
Cutaneous: irritant dermatitis, hypertrichosis

Serious side effects
None

Drug interactions
None

Contraindications/precautions
Hypersensitivity to drug class or component; caution in patients over 50 years old

References

Price VH (1999) Treatment of hair loss. New England Journal of Medicine 341(13):964–973

Mixed connective tissue disease

Synonym(s)
Sharp syndrome; Sharp's syndrome

Definition
Disorder characterized by elements of several connective tissue diseases, such as: systemic lupus erythematosus, systemic sclerosis, dermatomyositis, polymyositis, and Sjögren syndrome

Pathogenesis
Probable autoimmune phenomenon with antibodies against the U1-RNP complex in genetically predisposed individuals

Clinical manifestation
Skin findings: Raynaud phenomenon; sausage-shaped fingers; swelling of the dorsa of the hands; abnormal capillaries in the nail fold; with palpable red papules or plaques similar to chronic cutaneous lupus erythematosus; alopecia; facial erythema; periungual telangiectasia
Musculoskeletal: arthralgia and arthritis; myalgia; myositis; muscle weakness

Minoxidil, topical. Dermatologic indications and dosage

Disease	Adult dosage	Child dosage
Androgenetic alopecia	Apply twice daily	Not indicated
Anagen effluvium	Apply twice daily	Not indicated

Gastrointestinal: dysphagia and dysfunction of esophageal motility

Pulmonary: pleural effusion; interstitial pulmonary fibrosis; pulmonary arterial hypertension; vasculitis; pulmonary thromboembolism; aspiration pneumonia

Serositis; occasional nephritis, cardiac dysfunction; neurologic involvement

Differential diagnosis
Lupus erythematosus; dermatomyositis; progressive systemic sclerosis

Therapy
Severe involvement with evidence of organ dysfunction: prednisone*; steroid sparing agents: cyclosporine; azathioprine; cyclophosphamide

References
Farhey Y, Hess EV (1997) Mixed connective tissue disease. Arthritis Care & Research 10(5):333–342

Mixed cryoglobulinemia

▶ Cryoglobulinemia

Mixed porphyria

▶ Variegate porphyria

Moeller's disease

▶ Barlow's disease

Mole

▶ Nevus, melanocytic

Möller-Barlow disease

▶ Barlow's disease

Molluscum

▶ Molluscum contagiosum

Molluscum contagiosum

Synonym(s)
Water wart; molluscum; molluscum sebaceum; epithelioma contagiosum

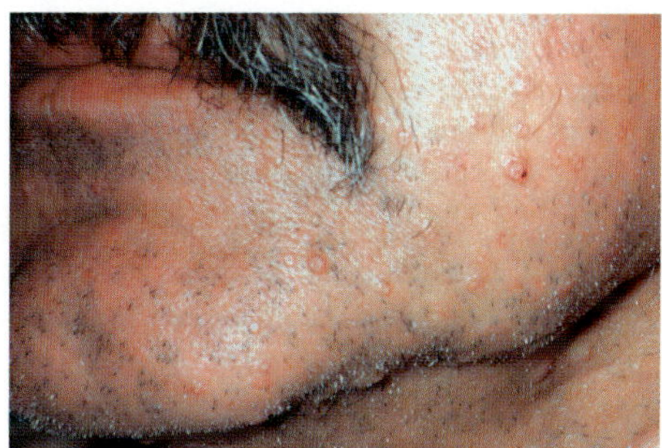

Molluscum contagiosum. Crystalline papules with central dell on the face

Definition
Viral skin infection that produces papules and nodules

Pathogenesis
Caused by large DNA poxvirus, Molluscipoxvirus; replicate in the cytoplasm of epithelial cells and produce cytoplasmic inclusions and enlargement of infected cells

Clinical manifestation
Solitary or grouped, asymptomatic, firm, smooth, umbilicated papules, on the skin and mucosal surfaces; may coalesce into

plaques; self-limited, but sometimes persists for months to years; multiple, widespread, persistent lesions occurring in immunocompromised patients, particularly those with HIV disease

Differential diagnosis
Wart; nevocellular nevus; varicella; fibrous papule of the face; basal cell carcinoma; sebaceous gland hyperplasia; xanthoma; milia; syringoma; juvenile xanthogranuloma; epidermoid cyst; granuloma annulare; cryptococcosis; histoplasmosis

Therapy
Cryotherapy; curettage; tretinoin; benzoyl peroxide; disseminated disease in immunocompromised patients: cidofovir 0.3% gel applied twice daily for 7–14 days

References
Smith KJ, Skelton H (2002) Molluscum contagiosum: recent advances in pathogenic mechanisms, and new therapies. American Journal of Clinical Dermatology 3(8):535–545

Molluscum sebaceum

▶ **Molluscum contagiosum**

Mometasone furoate

▶ **Corticosteroids, topical, medium potency**

Mondor's disease

Synonym(s)
Subcutaneous phlebitis of the breast and chest wall; sclerosing periphlebitis of the lateral chest wall

Definition
Thrombophlebitis of the superficial veins of the anterior chest wall

Pathogenesis
Unknown

Clinical manifestation
Pain and tenderness of lateral chest wall and/or breast, followed within hours to days by subcutaneous cord, with skin retraction

Differential diagnosis
Breast carcinoma; breast abscess; foreign body reaction; insect bite reaction

Therapy
Warm compresses for symptomatic relief

References
Mayor M, Buron I, de Mora JC, Lazaro TE, Hernandez-Cano N, Rubio FA, Casado M (2000) Mondor's disease. International Journal of Dermatology 39(12):922–925

Mongolian spot

Synonym(s)
Congenital dermal melanocytosis

Definition
Macular, blue-gray pigmentation usually on the sacral area and back of neonates

Pathogenesis
Results from arrested migration of melanocytes in the dermis during migration from the neural crest into the epidermis

Clinical manifestation
Congenital, asymptomatic, blue-gray, macular hyperpigmentation, most commonly involving the lumbosacral area, but also buttocks, flanks, and shoulders; most lesions resolve in early childhood, but some persist for many years

Differential diagnosis
Nevus of Ota/Ito; blue nevus; child abuse

Therapy
None indicated

References
Mallory SB (1991) Neonatal skin disorders. Pediatric Clinics of North America 38(4):745–761

Monilethrix

Definition
Beaded pattern on the hair shaft

References
Landau M, Brenner S, Metzker A (2002) Medical pearl: an easy way to diagnose severe neonatal monilethrix. Journal of the American Academy of Dermatology 46(1):111–112

Moniliasis

▶ Candidiasis

Morbid hair pulling

▶ Trichotillomania

Morphea

Synonym(s)
Localized scleroderma; circumscribed scleroderma

Definition
Disorder characterized by skin and subcutaneous tissue induration and thickening due to excessive collagen deposition

Pathogenesis
Multiple theories of causation, including endothelial cell injury, autoimmune problems, and dysregulation of collagen production

Clinical manifestation
Poorly defined areas of nonpitting edema, with sclerosis developing as disease progresses; skin surface becomes smooth and shiny, with loss of hair follicles and decreased ability to sweat; after months to years, skin softens and become atrophic
Guttate variant: small, white, minimally indurated papules
Linear variant: discrete, indurated, linear, hypopigmented, sclerotic bands
Frontoparietal linear morphea (en coup de sabre): linear, atrophic plaque, suggestive of a stroke from a sword, sometimes eventuating in hemifacial atrophy
Progressive hemifacial atrophy (Romberg-Perry syndrome): primary lesion occurring in the subcutaneous tissue, muscle, and bone; dermis affected only secondarily and skin not sclerotic
Eosinophilic fasciitis: involves primarily the fascia; characterized by acute onset of painful, indurated skin, usually of the upper extremity, with orange-peel appearance and swelling of the affected extremity
Diffuse variant: widespread hypopigmented, sclerotic plaques, often involving the upper trunk, abdomen, buttocks, and thighs

Differential diagnosis
Lichen sclerosus, necrobiosis lipoidica; granuloma annulare; graft versus host disease; porphyria cutanea tarda; hypertrophic scar; progressive systemic sclerosis; mixed connective tissue disease; lipodermatosclerosis; phenylketonuria; radiation fibrosis; scleromyxedema; Werner syndrome; medication- or chemical-induced scleroderma

Therapy
Localized disease: no effective therapy; diffuse or symptomatic disease: phototherapy; physical therapy; prednisone; plas-

M

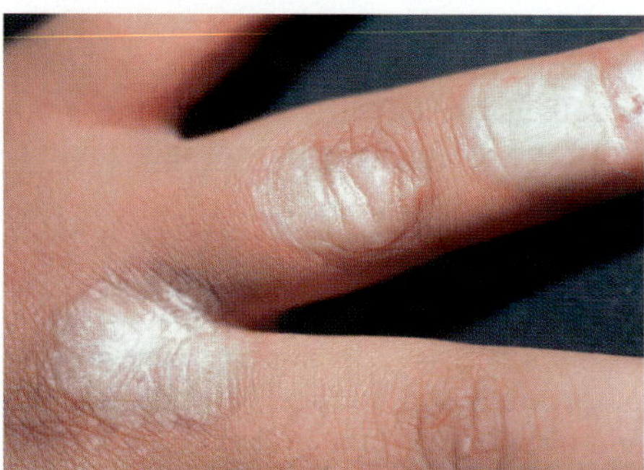

Morphea. Sclerotic, white plaques on the hand

mapheresis; D-penicillamine: 2.5 mg per kg
PO daily

References
Hawk A, English JC 3rd (2001) Localized and sys-
temic scleroderma. Seminars in Cutaneous
Medicine & Surgery 20(1):27–37

Morquio syndrome

Synonym(s)
Mucopolysaccharidosis type IV-A

Definition
Inherited metabolic storage disease arising
from a deficiency of N-acetylgalactosamine-
6-sulfatase (type IV-A) or beta-galactosidase deficiency (type IV-B)

Pathogenesis
Autosomal recessive trait; deficiency of N-
acetylgalactosamine-6-sulfatase, resulting
in accumulation of keratan sulfate (type IV-
A) or beta-galactosidase deficiency
(type IV-B), leading to accumulation of
chondroitin-6-sulfate (type IV-B) in the
connective tissue, the skeletal system, and
the teeth

Clinical manifestation
Abnormalities of the skeletal system (e.g.,
kyphoscoliosis, pectus carinatum, luxation
of the hips); aortic valvular disease; dental
abnormalities; odontoid hypoplasia, with
subsequent atlantoaxial instability; hearing
deficit; diffuse corneal opacification and
alterations of the trabecular meshwork;
occasional glaucoma; type IV-B: hearing
deficits, dental abnormalities; cardiac murmurs; hepatomegaly; no joint laxity

Differential diagnosis
Hurler syndrome; Hunter syndrome; Gaucher's disease; Niemann-Pick diseae; osteogenesis imperfecta

Therapy
Investigational enzyme replacement with
galactose-6-sulfatase

References
Northover H, Cowie RA, Wraith JE (1996) Mucopolysaccharidosis type IVA (Morquio syndrome): a clinical review. Journal of Inherited
Metabolic Disease 19(3):357–365

Mortification

▶ **Gangrene**

Morve

▶ **Glanders and melioidosis**

Mosaic speckled lentiginous nevus

▶ **Nevus spilus**

Mucha-Habermann disease

▶ **Pityriasis lichenoides**

Mucocutaneous lymph node syndrome

▶ Kawasaki disease

Mucopolysaccharidosis type I-H

▶ Hurler syndrome

Mucopolysaccharidosis type I-H/S

▶ Scheie syndrome

Mucopolysaccharidosis type I-S

▶ Scheie syndrome

Mucopolysaccharidosis type II

▶ Hunter syndrome

Mucopolysaccharidosis type III-A

▶ Sanfilippo syndrome

Mucopolysaccharidosis type III-B

▶ Sanfilippo syndrome

Mucopolysaccharidosis type III-C

▶ Sanfilippo syndrome

Mucopolysaccharidosis type IV-A

▶ Morquio syndrome

Mucormycosis

Synonym(s)
Phycomycosis; zygomycosis

Definition
Infection with fungi of the order Mucorales, of which Rhizopus species are the most common causative organisms, that affects otherwise chronically ill or immunosupressed patients

Pathogenesis
Inhalation of airborne mucorales spores, which settle in sinuses or lungs; local extension, lymphatic, or hematogenous spread from original site; invasion of blood vessel walls, thrombosis, and infarction produce signs and symptoms of disease

Clinical manifestation
Cutaneous variant: secondary infection in burns or other trauma

Superficial variety: occurs in healthy people after trauma; vesicles, pustules, and plaques

Gangrenous variant: solitary, violaceous, painful, papule or plaque, with ecchymotic center; may ulcerate and disseminate; occurs in immunosuppressed patients

Rhinocerebral variant: progressive orbital swelling and facial cellulitis, with discharge of black pus from the necrotic palatine or nasal eschars; proptosis; chemosis; ophthalmoplegia; blindness; decreased consciousness suggests spread to brain; non-specific gastrointestinal and pulmonary signs and symptoms

Differential diagnosis
Aspergillosis; nocardiosis; anthrax; orbital cellulitis; pseudallescheria boydii infection; disseminated Fusarium infection; ecthyma gangrenosum

Therapy
Amphotericin B*: 1–1.5 mg per kg IV daily infused over 4–6 hours

References
Eucker J, Sezer O, Graf B, Possinger K (2001) Mucormycoses. Mycoses 44(7-8):253–260

Mucosal neuroma syndrome

Synonym(s)
MEN III syndrome; MEN IIB syndrome; multiple mucosal neuroma syndrome; Sipple syndrome

Definition
One of the multiple endocrine neoplasia (MEN) syndromes, characterized by tumors of neuroendocrine origin

Pathogenesis
Autosomal dominant trait; gene mutations on chromosome 10

Clinical manifestation
Oral mucosal neuroma: yellow-white, sessile, painless papule of the lips, anterior tongue, and buccal commissures; similar lesions seen on the eyelids, sometimes producing eversion of the lid, and on the sclera; facial skin, especially around the nose, sometimes involved; lesions develop in first decade of life; tall, lanky, marfanoid body type, with a narrow face and muscle wasting; adrenal and thyroid tumors present after puberty; associated with adrenal pheochromocytoma, medullary thyroid carcinoma, diffuse alimentary tract ganglioneuromatosis, and multiple, small, submucosal neuroma nodules of the upper aerodigestive tract

Differential diagnosis
Granular cell tumor; neurofibroma; fibroma; squamous cell carcinoma; Gardner's syndrome; tuberous sclerosis

Therapy
Surgical removal for esthetic purposes or if repeatedly traumatized

References
Lee NC, Norton JA (2000) Multiple endocrine neoplasia type 2B-genetic basis and clinical expression. Surgical Oncology 9(3):111–118

Mucosal pemphigoid

► Cicatricial pemphigoid

Mucosal sebaceous cysts

► Fordyce's disease

Mucous cyst

► Digital mucous cyst

Mud fever

▶ **Leptospirosis**

Muir-Torre syndrome

Synonym(s)
Torre syndrome

Definition
Familial cancer syndrome consisting of at least one sebaceous neoplasm (sebaceous adenoma, sebaceous epithelioma, or sebaceous carcinoma) and at least one visceral malignancy, usually gastrointestinal or genitourinary carcinoma

Pathogenesis
Autosomal dominant trait involving mutations in mismatched repair genes, mostly the *MSH2* gene, located on chromosome arm 2p

Clinical manifestation
One or more sebaceous neoplasms, including sebaceous adenoma, sebaceous epithelioma, or sebaceous carcinoma, often on the face; other cutaneous neoplasms include keratoacanthoma, squamous cell carcinoma, and multiple follicular cysts; one or more visceral malignancies, most commonly colorectal cancer or genitourinary malignancies, either preceding or following the sebaceous tumors

Differential diagnosis
Gardner syndrome; Cowden syndrome; multiple trichoepitheliomas; basal cell nevus syndrome; basal cell carcinoma; squamous cell carcinoma; eruptive keratoacanthomas; tuberous sclerosis

Therapy
Surgical excision of sebaceous neoplasms[*]; isotretinoin as prophylactic agent

References
Omura NE, Collison DW, Perry AE, Myers LM (2002) Sebaceous carcinoma in children. Journal of the American Academy of Dermatology 47(6):950–953

Multicentric reticulohistiocytosis

Synonym(s)
Lipoid dermatoarthritis; lipoid rheumatism; giant cell reticulohistiocytosis

Definition
Disorder characterized by dermal papules and nodules consisting of histiocytic proliferation, associated with arthritis

Pathogenesis
May be a paraneoplastic response to underlying malignancy in some cases

Clinical manifestation
Asymptomatic to slightly pruritic, skin-colored to reddish-brown papules or nodules, usually on the upper potion of the body; may be isolated from one another or may be clustered, sometimes giving a cobblestone appearance; polyarthritis may precede or follow onset of skin lesions; remission may occur after years

Differential diagnosis
Rheumatoid nodule; xanthoma; dermatofibroma; progressive nodular histiocytoma; xanthoma; juvenile xanthogranuloma; leprosy; granuloma annulare; Jessner's lymphocytic infiltration; lupus erythematosus; Langerhans cell histiocytosis; lipogranulomatosis; gouty tophi; sarcoidosis; osteoarthritis, psoriatic arthritis, Reiter disease

Therapy
Prednisone; triamcinolone, intralesional; hydroxychloroquine; methotrexate; photochemotherapy

References

Rapini RP (1993) Multicentric reticulohistiocytosis. Clinics in Dermatology 11(1):107–111

Multiple hamartoma syndrome

▶ Cowden disease

Multiple hemangiomata syndrome

▶ Bannayan-Riley-Ruvalcaba syndrome

Multiple idiopathic hemorrhagic sarcoma

▶ Kaposi's sarcoma

Multiple lentigines syndrome

▶ LEOPARD syndrome

Multiple mucosal neuroma syndrome

▶ Mucosal neuroma syndrome

Multiple symmetrical lipomatosis

▶ Benign symmetric lipomatosis

Mupirocin

Trade name(s)
Bactroban

Generic available
No

Drug class
Topical antibiotic

Mechanism of action
Selective binding to bacterial isoleucyl transfer-RNA synthetase, causing inhibition of protein synthesis

Dosage form
2% cream, ointment

Dermatologic indications and dosage
See table

Common side effects
Cutaneous: burning sensation, dryness, pruritus; redness

Serious side effects
Cutaneous: superinfection after prolonged use

Drug interactions
None

Mupirocin. Dermatologic indications and dosage

Disease	Adult dosage	Child dosage
Impetigo	Apply 3 times daily for 7–14 days	Apply 3 times daily for 7–14 days

Contraindications/precautions
Hypersensitivity to drug class or component; caution when using in large open wounds

References
Williford PM (1999) Opportunities for mupirocin calcium cream in the emergency department. Journal of Emergency Medicine 17(1):211–220

Murrain

▶ Anthrax, cutaneous

Musculoaponeurotic fibromatosis

▶ Desmoid tumor

Mycetoma

Synonym(s)
Madura foot; maduromycosis

Definition
Chronic granulomatous disease of the skin and subcutaneous tissue, characterized by tumefaction, abscess formation, and fistulae

Pathogenesis
Caused by true fungi (eumycetoma) or by aerobic bacterial actinomycetes (actinomycetoma)

Organisms producing eumycetoma: Pseudallescheria boydii (the most common cause in the United States); Madurella mycetomatis; Madurella grisea; Phialophora jeanselmei; Pyrenochaeta romeroi; Lept-

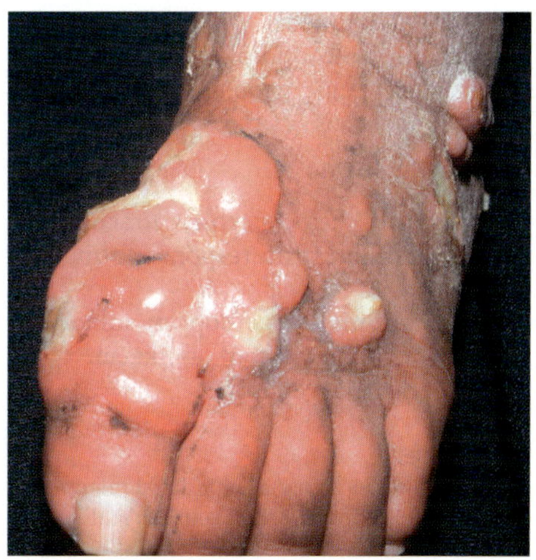

Mycetoma. Multiple, infiltrated nodules on the foot

osphaeria senegaliensis; Curvularia lunata; Neotestudina rosatii; Aspergillus nidulans; Aspergillus flavus; species of Fusarium: Cylindrocarpon and Acremonium

Organisms causing actinomycetoma: Actinomadura madurae and A. pelletieri; Streptomyces somaliensis; several species and varieties of Nocardia, particularly N. brasiliensis; organisms introduced via localized trauma of the skin with thorns, wood splinters, or implantation with solid objects

Clinical manifestation
Occurs most commonly in people that work in rural areas where they are exposed to acacia trees or cactus thorns containing the etiologic agents; slow-growing, painless, suppurative papules and nodules, abscesses and fistulae drain clear, viscous, or purulent exudate or grains; affects upper and lower limbs, particularly the feet and lower legs; progressive extension and formation of multiple sinus tracts; extensive tissue swelling, induration, and destruction; chronic lesions contain healed, scarred, sometimes closed sinus tracts with new, open, suppurative tracts in other adjacent areas; invasion of bone cortex results in replacement of osseous tissues and marrow by masses of grains

Differential diagnosis
Sporotrichosis; coccidioidomycosis; tuberculosis; osteogenic neoplasms; osteomyelitis; botryomycosis

Therapy
Eumycetoma: ketoconazole, itraconazole; surgical excision if no response to medical therapy
Actinomycetoma: trimethoprim-sulfamethoxazole, with or without amikacin, 15 mg per kg per day IM; dapsone

References
Rivitti EA, Aoki V (1999) Deep fungal infections in tropical countries. Clinics in Dermatology 17(2):171–190

Mycobacterium marinum infection

Synonym(s)
Fish tank granuloma; swimming pool granuloma; fish fancier's finger

Definition
Atypical mycobacterial infection following skin trauma in fresh or salt water, characterized by localized granuloma or sporotrichotic lymphangitis

Pathogenesis
Caused by inoculation by Mycobacterium marinum, occurring following trauma to skin in contact with an aquarium, salt water, or marine animals

Clinical manifestation
After 2–3 week incubation period, papule or bluish nodule appears at inoculation site, with subsequent ulceration; new lesions may occur along path of lymphatic drainage

Differential diagnosis
Other atypical mycobacterial pathogens, such as M. chelonae, M. fortuitum, or M. gordonae; bacterial pyoderma; herpetic whitlow; sporotrichosis; nocardiosis; inoculation coccidioidomycosis; orf; milker's nodule; cutaneous tuberculosis; anthrax; listeriosis; leishmaniasis; squamous cell carcinoma; foreign body granuloma

Therapy
Clarithromycin; minocycline; ciprofloxacin; trimethoprim-sulfamethoxazole; surgical hyperthermia; surgical excision

References
Aubry A, Chosidow O, Caumes E, Robert J, Cambau E (2002) Sixty-three cases of Mycobacterium marinum infection: clinical features, treatment, and antibiotic susceptibility of causative isolates. Archives of Internal Medicine 162(15):1746–1752

Mycobacterium ulcerans infection

▶ Buruli ulcer

Mycophenolate mofetil

Trade name(s)
CellCept

Generic available
No

Drug class
Immunosuppressive

Mechanism of action
Inhibits T-cell and B-cell proliferation by blocking de novo purine synthesis; noncompetitive inhibitor of inosine monophosphate dehydrogenase

Dosage form
250 mg, 500 mg tablet

Mycophenolate mofetil. Dermatologic indications and dosage

Disease	Adult dosage	Child dosage
Bullous pemphigoid	1–1.5 gm PO twice daily	600 mg per m^2 PO twice daily
Paraneoplastic pemphigus	1–1.5 gm PO twice daily	600 mg per m^2 PO twice daily
Pemphigus foliaceus, including fogo selvagem	1–1.5 gm PO twice daily	600 mg per m^2 PO twice daily
Pemphigus vulgaris	1–1.5 gm PO twice daily	600 mg per m^2 PO twice daily
Psoriasis	1–1.5 gm PO twice daily	600 mg per m^2 PO twice daily
Pyoderma gangrenosum	1–1.5 gm PO twice daily	600 mg per m^2 PO twice daily
Reiter syndrome	1–1.5 gm PO twice daily	600 mg per m^2 PO twice daily
Weber-Christian disease	1–1.5 gm PO twice daily	Not applicable

Dermatologic indications and dosage
See table

Common side effects
Cardiovascular: peripheral edema
Gastrointestinal: diarrhea, abdominal pain, nausea and vomiting
Genitourinary: urinary urgency, frequency, and dysuria
Hematologic: leukopenia
Laboratory: hypokalemia, hypercholesterolemia
Neurologic: headache
Pulmonary: cough

Serious side effects
Gastrointestinal: bleeding, ulceration, or perforation
Hematologic: bone marrow suppression, immunosuppression
Infectious: susceptibility to infection, malignancy

Drug interactions
Acyclovir; azathioprine; oral contraceptives; ganciclovir; iron salts; probenecid

Contraindications/precautions
Hypersensitivity to drug class or component; pregnancy; caution in patients with severe renal or gastrointestinal disease; caution with bone marrow suppression

References
Kitchin JE, Pomeranz MK, Pak G, Washenik K, Shupack JL (1997) Rediscovering mycophenolic acid: a review of its mechanism, side effects, and potential uses. Journal of the American Academy of Dermatology 37(3 Pt.1):445–449

Mycosis fungoides

▶ T-cell lymphoma, cutaneous

Myiasis

Synonym(s)
None

Definition
Invasion of living tissue by the larvae (maggots) of two-winged flies (Diptera)

Pathogenesis
Fly eggs deposited on the skin; larvae feed on wound debris, penetrate skin, and cause inflammatory response

Clinical manifestation
Wound variant: superficial inflammatory reaction on surface; furuncular (follicular) variant: larvae penetrate skin; pruritic inflammatory papule with volcano-like central punctum; intermittent sanguineous or serosanguineous discharge

Differential diagnosis
Tungiasis; furuncle; infected epidermoid cyst; insect bite reaction; foreign body granuloma; atypical mycobacterial infection; anthrax; nocardia infection; leishmaniasis

Therapy
Surgical excision; lidocaine injection beneath furuncle, then push organism into the punctum.; superficial incision followed by gentle pressure, inward and downward; bacon fat applied adjacent to the punctum; petroleum jelly applied over punctum

References
Sampson CE, MaGuire J, Eriksson E (2001) Botfly myiasis: case report and brief review. Annals of Plastic Surgery 46(2):150–152

Myxedema

Definition
Non-pitting edema of the skin due to infiltration of the subcutaneous tissues by metachromatic proteoglycans in patients with hypothyroidism

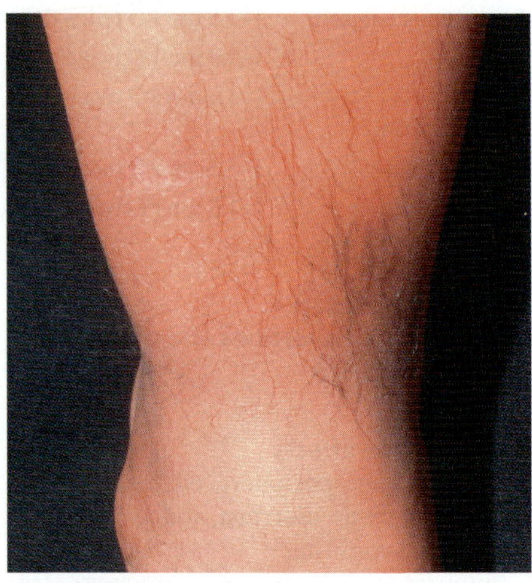

Myxedema. Minimally infiltrated plaque on the anterior leg

References
Guha B, Krishnaswamy G, Peiris A (2002) The diagnosis and management of hypothyroidism. Southern Medical Association Journal 95(5):475–480

Myoepithelioma

▶ **Eccrine acrospiroma**

Myosarcoma

▶ **Rhabdomyosarcoma**

Myxedematosus

▶ **Papular mucinosis**

Myxoid cyst

▶ **Digital mucous cyst**

Myxoma-spotty pigmentation-endocrine overactivity

▶ Carney's syndrome

Myxomatous cutaneous cyst

▶ Digital mucous cyst

Myxomatous degenerative cyst

▶ Digital mucous cyst

M

Naegeli-Franceschetti-Jadassohn syndrome

Synonym(s)
None

Definition
Form of ectodermal dysplasia characterized by reticulate pigmentation and keratoderma

Pathogenesis
Autosomal dominant trait; possibly associated with markers located near the type I keratin gene

Clinical manifestation
Reticulate hyperpigmentation beginning at age 1–5 years and improving after puberty; palmar and plantar hyperkeratosis with lack of dermatoglyphics; hypohidrosis with heat intolerance, worsened by reduced sweating; dental abnormalities including defective dentures with yellow spots on the enamel

Differential diagnosis
Incontinentia pigmenti; X-linked reticulate pigmentary disorder; dermatopathia pigmentosa reticularis; Dowling-Degos disease; confluent and reticulated papillomatosis of Gougerot and Carteaud; reticulated acropigmentation of Kitamura; hereditary bullous acrokeratotic poikiloderma of Weary-Kindler; acromelanosis progressiva; dyschromia universalis hereditaria; hidrotic ectodermal dysplasia; hereditary bullous acrokeratotic poikiloderma

Therapy
No effective therapy

References
Schnur RE, Heymann WR (1997) Reticulate hyperpigmentation. Seminars in Cutaneous Medicine & Surgery 16(1):72–80

Naevus a pernione

▶ **Angiokeratoma of Mibelli**

Naevus maternus

▶ **Nevus flammeus**

Naftifine

Trade name(s)
Naftin

Generic available
No

Naftifine. Dermatologic indications and dosage

Disease	Adult dosage	Child dosage
Cutaneous candidiasis	Apply daily for 3–6 weeks	Apply daily for 3–6 weeks
Tinea capitis	Apply daily for 3–6 weeks	Apply daily for 3–6 weeks
Tinea corporis	Apply daily for 3–6 weeks	Apply daily for 3–6 weeks
Tinea cruris	Apply daily for 3–6 weeks	Apply daily for 3–6 weeks
Tinea pedis	Apply daily for 3–6 weeks	Apply daily for 3–6 weeks

Drug class
Allylamine antifungal agent

Mechanism of action
Inhibition of squalene epoxidase, with subsequent reduction of cell wall ergosterol synthesis

Dosage form
1% cream; 1% gel

Dermatologic indications and dosage
See table

Common side effects
Cutaneous: burning sensation, pruritus, erythema, dryness

Serious side effects
None

Drug interactions
None

Contraindications/precautions
Hypersensitivity to drug class or component

References
Muhlbacher JM (1991) Naftifine: a topical allylamine antifungal agent. Clinics in Dermatology 9(4):479–485

Nail biting

▶ Onychophagia

Nail-patella syndrome

Synonym(s)
Hereditary osteo-onychodysplasia; Fong disease; onychoosteodysplasia; Turner-Kieser syndrome

Definition
Hereditary disorder characterized by fingernail dysplasia, absent or hypoplastic patellae, posterior conical iliac horns, deformation or luxation of the radial heads, and occasional nephropathy

Pathogenesis
Autosomal dominant trait; gene located on chromosome 9 at locus linked to that of the ABO blood group adenylate kinase and locus of the alpha 1 chain of type 5 collagen; altered connective tissue metabolism with widespread structural defects in collagen; abnormal collagen deposition in the glomeruli may cause nephropathy

Clinical manifestation
Nail changes: absent or short nail plate; V-shaped triangular lunulae with a distal peak in the midline; other abnormalities include: splitting, longitudinal ridging, koilonychia, poor lunula formation, and discoloration
Skeletal changes: small or absent patella; elbows may have limited motion; subluxation of the radial head; arthrodysplasia of the elbows; hyperextension of the joints; exostoses
Kidney changes: usually only asymptomatic proteinuria, but hematuria, nephrotic syndrome, and renal failure may occur

Differential diagnosis
Pachonychia congenita; other congenital ectodermal defects

Therapy
No effective therapy for skin defects

References
Ogden JA, Cross GL, Guidera KJ, Ganey TM (2002) Nail patella syndrome. A 55-year follow-up of the original description. Journal of Pediatric Orthopaedics, Part B 11(4):333–338

Nakagawa's angioblastoma

▶ Tufted angioma

Nakagawa's angioma

▶ Tufted angioma

NAME syndrome

▶ Carney's syndrome

Necrobiosis lipoidica

Synonym(s)
Necrobiosis lipoidica diabeticorum

Definition
Localized disorder of collagen, with connective tissue degeneration, granulomatous reaction, thickening of blood vessel walls, and deposition of fat

Pathogenesis
Theories of causation: microangiopathy; trauma; metabolic derangement; antibody-mediated vasculitis

Clinical manifestation
Well-circumscribed papule or nodule with active border, usually over pretibial area, but sometimes arising on face, trunk, or extremities; evolves into waxy, atrophic, round plaque beginning with red-brown color but progressing to yellow-brown color; painful ulcerations after weeks to months

Differential diagnosis
Morphea; lichen sclerosus; nodular vasculitis; Weber-Christian disease; factitial disease; granuloma annulare; sarcoidosis; necrobiotic xanthogranuloma; xanthoma

Therapy
Corticosteroids, topical, super potent; triamcinolone 3–4 mg per ml intralesional; tretinoin; aspirin/dipyrimidine; pentoxifylline: 400 mg PO 3 times daily

References
Sibbald RG, Landolt SJ, Toth D (1996) Skin and diabetes. Endocrinology & Metabolism Clinics of North America 25(2):463–472

Necrobiosis lipoidica diabeticorum

▶ Necrobiosis lipoidica

Necrobiotic xanthogranuloma

Synonym(s)
None

Definition
Inflammatory histiocytic granulomatosis, characterized by slowly enlarging papules and plaques

Pathogenesis
Associated with paraproteinemia and cryoglobulinemia in some cases; associated with myeloma

Clinical manifestation
Asymptomatic, firm, red-to-orange papules or nodules, coalescing into plaques that may ulcerate; lesions become yellowish as they evolve; located on face, trunk or extremities; hepatosplenomegaly; arthropathy

Differential diagnosis
Necrobiosis lipoidica; granuloma annulare; xanthoma; multicentric reticulohistiocytosis; squamous cell carcinoma; atypical fibroxanthoma

Therapy
Prednisone; radiation therapy; chlorambucil: 2 mg PO daily; plasmapheresis

References
Mehregan DA, Winkelmann RK (1992) Necrobiotic xanthogranuloma. Archives of Dermatology 128(1):94–100

Necrolytic migratory erythema

▶ Glucagonoma syndrome

Necrotic arachnidism

▶ Brown recluse spider bite

Necrotizing erysipelas

▶ Necrotizing fasciitis

Necrotizing fasciitis

Synonym(s)
Hospital gangrene; acute infective gangrene; necrotizing erysipelas; suppurative fasciitis

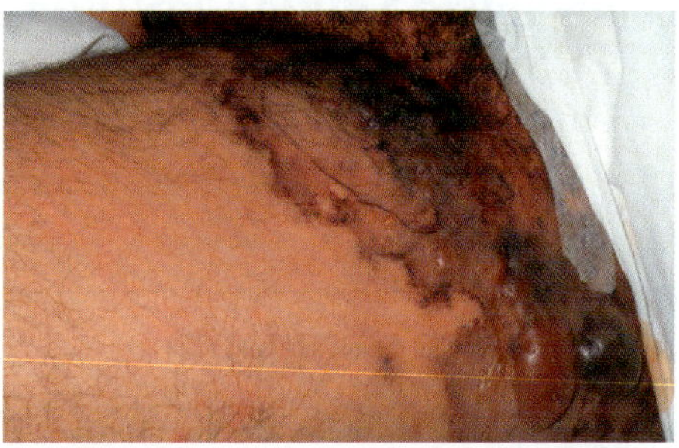

Necrotizing fasciitis. Necrotic plaque with bullae in the groin area

Definition
Bacterial soft tissue infection characterized by fascial necrosis

Pathogenesis
Subcutaneous bacterial invasion causes decreased oxygen tension, which reduces neutrophil function; multiple bacterial pathogens, including: Group A beta-hemolytic streptococci (most common organism), Haemophilus aphrophilus, Staphylococcus aureus, Clostridium perfringens and synergistic anaerobic and facultative bacteria; bacterial superantigens produce extreme immunologic response and subsequent tissue injury

Clinical manifestation
Most commonly involves extremities or trunk, but may involve perineum (Fornier's

gangrene); often follows trauma, surgical wound or hematogenous seeding from another site; early, severe, local pain, out of proportion to visible findings; poorly marginated red plaque with subcutaneous edema, which progresses to dusky plaque with vesiculation and occasional crepitus; marked constitutional changes, including fever, prostration, decreased sensorium, and hypotension

Differential diagnosis
Cellulitis; polyarteritis nodosa or other vasculitides; insect envenomation; pyoderma gangrenosum; acute febrile neutrophilic dermatosis; vascular insufficiency

Therapy
Emergency surgical debridement*; penicillin G 8–10 million units per day IV, given every 4–6 hours; clindamycin

References
Levine N, Kunkel M, Nguyen T, Ackerman L (2002) Emergency Department Dermatology. Current Problems in Dermatology 14(6):183–220

Necrotizing glomerulonephritis

▶ Wegener's granulomatosis

Necrotizing granulomatous inflammation of the respiratory tract

▶ Wegener's granulomatosis

Necrotizing livedo reticularis

▶ Calciphylaxis

Necrotizing lymphadenitis

▶ Kikuchi's syndrome

Necrotizing lymphocytic folliculitis

▶ Acne necrotica

Neonatal pustular melanosis

▶ Transient neonatal pustular melanosis

Nephrogenic fibrosing dermopathy

Synonym(s)
Scleromyxedema-like illness of hemodialysis; scleromyxedema-like illness of renal disease

Definition
Disorder of patients with renal disease, characterized by thickening and hardening of the skin

Pathogenesis
Involves mucin deposition in the skin

Clinical manifestation
Thickening and hardening of skin, most commonly over extremities and trunk, while sparing face; hyperpigmentation in sclerotic areas; flexion contractures; firm, yellowish papules and nodules; occurs in chronic renal failure, during hemodialysis or after renal transplantation

Differential diagnosis
Scleromyxedema; progressive systemic sclerosis; morphea; porphyria cutanea tarda; eosinophilic fasciitis; eosinophilia-myalgia syndrome; toxic oil syndrome; amyloidosis

Therapy
No effective therapy

References
Streams BN, Liu V, Liegeois N, Moschella SM (2003) Clinical and pathologic features of nephrogenic fibrosing dermopathy: a report of two cases. Journal of the American Academy of Dermatology 48(1):42–47

Netherton syndrome

Synonym(s)
Netherton's syndrome; Còmel-Netherton syndrome

Definition
Hereditary syndrome characterized by congenital erythroderma, trichorrhexis invaginata, ichthyosis linearis circumflexa, atopic diathesis, and failure to thrive

Pathogenesis
Autosomal recessive trait, with gene localization to chromosome 5q32; intermittent keratinizing defect of the hair cortex resulting from incomplete conversion of sulfhydryl –SH group into S-S disulfide bonds in the protein of the cortical fibers, which causes cortical softness, bulging, and bamboo deformity

Clinical manifestation
Congenital erythroderma; bamboo hair abnormality (trichorrhexis invaginata), leading to sparse, short, spiky, lusterless, and brittle hair; intermitent serpiginous migratory annular/polycyclic eruption with double-edged scale (ichthyosis linearis circumflexa), lasting for weeks to months; atopic diathesis, with multiple food allergies; early failure to thrive, with diarrhea and symptoms of malabsorption, which improves with age

Differential diagnosis
Other causes of congenital erythroderma, including lamellar ichthyosis; erythrokeratoderma variabilis; acrodermatitis enteropathica; seborrheic dermatitis; Leiner disease

Therapy
Emollients; corticosteroids, topical, low potency

References
Siegel DH, Howard R (2002) Molecular advances in genetic skin diseases. Current Opinion in Pediatrics 14(4):419–25

Netherton's syndrome

▶ Netherton syndrome

Neurilemmoma

Synonym(s)
Benign schwannoma; neurinoma; neurolemmoma; perineural fibroblastoma

Definition
Benign nerve sheath tumor derived from Schwann cells

Pathogenesis
Alteration or loss of the NF2 tumor suppressor gene may be partially responsible for tumor formation

Clinical manifestation
Asymptomatic, slow-growing, solitary or multiple, flesh-colored papules or nodules, with predilection for head, neck, and flexor surfaces of the upper and lower extremities; neurilemmomatosis (schwannomatosis) variant: subset of neurofibromatosis type 2 (NF2); autosomal dominant disor-

der; multiple, encapsulated nodules, located in the subcutaneous tissue

Differential diagnosis
Neurofibroma; neuroma; leiomyoma; myoblastoma; epidermoid cyst; lipoma

Therapy
Surgical excision*

References
Smith JT, Yandow SM (1996) Benign soft-tissue lesions in children. Orthopedic Clinics of North America 27(3):645–654

Neurinoma

▶ **Neurilemmoma**

Neurocysticercosis

▶ **Cysticercosis**

Neurodermatitis

▶ **Lichen simplex chronicus**

Neurodermatitis circumscripta

▶ **Lichen simplex chronicus**

Neurofibroma

▶ **Neurofibromatosis**

Neurofibromatosis

Synonym(s)
Von Recklinghausen's disease; Von Recklinghausen disease

Definition
Hereditary disorder with multiple phenotypes, affecting skin, bone, nervous system, and soft tissue, most characteristic finding of which is mulitple neurofibromas

Pathogenesis
Autosomal dominant trait, but many spontaneous mutations; NF-1 variant: linked to large gene on band 17q11.2, which encodes tumor suppressor protein, neurofibromin; NF-2 variant: mutation of unknown tumor suppressor protein; segmental variant: may be related to mosaicism or segmental hyperexpression

Clinical manifestation
NF-1 variant: 6 or more café au lait macules larger than 0.5 cm in prepubertal individuals and those larger than 1.5 cm in postpubertal individuals; two or more neurofibromas of any type or 1 plexiform neurofibroma; axillary freckling; optic glioma; iris hamartomas (Lisch nodules); osseous lesions
NF-2 variant: 8th cranial nerve tumors; neurofibromas; meningiomas; gliomas; schwannomas
Segmental variant: multiple soft papules (neurofibromas) in a nerve segment distribution

Differential diagnosis
Proteus syndrome; McCune-Albright syndrome LEOPARD syndrome; Carney's syndrome; Watson syndrome; tuberous sclerosis; Noonan's syndrome

Therapy
Surgical excision of symptomatic tumors*

N

References

Lynch TM, Gutmann DH (2002) Neurofibromatosis 1. Neurologic Clinics 20(3):841–865

Neurofibromatosis with Noonan phenotype

▶ Watson syndrome

Neurofibromatosis-Noonan syndrome

▶ Watson syndrome

Neurofollicular hamartoma

▶ Trichodiscoma

Neurolemmoma

▶ Neurilemmoma

Neurothekeoma

Synonym(s)

Neurothekeoma of Gallager and Helwig; benign nerve sheath tumor; perineural myxoma

Definition

Benign skin or mucous membrane tumor of nerve sheath origin

Pathogenesis

Unknown

Clinical manifestation

Asymptomatic, soft, flesh-colored-to-red papule, usually on the face or proximal upper extremities, but occasionally in oral mucous membrane; appears in the first two decades of life

Differential diagnosis

Dermal nerve sheath myxoma; neurofibroma; neural nevus; schwannoma

Therapy

Surgical excision★

References

Tomasini C, Aloi F, Pippione M (1996) Cellular neurothekeoma. Dermatology 192(2):160–163

Neurothekeoma of Gallager and Helwig

▶ Neurothekeoma

Neutral lipid storage disease

▶ Chanarin-Dorfman syndrome

Neutrophilic dermatitis

▶ Acute febrile neutrophilic dermatosis

Nevocellular nevus

▶ Nevus, melanocytic

Nevoid basal cell carcinoma syndrome

▶ Basal cell nevus syndrome

Nevoid hypermelanosis

Synonym(s)
Lentiginous hyperpigmentation; linear and whorled nevoid hypermelanosis

Definition
Congenital disorder characterized by streaks and whorls of macular hyperpigmentation along Blaschko's lines

Pathogenesis
Presumed to represent somatic mosaicism

Clinical manifestation
Onset in first few weeks of life; irregular swirls of macular hyperpigmentation, following Blaschko's lines; may cross the midline and be discontinuous; may fade somewhat as child ages

Differential diagnosis
Incontinentia pigmenti; hypomelanosis of Ito; Nevus of Ota and Ito; post-inflammatory hyperpigmentation; nevus spilus

Therapy
No effective therapy

References
Schepis C, Siragusa M, Alberti A, Cavallari V (1996) Linear and whorled nevoid hypermelanosis in a boy with mental retardation and congenital defects. International Journal of Dermatology 35(9):654–655

Nevoid hypertrichosis

Synonym(s)
Nevoid hypertrichosis; faun-tail nevus

Definition
Disorder characterized by solitary or few circumscribed areas of terminal hair growth, which is abnormal in length, shaft diameter, or color

Pathogenesis
Unknown

Clinical manifestation
Patches of terminal hair growth, occurring anywhere from the neck or legs to the palms; usually present at birth or in early infancy; when present in lumbosacral area (faun-tail nevus), associated with underlying kyphoscoliosis or partial spinal cord duplication

Differential diagnosis
Becker's nevus; Cornelia de Lange syndrome; congenital hemihypertrophy with hypertrichosis; hypertrichosis lanuginosa; hypertrichosis associated with neurologic disorders

Therapy
No therapy indicated

References
Chang SN, Hong CE, Kim DK, Park WH (1997) A case of multiple nevoid hypertrichosis. Journal of Dermatology 24(5):337–341

Nevoxanthoendothelioma

▶ Juvenile xanthogranuloma

Nevus anemicus

Synonym(s)
None

Definition
Congenital vascular anomaly, character-ized by a pale-colored patch resulting from localized reduced blood flow

Pathogenesis
Pharmacologic anomaly caused by increased vascular sensitivity to catecho-lamines

Clinical manifestation
Permanent, irregularly shaped, pale colored patch, with stellate margins; usually located on the upper trunk; present at birth, but sometimes difficult to discern because of similarity of color to background; increased frequency in patients with neurofibromato-sis

Differential diagnosis
Nevus depigmentosus; hypomelanosis of Ito; segmental vitiligo; tinea versicolor; post-inflammatory hypopigmentation; lep-rosy; tuberous sclerosis

Therapy
No effective therapy

References
Ahkami RN, Schwartz RA (1999) Nevus anemi-cus. Dermatology 198(4):327–329

Nevus araneus

▶ Spider angioma

Nevus, Becker's

▶ Becker's nevus

Nevus comedonicus

▶ Epidermal nevus

Nevus, connective tissue

▶ Connective tissue nevus

Nevus depigmentosus

Synonym(s)
Achromic nevus

Definition
Congenital and stable localized area of hypopigmentation or depigmentation

Pathogenesis
May involve defective melanin transfer from melanocytes to keratinocytes

Clinical manifestation
Pale-colored patch, with streaks, whorls; round in contour; no change with age

Differential diagnosis
Hypomelanosis of Ito; tinea versicolor; vitiligo; leprosy; nevus anemicus; post-inflammatory hypopigmentation; tuberous sclerosis

Therapy
No effective therapy

References
Pinto FJ, Bolognia JL (1991) Disorders of hypopig-mentation in children. Pediatric Clinics of North America 38(4):991–1017

Nevus flammeus

Synonym(s)
Nevus flammeus neonatorum; port-wine stain; port-wine mark; strawberry patch; naevus maternus

Definition
Congenital malformation of the upper dermal blood vessels producing a permanent, localized, red patch

Pathogenesis
Decreased local innervation may produce decreased vascular tone and progressive vascular dilatation

Clinical manifestation
Pink-to-violaceous patch, with variable blanching after external pressure; present from birth; usually located over the head and neck area; surface sometimes becomes thickened with a cobblestone-like contour and vascular papules or nodules or pyogenic granulomas, usually in adulthood; skin and underlying soft tissue or bony hypertrophy may occur.

Sturge-Weber (encephalofacial or encephalotrigeminal angiomatosis) variant: vascular malformation involving the upper facial area supplied by ophthalmic branch (CN V1) of the trigeminal nerve, the ipsilateral leptomeninges, and the ipsilateral cerebral cortex; more extensive than in isolated nevus flammeus; complications include glaucoma, seizures, hemiplegia, mental retardation, cerebral calcifications, subdural hemorrhage, and underlying soft tissue hypertrophy

Differential diagnosis
Capillary hemangioma; salmon patch; Beckwith-Wiedemann syndrome; Coats disease; Cobb syndrome; Parkes-Weber syndrome; phakomatosis pigmentovascularis; von Hippel-Lindau disease; Wyburn-Mason syndrome

Therapy
Flashlamp-pumped pulse dye laser*

References
Travelute Ammirati C, Carniol PJ, Hruza GJ (2001) Laser treatment of facial vascular lesions. Facial Plastic Surgery 17(3):193–201

Nevus flammeus neonatorum

▶ Nevus flammeus

Nevus fuscoceruleus acromiodeltoideus

▶ Nevus of Ota and Ito

Nevus fuscoceruleus ophtalmomaxillaris

▶ Nevus of Ota and Ito

Nevus fuscoceruleus zygomaticus

▶ Nevus of Ota and Ito

Nevus lipomatosis

Synonym(s)
Nevus lipomatosis of Hoffmann-Zurhelle; nevus lipomatosus cutaneous superficialis

Definition
Disorder characterized by solitary or grouped hamartomatous proliferations of fatty tissue

Pathogenesis
Unknown

Clinical manifestation
Asymptomatic, soft, skin colored to yellow papules and nodules, which often coalesce into plaques; surface is either smooth, wrinkled, cerebriform, or verrucoid, with comedones; distribution usually linear, systematized, zosteriform, or along the lines of skin folds, with predilection for the pelvic girdle, lumbar area, buttocks, and the upper thighs; solitary type consists of papule or nodule with no favored location, usually appearing during the third to sixth decades of life

Differential diagnosis
Focal dermal hypoplasia; lipoma; epidermal nevus, melanocytic nevus; nevus sebaceous; skin tags; connective tissue nevus; accessory nipple; neurofibroma; angiolipoma; trichoepithelioma; cylindroma; localized scleroderma

Therapy
Surgical excision for cosmesis only

References
Ioannidou DJ, Stefanidou, M P, Panayiotides, JG, Tosca, A D (2001) Nevus lipomatosus cutaneous superficialis (Hoffmann-Zurhelle) with localized scleroderma like appearance. International Journal of Dermatology 40(1):54–57

Nevus lipomatosis of Hoffmann-Zurhelle

▶ Nevus lipomatosis

Nevus lipomatosus cutaneous superficialis

▶ Nevus lipomatosis

Nevus, melanocytic

Synonym(s)
Nevocellular nevus; mole

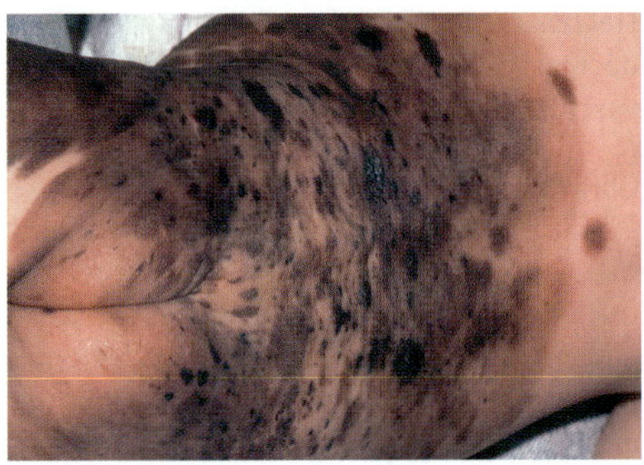

Nevus, melanocytic. Large, irregular hyperpigmented plaque over the trunk and buttocks

Definition
Benign neoplasm composed of melanocytes

Pathogenesis
Propensity to develop multiple lesions, particularly atypical moles; may be autosomal dominant trait; ultraviolet radiation may be cofactor

Clinical manifestation
Congenital variant: size ranging from <1 cm to lesions covering most of the integument; range in color from tan to deep blue-black; may begin as patch and become palpable as child ages; associated satellite pigmented papules, especially in patients with giant congenital nevus (>20 cm in diameter); melanoma risk increases with size of congenital lesion

Acquired variant: sharply marginated, uniform tan to brown, smooth to verrucous papule or macule, usually <1 cm in diameter

Spitz (spindle cell) nevus variant: uniform, smooth, reddish-brown papule, often with fine overlying scale, usually occurring in childhood

Blue nevus variant: uniform, firm, blue papule

Clark's nevus (atypical mole, dysplastic nevus) variant: reddish-brown flat papule, with central elevation and feathered red border ("fried egg appearance"), often >0.5 cm in diameter; sometimes marker of risk for melanoma, particularly with family history of melanoma or presence of multiple lesions

Differential diagnosis

Melanoma; seborrheic keratosis; nevus of Ota and Ito; lentigo; freckle; mastocytoma; juvenile xanthogranuloma; basal cell carcinoma; actinic keratosis; benign tumor of sweat gland or hair follicle

Therapy

Biopsy of all lesions in which melanoma is in the differential diagnosis[*]; congenital nevus: surgical excision, particularly larger lesions[*]; acquired nevus, blue nevus, or Spitz nevus: surgical excision for cosmesis only; Clark's nevus: controversial whether surgical excision is indicated

References

Makkar HS, Frieden IJ (2002) Congenital melanocytic nevi: an update for the pediatrician. Current Opinion in Pediatrics 14(4):397–403

Schaffer JV, Bolognia JL (2000) The clinical spectrum of pigmented lesions. Clinics in Plastic Surgery 27(3):391–408

Nevus mucinosis

▶ **Connective tissue nevus**

Nevus of Cannon

▶ **White sponge nevus**

Nevus of Ito

▶ **Nevus of Ota and Ito**

Nevus of Jadassohn and Tieche

▶ **Blue nevus**

Nevus of Ota and Ito

N

Synonym(s)

Nevus fuscoceruleus zygomaticus; Hori's nevus; Hori nevus; nevus fuscoceruleus acromiodeltoideus; oculodermal melanosis; nevus fuscoceruleus ophtalmomaxillaris; oculodermal melanocytosis

Definition

Melanin pigmentation of the facial skin, the sclera of the eye, and the oral mucosa (Ota variant), or over the shoulder (Ito variant)

Pathogenesis

May represent embryonic melanocytes that have not migrated completely from the neural crest to the epidermis

Clinical manifestation

Nevus of Ota: usually unilateral, poorly demarcated, gray-blue patch over the cheek, forehead, eyelid, temple, and gingiva; sclera blue and shiny; often follows distribution of the two first branches of the trigeminal nerve; sometimes slowly and progressively enlarges and darkens; usually stable once adulthood reached

Nevus of Ito: same appearance and course as nevus of Ota, but located over shoulder and upper arm areas

Differential diagnosis
Blue nevus; melasma; ochronosis; melanoma; lentigo; traumatic tattoo

Therapy
Q-switched ruby, Q-switched alexandrite or Q-switched Nd:YAG laser

References
Mishriki YY (2001) Are these pigmentary changes only cosmetic? Oculodermal melanocytosis (nevus of Ota). Postgraduate Medicine 110(6):43–46

Nevus of Sutton

▶ Halo nevus

Nevus on nevus

▶ Nevus spilus

Nevus sebaceous

▶ Epidermal nevus

Nevus simplex

▶ Salmon patch

Nevus spilus

Synonym(s)
Speckled lentiginous nevus; mosaic speckled lentiginous nevus; nevus on nevus; speckled nevus spilus

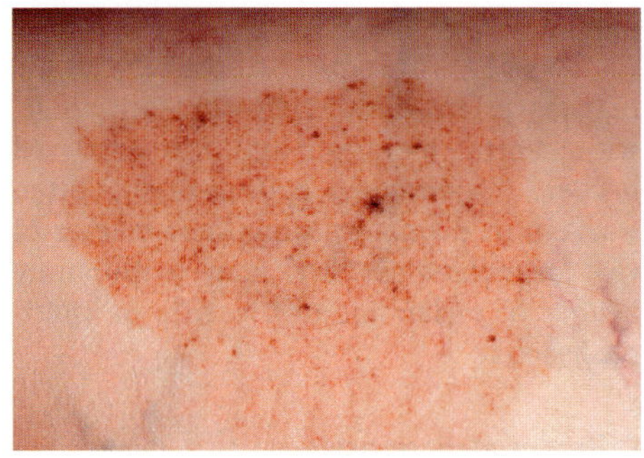

Nevus spilus. Speckled brown patch on the trunk

Definition
Lesions characterized by tan patches containing numerous darker macules or papules

Pathogenesis
May represent localized defect of melanoblast migration populating a particular area of skin; mosaicism possible cause of zosteriform variant

Clinical manifestation
Variable number of black, brown, or red-brown macules and papules seen within oval or linear (zosteriform) patch of tan to brown hyperpigmentation, often present at birth; some follow lines of Blaschko

Differential diagnosis
Congenital nevus; Spitz nevus; NAME syndrome; LEOPARD syndrome; Carney's syndrome

Therapy
Surgical excision for cosmesis only; Q-switched ruby or Q-switched Nd:YAG laser ablation for cosmesis only

References
Carpo BG, Grevelink JM, Grevelink SV (1999) Laser treatment of pigmented lesions in children. Seminars in Cutaneous Medicine & Surgery 18(3):233–243

Nevus spilus tardus

▶ Becker's nevus

Nevus syringadenoma papilliferum

▶ Syringocystadenoma papilliferum

Nevus unius lateris

▶ Epidermal nevus

Nevus varicousus osteohypertrophicus syndrome

▶ Klippel-Trenaunay-Weber syndrome

Nevus verrucosus

▶ Epidermal nevus

Nevus verrucosus hypertrophicans

▶ Klippel-Trenaunay-Weber syndrome

New World spotted fever

▶ Rocky Mountain spotted fever

Niacin deficiency

▶ Pellagra

Niacinamide (nicotinamide)

Trade name(s)
None

Generic available
Yes

Drug class
Vitamin

Mechanism of action
Suppression of antigen-induced lymphoblast transformation; mast cell stabilization

Dosage form
500 mg tablet

Dermatologic indications and dosage
See table

Common side effects
Neurologic: headache; dyspepsia

Serious side effects
Gastrointestinal: hepatotoxicity

Drug interactions
None

Contraindications/precautions
Hypersensitivity to drug class or component

Niacinamide (nicotinamide). Dermatologic indications and dosage

Disease	Adult dosage	Child dosage
Bullous pemphigoid	500 mg PO 2–3 times daily, often given concomitantly with tetracycline, doxycycline, or minocycline	500 mg PO 2–3 times daily, often given concomitantly with tetracycline, doxycycline, or minocycline
Linear IgA bullous dermatosis	500 mg PO 2–3 times daily, often given concomitantly with tetracycline, doxycycline, or minocycline	500 mg PO 2–3 times daily, often given concomitantly with tetracycline, doxycycline, or minocycline
Pellagra	100 mg PO every 6 hours for several days or until major acute symptoms resolve, followed by 50 mg PO 2–3 times daily until skin lesions heal	100 mg PO every 6 hours for several days or until major acute symptoms resolve, followed by 50 mg PO 2–3 times daily until skin lesions heal

References

Chaidemenos GC (2001) Tetracycline and niacinamide in the treatment of blistering skin diseases. Clinics in Dermatology 19(6):781–785001

References

Nousari HC, Anhalt GJ (1999) Pemphigus and bullous pemphigoid. Lancet 354(9179):667–672

Nicholas Favre disease

▶ Lymphogranuloma venereum

Niemann disease

▶ Niemann-Pick disease

Niemann's disease

▶ Niemann-Pick disease

Nikolsky sign

Definition
Condition where the epidermal layer of skin slips free from the lower layers with a slight rubbing pressure

Nocardia infection

▶ Nocardiosis

Nodose fever

▶ Erythema nodosum

Nodular cutaneous elastoidosis with cysts and comedones

▶ Favre-Racouchot syndrome

Nodular nonsuppurative panniculitis

▶ Weber-Christian disease

Nodular subepidermal fibrosis

▶ Dermatofibroma

Nodular vasculitis

Synonym(s)
Bazin's disease; erythema induratum

Definition
Nodular eruption on the lower legs, with histopathologic changes similar to erythema induratum (i.e., vasculitis of larger vessels and panniculitis)

Pathogenesis
Hypersensitivity reaction to endogenous or exogenous antigens, which include tubercle bacillus

Clinical manifestation
Chronic, recurrent crops of small, tender, erythematous nodules on the legs; depressed scars, or pigmentation from previously active lesions

Differential diagnosis
Erythema nodosum; chilblains; T-cell lymphoma; erythema nodosum leprosum; factitial panniculitis; panniculitis associated with alpha-1 antitrypsin deficiency; pancreatic panniculitis; lupus panniculitis; superficial thrombophlebitis

Therapy
Antituberculous therapy if associated with tuberculosis*; potassium iodide 300–500 mg PO three times daily; prednisone; bed rest

References
Phelps RG, Shoji T (2001) Update on panniculitis. Mount Sinai Journal of Medicine 68(4-5):262–267

Non-metastasizing fibrosarcoma

▶ Desmoid tumor

Non-venereal syphilis of children

▶ Bejel

Nonbullous congenital ichthyosiform erythroderma

▶ Lamellar ichthyosis

Noonan's syndrome

Synonym(s)
Familial Turner syndrome; female pseudo Turner syndrome; pseudo Turner syndrome; male Turner syndrome; pseudo Ullrich-Turner syndrome; Turner-like syndrome; Ullrich-Noonan syndrome; Turner phenotype syndrome

Definition
Familial syndrome characterized by short stature, low-set ears, and many minor skeletal deformities, of which the commonest are pectus excavatum and cubitus valgus

Pathogenesis
Autosomal dominant trait; unknown gene defect

Clinical manifestation
Short stature; low set ears; skeletal anomalies, including pectus excavatum and cubitus valgus; intelligence often below average; cardiac abnormalities including pul-

monary valve stenosis, right heart anomalies, and left ventricular cardiomyopathy

Differential diagnosis
Turner's syndrome; neurofibromatosis; edema neonatorum; Aarskog's syndrome; Watson's syndrome; LEOPARD syndrome; fetal alcohol syndrome

Therapy
Growth hormone therapy for short stature

References
Kelnar CJ (2000) Growth hormone therapy in Noonan syndrome. Hormone Research 53 Suppl 1:77–81

North American blastomycosis

Synonym(s)
Blastomycosis

Definition
Endemic systemic mycotic infection caused by the thermally dimorphic fungus, Blastomyces dermatitidis

Pathogenesis
Inhalation of the microconidia from the mold form of B dermatitidis into the lungs causes infection; transition from mold form to yeast form after deposition in distal airways; in the absence of nonspecific host defense mechanisms, cells increases in number in the lungs; subsequent lymphohematogenous spread to the other organs; rarely occurs in skin after direct innoculation

Clinical manifestation
Usually starts with pulmonary infection followed by cutaneous, osseous, genitourinary, or central nervous system involvement; skin findings: most common manifestation of extrapulmonary disease; lesions favor exposed areas; minimally tender papules or pustules evolve into purulent, verrucous, or ulcerative nodules or plaques, characterized by sharp and heaped-up borders with centrally located granulation tissue and exudate; pulmonary findings: signs of acute pneumonia, including fever, night sweats, wheezing and dyspnea; signs and symptoms of chronic pneumonia last for 2–6 months, including weight loss, night sweats, fever, cough, and chest pain; osteolytic bone lesions; prostatitis or epididymitis

Differential diagnosis
Basal cell carcinoma; squamous cell carcinoma; pyoderma gangrenosum; keratoacanthoma; wart; leishmaniasis; anthrax; coccidioidomycosis; nocardiosis; atypical mycobacterial infection; cutaneous tuberculosis; sarcoidosis

Therapy
Amphotericin B: 0.7–1 mg per kg IV per day; total dose 1.5–2.5 g; itraconazole; ketoconazole

References
Bradsher RW (1997) Therapy of blastomycosis. Seminars in Respiratory Infections 12(3):263–267

Notalgia paresthetica

Synonym(s)
Paresthetic notalgia

Definition
Sensory neuropathy involving dorsal spinal nerves causing proxysmal pruritus of the upper back

Pathogenesis
Form of peripheral neuropathy of unknown cause

Clinical manifestation
Pruritus, pain, and/or paresthesia occurring principally between the scapulas,

sometimes attacking either side of the midline or posterolateral aspect of the shoulder; onset in early to middle adulthood; sometimes persists for decades; hyperpigmentation secondary to chronic rubbing and scratching; rare early clinical marker of multiple endocrine neoplasia type IIA

Differential diagnosis
Intercostal neuralgia; thoracic outlet syndrome; lichen amyloidosis; atopic neurodermatitis; post-herpetic neuralgia; xerosis; contact dermatitis

Therapy
Capsaicin; oxcarbazepine 300 mg PO twice daily; titration of dose to effect; local nerve block

References
Massey EW (1998) Sensory mononeuropathies. Seminars in Neurology 18(2):177–183

Nummular dermatitis

▶ Nummular eczema

Nummular eczema

Synonym(s)
Nummular dermatitis; discoid eczema

Definition
Chronic disorder characterized by pruritic, coin-shaped papules and plaques

Pathogenesis
Associated with xerosis, atopy, and venous stasis

Clinical manifestation
Papules or vesicles that coalesce to form confluent plaques on erythematous base; early lesions sometimes exudative and crusted; secondary infection may occur; necessitating systemic antibiotics; older lesions are dry, scaly, and excoriated from scratching; lower extremities and dorsum of hand most frequently affected areas

Differential diagnosis
Atopic dermatitis; tinea corporis; psoriasis; stasis dermatitis; pityriasis lichenoides; contact dermatitis; lichen simplex chronicus

Therapy
Corticosteroids, topical, high potency[*]; prednisone for severe flares

References
Aoyama H, Tanaka M, Hara M, Tabata N, Tagami H (1999) Nummular eczema: An addition of senile xerosis and unique cutaneous reactivities to environmental aeroallergens. Dermatology 199(2):135–139

Obliterative calcific-thrombotic arteriolopathy

▶ Calciphylaxis

OCA

▶ Oculocutaneous albinism

Occupational acne

▶ Chloracne

Ochroid mycetoma

▶ Eumycetoma

Ochronosis

Synonym(s)
Alcaptonuria; alkaptonuria; homogentisic acid oxidase deficiency

Definition
Inherited metabolic disorder characterized by blue-black discoloration of certain tissues, including ear cartilage and ocular tissue

Pathogenesis
Autosomal recessive trait; caused by deficiency of homogentisic acid; deficiency results in accumulation and deposition of homogentisic acid in cartilage, causing diffuse bluish-black pigmentation

Clinical manifestation
Dark urine in diapers usual first sign of disease; gray-black scleral pigmentation in configuration of small, dark rings; ear cartilage discoloration with a grayish-blue hue, followed by structural changes with stiffness, contour irregularities, and calcification; discoloration on nasal tip, costochondral junctions, extensor tendons of the hands, cheeks, fingernails, and buccal mucosa; ochronotic arthropathy; ochronosis-like pigmentation as idiosyncratic reaction to application of hydroquinone or phenol

Differential diagnosis
Argyria; medication-related hyperpigmentation; arsenical keratosis

Therapy
No effective therapy

▶ Alcaptonuria

References
Kneebone TS, Selner AJ (1995) Ochronosis and alkaptonuria. Case report and literature review. Journal of the American Podiatric Medical Association 85(10):554–555

Ocular albinism

▶ Oculocutaneous albinism

Oculocutaneous albinism

Synonym(s)
Albinism; OCA

Definition
Group of disorders characterized by an abnormality in melanin synthesis due to dysfunction of melanocytes in the skin, eyes, and/or ears

Pathogenesis
Autosomal recessive disorders; mutation in genes that regulate the process of melanin synthesis and distribution by the melanocyte
OCA Type 1: mutation in the tyrosinase gene
OCA Type 2: mutation in the P gene
OCA Type 3: mutation in the tyrosinase-related protein-1 (TRP-1) gene

Clinical manifestation
Three forms:
OCA1: complete absence of pigment in the skin, hair, and eyes; photophobia; reduced visual acuity; and nystagmus
OCA2: minimal to moderate pigment in the skin, hair, and eyes; in some patients, pigmented freckles, lentigines, and/or nevi; photophobia; reduced visual acuity; and nystagmus
OCA3: minimal pigment reduction in the skin, hair, and eyes; mild photophobia; reduced visual acuity; and nystagmus

Ocular albinism: ocular depigmentation and iris translucency; motor nystagmus; reduced visual acuity; fundus hypopigmentation

Differential diagnosis
Hermansky-Pudlak syndrome; phenylketonuria; Chediak-Higashi syndrome; histidinemia; homocystinuria; Menkes steely hair disease; Tietz syndrome; Prader-Willi syndrome; Angelman syndrome

Therapy
Sun protection with protective clothing and sunscreens; corrective lenses for visual impairment

References
Carden SM, Boissy RE, Schoettker PJ (1998) Albinism: Modern molecular diagnosis. British Journal of Ophthalmology (2):189–195

Oculodermal melanocytosis

▶ Nevus of Ota and Ito

Oculodermal melanosis

▶ Nevus of Ota and Ito

Oculomandibulodyscephaly with hypotrichosis

▶ Hallermann-Streiff syndrome

Oculomandibulofacial syndrome

▶ Hallermann-Streiff syndrome

Ofuji disease

▶ Eosinophilic pustular folliculitis

Ofuji's disease

▶ Eosinophilic pustular folliculitis

Ofuji's papuloerythroderma

▶ Eosinophilic pustular folliculitis

Olmsted syndrome

Synonym(s)
Olmsted's syndrome; pluriorificial keratosis of Olmsted; congenital palmoplantar and periorificial keratoderma

Definition
Congenital palmoplantar keratoderma with progressive palmoplantar hyperkeratosis and periorificial hyperkeratotic papules and plaques

Pathogenesis
Unknown

Clinical manifestation
At birth, sharply demarcated keratotic plaques involving periorificial sites; slow, progressive palmar and plantar keratoderma, producing flexion deformities and autoamputation

Differential diagnosis
Acrodermatitis enteropathica; pachonychia congenita; mutilating palmoplantar keratoderma

Therapy
Acitretin

References
Kress DW, Seraly MP, Falo L, Kim B, Jegasothy BV, Cohen B (1996) Olmsted syndrome. Case report and identification of a keratin abnormality. Archives of Dermatology 132(7):797–800

Olmsted's syndrome

▶ Olmsted Syndrome

Omnipen

▶ Ampicillin

Onchocerciasis

▶ Filariasis

Onychocryptosis

Definition
Ingrowing of the nail plate

References
Ikard RW (1998) Onychocryptosis. Journal of the American College of Surgeons 187(1):96–102

Onychogryphosis

Definition
Nail plate enlargement with increased thickening and curvature

References

Mohrenschlager M, Wicke-Wittenius K, Brockow K, Bruckbauer H, Ring J (2001) Onychogryphosis in elderly persons: an indicator of longstanding poor nursing care? Report of one case and review of the literature. Cutis 68(3):233–235

Onycholysis

Definition

Separation of the nail plate from the underlying nail bed at distal and lateral attachments

References

Mohrenschlager M, Wicke-Wittenius K, Brockow K, Bruckbauer H, Ring J (2001) Onychogryphosis in elderly persons: an indicator of longstanding poor nursing care? Report of one case and review of the literature. Cutis. 68(3):233–235

Onychomadesis

Definition

Complete separation of nail plate from underlying nail bed

References

Tosti A, Piraccini BM (2000) Treatment of common nail disorders. Dermatologic Clinics 18(2):339

Onychomycosis

Synonym(s)

Fungal nail infection

Definition

Fungal infection affecting the toenails or the fingernails

Pathogenesis

Caused by 3 classes of fungi: dermatophytes (usually Trichophyton rubrum), yeasts, and nondermatophyte molds; spread from plantar skin to underside of nail via the hyponychium or distal lateral nail bed

Clinical manifestation

Distal lateral subungual variant: thickened and opacified nail plate, nail bed hyperkeratosis, and onycholysis; endonyx variant: milky-white discoloration of the nail plate without subungual hyperkeratosis or onycholysis.

Superficial white variant: confined to the toenails, with small, white speckled or powdery patches on the surface of the nail plate; nail is roughened and crumbles easily

Proximal subungual variant: leukonychia in the proximal nail fold

Candidal infection: paronychia; onycholysis; hyperkeratosis of nail bed and inflammation of the nail fold in chronic mucocutaneous disease

Differential diagnosis

Psoriasis; pityriasis rubra pilaris; twenty nail dystrophy; lichen planus; traumatic nail dystrophy; contact dermatitis; pachonychia congenita; Darier disease; nail patella syndrome; melanoma; bacterial paronychia; yellow nail syndrome; drug-related nail dystrophy

Therapy

Terbinafine; itraconazole; griseofulvin; fluconazole; ciclopirox nail lacquer; surgical nail avulsion and matrixectomy by chemical or mechanical means

References

Crawford F, Young P, Godfrey C, Bell-Syer SE, Hart R, Brunt E, Russell I (2002) Oral treatments for toenail onychomycosis: a systematic review. Archives of Dermatology 138(6):811–816

Onychoosteodysplasia

▶ Nail-patella syndrome

Onychophagia

Definition
Compulsive biting or chewing of the nails

References
Wells JH, Haines J, Williams CL (1998) Severe morbid onychophagia: the classification as self-mutilation and a proposed model of maintenance. Australian & New Zealand Journal of Psychiatry 32(4):534–545

Onychorrhexis

Definition
Superficial splitting of the free edge of the nail

References
Bodman MA. (1995) Miscellaneous nail presentations. Clinics in Podiatric Medicine & Surgery 12(2):327–346

Onychoschizia

Definition
Splitting of the fingernails at the distal tip

References
Bodman MA (1995) Miscellaneous nail presentations. Clinics in Podiatric Medicine & Surgery 12(2):327–346

Onychotillomania

Definition
Compulsive picking at fingernails and/or toenails

References
Colver GB (1987) Onychotillomania. British Journal of Dermatology 117(3):397–399

Oral cutaneous fistula

Synonym(s)
Orofacial fistula; intra-oral fistula; dental abscess with sinus tract formation; dental sinus

Definition
Dental periapical inflammation, with development of a fistulous tract exiting through the face or neck

Pathogenesis
Direct extension or continuity from an acute irreversible pulpitis spreading beyond the apex of the tooth or an acute exacerbation of a chronic apical periodontitis or periapical granuloma; often associated with poor oral hygiene and trauma; bacteria such as Streptococcus mutans, Staphylococcus epidermidis, Staphylococcus aureus, and Porphyromonas, Actinomycoses, Bacteroides, and Fusobacterium species found at the site of the fistula

Clinical manifestation
Reddish-brown nodule sometimes exuding serous or purulent material; most commonly involves the mandible and chin region; site of fistulation sometimes distant from the intraoral infection site

Differential diagnosis
Pyogenic granuloma; melanoma; squamous cell carcinoma; basal cell carcinoma;

nocardiosis, sporotrichosis; South American blastomycosis; granuloma faciale; lupus erythematosus; epidermoid cyst

Therapy
Penicillin*; amoxicillin; doxycycline; incision and drainage often necessary; extraction of the affected tooth; pulpotomy, or pulp removal and drainage; surgical removal of sequestered or necrotic bone*

References
Fernandez JM, Metlich MA, Bravo JM, Freyre IC (1982) Oral-cutaneous fistula of dental origin. Journal of Oral & Maxillofacial Surgery 40(3):183–185

Oral epithelial nevus

▶ White sponge nevus

Oral fibroma

▶ Angiofibroma

Oral florid papillomatosis

▶ Verrucous carcinoma

Oral hairy leukoplakia

▶ Hairy leukoplakia

Orf

Synonym(s)
Contagious ecthyma; ecthyma contagiosum; ecthyma infectiosum; contagious pustular dermatitis; sheep pox

Definition
Viral disease of goats and sheep that can be transmitted to humans and produce self-healing cutaneous nodules

Pathogenesis
Caused by DNA virus belonging to Parapoxvirus genus; infection from contact with infected animals, carcasses, or nonliving material

Clinical manifestation
Small, firm, red-to-blue papule which form hemorrhagic, flat-topped pustule or bulla, with crust or central umbilication, on the fingers, hands, or forearms; resolves after 30–40 days

Differential diagnosis
Tularemia; anthrax; milker's nodule; acute febrile neutrophilic dermatosis; leishmaniasis; bacterial ecthyma; cutaneous tuberculosis; sporotrichosis; nocardiosis; squamous cell carcinoma; keratoacanthoma

Therapy
No medical therapy; surgical excision or destruction by electrodesiccation and curettage for persistent lesion

References
Huerter CJ, Alvarez L, Stinson R (1991) Orf: case report and literature review. Cleveland Clinic Journal of Medicine 58(6):531–534

Organoid nevus

▶ Epidermal nevus

Oriental sore

▶ Leishmaniasis, cutaneous

Orofacial fistula

▶ Oral cutaneous fistula

Orofacial granulomatosis

▶ Cheilitis granulomatosa

Oroya fever

▶ Bartonellosis

Osler disease

▶ Osler-Weber-Rendu syndrome

Osler's disease

▶ Osler-Weber-Rendu syndrome

Osler-Weber-Rendu syndrome

Synonym(s)
Hereditary hemorrhagic telangiectasia; Rendu-Osler syndrome; Osler's disease; Osler disease; heredofamilial angiomatosis; familial hemorrhagic angiomatosis

Definition
Hereditary disorder characterized by telangiectasia and recurrent epistaxis

Pathogenesis
Mutation of the protein endoglin, a receptor for transforming growth factor beta, with a role in tissue repair and angiogenesis; defects in the endothelial cell junctions, endothelial cell degeneration, and weakness of the perivascular connective tissue cause dilation of capillaries and post-capillary venules, manifested as telangiectases

Clinical manifestation
Telangiectases, found on the oral mucosa, nasal mucosa, skin, and conjunctiva; pinhead-sized macules or barely palpable papules, partially blanching with pressure; color ranges from bright red to violaceous to purple; face, lips and mouth, nares, tongue, ears, hands, chest, and feet most commonly affected sites; cyanosis and clubbing in patients with pulmonary arterio-venous malformations; stroke, brain abscess, or intracerebral hematoma; pulmonary arterio-venous malformations, tachypnea; cyanosis; clubbing; retinal telangiectasias and hemorrhages; gastrointestinal bleeding; arterio-venous fistulas of the liver

Differential diagnosis
CREST syndrome; Louis-Bar syndrome; ataxia-telangiectasia; benign essential telangiectasia; rosacea; actinically damaged skin; dermatomyositis; Rothmund-Thomson syndrome; scleroderma; Cockayne syndrome; angiokeratoma corporis diffusum

Therapy

ND:YAG laser ablation of symptomatic vascular lesions; recurrent, uncontrollable epistaxis: septal dermoplasty; bleeding prophylaxis: estradiol: 0.6 mg PO per day or via transdermal patch

References

Haitjema T, Westermann CJ, Overtoom TT, Timmer R, Disch F, Mauser H, Lammers JW (1996) Hereditary hemorrhagic telangiectasia (Osler-Weber-Rendu disease): new insights in pathogenesis, complications, and treatment. Archives of Internal Medicine 156(7):714–719

Osmidrosis

▶ Bromhidrosis

Osteitis fibrosa cystica

▶ McCune-Albright syndrome

Osteitis fibrosa disseminata

▶ McCune-Albright syndrome

Osteogenesis imperfecta

Synonym(s)

None

Definition

Group of heritable disorders of collagen synthesis characterized by fragile bones

Pathogenesis

Autosomal dominant trait; mutation in protein that codes for pro-α1 and pro-α2 collagen chains, producing both qualitative and quantitative collagen defects

Clinical manifestation

Type 1: blue sclera; in-utero fractures; mild-to-moderate bone fragility; kyphoscoliosis; hearing loss; premature arcus senilis; easy bruising; short stature

Type 2: abnormal dentition; blue sclera; small nose; micrognathia; connective tissue fragility; short trunk

Type 3: abnormal dentition; sclera of variable hue; in-utero fractures; limb shortening and progressive deformities; triangular facies with frontal bossing; pulmonary hypertension

Type 4: normal sclera; normal hearing; fractures beginning in infancy; mild angulation and shortening of long bones

Differential diagnosis

Turner syndrome; Paget disease; osteopetrosis; camptomelic dysplasia; achondrogenesis type I; congenital hypophosphatasia; steroid-induced osteoporosis; battered child syndrome; copper deficiency

Therapy

Intravenous aminohydroxypropylidene for increasing bone mineral density

References

Cole WG (2002) Advances in osteogenesis imperfecta. Clinical Orthopaedics & Related Research (401):6–16

Osteoma cutis

Synonym(s)

None

Definition

Presence of bone within the skin without preexisting or associated lesion

Pathogenesis

Unknown

Clinical manifestation
Single or multiple, extremely hard papules, plaques, or nodules, usually on face, extremities, scalp, digits, and subungual regions; seen in Albright hereditary osteodystrophy, fibrodysplasia ossificans heteroplasia, and fibrodysplasia ossificans progressiva

Differential diagnosis
Calcinosis cutis; pilomatricoma; metastasis; cartilaginous skin tumors; foreign body reaction; gouty tophus; myositis ossificans; secondary ossification

Therapy
Surgical excision*

References
Orlow SJ, Watsky KL, Bolognia JL (1991) Skin and bones. II. Journal of the American Academy of Dermatology 25(3):447–462

Ostiderm

▶ **Aluminium chlorohydrate**

Otitis externa

Synonym(s)
External otitis; swimmer's ear

Definition
Inflammation of the skin of the ear canal, characterized by pain, redness, swelling, and discharge

Pathogenesis
No single causative agent; often a combination of infection with bacterial pathogens (Pseudomonas species or other gram-negative organisms, S. aureus) or fungi (candida and aspergillus species) and irritation; predisposing factors are moisture with maceration and trauma to mucosa

Clinical manifestation
Painful tragus when applying traction to the pinna; edema and redness of ear canal; purulent or serous discharge; conductive hearing loss; cellulitis of the face or neck; lymphadenopathy; fungal infections resulting in severe itch but less pain than bacterial infection; thick discharge
Necrotizing (malignant) otitis externa variant: pain out of proportion to clinical findings; granulation tissue in the ear canal

Differential diagnosis
Otitis media; foreign body in ear canal; squamous cell carcinoma of ear canal; ear canal trauma; erysipelas

Therapy
Neomycin, polymyxin B, hydrocortisone otic solution applied 4 times daily for 10–14 days*; hydrocortisone and acetic acid otic solution applied on cotton wick 4 times daily for 10–14 days; acetic acid 5% in aluminium acetate solution applied on cotton wick 3–4 times daily until symptoms abate; prednisone for severe inflammation; surgical debridement in individuals with necrotizing (i.e., malignant) variant

References
Sander R (2001) Otitis externa: a practical guide to treatment and prevention. American Family Physician 63(5):927-936, 941–942

Ota, nevus of

▶ **Nevus of Ota and Ito**

Oudtshoorn skin

▶ **Keratolytic winter erythema**

P

Pachydermia verticis gyrata

▶ Cutis verticis gyrata

Pachydermodactyly

Synonym(s)
None

Definition
Form of acquired digital fibromatosis, characterized by non-inflammatory bulbous swelling of the dorsal and lateral surfaces of the fingers at the level of proxymal phalanges and interphalangeal joints

Pathogenesis
Possible role of repeated trauma, sometimes in the background of neurotic behavior

Clinical manifestation
Asymptomatic, persistent, symmetrical swellings on the lateral and medial aspects of fingers; second, third, and fourth digits affected bilaterally; almost always in men

Differential diagnosis
Knuckle pad; post-traumatic callosity; foreign-body granuloma; fibroma; infantile digital fibromatosis; rheumatoid and pseudo-rheumatoid nodule; arthritis; pachydermoperiostosis; proteus syndrome

Therapy
Triamcinolone 3–5 mg per ml intralesional

References
Tompkins SD, McNutt NS, Shea CR (1998) Distal pachydermodactyly. Journal of the American Academy of Dermatology 38(2 Pt 2):359–362

Pachydermoperiostosis

Synonym(s)
Primary hypertrophic osteoarthropathy; idiopathic hypertrophic osteoarthropathy; Touraine-Solente-Gole syndrome

Definition
Syndrome characterized by digital clubbing and subperiosteal new bone formation, associated with pain, polyarthritis, cutis verticis gyrata, seborrheic dermatitis, and hyperhidrosis

Pathogenesis
Autosomal dominant trait with variable penetrance; unknown gene defect

Clinical manifestation
Digital clubbing and/or paronychial thickening; coarse facial features similar to those of acromegaly; scleroderma-like thickening and furrowing of the skin on the forehead and cheeks, with leonine facies in advanced stages; cutis verticis gyrata; seborrheic dermatitis of the face and the scalp; palmo-

plantar hyperhidrosis or generalized hyperhidrosis with secondary dermatitis

Differential diagnosis
Acromegaly; thyroid acropachy; psoriatic arthritis; secondary hypertrophic pulmonary osteoarthropathy

Therapy
No effective therapy

References
Sinha GP, Curtis P, Haigh D, Lealman GT, Dodds W, Bennett CP (1997) Pachydermoperiostosis in childhood. British Journal of Rheumatology 36(11):1224–1227

Pachyonychia congenita

Synonym(s)
Jadassohn-Lewandowsky syndrome; polykeratosis congenita

Definition
Hereditary palmoplantar keratoderma characterized by keratoderma of the palms and soles and thickened nail plates

Pathogenesis
Usually autosomal recessive trait; mutations in the genes encoding epidermal keratinocyte keratins, specifically K6a, K6b, K16, and K17, which disrupt keratin filament assembly

Clinical manifestation
Jadassohn-Lewandowsky type (PC-1): present at birth or from early childhood; thickened, brown-to-gray nail plates with rough surface; usually affects all fingers; toenails sometimes also involved; thickened fingernails may extend into periungual tissue, causing paronychia; circumscribed or diffuse hyperkeratoses of palms and soles; follicular hyperkeratosis on the face and on extensor aspect of proximal extremities; leukokeratosis of oral mucosa

Jackson-Lawler type (PC-2): thickened nail plates and other features of PC-1 type; natal teeth; unruly hair

Differential diagnosis
Psoriasis; pityriasis rubra pilaris; onychomycosis; Darier disease; epidermolysis bullosa; mucocutaneous candidiasis

Therapy
Acitretin★

References
Su WP, Chun SI, Hammond DE, Gordon H (1990) Pachyonychia congenita: a clinical study of 12 cases and review of the literature. Pediatric Dermatology 7(1):33–38

Paddy-field foot

▶ **Immersion foot**

Paget's disease

Synonym(s)
Paget's disease of the nipple and areola; Paget's disease of the skin, apocrine type; eczematoid epitheliomatous dermatosis; malignant papillary dermatosis; intraepidermal adenocarcinoma

Definition
Form of ductal carcinoma of either the breast (mammary Paget's disease) or the anogenital axillary, or other skin site (extramammary Paget's disease)

Pathogenesis
Mammary variant: underlying intraductal carcinoma of the breast with retrograde extension into the overlying epidermis through mammary duct epithelium; tumor cells derive from luminal lactiferous ductal epithelium of the breast tissue
Extramammary variant: in most cases, arises as a primary cutaneous adenocarci-

noma; epidermis is infiltrated with neoplastic cells showing glandular differentiation; tumor cells sometimes originate from apocrine gland ducts or from keratinocytic stem cells

Clinical manifestation
Mammary variant: may occur after long history of an eczematous skin lesion in the nipple and adjacent areas; sharply demarcated, scaly, red, crusted, and thickened plaques on the nipple, spreading to the surrounding areolar areas; may have retraction of the nipple or palpable nodules, indicating an underlying breast cancer; serosanguinous nipple discharge
Extramammary variant: chronic, pruritic eczematous lesions in the groin, genitalia, perineum, or perianal area; unilateral, sharply marginated plaque with peripheral erythema; erosion or scaling sometimes occurs in mature lesions

Differential diagnosis
Mammary variant: irritant contact dermatitis; atopic dermatitis; fixed medication reaction; nipple duct adenoma; erosive adenomatosis of the nipple; melanoma; Bowen's disease
Extramammary variant: Bowen's disease; basal cell carcinoma; melanoma; candidiasis; intertrigo; contact dermatitis; seborrheic dermatitis; psoriasis; lichen simplex chronicus

Therapy
Mammary variant: mastectomy and lymph node clearance*
Extramammary variant: Mohs micrographic surgery*; wide local excision; imiquimod

References
Fu W, Mittel VK, Young SC (2001) Paget disease of the breast: analysis of 41 patients. American Journal of Clinical Oncology 24(4):397–400
Mehta NJ, Torno R, Sorra T (2000) Extramammary Paget's disease. Southern Medical Association Journal 93(7):713–715

Paget's disease, extramammary

▶ Paget's disease

Paget's disease of the nipple and areola

▶ Paget's disease

Paget's disease of the skin, apocrine type

▶ Paget's disease

Painful papule

▶ Piezogenic papule

Palmar fasciitis

▶ Dupuytren's contracture

Palmoplantar fibromatosis

▶ Dupuytren's contracture

Palmoplantar hyperhidrosis

Definition
Excess sweating of the palms and soles

References

Togel B, Greve B, Raulin C (2002) Current therapeutic strategies for hyperhidrosis: a review. European Journal of Dermatology 12(3):219–223

Palmoplantar keratoderma

Definition
Pathologic condition characterized by diffuse or localized thickening of the stratum corneum, sometimes part of a generalized condition or a disorder primarily involving the hands and feet

▶ **Keratosis palmaris et plantaris**

References

Zemtsov A, Veitschegger M (1993) Keratodermas. International Journal of Dermatology 32(7):493–498

Palmoplantar keratoderma areata

▶ **Striate keratoderma**

Palmoplantar keratoderma diffusa circumscripta

▶ **Unna-Thost palmoplantar keratoderma**

Palmoplantar keratoderma mutilans

▶ **Vohwinkel syndrome**

Palmoplantar keratoderma striata

▶ **Striate keratoderma**

Palmoplantar keratoderma with periodontitis

▶ **Papillon-Lefèvre syndrome**

Palmoplantar pustulosis

▶ **Psoriasis**

Panatrophy of Gowers

Synonym(s)
Gowers' panatrophy; Gowers' local panatrophy

Definition
Disorder characterized by plaques of morphea-like, cutaneous atrophy due to partial or total loss of subcutaneous fat and atrophy of overlying skin, sometimes associated with atrophy or impaired growth of underlying muscle or bone

Pathogenesis
May be the end result of more than one pathologic process; reduced sympathetic skin response and aberrant production of non-esterified fatty acids after stimulation with epinephrine in lesional skin

Clinical manifestation
Sharply defined, irregular area of atrophy, developing over a period of a few weeks

without preceding inflammation; subcutaneous fatty tissue regresses and overlying skin appears atrophic, but otherwise normal; atrophy reaches maximum extent within a few months and then stabilizes indefinitely

Differential diagnosis
Sclerotic panatrophy; facial hemiatrophy (Romberg's syndrome); morphea; panniculitis

Therapy
No effective therapy

References
Sakamoto T, Oku T, Takagawa M (1998) Gowers' local panatrophy. Europeon Journal of Dermatology 8(2):116–117

Panniculitis, cold

▶ Cold panniculitis

Panniculitis of the newborn

▶ Subcutaneous fat necrosis of newborn

Papillary adenoma of the nipple

▶ Erosive adenomatosis of the nipple

Papillary hidradenoma

▶ Hidradenoma papilliferum

Papillary intralymphatic angioendothelioma

▶ Endovascular papillary angioendothelioma of childhood

Papillary syringadenoma

▶ Syringocystadenoma papilliferum

Papillomatosis of the subareolar ducts

▶ Erosive adenomatosis of the nipple

Papillon-Lefèvre syndrome

Synonym(s)
Palmoplantar keratoderma with periodontitis; keratoderma palmoplantaris diffusa with periodontosis

Definition
Hereditary disorder characterized by palmoplantar keratoderma and periodontosis

Pathogenesis
Autosomal recessive trait; gene locus mapped to 11q14-q21; possible dysfunction of cathepsin C gene; possible defect in leukocyte function

Clinical manifestation
Diffuse palmoplantar keratosis; scaly erythematous plaques over knees, elbows, and interphalangeal joints; hyperhidrosis and malodor; periodontosis with severe gingivi-

tis and loss of teeth by age 5 years; increased susceptibility to infection

Differential diagnosis
Olmsted syndrome; Richner-Hanhart syndrome; Vohwinkel syndrome; mal de Meleda

Therapy
Acitretin*; aggressive dental care

References
Siragusa M, Romano C, Batticane N, Batolo D, Schepis C (2000) A new family with Papillon-Lefevre syndrome: effectiveness of etretinate treatment. Cutis 65(3):151–155

Papular acrodermatitis

▶ Gianotti-Crosti syndrome

Papular acrodermatitis of childhood

▶ Gianotti-Crosti syndrome

Papular angioplasia

▶ **Angiolymphoid hyperplasia with eosinophilia**

Papular dermatitis of pregnancy

▶ **Prurigo of pregnancy**

Papular infantile acrodermatitis

▶ Gianotti-Crosti syndrome

Papular mucinosis

Synonym(s)
Lichen myxedematosus; myxedematosus; scleromyxedema

Definition
Spectrum of disease characterized by generalized, densely grouped, dome-shaped papules with increased mucin deposition in the dermis, sometimes associated with a monoclonal gammopathy

Pathogenesis
May be a fibroblast disorder, causing increased mucin deposition in the skin

Clinical manifestation
Papular mucinosis (lichen myxedematosus) variant: dome-shaped and flesh-colored or erythematous papules, often in a pattern of parallel ridges, sometimes coalescing into grouped lichenoid papules, on dorsal hands, face, or extensor surfaces of the arms and legs; with extensive involvement, leonine faces and difficulty opening the mouth

Scleromyxedema variant: widespread, erythematous, indurated skin resembling scleroderma, with diffuse tightness and decreased range of motion; systemic manifestations include restrictive and obstructive pulmonary dysfunction, cardiovascular abnormalities, and polyarthritis; gastrointestinal symptoms (most commonly dysphagia) related to deficient esophageal peristalsis; proximal muscle weakness, polyarthritis; organic brain syndrome; ectropion and corneal opacities; cardiovascular abnormalities

Differential diagnosis
Persistent acral papular mucinosis; malignant atrophic papulosis; scleroderma; lymphoma; scleredema; leprosy; sarcoidosis; follicular mucinosis; Darier disease; Grover's disease; colloid milium; granuloma annulare; lipoid proteinosis; progressive nodular histiocytosis

Therapy
Acetretin; prednisone; orthovoltage radiation; electron beam radiation; photochemotherapy; plasmapheresis; extracorporeal photophoresis; dermabrasion; carbon dioxide laser ablation

References
Rongioletti F, Rebora A (2001) Updated classification of papular mucinosis, lichen myxedematosus, and scleromyxedema. Journal of the American Academy of Dermatology 44(2):273–281

Papular urticaria

Synonym(s)
Insect bite reaction

Definition
Pruritic eruption occurring in some children after insect bites, most often from fleas, chiggers, or mosquitoes

Pathogenesis
May be autosensitization response to arthropod bite

Clinical manifestation
Small, firm, red, pruritic papules often appearing in tight clusters and lasting for 2–12 days, at sites of insect bites; few new bites may cause reaction in old bite sites; post-inflammatory hyperpigmentation

Differential diagnosis
Urticaria; mastocytosis; acral papular dermatitis of childhood; drug eruption; dermatitis herpetiformis; scabies; atopic dermatitis; prurigo nodularis

Therapy
Ice water soaks; insect repellants for prophylaxis

References
Howard R, Frieden IJ (1996) Papular urticaria in children. Pediatric Dermatology 13(3):246–249

Papulopustular facial dermatitis

▶ **Perioral dermatitis**

Papulosis atrophicans maligna

▶ **Malignant atrophic papulosis**

Papulovesicular acrolocated syndrome

▶ **Gianotti-Crosti syndrome**

Paracoccidioidomycosis

▶ **South American blastomycosis**

Paradoxical fibrosarcoma

▶ **Atypical fibroxanthoma**

Parakeratose brilliante

▶ **Confluent and reticulated papillomatosis**

Paraneoplastic acrokeratosis

Synonym(s)
Acrokeratosis paraneoplastica of Bazex; acrokeratosis paraneoplastica

Definition
Scaly acral papules, paronychia, nail dystrophy, and keratoderma as signs of upper airway and upper digestive tract cancer

Pathogenesis
Possible circulating antibodies to tumor antigens

Clinical manifestation
Stage 1: eruption confined to fingers and toes, nasal bridge, and tips of ears; red, scaly papules; tender nail folds; nail plate dystrophy
Stage 2: palms and soles scaly and red; honeycomb-like thickening of palms and fingers; facial eruption involving the cheeks and entire ear
Stage 3: eruption extends to the proximal extremities; diffuse scalp scaling

Differential diagnosis
Contact dermatitis; lupus erythematosus; dermatomyositis; photosensitivity reaction; medication reaction

Therapy
Treatment of the underlying neoplasm; no specific therapy for cutaneous disease

References
Bolognia JL (1995) Bazex syndrome: Acrokeratosis paraneoplastica. Seminars in Dermatology 14(2):84–89

Paraneoplastic pemphigus

Synonym(s)
None

Definition
Disorder characterized by oral erosions and bullous skin lesions in patients with underlying neoplastic disease

Pathogenesis
Tumor antigens evoke immune response to plakins, molecules found in desmosomes and hemidesmosomes playing key role in intermediate filament attachment; target antigens: desmoplakins I and II, bullous pemphigoid antigen I (BP230 kd or BPAG1), envoplakin, periplakin, and HD1/plectin

Clinical manifestation
Oral erosions or ulcerations, occurring anywhere in the mouth, usually as first sign of disease; similar lesions in nose, pharynx, tonsils, gastrointestinal tract, respiratory tract, genital mucosal surfaces; variable skin eruptions include diffuse erythema, vesiculobullous lesions, papules, scaly plaques, exfoliative erythroderma, erosions, or ulcerations; ocular involvement varies from conjunctivitis to symblepharon with corneal scarring; most common associated malignancy: non-Hodgkin's lymphoma; others: chronic lymphocytic leukemia, Castleman tumor, giant cell lymphoma, Waldenström macroglobulinemia, thymoma, bronchogenic squamous cell carcinoma, and follicular dendritic cell sarcoma

Differential diagnosis
Erythema multiforme; Stevens-Johnson syndrome; toxic epidermal necrolysis; pemphigus vulgaris; bullous pemphigoid; cicatricial pemphigoid; epidermolysis bullosa acquisita; lichen planus

Therapy

Prednisone; steroid-sparing drugs: azathioprine; cyclosporine; mycophenolate mofetil; cyclophosphamide; plasmapheresis

References

Kimyai-Asadi A, Jih MH (2001) Paraneoplastic pemphigus. International Journal of Dermatology 40(6):367–372

Parangi

▶ Yaws

Parapsoriasis

Synonym(s)

None

Definition

Group of cutaneous diseases characterized by scaly plaques having a resemblance to psoriasis

References

Lambert WC, Everett MA (1981) The nosology of parapsoriasis. Journal of the American Academy of Dermatology 5(4):373–395

Parapsoriasis en plaque

▶ Large plaque parapsoriasis

Parapsoriasis guttata

▶ Small plaque parapsoriasis

Paratyphoid fever

▶ Salmonellosis

Paresthetic notalgia

▶ Notalgia paresthetica

Parinaud oculoglandular syndrome

▶ Bartonellosis

Parinaud's oculoglandular syndrome

▶ Bartonellosis

Parkes-Weber syndrome

▶ Klippel-Trenaunay-Weber syndrome

Paronychia

Synonym(s)

Finger infection; runaround abscess; fingernail infection; runaround infection

Definition

Soft-tissue infection in the area around fingernail

Pathogenesis
Breakdown of protective barrier between nail plate and nail fold; entry of organisms into nail crevice allow bacterial or fungal colonization; acute variant: Staphylococcus aureus most common organism; chronic variant: Candida albicans most common pathogen; other causes: bacterial, mycobacterial, or viral infection; metastatic cancer; subungual melanoma; squamous cell carcinoma

Clinical manifestation
Acute variant: history of minor trauma or nail manipulation; pain, tenderness, and swelling in lateral nail fold; erythematous, edematous distal finger, sometimes with purulent exudate, most prominent in proximal and lateral nail fold area, with extension into eponychium; purulence of the nail bed; onycholysis
Chronic variant: inflammation, pain, and swelling occur episodically, often after exposure to moist environment; edematous, erythematous, tender nail folds without fluctuance; thickened and discolored nail plates, with transverse ridges

Differential diagnosis
Mucocutaneous candidiasis; herpetic whitlow; contact dermatitis; periungual wart; squamous cell carcinoma; melanoma; onychomycosis

Therapy
Acute variant: warm water soaks; amoxicillin; surgical incision and drainage if abscess forms; chronic variant: avoidance of inciting factors such as exposure to moist environments or skin irritants; avoidance of nail manipulation; if Candida is causative, topical clotrimazole and/or fluconazole; in recalcitrant cases, eponychial marsupialization

References
Rockwell PG (2001) Acute and chronic paronychia. American Family Physician 63(6):1113–1116

Paroxysmal nocturnal hemoglobinuria

Synonym(s)
Marchiafava-Micheli syndrome; Strübing-Marchiafava-Micheli syndrome

Definition
Clinical manifestation of red cell breakdown with release of hemoglobin into the urine manifested by dark-colored urine in the morning

Pathogenesis
Genetic mutation leading to inability to synthesize glycosyl-phosphatidylinositol (GPI) anchor that binds proteins to cell membranes; deficient hematopoiesis from diminished blood cell production with hypoplastic bone marrow

Clinical manifestation
Anemia associated with cola-colored urine; venous thrombosis: vein thrombosis manifested as raised, painful, red papules and nodules affecting large areas, subsiding within a few weeks, occasionally with necrosis and ulceration; hepatic vein thrombosis resulting in Budd-Chiari syndrome; abdominal vein thrombosis producing upper abdominal pain; cerebral vein thrombosis causing headache, papilledema, or pseudotumor cerebri

Differential diagnosis
Septic vasculitis; leukemia cutis; lymphoma; Wegener's granulomatosis; polyarteritis nodosa; cryoglobulinemia; Sweet syndrome; pyoderma gangrenosum

Therapy
Thrombotic complications: heparin emergently; then maintenance with an oral anticoagulant, such as warfarin; severe disease: bone marrow transplantation

References
Packman CH (1998) Pathogenesis and management of paroxysmal nocturnal haemoglobinuria. Blood Reviews 12(1):1–11

Partial albinism

▸ Piebaldism

Partial albinism with immunodeficiency

▸ Griscelli syndrome

Paru

▸ Yaws

Pasini and Pierini, atrophoderma of

▸ Atrophoderma of Pasini and Pierini

Pathergy

Definition
Erythematous papule, >2 mm, at the prick site 48 hours after superficial penetration with sterile needle

References
Lee LA (2001) Behcet disease. Seminars in Cutaneous Medicine & Surgery 20(1):53–57

Pattern baldness

▸ Androgenetic alopecia

Pearly penile papules

▸ Angiofibroma

Peat moss disease

▸ Sporotrichosis

Pediculosis

Synonym(s)
Lice; phthiriasis

Definition
Infestation with lice

Pathogenesis
Three types of human lice all belonging to order Anoplura; body lice infest clothing, laying their eggs on fibers in the fabric seams; head and pubic lice infest hair, laying eggs at base of hair fibers; organisms take blood meals by piercing host skin

Clinical manifestation
Pediculosis capitis (head lice): organisms most commonly found in retroauricular scalp; nits attach to hair shafts just above level of the scalp; pruritus with evidence of excoriation, particularly on the upper neck
Pediculosis corporis (body lice): nits found in the seams of clothing, not on body of host; hemosiderin-stained purpuric spots where lice have fed (maculae ceruleae)
Pediculosis pubis (pubic lice): lice and nits visible throughout pubic hair, extending onto adjacent hair-bearing areas; same organism also infests eyelashes

Differential diagnosis
Hair casts; seborrheic dermatitis; scabies; impetigo; benign pigmented purpura; folliculitis decalvans; acne keloidalis

Therapy
Permethrin 1% cream rinse[*]; complete nit removal with nit comb or chemical remover such as Step 2

References

Roberts RJ (2002) Clinical practice. Head lice. New England Journal of Medicine 346(21):1645–1650

Pediculosis capitis

▶ Pediculosis

Pediculosis corporis

▶ Pediculosis

Pediculosis palpebrum

▶ Pediculosis

Pediculosis pubis

▶ Pediculosis

Pellagra

Synonym(s)
Niacin deficiency; vitamin B_3 deficiency

Definition
Disease caused by a deficient diet or failure of the body to absorb niacin or tryptophan, characterized by photosensitive dermatitis, diarrhea, dementia, and ultimately death if untreated

Pathogenesis
Late stage of severe and prolonged niacin deficiency, vitamin required for adequate cellular function and metabolism as an essential component in coenzyme I and coenzyme II, which either donate or accept hydrogen ions in vital oxidation-reduction reactions; primary disease: inadequate nicotinic acid (i.e., niacin) and/or tryptophan intake in diet; secondary disease: adequate amounts of niacin present in the diet, but other diseases or conditions interfere with absorption and/or processing, such as chronic diarrhea, carcinoid syndrome, or Hartnup syndrome

Clinical manifestation
Cutaneous findings: symmetrical areas of involvement including dorsal surfaces of hands, face, neck (Casal necklace), arms, and feet
Early skin changes: edematous, exudative plaques, evolving to erythema on dorsa of hands, with pruritus and burning sensation; erythema sometimes evolves to cinnamon brown in color; coalescent bullae in some patients; dry brown scales and crusts, resulting from hemorrhage, scale, and erythema on sun-exposed skin
Late skin changes: darkly pigmented, thickened, dry, scaly, hard, rough, and cracked skin; glossitis with soreness of the mouth
Gastrointestinal findings: poor appetite; nausea; vomiting; diarrhea; epigastric discomfort; abdominal pain; increased salivation
Neuropsychiatric changes: headache, irritability; poor concentration; anxiety; delusional state; hallucinations; stupor; apathy; tremor; ataxia; spastic paresis

Differential diagnosis
Drug reaction; polymorphous light eruption; lupus erythematosus; erythropoietic protoporphyria; porphyria cutanea tarda; variegate porphyria; contact dermatitis; actinic reticuloid; leprosy; Hartnup syndrome

Therapy
Niacinamide[*]

References
Hendricks WM (1991) Pellagra and pellagralike dermatoses: etiology, differential diagnosis, dermatopathology, and treatment. Seminars in Dermatology 10(4):282–292

Pemphigoid

▶ Bullous pemphigoid

Pemphigoid gestationis

▶ Herpes gestationis

Pemphigoid vegetans

▶ Bullous pemphigoid

Pemphigus circinatus

▶ Dermatitis herpetiformis

Pemphigus erythematosus

▶ Pemphigus foliaceus

Pemphigus foliaceus

Synonym(s)
Superficial pemphigus

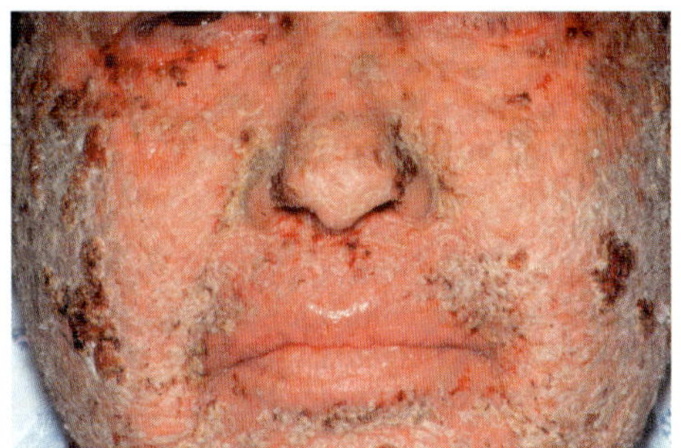

Pemphigus foliaceus Scaly, eroded plaques on the face

Definition
Autoimmune skin disorder characterized by formation of superficial blisters in normal-appearing skin

Pathogenesis
IgG (mainly IgG4 subclass) autoantibodies directed against desmoglein 1 (160 kDa), expressed mainly in the granular layer of the epidermis; medications and sunlight exposure may be precipitating factors

Clinical manifestation
Transient, superficial vesicles and bullae, transforming into crusted or scaly eroded plaques on an erythematous base, mainly in seborrhoic areas, with little or no involvement of mucous membranes; pemphigus erythematosus (Senear-Usher) variant: features of cutaneous lupus erythematosus and pemphigus foliaceus; red scaly plaques on the bridge of the nose and malar area; exfoliative erythroderma with extensive involvement; pemphigus herpetiformis variant: pruritic grouped papules and vesicles, suggestive of dermatitis herpetiformis; occasional oral erosions; drug-induced variant: may occur with penicillamine or captopril therapy, usually after at least 2 months of use; relatively mild signs and symptoms

Differential diagnosis
Pemphigus vulgaris; paraneoplastic pemphigus; bullous pemphigoid; erythema multiforme; dermatitis herpetiformis; lin-

ear IgA dermatosis; lupus erythematosus; impetigo; Darier disease; transient acantholytic dermatosis; Hailey-Hailey disease; subcorneal pustular dermatosis

Therapy
Corticosteroids, topical, super potent; prednisone; hydroxychloroquine; minocycline; steroid sparing agents: azathioprine; dapsone; cyclophosphamide

References
Huilgol SC, Black MM (1995) Management of the immunobullous disorders. II. Pemphigus. Clinical & Experimental Dermatology 20(4):283–293

Pemphigus neonatorum

► **Staphylococcal scalded skin syndrome**

Pemphigus paraneoplastica

► **Paraneoplastic pemphigus**

Pemphigus vegetans

► **Vegetans pemphigus**

Pemphigus vulgaris

Synonym(s)
None

Definition
Autoimmune blistering disease characterized by superficial vesicles and bullae of the skin and mucous membranes

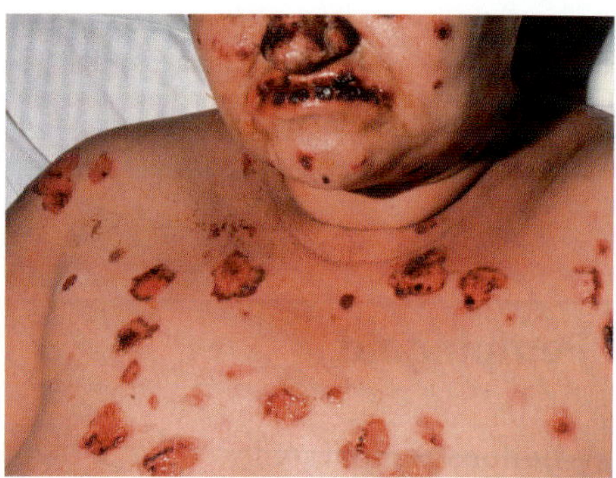

Pemphigus vulgaris. Eroded papules and plaques on the lip, face, and trunk

Pathogenesis
Mediated by circulating autoantibodies directed against keratinocyte cell surface antigens, desmoglein 1 and desmoglein 3, which may have direct effect on desmosomal function or may trigger cellular process resulting in acantholysis; may occur in patients with other autoimmune diseases, particularly myasthenia gravis and thymoma

Clinical manifestation
Mucous membrane lesions: painful, ill-defined, irregularly shaped, gingival, buccal, or palatine erosions; erosions sometimes spread to larynx with subsequent hoarseness; other sites of mucous membrane involvement: conjunctiva, esophagus, labia, vagina, cervix, penis, urethra, and anus

Skin lesions: fragile, flaccid vesicle or bulla filled with clear fluid, arising on normal skin or on an erythematous base; large erosions with lateral spread of blisters

Vegetating (vegetans) variant: lesions in skin folds form vegetating plaques with excessive granulation tissue and crusting; occur more frequently in intertriginous areas and on scalp and face

Differential diagnosis
Pemphigus foliaceus; paraneoplastic pemphigus; bullous pemphigoid; erythema multiforme; dermatitis herpetiformis; Hai-

ley-Hailey disease; aphthous stomatitis; herpetic stomatitis; erosive lichen planus

Therapy
Prednisone*; steroid sparing agents: azathioprine; dapsone; cyclophosphamide; mycophenolate mofetil; cyclosporine; auranofin; corticosteroids, topical, super potent; intravenous immunoglobulin (IVIG): 2 gm IV divided over 3 days every 4–8 weeks

References
Toth GG, Jonkman MF (2001) Therapy of pemphigus. Clinics in Dermatology 19(6):761–767

Pemphigus vulgaris chronicus

▶ Bullous pemphigoid

Penicillin G benzathine

Trade name(s)
Bicillin LA

Generic available
Yes

Drug class
Antibiotic

Mechanism of action
Inhibits penicillin-binding proteins, which cause inhibition of bacterial cell wall synthesis

Dosage form
300,000 units per ml; 600,000 units per ml for intramuscular injection

Dermatologic indications and dosage
See table

Common side effects
Cutaneous: urticaria and other skin eruptions
Gastrointestinal: nausea, vomiting, diarrhea

Serious side effects
Bone marrow: thrombocytopenia
Cutaneous: anaphylaxis
Gastrointestinal: pseudomembranous colitis
Renal: interstitial nephritis

Drug interactions
Aminoglycosides; oral contraceptives; methotrexate; probenecid

Contraindications/precautions
Hypersensitivity to drug class or component; caution in patients with cephalosporin allergy, seizure disorder, impaired renal function

References
Salkind AR, Cuddy PG Foxworth JW (2001) The rational clinical examination. Is this patient allergic to penicillin? An evidence-based analysis of the likelihood of penicillin allergy. Journal of the American Medical Association 285(19):2498–2950

Penicillin VK

Trade name(s)
Pen-Vee K; Veetids

Generic available
Yes

Drug class
Antibiotic

Mechanism of action
Inhibits penicillin-binding proteins, which cause inhibition of bacterial cell wall synthesis

Dosage form
250 mg, 500 mg tablets; 125 mg per 5 ml suspension; 250 mg per 5 ml suspension

Penicillin G benzathine. Dermatologic indications and dosage

Disease	Adult dosage	Child dosage
Bejel	2.4 million units IM (over age 10 years)	600,000 units IM as single injection
Blistering distal dactylitis	1.2 million units IM as single injection	0.3–0.6 million units IM for children < 27 kg; 0.9 million units IM for children > 27 kg
Erysipelas	1.2 million units IM as single injection	< 30 kg 300,000 units IM daily for 10–14 days
Impetigo	1.2 million units IM as single injection	0.3–0.6 million units IM for children < 27 kg; 0.9 million units IM for children > 27 kg
Pinta	2.4 million units IM (over age 10 years)	50,000 units IM as single dose
Scarlet fever	1.2 million units IM as single injection	300,000–600,00 units IM as single injection
Syphilis (primary, secondary, early latent)	2.4 million units IM (over age 10 years)	0.05 million units per kg IM weekly for 3 weeks; neonates > 1200 gm – 0.05 million units per kg IM for 1 dose
Tropical phagedenic ulcer	800,000–1,000,000 million units IM for a total dose of 6–10 million units	400,000–600,000 million units IM daily for a total dose of 3–5 million units
Yaws	1.2 million units IM as single injection	600,000 units IM as single injection

Dermatologic indications and dosage
See table

Common side effects
Cutaneous: urticaria and other skin eruptions
Gastrointestinal: nausea, vomiting, diarrhea

Serious side effects
Bone marrow: thrombocytopenia
Cutaneous: anaphylaxis, Stevens-Johnson syndrome, toxic epidermal necrolysis
Gastrointestinal: pseudomembranous colitis
Renal: interstitial nephritis

Drug interactions
Aminoglycosides; oral contraceptives; methotrexate; probenecid

Contraindications/precautions
Hypersensitivity to drug class or component; caution in patients with cephalosporin allergy, seizure disorder, impaired renal function

References
Salkind AR, Cuddy PG Foxworth JW (2001) The rational clinical examination. Is this patient allergic to penicillin? An evidence-based analysis of the likelihood of penicillin allergy. Journal of the American Medical Association 285(19):2498–2950

Penile fibromatosis

▶ **Peyronie's disease**

Penicillin VK. Dermatologic indications and dosage

Disease	Adult dosage	Child dosage
Acute necrotizing gingivitis	250–500 mg PO 4 times daily for 10 days	25–50 mg per kg PO divided into 4 doses daily for 10 days
Anthrax	250–500 mg PO for up to 60 days in bioterrorism situation	25–50 mg per kg PO divided into 4 doses daily for up to 60 days in bioterrorism situation
Blistering distal dactylitis	250–500 mg PO 4 times daily for 10 days	25–50 mg per kg PO divided into 4 doses daily for 10 days
Erysipelas	250–500 mg PO 4 times daily for 10–14 days	25–50 mg per kg daily PO divided into 4 doses for 10–14 days
Erysipeloid	250–500 mg PO 4 times daily for 10 days	25–50 mg per kg PO divided into 4 doses daily for 10 days
Impetigo	250–500 mg PO 4 times daily for 10 days	25–50 mg per kg PO divided into 4 doses daily for 10 days
Scarlet fever	500 mg PO for 10 days	25–50 mg per kg daily divided into 4 doses PO for 10 days

Penile lichen sclerosus

▶ Balanitis xerotica obliterans

Perforating folliculitis

Synonym(s)
Acquired perforating dermatosis; acquired perforating dermatitis

Definition
Disease characterized by disruption of the infundibular portion of the follicular wall, with transepidermal elimination of connective tissue elements and cellular debris

Pathogenesis
Theories of causation: premature follicular keratinization; primary alteration of connective tissue or deposition of foreign material within the superficial dermis, with subsequent engulfment and elimination by proliferative follicular epithelium; coiled hairs which disrupt the follicular epithelium

Clinical manifestation
Association with diabetes mellitus and renal failure; papules concentrated on hair-bearing portions of the extremities and buttocks; chronic, recurrent, asymptomatic, or mildly pruritic, scaly papules, often folliculocentric, with small central keratotic plugs and varying degrees of erythema; spontaneous remission may occurr

Differential diagnosis
Folliculitis; acne; pseudofolliculitis barbae; elastosis perforans serpiginosa; Kyrle disease; reactive perforating collagenosis; perforating granuloma annulare; prurigo nodularis; insect bite reaction

Therapy
Tretinoin

References
Chang P, Fernandez V (1993) Acquired perforating disease: report of nine cases. International Journal of Dermatology 32(12):874–876

Perfume phototoxicity

▶ Berloque dermatitis

Periadenitis mucosa necrotica recurrens

▶ Aphthous stomatitis

Perianal dermatitis

▶ Diaper dermatitis

Periarteritis nodosa

▶ Polyarteritis nodosa

Perifolliculitis capitis abscedens et suffodiens

▶ Dissecting cellulitis of scalp

Perineural fibroblastoma

▶ Neurilemmoma

Perineural myxoma

▶ Neurothekeoma

Perioral dermatitis

Synonym(s)
Rosacea-like dermatitis; periorificial dermatitis; light-sensitive seborrheid; chronic papulopustular facial dermatitis; granulomatous perioral dermatitis; steroid rosacea

Definition
Chronic facial dermatitis, occurring mostly in young women, characterized by small red papules and pustules around the mouth, nose, and eyes

Pathogenesis
Associated with topical corticosteroid use on the face

Clinical manifestation
Grouped follicular papules, papulovesicles, and papulopustules on an erythematous base, may evolve into plaques; located mainly in perioral area, but also in nasolabial fold and lateral portions of the lower eyelids

Differential diagnosis
Haber syndrome; acne vulgaris; rosacea; seborrheic dermatitis; lupus erythematosus; tinea faciei; contact dermatitis

Therapy
Discontinuance of all topical steroid use to the face[*]; tetracycline; doxycycline; minocycline; erythromycin

References
Kuflik JH, Janniger CK, Piela Z (2001) Perioral dermatitis: an acneiform eruption. Cutis 67(1):21–22

Periorificial dermatitis

▶ Perioral dermatitis

Perleche

▶ **Candidiasis**

Permethrin

Trade name(s)
Elimite; Nix

Generic available
No

Drug class
Anti-parasitic agent

Mechanism of action
Neural transmission blockade

Dosage form
5% cream; 1% cream rinse

Dermatologic indications and dosage
See table

Common side effects
Cutaneous: pruritus, redness, scalp swelling

Serious side effects
None

Drug interactions
None

Contraindications/precautions
Hypersensitivity to drug class or component

References
Wendel K, Rompalo A (2002) Scabies and pediculosis pubis: an update of treatment regimens and general review. Clinical Infectious Diseases 35(Suppl 2):S146–151

Pernio

▶ **Chilblains**

Perniosis

▶ **Chilblains**

Persistent light reaction

▶ **Chronic actinic dermatitis**

Persistent light reactivity

▶ **Chronic actinic dermatitis**

Permethrin. Dermatologic indications and dosage

Dosage	Adult dosage	Child dosage
Pediculosis capitis and pubis	Apply 1% cream rinse for 10 minutes; remove nits with comb provided with medication	Apply 1% cream rinse for 10 minutes; remove nits with comb provided with medication
Scabies	Apply 5% cream over whole skin surface below the neck; repeat in 7 days	Apply 5% cream over whole skin surface below the neck; repeat in 7 days

Peutz-Jeghers syndrome

Synonym(s)
None

Definition
Hereditary syndrome characterized by multiple gastrointestinal polyps and mucocutaneous pigmentation

Pathogenesis
Autosomal dominant trait; germline mutation of STK11 (serine threonine kinase 11) gene; protein likely regulated by phosphorylation by cAMP-dependent protein kinase A

Clinical manifestation
Dozens to thousands of hamartomatous polyps in stomach and intestines, primarily in the small intestine; macular hyperpigmentation on inner lining of the mouth, gums, lips, around the mouth, around the eyes, fingers or toes, and genitalia; pigmentation varying in color from bluish black to dark brown to blue; lesions may fade over time

Differential diagnosis
Familial adenomatous polyposis; Cowden disease; juvenile polyposis; Ruvalcaba-Myhre-Smith; Turcot syndrome; Carney's syndrome; Cronkhite-Canada syndrome

Therapy
No treatment for mucocutaneous pigmentation; repeated gastrointestinal endoscopic examinations with surgical removal of polyps suspicious for malignancy

References
McGarrity TJ, Kulin HE, Zaino RJ (2000) Peutz-Jeghers syndrome. American Journal of Gastroenterology 95(3):596–604

Peyronie disease

▶ Peyronie's disease

Peyronie's disease

Synonym(s)
Peyronie disease; plastic induration of the penis; penile fibromatosis; fibrous sclerosis of the penis; Van Buren's disease

Definition
Syndrome characterized by penile deformity and painful erection secondary to fibrosis of the tunica albuginea

Pathogenesis
Microtraumatic events during intercourse may be part of the cause; associated with Dupeytron's contracture in some patients; possibly associated with erectile dysfunction, diabetes mellitus, and hypertension, with partial erections leading to buckling during intercourse

Clinical manifestation
Penile pain and curvature during erection; fibrotic plaque over the midline of the penile shaft, either ventrally or dorsally; stabilization of signs and symptoms over time in many patients

Differential diagnosis
Scleroderma; lichen sclerosus; congenital penile curvature; penile fracture; penile dorsal vein thrombosis; leukemic infiltrate of the penis; syphilis; lymphogranuloma venereum

Therapy
Surgical correction[*]

References
Kadioglu A, Tefekli A, Erol B, Oktar T, Tunc M, Tellaloglu S (2002) A retrospective review of 307 men with Peyronie's disease. Journal of Urology 168(3):1075–1079

Pfeifer-Weber-Christian syndrome

▶ Weber-Christian disease

Pfeiffer's syndrome

▶ Acrocephalosyndactyly

Phaeohyphomycosis

▶ Chromoblastomycosis

Photochemotherapy

▶ Methoxsalen

Photodermatitis pigmentaria

▶ Berloque dermatitis

Photosensitive eczema

▶ Chronic actinic dermatitis

Photosensitivity dermatitis

▶ Chronic actinic dermatitis

Phototoxic dermatitis

▶ Contact dermatitis

Phthiriasis

▶ Pediculosis

Phycomycosis

▶ Mucormycosis

Phytosterolemia

Synonym(s)
Sitosterolemia; pseudohomozygous familial hypercholesterolemia

Definition
Inherited plant sterol storage disease, characterized by tendon and tuberous xanthomas and a strong tendency to develop premature coronary atherosclerosis

Pathogenesis
Autosomal recessive disorder; mutations in either of the genes for two proteins (ABCG5 or ABCG8) that preferentially pump plant sterols out of intestinal cells into the gut lumen and out of liver cells into the bile ducts, thereby decreasing sterol absorption; hyperabsorption of sitosterol from the gastrointestinal tract; decreased hepatic secretion of sitosterol with subsequent decreased elimination; dysfunctional cholesterol synthesis

Clinical manifestation
Xanthomas at any age, even in childhood; xanthelasma and corneal arcus; signs of premature coronary vascular disease, such as congestive heart failure; decreased range of motion and/or redness, swelling, and warmth of joints due to arthritis; splenomegaly

Differential diagnosis
Familial hypercholesterolemia; pseudo-homozygous familial hypercholesterolemia; cerebrotendinous xanthomatosis; lipid storage disorders

Therapy
Diet low in plant sterols*; cholestyramine: 3–4 g/d PO tid; ileal bypass surgery

References
Ling WH, Jones PJ (1995) Dietary phytosterols: a review of metabolism, benefits and side effects. Life Sciences 57(3):195–206

Pian

▶ Yaws

Pick disease

▶ Niemann-Pick disease

Pick's disease

▶ Niemann-Pick disease

Picker's acne

▶ Acne excoriée

Piebaldism

Synonym(s)
Partial albinism; familial white spotting

Definition
Familial disorder characterized by congenital white forelock and multiple symmetrical hypopigmented or depigmented macules and patches

Pathogenesis
Autosomal trait; mutations of the KIT proto-oncogene

Clinical manifestation
White forelock, with both hair and skin in the central frontal scalp often in triangular shape; permanently white from birth or when hair color first becomes apparent; may affect eyebrow and eyelash hair; symmetrical, irregular, hypopigmented macules and patches on face, trunk, and extremities; depigmented skin, sometimes showing narrow border of hyperpigmentation or island of pigmentation

Differential diagnosis
Vitiligo; albinism; nevus depigmentosus; hypomelanosis of Ito; Waardenburg's syndrome; chemical leukoderma; onchocerciasis; preus syndrome; pinta; Vogt-Koyanagi-Harada syndrome; leprosy; tinea versicolor; pityriasis alba

Therapy
No effective therapy

References
Le Poole C, Boissy RE (1997) Vitiligo. Seminars in Cutaneous Medicine & Surgery 16(1):3–14

Piedra

Synonym(s)
Black piedra, white piedra, trichosporosis, tinea nodosa; trichomycosis nodularis

Definition
Superficial fungal infection of the hair shafts, resulting in the formation of small nodules

Pathogenesis
Two pathogenic fungal organisms: Piedraia hortae causing black piedra; Trichosporon beigelii causing white piedra

Clinical manifestation
Black piedra: firmly adherent, black, firm, oval or elongated papules, composed of a mass of fungus cells; scalp most common site of involvement, but also seen in the beard and pubic areas
White piedra: soft, white or light-brown papules loosely adherent to or within the hair shaft; scalp most common site of involvement, but also seen in the beard and pubic areas; increased carriage rate in HIV-positive patients; may be sexually transmitted

Differential diagnosis
Pediculosis; tinea capitis; tinea corporis; trichomycosis axillaris

Therapy
Shaving or cutting the affected hair[*]
Black piedra: terbinafine
White piedra: topical azole antifungal agents; ciclopirox cream; itraconazole for recalcitrant disease

References
Drake L, Dinehart S, Farmer E, Goltz RW, et al. (1996) Guidelines for care for superficial mycotic infections of the skin: piedra. Journal of the American Academy of Dermatology 34(1):122–124

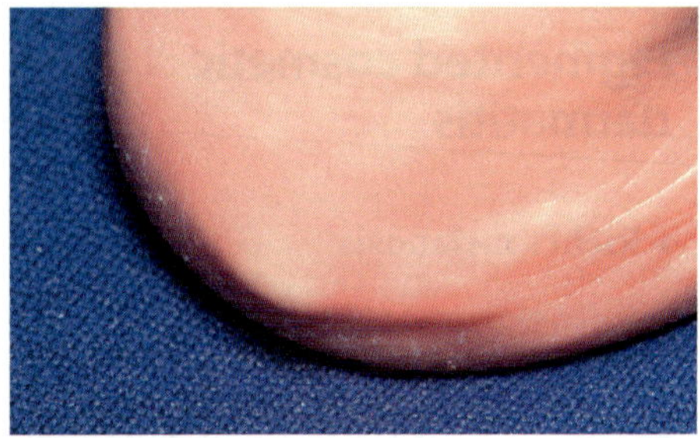

Piezogenic papule. Flesh-colored papules on the heel of the foot

Clinical manifestation
Asymptomatic or painful, flesh-colored papules over medial, posterior, and lateral aspects of the heels, usually occurring bilaterally; more common in overweight people, those with flat feet, with Ehlers-Danlos syndrome, or those who spend significant time on their feet

Differential diagnosis
Wart; benign adnexal tumor; foreign body granuloma

Therapy
No effective curative therapy; heel cup in shoe to minimize herniation

References
Pontious J, Lasday S, Mele R (1990) Piezogenic pedal papules extending into the arch. Case report and discussion. Journal of the American Podiatric Medical Association 80(8):444–445

Piezogenic papule

Synonym(s)
Piezogenic pedal papule; painful piezogenic papule

Definition
Papules of the feet resulting from herniation of fat through the dermis

Pathogenesis
Results from fat herniation into the dermis

Piezogenic pedal papule

▶ Piezogenic papule

Pigmented contact dermatitis

▶ Riehl's melanosis

Pigmented cosmetic dermatitis

▶ Riehl's melanosis

Pigmented hairy epidermal nevus

▶ Becker's nevus

Pigmented pretibial patches

▶ Diabetic dermopathy

Pigmented purpuric dermatitis

▶ Benign pigmented purpura

Pigmented purpuric eruption

▶ Benign pigmented purpura

Pigmented purpuric lichenoid dermatosis of Gougerot and Blum

▶ Benign pigmented purpura

Pigmented reticular dermatosis of the flexures

▶ Confluent and reticulated papillomatosis

Pilar cyst

Synonym(s)
Trichilemmal cyst; scalp cyst; wen; keratinous cyst

Definition
Keratin-producing cyst, derived from the hair follicle outer root sheath, usually appearing on the scalp

Pathogenesis
Derived from outer root sheath of hair follicle; may begin as budding from external root sheath as a genetically determined structural aberration

Clinical manifestation
Smooth, firm, subcutaneous nodule, usually on the scalp, without punctum, containing keratinous material

Differential diagnosis
Epidermoid cyst; pilomatricoma; dermoid cyst; lipoma; organized hematoma

Therapy
Surgical excision★

References
Bulengo-Ransby SM, Johnson C, Metcalf JS (1995) Enlarging scalp nodule. Proliferating trichilemmal cyst (PTC). Archives of Dermatology 131(6):721,724

Pilar tumor

Synonym(s)
Proliferating pilar tumor; proliferating trichilemmal cyst

Definition
Neoplasm derived from follicular outer root sheath, characterized by a large exophytic nodule, usually on the scalp

Pathogenesis
Arises as neoplastic transformation of pilar cyst; may be associated with trauma, irritation, or inflammation

Clinical manifestation
Asymptomatic, large, flesh-colored nodule; sometimes having inflammation, ulceration, bleeding, and/or yellowish discharge; occasional malignant degeneration

Differential diagnosis
Pilar cyst; lipoma; cylindroma; squamous cell carcinoma; cutaneous metastasis

Therapy
Complete surgical excision★

References
Mathis ED, Honningford JB, Rodriguez HE, Wind KP, Connolly MM, Podbielski FJ (2001) Malignant proliferating trichilemmal tumor. American Journal of Clinical Oncology 24(4):351–353

Pili annulati (ringed hairs)

Definition
Hair with alternating light and dark bands

References
Moffitt DL, Lear JT, de Berker DA. Peachey RD (1998) Pili annulati coincident with alopecia areata. Pediatric Dermatology 15(4):271–273

Pili bifurcati

Definition
Hairs arising from single papilla and then dividing into separate shafts

References
Camacho FM, Happle R, Tosti A, Whiting D (2000) The different faces of pili bifurcati. A review. European Journal of Dermatology 10(5):337–340

Pili incarnati

▶ **Pseudofolliculitis barbae**

Pili torti

Definition
Hair shaft that is flattened and twisted on its own axis, usually through 180° angle

References
Rogers M (1995) Hair shaft abnormalities: Part I. Australasian Journal of Dermatology 36(4):179–184

Pili trianguli canaculi

Definition
Uncombable hair syndrome characterized by hair shafts that are triangular in cross-section

References
Hicks J, Metry DW, Barrish J, Levy M (2001) Uncombable hair (cheveux incoiffables, pili trianguli et canaliculi) syndrome: brief review and role of scanning electron microscopy in diagnosis. Ultrastructural Pathology 25(2):99–103

Pili trianguli et canaliculi

▶ Uncombable hair syndrome

Pilomatricoma

Synonym(s)
Pilomatrixoma; calcifying epithelioma of Malherbe; trichomatrioma; benign calcifying epithelioma of Malherbe

Definition
Benign tumor of skin appendage, with differentiation toward hair matrix cells

Pathogenesis
May involve faulty suppression of apoptosis, with beta-catenin/LEF dysregulation

Clinical manifestation
Flesh-colored, firm nodule, often in the head and neck area; usually asymptomatic, but sometimes painful during episodes of inflammation

Differential diagnosis
Epidermoid cyst; basal cell carcinoma; trichilemmoma; trichoepithelioma; calcinosis cutis; cutaneous tuberculosis; granuloma annulare; sarcoidosis; cutaneous metastasis; Merkel cell carcinoma; osteoma cutis; dermatofibrosarcoma protuberans

Therapy
Surgical excision[*]

References
Sassmannshausen J, Chaffins M (2001) Pilomatrix carcinoma: a report of a case arising from a previously excised pilomatrixoma and a review of the literature. Journal of the American Academy of Dermatology 44(2 Suppl):358–361

Pilomatrixoma

▶ Pilomatricoma

Pincer nail

Definition
Excessive transverse curvature of the nail plate, often of the great toe, with grooving into the lateral and medial nail fold

References
Baran R, Haneke E, Richert B (2001) Pincer nails: definition and surgical treatment. Dermatologic Surgery 27(3):261–266

Pink disease

▶ Acrodynia

Pinkus tumor

▶ Fibroepithelioma of Pinkus

Pinta

Synonym(s)
Azul; carate; endemic treponematosis; mal de pinto

Definition
Bacterial infection of the skin caused by a treponemal pathogen, characterized by

papules and plaques in the early stage and dyschromic patches in the late stage

Pathogenesis
Treponema carateum is causative agent, separate species from Treponema pallidum, the cause of syphilis; unclear mode of transmission; possibly transmitted by skin-to-skin contact

Clinical manifestation
Papule that slowly enlarges to become pruritic plaque; dorsum of foot and legs most common sites; regional lymphadenopathy; lesions become pigmented with age; sometimes copper to gray to slate; late lesions are achromic or hyperpigmented

Differential diagnosis
Syphilis; yaws; leprosy; tinea corporis; tinea versicolor; vitiligo; post-inflammatory hypopigmentation; pityriasis alba

Therapy
Penicillin G*; therapy for penicillin-allergic patients: tetracycline; erythromycin

References
Parish JL (2000) Treponemal infections in the pediatric population. Clinics in Dermatology 18(6):687–700

Pitted keratolysis

Synonym(s)
Keratoma plantarum sulcatum; keratolysis plantaris sulcatum; ringed keratolysis

Definition
Bacterial infection characterized by crateriform pitting primarily affecting the pressure-bearing aspects of the plantar surface of the feet

Pathogenesis
Infection with Micrococcus sedentarius, Dermatophilus congolensis, or species of

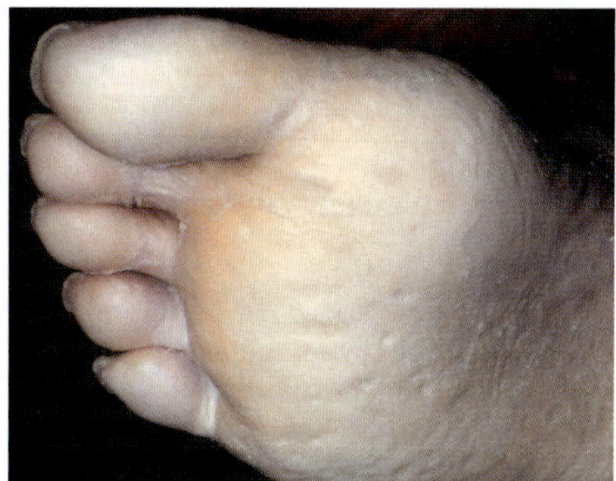

Pitted keratolysis. Pits on the plantar aspect of the foot

Corynebacterium or Actinomyces; under appropriate conditions (i.e., prolonged occlusion, hyperhidrosis, increased skin surface pH), bacterial proliferate and produce proteinases that destroy stratum corneum, creating pits; malodor secondary to production of sulfur-compound by-products

Clinical manifestation
Pits in stratum corneum, with some confluence, irregular erosions, or sulci, most often on plantar aspects of feet; usually asymptomatic, but may have malodor, hyperhidrosis, sliminess, and occasionally soreness or itching

Differential diagnosis
Plantar warts; tinea pedis; essential hyperhidrosis; basal cell nevus syndrome; keratolysis exfoliativa; punctate keratoderma; arsenical keratoses

Therapy
Erythromycin, topical; clindamycin, topical; erythromycin, oral; limited use of occlusive footwear; reduced foot friction with properly fitting shoes; absorbent cotton socks, changed frequently

References
Omura EF, Rye B (1994) Dermatologic disorders of the foot. Clinics in Sports Medicine 13(4):825–841

Pityriasis alba

Synonym(s)
Pityriasis simplex; pityriasis sicca faciei

Definition
Disorder characterized by asymptomatic, scaly, variably hypopigmented plaques, mostly occurring in children

Pathogenesis
Associated with atopic diathesis; may represent post-inflammatory change

Clinical manifestation
Solitary or multiple, rounded, oval, or irregular plaques that are red, pink, or skin colored, with pityriasiform scale, most often on the face, neck, and lateral arms; occurs mainly in children

Differential diagnosis
Tinea corporis; tinea versicolor; sarcoidosis; vitiligo; psoriasis; leprosy; mycosis fungoides; seborrheic dermatitis; nummular eczema

Therapy
Corticosteroids, topical, low potency[*]; emollients

References
Galan EB, Janniger CK (1998) Pityriasis alba. Cutis 61(1):11–13

Pityriasis corporis

▶ Seborrheic dermatitis

Pityriasis lichenoides

Synonym(s)
Mucha-Habermann disease; guttate parapsoriasis; pityriasis lichenoides chronica; pityriasis lichenoides et varioliformis acuta

Definition
Disease spectrum ranging from an acute papulovesicular eruption to a chronic eruption consisting of small, scaly, red papules

Pathogenesis
Unclear whether two distinct diseases or variants of same process; acute disease (Mucha-Habermann disease) may be hypersensitivity reaction to infectious agent or some other environmental insult

Clinical manifestation
Acute variant (Mucha-Habermann disease): abrupt appearance of multiple pruritic papules on the trunk, buttocks, and proximal extremities, evolving to vesicles which rupture and produce hemorrhagic crusts; lesions heal with postinflammatory leukoderma or hyperpigmentation; may have lesions identical to those of chronic variant

Chronic variant (pityriasis lichenoides chronica): at the subacute end of spectrum, may develop over days; distributed over the trunk, buttocks, and proximal extremities; small, erythematous-to-reddish brown papules, with fine scale; often polymorphic, with lesions at different stages of evolution

Differential diagnosis
Acute variant: varicella; vasculitis; scabies; dermatitis herpetiformis; external trauma; insect bite reaction

Chronic variant: psoriasis; small plaque parapsoriasis; mycosis fungoides; tinea corporis; lupus erythematosus; pityriasis rosea; syphilis; viral exanthem

Therapy
Acute variant: methotrexate; tetracycline; erythromycin; photochemotherapy

Chronic variant: phototherapy; photochemotherapy; corticosteroids, topical, high potency

References
Patel DG, Kihiczak G, Schwartz RA, Janniger CK Lambert WC (2000) Pityriasis lichenoides. Cutis 65(1):17–20,23

Pityriasis lichenoides chronica

▶ Pityriasis lichenoides

Pityriasis lichenoides et varioliformis acuta

▶ Pityriasis lichenoides

Pityriasis oleosa

▶ Seborrheic dermatitis

Pityriasis pilaris

▶ Keratosis pilaris

Pityriasis rosea

Synonym(s)
None

Definition
Self-limited eruption consisting of multiple, oval, scaling papules often preceded by a single larger plaque known as "herald patch"

Pathogenesis
May be viral exanthem, although no virus consistently isolated

Clinical manifestation
Herald patch: single (or few) annular, scaly plaque(s), on neck or trunk; several days after herald patch, onset of multiple, salmon-colored, scaly papules; long axes of the lesions oriented in parallel fashion along cleavage lines; occurs on the trunk, abdomen, back, and the proximal upper extremities; eruption clears in 6–12 weeks, with only rare recurrences

Differential diagnosis
Syphilis; pityriasis lichenoides; tinea corporis; mycosis fungoides; lupus erythematosus; drug eruption; viral exanthem; nummular eczema; seborrheic keratosis

Therapy
Erythromycin; UVB phototherapy

References
Nelson JS, Stone MS (2000) Update on selected viral exanthems. Current Opinion in Pediatrics 12(4):359–364

Pityriasis rubra pilaris

Synonym(s)
None

Definition
Chronic disorder characterized by reddish-orange scaling plaques, palmoplantar keratoderma, and keratotic follicular papules

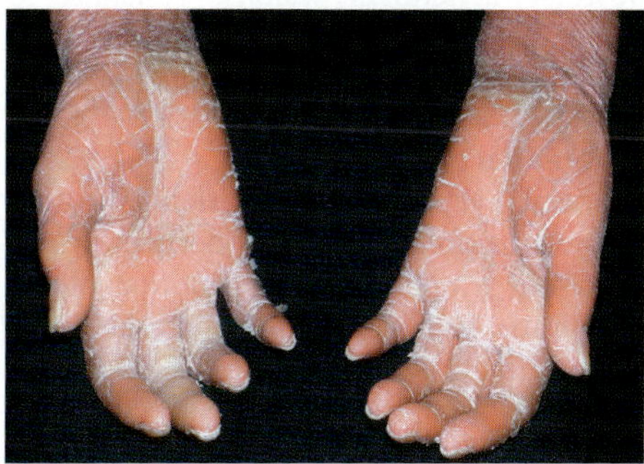

Pityriasis rubra pilaris. Marked scale and erythema of the palms

Pathogenesis
Unknown

Clinical manifestation
Orange-red or salmon-colored scaling plaques with sharp borders, which may expand to become whole body erythroderma, with islands of sparing; follicular hyperkeratosis on the dorsal aspects of the proximal phalanges, elbows, and wrists; palmoplantar hyperkeratosis; nails with distal yellow-brown discoloration, subungual hyperkeratosis, longitudinal ridging, nail plate thickening, and splinter hemorrhages

Subtypes:

Type I: most common form; acute onset of erythroderma with islands of sparing, palmoplantar keratoderma, and follicular hyperkeratosis; 80% of patients have remission in about 3 years

Type II: ichthyosiform lesions; areas of eczematous change; alopecia; long duration of disease

Type III: very similar to type I, but onset within the first 2 years of life

Type IV: occurs in prepubertal children; sharply demarcated areas of follicular hyperkeratosis and erythema of the knees and elbows, without progression

Type V: most cases of familial disease belong to this group; early onset and chronic course; prominent follicular hyperkeratosis; scleroderma-like changes on the palms and soles; infrequent erythema

Type VI: HIV-associated; nodulocystic and pustular acneiform lesions; resistant to standard treatments but sometimes responds to antiretroviral therapies

Differential diagnosis
Psoriasis; erythroderma variabilis; other causes of exfoliative erythroderma, including T-cell lymphoma, drug eruption, atopic dermatitis, pemphigus foliaceus, and seborrheic dermatitis

Therapy
Methotrexate; cyclosporine; acitretin; thioguanine

References
Albert MR, Mackool BT (1999) Pityriasis rubra pilaris. International Journal of Dermatology 38(1):1–11

Pityriasis sicca

▶ Seborrheic dermatitis

Pityriasis sicca faciei

▶ Pityriasis alba

Pityriasis simplex

▶ Pityriasis alba

Pityriasis simplex capitis

▶ Seborrheic dermatitis

Pityriasis versicolor

▶ Tinea versicolor

Pityriasis vulgaris

▶ Ichthyosis vulgaris

Pityrosporom folliculitis

▶ Folliculitis

Planar xanthoma

▶ Xanthoma

Plane xanthoma

▶ Xanthoma

Plantar fibromatosis

Synonym(s)
Ledderhose disease

Definition
Heterogeneous group of conditions in plantar location with histologic features of mature collagen and fibroblasts with no malignant cytologic features

Pathogenesis
Associated with repeated trauma, long-term alcohol consumption, chronic liver disease, diabetes mellitus; may have other fibrosing conditions such as Dupeytron's contracture, knuckle pads, or Peyronie disease

Clinical manifestation
One or more small, asymptomatic, slowly progressive, round or flattened, hard nodules generally located on the medial side of the sole, often bilaterally symmetrical

Differential diagnosis
Desmoid tumor; keloid/hypertrophic scar; granuloma annulare; calcinosis cutis; mucocoele; dermatofibrosarcoma protuberans; neurofibroma; neuroid nevus; melanoma; osteoma; gout

Therapy
Fasciotomy and excision of the fibrous tissue for symptomatic lesions

References
Godette GA, O'Sullivan M, Menelaus MB (1997) Plantar fibromatosis of the heel in children: a report of 14 cases. Journal of Pediatric Orthopedics 17(1):16–17

Plantar wart

▶ Wart

Plaque-like dermal fibromatosis

▶ Dermatomyofibroma

Plasma cell balanitis

▶ Zoon balanitis

Plasma cell balanitis of Zoon

▶ Zoon balanitis

Plasma cell mucositis

▶ Zoon balanitis

Plastic induration of the penis

▶ Peyronie's disease

Plumber's itch

▶ Cutaneous larva migrans

Pluriorificial keratosis of Olmsted

▶ Olmsted syndrome

Podofilox

Trade name(s)
Condylox

Generic available
No

Drug class
Podophyllum resin (podophyllin)

Mechanism of action
Inhibits microtubular function by combining with a component of microtubules

Dosage form
0.5% solution, gel

Dermatologic indications and dosage
See table

Common side effects
Cutaneous: burning sensation, irritant dermatitis

Serious side effects
None

Drug interactions
None

Contraindications/precautions
Hypersensitivity to drug class or component

References
Beutner KR (1996) Podophyllotoxin in the treatment of genital warts. Current Problems in Dermatology 24:227–232

Podophyllin

▶ Podofilox

POEMS syndrome

Synonym(s)
Crow-Fukase syndrome; Takatsuki syndrome

Definition
Multisystem disease consisting of polyneuropathy, organomegaly, endocrinologic disorders, monoclonal gammopathy, and various skin abnormalities

Pathogenesis
Plasma cell disorder central to other findings

Podofilox. Dermatologic indications and dosage

Disease	Adult dosage	Child dosage
Bowenoid papulosis	Apply twice daily for 3 consecutive days weekly, up to 4 weeks	Not indicated
Genital wart	Apply twice daily for 3 consecutive days weekly, up to 4 weeks	Not indicated

Clinical manifestation

Skin manifestations: diffuse hyperpigmentation; lower extremity edema; hypertrichosis, usually most pronounced over the face, limbs, and chest; sclerodermoid changes; angiomas; whitening of the proximal nails; hepatomegaly; splenomegaly; lymphadenopathy; abnormal estrogen levels with gynecomastia; hypothyroidism; hyperprolactinemia; hypoparathyroidism

Neurologic manifestations: progressive bilateral symmetric disturbances involving both motor and sensory nerves; begins distally and has progressive proximal spread; osteosclerotic myeloma or monoclonal gammopathy

Differential diagnosis

Scleroderma; Raynaud disease; multiple myeloma; Addison's disease

Therapy

Treatment of underlying plasma cell disorder with corticosteroids and chemotherapy and/or radiation therapy; surgical excision of isolated plasmacytoma

References

Koike H, Sobue G (2000) Crow-Fukase syndrome. Neuropathology. 20 Suppl:S69–72

Poikiloderma atrophicans vasculare

Synonym(s)

None

Definition

Term used to describe plaques with cigarette paper-like atrophy, telangiectasia, and mottled hyperpigmentation

▶ **Large plaque parapsoriasis**

References

Howard MS, Smoller BR (2000) Mycosis fungoides: classic disease and variant presentations. Seminars in Cutaneous Medicine & Surgery 19(2):91–99

Poikiloderma congenitale

▶ **Rothmund-Thomson syndrome**

Poikiloderma of Civatte

Synonym(s)

Berkshire neck

Definition

Erythema and mottled pigmentation seen on the sides of the neck, related to chronic sun exposure

Pathogenesis

Associated with chronic sun exposure in fair-skinned individuals

Clinical manifestation

Reddish-brown reticulate pigmentation with atrophy and telangiectasia, usually in symmetrical plaques on sides of the neck

Differential diagnosis

Poikiloderma atrophicans vasculare; Rothmund-Thomson syndrome; Bloom syndrome; lupus erythematosus; dermatomyositis; berloque dermatitis; Riehl's melanosis

Therapy

Intense pulsed-light (IPL) source; flashlamp-pumped pulse dye laser (FPDL, 585 nm); potassium-titanyl-phosphate (KTP) laser

References

Ross BS, Levine VJ, Ashinoff R (1997) Laser treatment of acquired vascular lesions. Dermatologic Clinics 15(3):385–396

Poikiloderma of Kindler

▶ **Kindler syndrome**

Poikiloderma vasculare atrophicans

▶ Large plaque parapsoriasis

Polyarteritis nodosa

Synonym(s)
Periarteritis nodosa

Definition
Systemic vasculitis characterized by necrotizing inflammatory lesions affecting predominately medium and small muscular arteries

Pathogenesis
May be immune complex-mediated process in hepatitis B-associated disease

Clinical manifestation
Constitutional signs and symptoms: fever; weight loss; myalgias; abdominal pain
Skin findings: palpable purpura; cutaneous infarctions with ulceration, discontinuous livedo reticularis (retiform purpura); ischemic changes of the distal digits; subcutaneous nodules; purely cutaneous involvement sometimes occurs; may have myalgias, arthralgias, and peripheral neuropathy
Systemic disease: mesenteric thrombosis and ischemia; renal vascular nephropathy; sensory and motor neuropathies; mononeuritis multiplex; coronary arteritis; tachycardia; retinal vasculitis

Differential diagnosis
Microscopic polyangiitis; septicemia, infective endocarditis, malignancy; atherosclerosis; rheumatoid arthritis; Sjögren syndrome; cryoglobulinemia; lupus erythematosus

Therapy
Prednisone★; cyclophosphamide; cyclosporine

References
Guillevin L (1999) Treatment of classic polyarteritis nodosa in 1999. Nephrology Dialysis Transplantation 14(9):2077–2079

Polychondropathy

▶ Relapsing polychondritis

Polykeratosis congenita

▶ Pachyonychia congenital

Polymorphic eruption of pregnancy

▶ Pruritic urticarial papules and plaques of pregnancy

Polymorphic light eruption

▶ Polymorphous light eruption

Polymorphic prurigo syndrome

▶ Sulzberger-Garbe syndrome

Polymorphic reticulosis

▶ Lymphomatoid granulomatosis

Polymorphous light eruption

Synonym(s)
Polymorphic light eruption

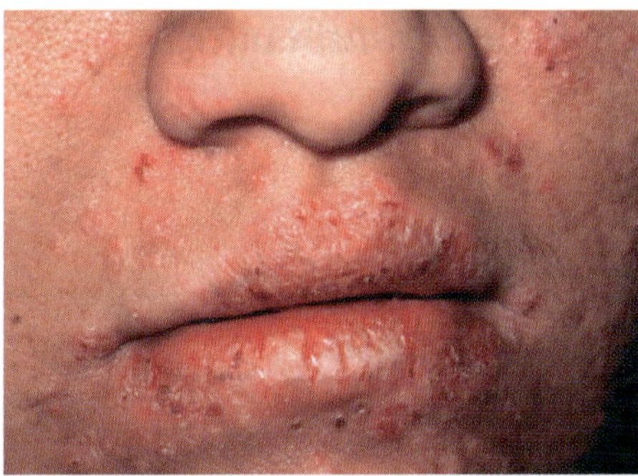

Polymorphous light eruption. Flesh-colored and eroded papules on the face and lips

Definition
Photodermatosis characterized by recurrent, abnormal, delayed reactions to sunlight, ranging from erythematous papules, papulovesicles, and plaques to erythema multiforme-like lesions

Pathogenesis
Ultraviolet A (UVA) light causative in most cases; mechanism of inflammatory response unclear; immunologic factors probably important

Clinical manifestation
Often seen at onset of a vacation in a sunny place or at high altitude; sun-exposed skin, especially that normally covered in winter, most commonly affected; improves as the summer progresses; eruption appears within hours to days of exposure and subsides over 1–7 days without scarring; pruritic papules (most common), plaques, papulovesicles, and erythema multiforme-like lesions, often combined in the same patient; small papular lesions sometimes coalesce to form eczematous plaque; autosensitization sometimes leads to a generalized involvement; cheilitis occurs mainly in Native American children with a combined polymorphous light and atopic dermatitis-like syndrome (actinic prurigo)

Differential diagnosis
Solar urticaria; lupus erythematosus; erythropoietic protoporphyria; actinic dermatitis; hydroa vacciniforme; drug-induced photosensitivity

Therapy
Prophylactic broadband UVB phototherapy before the onset of the sunny season; prophylactic photochemotherapy (PUVA) before the onset of the sunny season; prophylactic narrowband UVB phototherapy before the onset of the sunny season; hydroxychloroquine; thalidomide; beta carotene: 120–300 mg PO per day; niacinamide: 1000 mg PO 3 times daily for 2 weeks; corticosteroids, topical, high potency; prednisone for severe acute flares

References
Naleway AL. Polymorphous light eruption. International Journal of Dermatology 41(7):377–383

Polymorphous prurigo syndrome

▶ Sulzberger-Garbe syndrome

Polyostotic dysplasia

▶ McCune-Albright Syndrome

Polyostotic fibrous dysplasia

▶ McCune-Albright syndrome

Polythelia

▶ **Supernumerary nipple**

Pomade acne

Synonym(s)
None

Definition
Form of acne occurring in those using heavy pomades on the hair

Pathogenesis
Comedones caused by heavy oils in pomades, which plug sebaceous follicles; other chemicals in pomades may be irritating to skin

Clinical manifestation
Multiple comedones with few inflammatory papules on scalp, forehead, and temples

Differential diagnosis
Milia; nevus comedonicus; Favre-Racouchot disease; radiation acne; chloracne; flat warts; appendageal tumors (syringoma, etc.); sebaceous gland hyperplasia

Therapy
Tretinoin*; avoidance of comedogenic agents on scalp

References
Laude TA (1995) Approach to dermatologic disorders in black children. Seminars in Dermatology 14(1):15–20

Pompholyx

▶ **Dyshidrotic eczema**

Ponytail band alopecia

▶ **Traction alopecia**

Popsicle panniculitis

▶ **Cold panniculitis**

Porokeratosis

Synonym(s)
Porokeratosis of Mibelli; disseminated superficial actinic porokeratosis; DSAP; porokeratosis palmaris et plantaris disseminata; linear porokeratosis; punctate porokeratosis; hyperkeratosis eccentrica; hyperkeratosis figurata centrifuga atrophicans

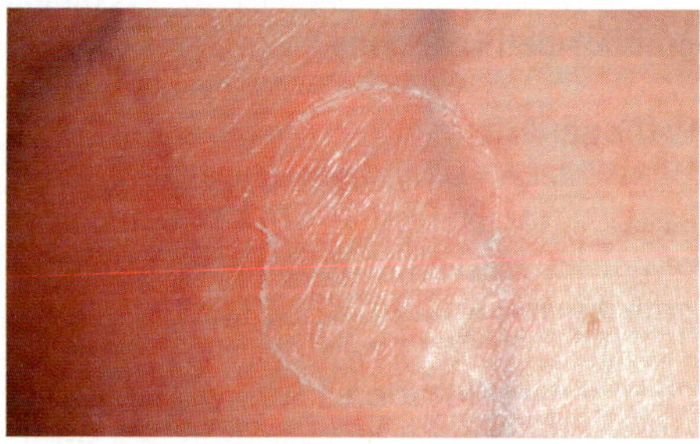

Porokeratosis. Plaque with thready border of scale

Definition
Keratotic lesion characterized by peripheral spread, a thin thready border, and an atrophic center

Pathogenesis
Clonal hyperproliferation of atypical keratinocytes leading to the formation of the cornoid lamella, which forms the boundary

between abnormal and normal keratinocytes; loss of heterozygosity may be mechanism for linear porokeratosis; genetic factors in disseminated superficial actinic porokeratosis

Clinical manifestation
Porokeratosis of Mibelli: slowly expanding, irregularly shaped plaque with a raised, thready border; lesion slightly hypopigmented or hyperpigmented, minimally scaly, hairless, slightly atrophic, and anhidrotic
Disseminated superficial actinic porokeratosis: multiple, small, indistinct, light brown papules with a threadlike border, on the extensor surface of upper and lower extremities
Linear porokeratosis: grouped, linear, annular papules and plaques with a raised peripheral ridge on an extremity, the trunk, and/or the head and neck area, often in a dermatomal distribution

Differential diagnosis
Actinic keratosis; squamous cell carcinoma; granuloma annulare; superficial basal cell carcinoma; annular lichen planus; elastosis perforans serpiginosa; flat warts

Therapy
Fluorouracil cream; imiquimod 5% cream applied 3 times weekly for 4–8 weeks; destruction by liquid nitrogen cryotherapy or by electrodesiccation and curettage; calcipotriene; isotretinoin; dermabrasion

References
Sehgal VN, Jain S, Singh N (1996) Porokeratosis. Journal of Dermatology 23(8):517–525

Porokeratosis of Mibelli

▶ Porokeratosis

Porokeratosis palmaris et plantaris disseminata

▶ Porokeratosis

Poroma

Synonym(s)
Eccrine poroma; apocrine poroma; juxtaepidermal poroma; hidroacanthoma simplex; dermal duct tumor

Definition
Adnexal neoplasm composed of benign epithelial cells that show tubular (usually ductal) differentiation of either eccrine or apocrine lineage

Pathogenesis
Unknown

Clinical manifestation
Asymptomatic, solitary, slow-growing, or stable papule or nodule; exophytic lesions sometimes have surface erosion or ulceration; may appear as if erupting through a collarette; eccrine variant almost always on the palm or sole

Differential diagnosis
Acrospiroma; pyogenic granuloma; melanoma; hidradenoma; wart; callus; foreign body reaction

Therapy
Surgical excision[*]

References
Kamiya H, Oyama Z, Kitajima Y (2001) "Apocrine" poroma: review of the literature and case report. Journal of Cutaneous Pathology 28(2):101–104

Porphyria

Synonym(s)
None

Definition
Group of inherited disorders involving abnormalities in the production of heme, resulting in abnormal accumulations of porphyrins

References
Sassa S (2002) The porphyrias. Photodermatology, Photoimmunology & Photomedicine 18(2):56–67

Porphyria cutanea tarda

Synonym(s)
Hepatic porphyria

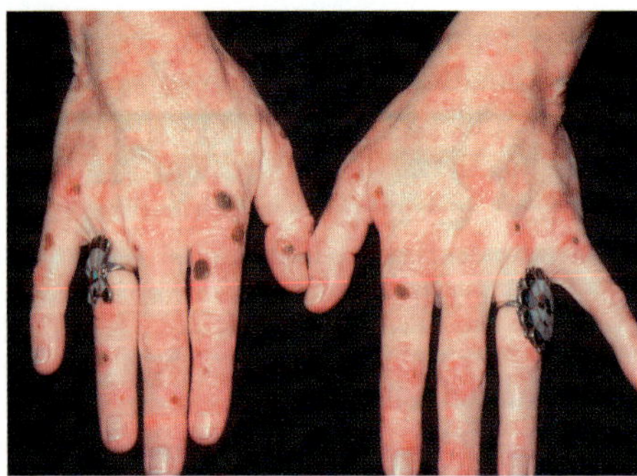

Porphyria cutanea tarda. Numerous eroded papules and scars over the dorsal aspects of the hands

Definition
Group of related disorders arising from deficient activity of the heme-synthetic enzyme uroporphyrinogen decarboxylase in the liver, characterized by photosensitivity eruption

Pathogenesis
Reduced activity of uroporphyrinogen decarboxylase in hepatic heme synthesis, resulting in overproduction of porphyrin by-products of the heme biosynthetic pathway; photoexcited porphyrins in the skin mediate oxidative damage to biomolecular targets, producing photosensitivity reaction

Clinical manifestation
Fragility in sun-exposed skin after mechanical trauma, leading to erosions and bullae, most commonly on dorsal hands, forearms, and face; healing of crusted erosions and blisters leaves scars, milia, and dyspigmentation; hypertrichosis, mostly over temporal and malar facial areas; melasmalike hyperpigmentation of face; erythematous suffusion of central face, neck, upper chest, and shoulder; scarring alopecia; photo-onycholysis; scleroderma-like papules on trunk and extremities

Differential diagnosis
Other forms of porphyria; pseudoporphyria; bullous pemphigoid; epidermolysis bullosa acquisita; bullous diabeticorum; bullous lupus erythematosus; polymorphous light eruption

Therapy
Therapeutic phlebotomy, 1 unit every 2–3 weeks until clinical response or until hemoglobin falls below 10.5–11 gm*; hydroxychloroquine; chelation therapy with desferrioxamine

References
Sarkany RP (2001) The management of porphyria cutanea tarda. Clinical & Experimental Dermatology 26(3):225–232

Porphyria erythropoietica

▶ Erythropoietic porphyria

Porphyria variegata

▶ Variegate porphyria

Port-wine mark

▶ Nevus flammeus

Port wine stain

▶ Nevus flammeus

Posterior lingual papillary atrophy

▶ Median rhomboid glossitis

Postinfectious cockade purpura of early childhood

▶ Acute hemorrhagic edema of infancy

Postinflammatory anetoderma of Jadassohn and Pellizzari

▶ Anetoderma

Postinflammatory hypermelanosis

▶ Postinflammatory hyperpigmentation

Postinflammatory hyperpigmentation

Synonym(s)
Postinflammatory hypermelanosis; melanotic hyperpigmentation

Definition
Sequela of inflammatory skin disorders and therapeutic interventions, characterized by macular hyperpigmentation

Pathogenesis
Epidermal hypermelanosis: inflammatory products stimulate epidermal melanocytes to increase melanin synthesis, with subsequent increased transfer of pigment to surrounding keratinocytes
Dermal melanosis: inflammation disrupts basal cell layer, causing melanin pigment to fall into dermis, with subsequent trapping by macrophages (pigmentary incontinence)

Clinical manifestation
Irregular, light brown-to-black macules and/or patches at sites of prior inflammation

Differential diagnosis
Tinea versicolor; acanthosis nigricans; lichen planus; lupus erythematosus; nevoid hypermelanosis; melasma; amyloidosis; ashy dermatosis

Therapy
Hydroquinone; tretinoin; azelaic acid

References

Pandya AG, Guevara IL (2000) Disorders of hyperpigmentation. Dermatologic Clinics 18(1):91–98

Prader-Willi syndrome

Synonym(s)
None

Definition
Developmental syndrome consisting of mental retardation, abnormal behavior, and hypopigmentation

Pathogenesis
Chromosomal and molecular changes of the proximal region of chromosome 5

Clinical manifestation
Neonatal hypotonia; hyperphagia and obesity; short stature; developmental delay; behavioral abnormalities; skin pigment dilution of the skin and eyes

Differential diagnosis
Angelman syndrome; oculocutaneous albinism

Therapy
Sun protection

References

Khan NL, Wood NW (1999) Prader-Willi and Angelman syndromes: update on genetic mechanisms and diagnostic complexities. Current Opinion in Neurology 12(2):149–154

Prednisone

Trade name(s)
Deltasone; Sterapred

Generic available
Yes

Drug class
Glucocorticoid

Mechanism of action
Nuclear glucocorticoid receptor binding and gene transcription; reduction of synthesis of inflammatory cells and access of those cells to sites of inflammation

Dosage form
1 mg, 2.5 mg, 5 mg, 10 mg, 20 mg, 50 mg tablet

Dermatologic indications and dosage
See table

Common side effects
Cardiovascular: hypertension, fluid retention
Cutaneous: skin fragility and ecchymoses, skin atrophy, impaired wound healing
Endocrine: Cushingoid features, hyperglycemia
Gastrointestinal: nausea, vomiting, dyspepsia, weight gain
Genitourinary: menstrual irregularities
Infectious: increased susceptibility to infection
Musculoskeletal: osteopenia
Neurologic: mood change, insomnia

Serious side effects
Cardiovascular: congestive heart failure
Endocrine: adrenal insufficiency upon withdrawal
Gastrointestinal: peptic ulcer
Genitourinary: menstrual irregularities
Infectious: increased susceptibility to infection
Musculoskeletal: aseptic hip necrosis
Neurologic: psychosis, pseudotumor cerebri

Drug interactions
Barbiturates; beta agonists; COX-2 inhibitors; cyclosporine; digoxin; thiazide diuretics; glyburide/metformin; non-steroidal anti-inflammatory agents; phenytoin; rifampin; warfarin; many others

Prednisone. Dermatologic indications and dosage

Disease	Adult dosage	Child dosage
Acne vulgaris	0.5–2 mg per kg daily PO as a single AM dose for 7–21 days	0.5–2 mg per kg daily PO as a single AM dose for 7–21 days
Acute febrile neutrophilic dermatosis	0.5–2 mg per kg daily PO as a single AM dose	0.5–2 mg per kg daily PO as a single AM dose
Acute generalized exanthematous pustular dermatitis	0.5–2 mg per kg daily PO as a single AM dose for 7–21 days	0.5–2 mg per kg daily PO as a single AM dose for 7–21 days
Acute graft versus host reaction	0.5–2 mg per kg daily PO as a single AM dose	0.5–2 mg per kg daily PO as a single AM dose
Alopecia areata	0.5–2 mg per kg daily PO as a single AM dose	0.5–2 mg per kg daily PO as a single AM dose
Aphthous stomatitis	0.5–2 mg per kg daily PO as a single AM dose for 7–21 days	0.5–2 mg per kg daily PO as a single AM dose for 7–21 days
Atopic dermatitis	0.5–2 mg per kg daily PO as a single AM dose for 7–21 days	0.5–2 mg per kg daily PO as a single AM dose for 7–21 days
Autoerythrocyte sensitization; erythema induratum	0.5–2 mg per kg daily PO as a single AM dose for 7–21 days	0.5–2 mg per kg daily PO as a single AM dose for 7–21 days
Behçet's disease	0.5–2 mg per kg daily PO as a single AM dose	0.5–2 mg per kg daily PO as a single AM dose
Brown recluse spider bite	0.5–2 mg per kg daily PO as a single AM dose	0.5–2 mg per kg daily PO as a single AM dose
Bullous pemphigoid	0.5–2 mg per kg daily PO as a single AM dose	0.5–2 mg per kg daily PO as a single AM dose
Churg-Strauss disease	0.5–2 mg per kg daily PO as a single AM dose	0.5–2 mg per kg daily PO as a single AM dose
Cicatricial pemphigoid	0.5–2 mg per kg daily PO as a single AM dose	0.5–2 mg per kg daily PO as a single AM dose
Contact dermatitis	0.5–2 mg per kg daily PO as a single AM dose for 7–21 days	0.5–2 mg per kg daily PO as a single AM dose for 7–21 days
Dyshidrotic eczema	0.5–2 mg per kg daily PO as a single AM dose for 7–21 days	0.5–2 mg per kg daily PO as a single AM dose for 7–21 days
Eosinophilic pustular folliculitis	0.5–2 mg per kg daily PO as a single AM dose for 7–21 days	0.5–2 mg per kg daily PO as a single AM dose for 7–21 days
Epidermolysis bullosa acquisita	0.5–2 mg per kg daily PO as a single AM dose	0.5–2 mg per kg daily PO as a single AM dose
Epidermolytic hyperkeratosis	0.5–2 mg per kg daily PO as a single AM dose	0.5–2 mg per kg daily PO as a single AM dose
Erythema annulare centrifugum	0.5–2 mg per kg daily PO as a single AM dose	0.5–2 mg per kg daily PO as a single AM dose
Erythema gyratum repens	0.5–2 mg per kg daily PO as a single AM dose	0.5–2 mg per kg daily PO as a single AM dose

P

Prednisone. Dermatologic indications and dosage (Continued)

Disease	Adult dosage	Child dosage
Erythema induratum	0.5–2 mg per kg daly PO as a single AM dose	0.5–2 mg per kg daily PO as a single AM dose
Erythema multiforme	0.5–2 mg per kg daily PO as a single AM dose for 7–21 days	0.5–2 mg per kg daily PO as a single AM dose for 7–21 days
Erythema nodosum	0.5–2 mg per kg daily PO as a single AM dose for 7–21 days	0.5–2 mg per kg daily PO as a single AM dose for 7–21 days
Fogo selvagem	0.5–2 mg per kg daly PO as a single AM dose	0.5–2 mg per kg daily PO as a single AM dose
Herpes gestationis	0.5–2 mg per kg daily PO as a single AM dose	0.5–2 mg per kg daily PO as a single AM dose
Herpes zoster	0.5–2 mg per kg daily PO as a single AM dose for 7–14 days	0.5–2 mg per kg daily PO as a single AM dose for 7–14 days
Hypereosinophilic syndrome	0.5–2 mg per kg daily PO as a single AM dose	0.5–2 mg per kg daily PO as a single AM dose
Jessner lymphocytic infiltration of skin	0.5–2 mg per kg daily PO as a single AM dose	0.5–2 mg per kg daily PO as a single AM dose
Kasabach-Merritt syndrome	2-4 mg per kg daily PO for 6-30 weeks	2-4 mg per kg daily PO for 6-30 weeks
Kerion	0.5–2 mg per kg daily PO as a single AM dose for 7–14 days	0.5–2 mg per kg daily PO as a single AM dose for 7–14 days
Kimura's syndrome	0.5–2 mg per kg daily PO as a single AM dose	0.5–2 mg per kg daily PO as a single AM dose
Leprosy reactional state	0.5–2 mg per kg daily PO as a single AM dose	0.5–2 mg per kg daily PO as a single AM dose
Lichen planus	0.5–2 mg per kg daily PO as a single AM dose	0.5–2 mg per kg daily PO as a single AM dose
Linear IgA bullous dermatosis	0.5–2 mg per kg daily PO as a single AM dose	0.5–2 mg per kg daily PO as a single AM dose
Lupus erythematosus, discoid	0.5–2 mg per kg daily PO as a single AM dose	0.5–2 mg per kg daily PO as a single AM dose
Lupus erythematosus, subacute	0.5–2 mg per kg daily PO as a single AM dose	0.5–2 mg per kg daily PO as a single AM dose
Mixed connective tissue disease	0.5–2 mg per kg daily PO as a single AM dose	0.5–2 mg per kg daily PO as a single AM dose
Morphea	0.5–2 mg per kg daily PO as a single AM dose	0.5–2 mg per kg daily PO as a single AM dose
Necrobiotic xanthogranuloma	0.5–2 mg per kg daily PO as a single AM dose	0.5–2 mg per kg daily PO as a single AM dose
Nummular eczema	0.5–2 mg per kg daily PO as a single AM dose for 7–21 days	0.5–2 mg per kg daily PO as a single AM dose for 7–21 days
Otitis externa	0.5–2 mg per kg daily PO as a single AM dose for 7–21 days	0.5–2 mg per kg daily PO as a single AM dose for 7–21 days

Prednisone. Dermatologic indications and dosage (Continued)

Disease	Adult dosage	Child dosage
Papular mucinosis	0.5–2 mg per kg daily PO as a single AM dose	0.5–2 mg per kg daily PO as a single AM dose
Paraneoplastic pemphigus	0.5–2 mg per kg daily PO as a single AM dose	0.5–2 mg per kg daily PO as a single AM dose
Pemphigus vulgaris	1–2 mg per kg daily PO as a single AM dose	1–2 mg per kg daily PO as a single AM dose
Pityriasis lichenoides	0.5–2 mg per kg daily PO as a single AM dose	0.5–2 mg per kg daily PO as a single AM dose
Polymorphous light eruption	1 mg per kg PO as a single AM dose for 7–14 days	1 mg per kg PO as a single AM dose for 7–14 days
Post-herpetic neuralgia prophylaxis	1 mg per kg PO daily for 14–21 days	Not indicated
Pruritic papules and plaques of pregnancy	1 mg per kg PO as a single AM dose for 7–14 days	Not applicable
Psoriasis	1 mg per kg PO as a single AM dose for 7–14 days	1 mg per kg PO as a single AM dose for 7–14 days
Pyoderma gangrenosum	1 mg per kg PO as a single AM dose	1 mg per kg PO as a single AM dose
Sarcoidosis	20–40 mg daily PO for 2–3 months, followed by slow taper to 10 mg every other day for up to 1 year	10–30 mg daily PO for 2–3 months, followed by slow taper to 5 mg every other day for up to 1 year
Scabies	1 mg per kg PO as a single AM dose for 7–14 days	1 mg per kg PO as a single AM dose for 7–14 days
Schnitzler syndrome	1 mg per kg PO daily for 14–21 days	1 mg per kg PO daily for 14–21 days
Seborrheic dermatitis	0.5–2 mg per kg daily PO as a single AM dose for 7–21 days	0.5–2 mg per kg daily PO as a single AM dose for 7–21 days
Serum sickness	0.5–1 mg per kg PO daily for 7–21 days	0.5–1 mg per kg PO daily for 7–21 days
Stasis dermatitis	1 mg per kg PO as a single AM dose for 7–14 days	1 mg per kg PO as a single AM dose for 7–14 days
Stevens-Johnson syndrome	1 mg per kg PO daily for 14–21 days	1 mg per kg PO daily for 14–21 days
Sulzberger-Garbe syndrome	1 mg per kg PO daily as a single AM dose	1 mg per kg PO daily as a single AM dose
Temporal arteritis	1–2 mg per kg PO daily as a single AM dose	1–2 mg per kg PO daily as a single AM dose
Urticaria	1 mg per kg PO daily for no longer than 21 days; to be used only in severe, recalcitrant disease	1 mg per kg PO daily for no longer than 21 days; to be used only in severe, recalcitrant disease
Vogt-Koyanagi-Harada syndrome - iritis	1–2 mg per kg PO daily as a single AM dose	1–2 mg per kg PO daily as a single AM dose

Prednisone. Dermatologic indications and dosage (Continued)

Disease	Adult dosage	Child dosage
Weber-Christian disease	1–2 mg per kg PO daily as a single AM dose	1–2 mg per kg PO daily as a single AM dose
Wegener's granulomatosis	1–2 mg per kg PO daily as a single AM dose	1–2 mg per kg PO daily as a single AM dose
Xerotic eczema	0.5–1 mg per kg daily PO as a single AM dose for 7–10 days	0.5–1 mg per kg daily PO as a single AM dose for 7–10 days

Contraindications/precautions
Hypersensitivity to drug class or component; systemic fungal infection; caution in patients with congestive heart failure, seizure disorder, hypertension, diabetes mellitus, tuberculosis; osteoporosis; impaired liver function

References
Williams LC, Nesbitt LT (2001) Update on systemic glucocorticosteroids in dermatology. Dermatologic Clinics 19(1):63–77

Pregnancy mask

► Melasma

Pregnancy-associated autoimmune disease

► Herpes gestationis

Premalignant fibroepithelial tumor

► Fibroepithelioma of Pinkus

Pressure alopecia

► Traction alopecia

Pressure sore

► Decubitus ulcer

Pressure ulcer

► Decubitus ulcer

Prickle cell carcinoma

► Squamous cell carcinoma

Prickly heat

► Miliaria

Primary adrenal insufficiency

▶ Addison's disease

Primary cutaneous neuroendocrine carcinoma

▶ Merkel cell carcinoma

Primary hemochromatosis

▶ Hemochromatosis

Primary hypertrophic osteoarthropathy

▶ Pachydermoperiostosis

Primary localized cutaneous amyloidosis

▶ Lichen amyloidosis

Primary Raynaud's

▶ Raynaud's disease

Primary varicella

▶ Varicella

Principen

▶ Ampicillin

Progressive and recurring dermatofibroma

▶ Dermatofibrosarcoma protuberans

Progressive capillary hemangioma

▶ Tufted angioma

Progressive cardiomyopathic lentiginosis

▶ LEOPARD syndrome

Progressive lipodystrophy

Synonym(s)
Progressive partial lipodystrophy; Barraquer-Simons syndrome; acquired partial lipodystrophy; cephalothoracic dystrophy; acquired progressive lipodystrophy

Definition
Disorder characterized by progressive and symmetric loss of subcutaneous fat

Pathogenesis
May be associated with glomerulonephritis, low C_3 levels, and the presence of a C_3 nephritic factor

Clinical manifestation
Onset between 5 and 15 years of age; slow, insidious loss of subcutaneous fat, initially limited to the face, sometimes extending to the upper portion of the body, giving the patient a cachetic appearance

Differential diagnosis
HIV-associated lipodystrophy; Cockayne syndrome; generalized lipodystrophies such as Berardinelli-Seip syndrome; Werner syndrome; hypothalamus tumor

Therapy
Subcutaneous fat injections from unaffected areas; temporal muscle flaps; silicone filling material

References
Ketterings C (1988) Lipodystrophy and its treatment. Annals of Plastic Surgery 21(6):536–543

Progressive partial lipodystrophy

▶ Progressive lipodystrophy

Progressive septic granulomatosis

▶ Chronic granulomatous disease

Progressive symmetric keratoderma

Synonym(s)
Erythrokeratodermia progressiva symmetrica

Definition
Hereditary keratoderma with slowly progressive, symmetric, and well-defined hyperkeratotic plaques

Pathogenesis
Autosomal dominant trait; defect in loricrin gene or in an unknown locus on chromosome 1

Clinical manifestation
Well demarcated, red, scaly plaques, distributed with almost perfect symmetry on the head, extremities, palms, soles, and buttocks; chest and abdomen usually spared; onset during the first year of life or shortly thereafter, progressing for a few years, and then stablilizing; some cases remit spontaneously

Differential diagnosis
Erythrokeratodermia variabilis; Giroux-Barbeau erythrokeratodermia with ataxia; Greither disease; erythrokeratolysis hiemalis; ichthyosis linearis circumflexa; psoriasis; lupus erythematosus; lamellar ichthyosis; gyrate erythema; atopic dermatitis

Therapy
Keratolytics such as alpha hydroxy acids; acitretin

References
Gray LC, Davis LS, Guill MA (1996) Progressive symmetric erythrokeratodermia. Journal of the American Academy of Dermatology 34(5 Pt 1):858–859

Progressive systemic sclerosis

Synonym(s)
Systemic sclerosis; scleroderma; systemic connective tissue disease; diffuse systemic sclerosis

Definition
Multisystem connective tissue disorder, characterized by vasomotor disturbances, fibrosis of the skin, subcutaneous tissue, muscles, and internal organs

Pathogenesis
Immunologic system abnormality and vascular changes; increased collagen production or disturbances in its degradation, causing excessive collagen deposition in tissues

Clinical manifestation
Skin: areas of hyperpigmentation alternating with hypopigmentation; overall appearance of tanned skin persists long after sun exposure; telangiectasias on face, neck, and periungual areas; skin of the hands sometimes edematous or indurated early, later sclerotic stage where skin is tight and shiny, with a loss of hair, decreased sweating, and loss of ability to make a skin fold; starts distally on the fingers; any area of the body ultimately may be involved; calcinosis on the fingers and extremities; reduced oral aperture (microstomia) from perioral involvement
Ears, nose and throat: xerostomia and xerophthalmia; vascular changes – Raynaud phenomenon triggered by cold, smoking, or emotional stress; infarction and dry gangrene sometimes results from severe vasospasm
Musculoskeletal system: arthralgias and morning stiffness sometimes mimicking other systemic autoimmune diseases; hand and joint function may decline from skin tightening; acroosteolysis (i.e., resorption or dissolution of the distal end of the phalanx) sometimes occurs; flexion contractures
Neurologic system: trigeminal neuralgia; carpal tunnel syndrome
Respiratory system: dry rales, indicating fibrosis
Esophageal sphincter incompetence
Gastrointestinal system: reflux; esophagitis Barrett metaplasia; candidiasis; watermelon stomach or gastric vascular antral ectasia; primary biliary cirrhosis; malabsorption; atrophy of smooth muscle and fibrotic changes leading to decreased peristalsis throughout the gastrointestinal tract
Renal system: renal failure; cardiac involvement: indicates poor prognosis; pericardial effusions with cor pulmonale; conduction abnormalities; infiltrative cardiomyopathy

Differential diagnosis
Morphea; linear scleroderma; bleomycin-induced scleroderma; toxic oil syndrome; porphyria cutanea tarda; digital sclerosis of diabetes mellitus; radiation exposure; intestinal obstruction from other causes; infiltrative cardiomyopathy from other causes; eosinophilia-myalgia syndrome; chronic graft versus host disease

Therapy
D-penicillamine: 250–1500 mg per day PO divided into 2 or 3 doses; methotrexate

References
Sapadin AN, Fleischmajer R (2002) Treatment of scleroderma. Archives of Dermatology 138(1): 99–105

Proliferating endotheliosis

▶ Angioendotheliomatosis

Proliferating pilar tumor

▶ Pilar tumor

Proliferating systematized endotheliosis

▶ Angioendotheliomatosis

Proliferating trichilemmal cyst

► Pilar tumor

Protein energy malnutrition

► Marasmus

Protocoproporphyria

► Variegate porphyria

Protoporphyria

► Erythropoietic protoporphyria

Protothecosis, cutaneous

Synonym(s)
Infection by achlorophillic algae

Definition
Infection caused by algae of the genus Prototheca

Pathogenesis
Usually caused by Prototheca wickerhamii; wide variety of aqueous sources, including lakes, streams, ponds; host immunsuppression is a risk factor

Clinical manifestation
History of trauma (e.g., abrasion, cut) to skin and subsequent exposure to contaminated water; extremities most common sites of involvement; ill-defined plaque or nodule, often with verrucous surface; bullae with rupture, drainage, and crusting

Differential diagnosis
Bacterial pyoderma; orf; milker's nodule; anthrax; atypical mycobacterial infection; nocardiosis; deep fungal infection, such as cryptococcosis, chromomycosis, coccidioidomycosis, or North American blastomycosis

Therapy
Combination of tetracycline and amphotericin B: 0.5 mg per kg IV daily for 1–6 weeks*; ketoconazole; itraconazole

References
Thiele D, Bergmann A (2002) Protothecosis in human medicine. International Journal of Hygiene & Environmental Health 204(5-6):297–302

Prurigo gestationis

► Prurigo of pregnancy

Prurigo of pregnancy

Synonym(s)
Pruritus of pregnancy; prurigo gestationis; early-onset prurigo of pregnancy; papular dermatitis of pregnancy; pruritic folliculitis of pregnancy

Definition
Disorder occurring in the second half of pregnancy, characterized by discrete, crusted papules located predominantly over the extensor aspects of the limbs, shoulders, and abdomen

Pathogenesis
Pruritus gravidarum variant may be associated with intrahepatic cholestasis, perhaps resulting from elevated estrogen and progesterone levels thought to interfere with the liver's ecretion of bile salts

Clinical manifestation
Pruritus with papules produced by scratching, usually occurring in last trimester of pregnancy; may have jaundice with cholestasis

Differential diagnosis
Scabies; insect bite reaction; impetigo herpetiformis; pemphigoid gestationis (herpes gestationis); pruritic urticarial papules and plaques of pregnancy

Therapy
Corticosteroids, topical, medium potency

References
Vaughan Jones SA, Hern S, Nelson-Piercy C, Seed PT, Black MM (1999) A prospective study of 200 women with dermatoses of pregnancy correlating clinical findings with hormonal and immunopathological profiles. British Journal of Dermatology 141(1):71–81

Pruritic folliculitis of pregnancy

▶ Prurigo of pregnancy

Pruritic urticarial papules and plaques of pregnancy

Synonym(s)
Polymorphic eruption of pregnancy; toxemic erythema of pregnancy; toxemic rash of pregnancy; late-onset prurigo of pregnancy; PUPPP

Definition
Dermatosis of pregnancy characterized by intensely pruritic red papules and plaques arising late in the third trimester

Pathogenesis
May be related to increased skin distension

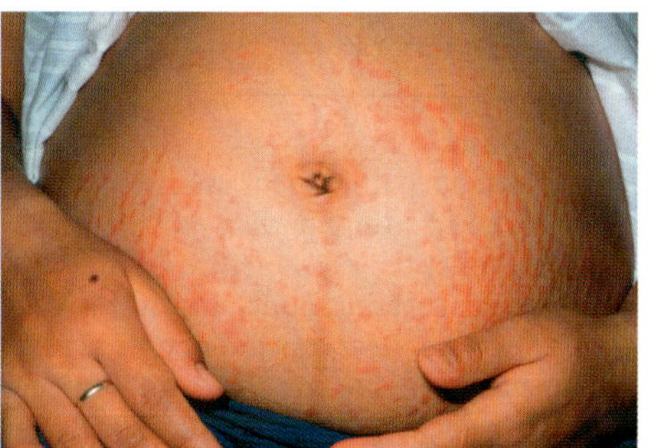

Pruritic urticarial papules and plaques of pregnancy. Erythematous papules and plaques on the abdomen of a pregnant woman, with accentuation in striae

Clinical manifestation
Erythematous urticarial papules and plaques of the trunk and extremities, most notably in striae; periumbilical area spared; usually arises in third trimester, particularly in first pregnancy; no fetal effects; resolves within weeks of partuition

Differential diagnosis
Urticaria; erythema multiforme; cholestasis of pregnancy; impetigo herpetiformis; herpes gestationis; papular dermatitis of pregnancy; prurigo gestationis; viral exanthem; drug eruption

Therapy
Corticosteroids, topical, high potency; prednisone for severe flares

References
Aronson IK, Bond S, Fiedler VC, Vomvouras S, Gruber D, Ruiz C (1998) Pruritic urticarial papules and plaques of pregnancy: clinical and immunopathologic observations in 57 patients. Journal of the American Academy of Dermatology 39(6):933–939

Pruritus ani

Synonym(s)
Anal itching

Definition
Pruritus involving the area around the anus

Pathogenesis
Final common pathway for multiple inciting factors, including: perfumes, chemicals, or dye on toilet paper; moisture from sweat or diarrhea; certain foods, including caffeine, chocolate, beer, nuts, dairy products, and spicy foods; infections or infestations such as pinworm infestation, candidiasis, or genital warts; hemorrhoids; recent antibiotic use

Clinical manifestation
Pruritus, often without obvious dermatosis; may have erythema with or without exudate, depending upon inciting factors

Differential diagnosis
Neurodermatitis; drug hypersensitivity reaction; anal carcinoma; contact dermatitis

Therapy
Careful attention to hygiene: gentle but thorough rectal cleansing after bowel movements; drying powders; sitz baths; corticosteroids, topical, low potency; cotton placed over anal orifice to minimize fecal leakage; lubricating cream or lotion to perianal area twice daily

References
Nagle D, Rolandelli RH (1996) Primary care office management of perianal and anal disease. Primary Care Clinics in Office Practice 23(3):609–620

Pruritus gravidarum

▶ Prurigo of pregnancy

Pruritus of pregnancy

▶ Prurigo of pregnancy

Pseudo Hodgkin's disease

▶ Cutaneous CD30+ (Ki-1) anaplastic large-cell lymphoma

Pseudo Kaposi's sarcoma

▶ Acroangiodermatitis
▶ Granuloma gluteale infantum

Pseudo Turner syndrome

▶ Noonan's syndrome

Pseudo Ullrich-Turner syndrome

▶ Noonan's syndrome

Pseudochromhidrosis plantaris

▶ Black heel

Pseudocolloid lip mucous membrane sebacous milia

▶ Fordyce's disease

Pseudocolloid of the buccal mucosa

▶ Fordyce's disease

Pseudocolloid of the lips

▶ Fordyce's disease

Pseudofolliculitis barbae

Synonym(s)
Pseudofolliculitis of the beard; pili incarnati; folliculitis barbae traumatica; shaving bumps; razor bumps

Definition
Foreign body reaction from ingrown curly hair characterized by papules and pustules in the beard area

Pathogenesis
Tightly curved hair from a recent shave briefly surfaces from the skin and reenters a short distance away, producing foreign body reaction; transfollicular penetration occurs when the sharp tip of hair pierces the follicle wall without emerging from skin

Clinical manifestation
Flesh-colored or erythematous papule with central hair shaft, seen in shaved areas adjacent to the follicular ostia; pustules and abscess formation from secondary infection; postinflammatory hyperpigmentation, scarring, and keloid formation after chronic involvement

Differential diagnosis
Folliculitis; acne vulgaris; tinea barbae; acne keloidalis; sarcoidosis; granuloma annulare; rosacea

Therapy
Shaving techniques: stop shaving for at least 3–4 weeks; clean beard with face cloth, wet sponge, or soft-bristled toothbrush with a mild soap for several minutes before shaving; shave with 3-headed, rotary electric razor with heads slightly off skin surface; shave in a slow circular motion; use chemical depilatories; laser destruction of hair follicles in affected areas

References
Perry PK, Cook-Bolden FE, Rahman Z, Jones E, Taylor SC (2002) Defining pseudofolliculitis barbae in 2001: a review of the literature and current trends. Journal of the American Academy of Dermatology 46(2 Suppl Understanding):S 113–119

Pseudofolliculitis of the beard

▶ Pseudofolliculitis barbae

Pseudohomozygous familial hypercholesterolemia

▶ Phytosterolemia

Pseudohypoparathyroidism

Synonym(s)
Albright hereditary osteodystrophy

Definition
Hereditary condition which resembles hypoparathyroidism, but caused by a lack of response to parathyroid hormone rather than a deficiency of the hormone

Pathogenesis
Molecular defects in the gene (GNAS1) encoding the alpha subunit of the stimulatory G protein; unresponsivieness of appropriate organs to the actions of parathyroid hormone

Clinical manifestation
Soft tissue calcifications; hypocalcemia; brachydactyly; dimples may replace knuck-

les on affected digits; short stature; mental retardation; basal ganglia calcifications; cataracts; tetany; hyperphosphatemia and hypocalcemia; normal parathyroid hormone levels

Differential diagnosis
Dystrophic calcification; hypoparathyroidism; secondary hyperparathyroidism; autoimmune polyglandular syndromes

Therapy
Calcium 1200 mg PO per day; 1-alpha-hydroxylated vitamin D metabolites 250 mg PO per day; surgical excision of symptomatic soft tissue calcifications

References
Bastepe M, Juppner H (2000) Pseudohypoparathyroidism. New insights into an old disease. Endocrinology and Metabolism Clinics of North America 29(3):569–589

Pseudolymphoma

Synonym(s)
Lymphocytoma cutis; cutaneous lymphomatous hyperplasia; lymphadenosis benigna cutis; cutaneous lymphoplasia; pseudolymphoma of Spiegler-Fendt; Spiegler-Fendt sarcoid

Definition
Group of disorders with a common trait of response to stimuli resulting in a lymphomatous-appearing but benign accumulation of inflammatory cells

Pathogenesis
Most cases with unknown inciting agent; some known agents: tattoo dye, jewelry, insect bite reaction, medications, folliculitis, trauma, vaccinations, irritants, cutaneous infection

Clinical manifestation
B cell variant: one or several firm, red-to-violaceous nodules, from one to several centimeters in diameter
T-cell variant: broad, erythematous patches and/or plaques

Differential diagnosis
Insect bite; inflamed epidermoid cyst; granuloma faciale; foreign body granuloma; granuloma annulare; granulomatous rosacea; Jessner's lymphocytic infiltration; lymphoma; metastasis; basal cell carcinoma; squamous cell carcinoma; Merkel cell carcinoma; actinic reticuloid; lymphomatoid papulosis

Therapy
Triamcinolone 3–4 mg per ml intralesional; superficial radiation; surgical excision; liquid nitrogen cryotherapy

References
Gilliam AC, Wood GS (2000) Cutaneous lymphoid hyperplasias. Seminars in Cutaneous Medicine & Surgery 19(2):133–141

Pseudolymphoma of Spiegler-Fendt

▶ Pseudolymphoma

Pseudomonas folliculitis

▶ Hot tub folliculitis

Pseudopapilledema

▶ Bannayan-Riley-Ruvalcaba syndrome

Pseudopelade

Synonym(s)
Pseudopelade of Brocq; Brocq pseudopelade

Definition
End stage or clinical variant of various forms of scarring alopecia

Pathogenesis
Linked to underlying disease, such as lupus erythematosus or lichen planus

Clinical manifestation
Randomly distributed, irregularly shaped areas of scarring alopecia of scalp ("footprints in the snow"), often with hypopigmentation and slight atrophy; few hairs sometimes remain in otherwise completely bald and scarred plaque; no clinical evidence of inflammation

Differential diagnosis
Lupus erythematosus; lichen planus; follicular degeneration syndrome; alopecia areata; post-traumatic alopecia; folliculitis decalvans; lichen sclerosus; androgenetic alopecia

Therapy
No effective therapy

References
Headington JT (1996) Cicatricial alopecia. Dermatologic Clinics 14(4):773–782

Pseudoporphyria

Synonym(s)
Drug-induced bullous photosensitivity; therapy-induced bullous photosensitivity

Definition
Bullous photosensitivity disorder mimicking porphyria cutanea tarda, without demonstrable porphyrin abnormalities

Pathogenesis
Associated with ingestion of certain medications and with hemodialysis

Clinical manifestation
Increased skin fragility; erythema; tense bullae and erosions on sun-exposed skin, without hypertrichosis or sclerodermoid skin changes; variant mimicking erythropoietic protoporpria in children on naproxen for juvenile rheumatoid arthritis

Differential diagnosis
Porphyria cutanea tarda; erythropoietic protoporphyria; epidermolysis bullosa acquisita; bullous pemphigoid; bullous lupus erythematosus

Therapy
Discontinued use of offending agent; reduced sun exposure until blistering eruption has cleared

References
Green JJ, Manders SM (2001) Pseudoporphyria. Journal of the American Academy of Dermatology 44(1):100–108

Pseudopelade of Brocq

▶ Pseudopelade

Pseudopyogenic granuloma

▶ Angiolymphoid hyperplasia with eosinophilia

Pseudosarcoma

▶ Atypical fibroxanthoma

Pseudosarcomatous dermatofibroma

▶ Atypical fibroxanthoma

Pseudosarcomatous reticulohistiocytoma

▶ Atypical fibroxanthoma

Pseudoxanthoma elasticum

Synonym(s)
Systematized elastorrhexis; Grönblad-Strandberg syndrome

Definition
Hereditary connective tissue disease characterized by symptoms and signs secondary to progressive calcification and fragmentation of elastic fibers in the skin, retina, and cardiovascular system

Pathogenesis
Dominant and recessive types, with unknown gene defects; may be related to abnormal glycosaminoglycan secretion, causing calcification and fragmentation of elastic fibers

Clinical manifestation
Skin findings: symmetrical, small, yellow papules, coalescing into plaques in a linear pattern, giving affected skin "plucked chicken" appearance; first noted on the lateral neck and later involving antecubital fossae, axillae, popliteal fossae, inguinal and periumbilical areas, oral, vaginal and rectal mucosa; with disease progression, skin sometimes becomes soft, lax, wrinkled, and hangs in folds; elastosis perforans serpiginosa may coexist

Ocular findings: bilaterally symmetrical angioid streaks of retina, noted several years after onset of cutaneous lesions; may have to retinal hemorrhages; progressive loss of central vision

Cardiovascular findings: usually the last lesions to be recognized; peripheral pulses often severely diminished; hypertension; coronary artery disease causes angina pectoris and subsequent myocardial infarction; mitral valve prolapse; gastrointestinal hemorrhage, usually gastric in origin; less commonly, hemorrhaging occurs in urinary tract or cerebrovascular system

Differential diagnosis
Marfan syndrome; Ehlers-Danlos syndrome; Buschke-Ollendorff syndrome; localized acquired cutaneous pseudoxanthoma elasticum; penicillamine therapy; actinic damage to the lateral neck

Therapy
Surgical correction of lax skin; diet and exercise to minimize risks associated with cardiovascular disease

References
Sherer DW, Sapadin AN, Lebwohl MG (1999) Pseudoxanthoma elasticum: an update. Dermatology 199(1):3–7

Psoriasis

Synonym(s)
None

Definition
Chronic inflammatory skin disorder characterized by scaly, red papules and plaques distributed over extensor body surfaces and the scalp

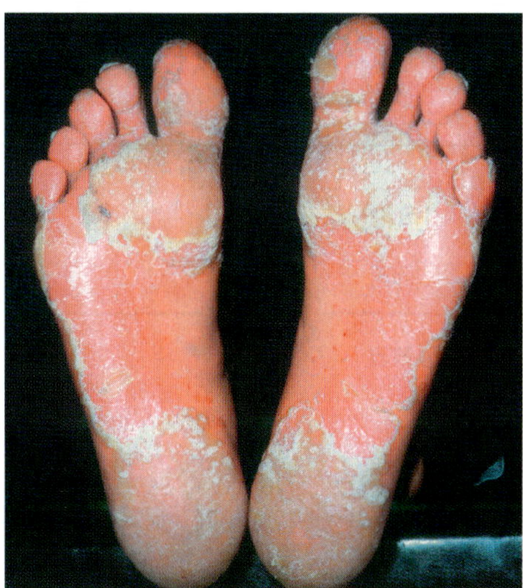

Psoriasis. Scaly, red plaques of the feet

Pathogenesis
Multifactorial, with genetic factors and environmental triggers, including infections (e.g., HIV and streptococcal), smoking, UV light, medications such as lithium, and emotional factors; T-cell immunologic reaction causes epidermal hyperproliferation

Clinical manifestation
Plaque variant: sharply demarcated, red papules and plaques, with silvery-white scale, most often located on scalp, trunk, and limbs, with predilection for extensor surfaces, such as the elbows and knees; tendency toward bilateral symmetry; development of lesions in traumatized skin (Koebner phenomenon); lesions encircled by a paler peripheral zone (Woronoff ring); nails with pitting, onycholysis, subungual hyperkeratosis, irregular and brown nail bed discoloration (oil-drop sign)
Pustular variant: may occur after withdrawal of systemic corticosteroids; patient sometimes systemically ill with fever, leucocytosis; generalized or patchy erythema studded with pustules in annular or nonspecific configuration; flexural and anogenital accentuation; may also appear on trunk or extremities and rarely on face; may involve one or few digits only (acrodermatitis continua of Hallopeau)
Guttate variant: may follow infection, most commonly streptococcal; multiple, discrete, salmon pink, scaly, droplike papules, beginning on trunk and proximal extremities and spreading to face, ears, and scalp; palms and soles rarely affected; all variants may include psoriatic arthritis

Differential diagnosis
Plaque and guttate variants: pityriasis rubra pilaris; seborrheic dermatitis; tinea corporis; lupus erythematosus; pityriasis rosea; syphilis; lichen planus; parapsoriasis; pityriasis lichenoides; cutaneous T-cell lymphoma; nummular eczema
Pustular variant: subcorneal pustular dermatosis; acute generalized exanthematous pustulosis; septicemia; generalized atopic and/or seborrheic dermatitis; dyshidrotic eczema; contact dermatitis; autosensitization reaction; vesicular dermatophyte infection

Therapy
Topical therapy: corticosteroids, topical, super potent; coal tar 1–5 % gel applied nightly; anthralin; calcipotriene; tazarotene
Scalp therapy: corticosteroids, topical, high potency in foam or lotion; anti-seborrheic shampoo used daily; phenol/saline lotion applied to wet scalp nightly under shower cap; UVB phototherapy; photochemotherapy; excimer laser therapy
Systemic therapy: methotrexate; acitretin; cyclosporine; thioguanine; mycophenolate mofetil; hydroxyurea; alefacept – 7.5 mg IM weekly for 12 weeks

References
Lui H (2002) Phototherapy of psoriasis: update with practical pearls. Journal of Cutaneous Medicine & Surgery 6(3 Suppl):17–21
Silvis N (2001) Antimetabolites and cytotoxic drugs. Dermatologic Clinics 19(1):105–118
Tremblay JF, Bissonnette R (2002) Topical agents for the treatment of psoriasis, past, present and future. Journal of Cutaneous Medicine & Surgery 6(3 Suppl):8–11

Psychogenic purpura

▶ Autoerythrocyte sensitization syndrome
▶ Gardner-Diamond syndrome

PTEN hamartoma tumor syndrome

▶ Bannayan-Riley-Ruvalcaba syndrome

Pulmonic stenosis

▶ Watson syndrome

Punctate keratoderma

Synonym(s)
None

Definition
Condition characterized by histologic punctate thickening of the stratum corneum, possibly as part of a generalized condition or a disorder primarily involving the hands and feet

References
Ratnavel RC, Griffiths WA (1997) The inherited palmoplantar keratodermas. British Journal of Dermatology 137(4):485–490

Punctate porokeratosis

▶ Porokeratosis

PUPPP

▶ Pruritic urticarial papules and plaques of pregnancy

Purpura

Definition
Superficial hemorrhage into the skin, up to 1 cm in diameter

References
Piette WW (1994) The differential diagnosis of purpura from a morphologic perspective. Advances in Dermatology 9:3–23

Purpura annularis telangiectodes

▶ Benign pigmented purpura

Purpura autoerythrocytica

▶ Autoerythrocyte sensitization syndrome

Purpura en cocarde avec oedema

▶ Acute hemorrhagic edema of infancy

Purpura fulminans

Definition
Rapidly developing, generalized purpura, associated with severe disturbance of the coagulation system, usually with disseminated intravascular coagulation

References
Darmstadt GL (1998) Acute infectious purpura fulminans: pathogenesis and medical management. Pediatric Dermatology 15(3):169–183

Pustular perifolliculitis

▶ Acne necrotica

Pyoderma

▶ Ecthyma

Pyoderma faciale

▶ Rosacea

Pyoderma gangrenosum

Synonym(s)
None

Definition
Disorder characterized by sudden onset of rapidly expanding cutaneous ulceration, often in patients with preexisting systemic disease such as rheumatoid arthritis, inflammatory bowel disease, or myelogenous leukemia

Pathogenesis
May be a hypersensitivity reaction to antigenic stimuli

Clinical manifestation
Classic subtype: small, red papule or pustule evolving into deep ulceration; often arising at site of minor trauma, with violaceous undermined border; occurs most commonly on legs, but may be seen on any skin surface, including around stoma sites (peristomal pyoderma gangrenosum); intraoral ulcerated plaques (pyostomatitis vegetans), primarily in patients with inflammatory bowel disease

Aytical subtype: vesiculopustular component only at the border, with erosion or superficial ulceration; most often occurs on dorsal aspect of hands, extensor surface of forearms or face

Pyoderma vegetans subtype: crusted, hyperplastic plaques without deep ulceration, similar to that seen in pyostomatitis vegetans; all subtypes may be associated with underlying polyarthritis, inflammatory bowel disease, myelogenous leukemia, or monoclonal gammopathy

Differential diagnosis
Vasculitis; Wegener's granulomatosis; spider bite reaction; squamous cell carcinoma; sporotrichosis; orf; milker's nodule; herpes simplex virus infection (particularly in immunosuppressed patient); antiphospholipid antibody syndrome; anthrax; vascular insufficiency; acute febrile neutrophilic dermatosis; North American blastomycosis; traumatic ulceration, including factitial disease; tuberculosis; syphilis

Therapy
Prednisone; steroid-sparing agents: azathioprine; dapsone; cyclophosphamide; mycophenolate mofetil; cyclosporine; hydrocolloid dressings

References
Powell FC, O'Kane M (2002) Management of pyoderma gangrenosum. Dermatologic Clinics 20(2):347–355

Pyoderma vegetans

▶ **Pyoderma gangrenosum**

Pyogenic granuloma

Synonym(s)
Lobular capillary hemangioma; granuloma pyogenicum; granuloma telangiectaticum

Definition
Vascular skin tumor characterized by solitary, glistening, red papule or nodule that bleeds easily and may ulcerate

Pathogenesis
Unknown

Clinical manifestation
Rapidly enlarging, bright red, friable, polypoid papule or nodule, sometimes spontaneously bleeding, eroding, or ulcerating; occurs most commonly on gingiva, lips, nasal mucosa, face, and distal extremities; may develop multiple recurrent lesions after prior attempts at removal; when occurring in pregnancy, found along the maxillary intraoral mucosal surface, but any intraoral, perioral, and nonoral tissue may be involved; associated with indinavir use

Differential diagnosis
Melanoma; squamous cell carcinoma; Kaposi's sarcoma; atypical fibroxanthoma; excess granulation tissue; glomus tumor; capillary hemangioma; angioendothelioma; angiolymphoid hyperplasia; angiosarcoma; hemangioendothelioma; intravascular angiomatosis; tufted hemangioma

Therapy
Surgical excision; destruction by electrodesiccation and curettage

References
Park YH, Houh D, Houh W (1996) Subcutaneous and superficial granuloma pyogenicum. International Journal of Dermatology 35(3):205–206

Pyostomatitis vegetans

▶ **Pyoderma gangrenosum**

Q

Quintan fever

▶ Trench fever

R

Rabbit fever

▶ Tularemia

Radiation dermatitis

Synonym(s)
Radiodermatitis

Definition
Skin disorder at the site of exposure to X-irradiation

Pathogenesis
Radiation effects on stem cells, preventing renewal of aging or injured cells

Clinical manifestation
Acute variant: occurs after single or few large doses of radiation; erythema and edema within 24 hours of dosing; secondary, progressive erythema 3–6 days after irradiation, with vesicles and bullae if dose is sufficiently high; desquamation followed by postinflammatory hyperpigmentation, often with atrophy
Chronic variant: atrophy, telangiectasia, and dryness, often with skin tethering to underlying tissue; ulceration in center of radiation scar, often 1–2 years after complete healing of skin following radiation therapy

Differential diagnosis
Contact dermatitis; basal cell carcinoma; squamous cell carcinoma; traumatic ulceration; decubitus ulceration; erythema ab igne; retiform purpura (discontinuous livedo reticularis)

Therapy
Biopsy of suspicious ulcerations to rule out skin cancer; protective padding to minimize trauma

References
Porock D, Nikoletti S, Kristjanson L (1999) Management of radiation skin reactions: literature review and clinical application. Plastic Surgical Nursing 19(4):185–192

Radiodermatitis

▶ Radiation dermatitis

Ramsay Hunt syndrome

▶ Herpes zoster

Raspberry lesion

▶ Capillary hemangioma

Rat-bite fever

Synonym(s)
Streptobacillary fever; Haverhill fever; epidemic arthritic erythema; spirillary fever; Sodoku

Definition
Systemic febrile illness transmitted in the secretions of the mouth, nose, or urine of an infected rodent, often by rat bite

Pathogenesis
Caused by two different organisms, Streptobacillus moniliformis and Spirillum minus; acquired through contact with urine or oral or conjunctival secretions from an infected animal, usually after bite

Clinical manifestation
Variant caused by Streptobacillus moniliformis: fever, chills, headache, and muscle pain, usually occurring within 10 days of exposure, followed within 3 days by diffuse erythematous eruption, primarily in the distal extremities; ulceration at site of bite; one or several large joints sometimes become swollen, red, and painful; occasional splenomegaly
Variant caused by Spirillum minus (Sodoku): red or purple plaques; previously healed wound at site of bite sometimes reactivate and ulcerate; rare joint involvement

Differential diagnosis
Viral exanthem; drug eruption; rickettsiosis; legionellosis; leptospirosis; Lyme disease

Therapy
Aqueous penicillin G: 1.2–2.4 million units per day IV for 7 days, followed by penicillin V 500 mg PO for 7 days*; tetracycline for penicillin-allergic patients

References
Cunningham BB, Paller AS, Katz BZ (1998) Rat bite fever in a pet lover. Journal of the American Academy of Dermatology 38(2 Pt 2):330–332

Raynaud disease

▶ Raynaud's disease

Raynaud syndrome

▶ Raynaud's disease

Raynaud's disease

Synonym(s)
Raynaud's syndrome; Raynaud disease; Raynaud syndrome; primary Raynaud's

Definition
Disorder characterized by paroxysmal vasospasm (Raynaud's phenomenon), without association with another illness

Pathogenesis
Abnormal blood flow to affected areas; abnormal recovery from cold stimuli; decreased blood flow may occur from increased blood viscosity or pathologic vessel constriction

Clinical manifestation
Paroxysmal color changes: white, blue, and then red; affected body part usually changes colors at least twice during an episode; completely reversible; rare extreme ischemia of the affected body part may result in necrosis and digital ulceration

Differential diagnosis
Raynaud's phenomenon associated with underlying disease, such as scleroderma, lupus erythematosus, dermatomyositis, rheumatoid arthritis, viral hepatitis or neoplastic disease; chilblains; frostbite; Buerger

disease; paroxysmal nocturnal hemoglobinuria; peripheral arterial occlusive disease; acrocyanosis; carpal tunnel syndrome; thoracic outlet syndrome

Therapy
Nifedipine: 30–90 mg PO daily; losartan – 50 mg PO daily

References
Wigley FM (2002) Clinical practice. Raynaud's phenomenon. New England Journal of Medicine 347(13):1001–1008

Raynaud's phenomenon

Definition
Reversible constriction of peripheral arterioles in response to a variety of stimuli, most commonly caused by exposure to cold or stressful circumstances

References
Wigley FM (2002) Clinical practice. Raynaud's phenomenon. New England Journal of Medicine 347(13):1001–1008

Raynaud's syndrome

▶ Raynaud's disease

Razor bumps

▶ Pseudofolliculitis barbae

Reactive angioendotheliomatosis

▶ Angioendotheliomatosis

Reactive inflammatory systematized angioendotheliomatosis

▶ Angioendotheliomatosis

Reactive perforating collagenosis

Synonym(s)
Acquired perforating disease; collagenoma perforant verruciforme; acquired reactive perforating dermatosis

Definition
Inherited and acquired dermatosis in which the skin eliminates keratotic debris and altered collagen fibers by the transepidermal route

Pathogenesis
Minor skin trauma causes focal damage to collagen, followed by elimination of the disrupted collagen through the epidermis

Clinical manifestation
Flesh-colored, dome-shaped papules with a central keratotic plug occurring at sites of minor trauma; most commonly found on the extensor surfaces of the limbs and dorsa of the hands; linear distribution (Koebner phenomenon); scarring occurs with healing

Differential diagnosis
Kyrle's disease; perforating folliculitis; elastosis perforans serpiginosa; prurigo nodularis; Ferguson-Smith type of keratoacanthoma

Therapy
Tretinoin 0.025% cream; adapalene 0.1% gel; photochemotherapy; isotretinoin; emollients to control pruritus

R

References

Faver IR, Daoud MS, Su WP (1994) Acquired reactive perforating collagenosis. Report of six cases and review of the literature. Journal of the American Academy of Dermatology 30:575–580

Reactive perforating elastosis

▶ Elastosis perforans serpiginosa

Recessive dystrophic epidermolysis bullosa

▶ Epidermolysis bullosa

Recurrent aphthous stomatitis

▶ Aphthous stomatitis

Recurrent aphthous ulcers

▶ Aphthous stomatitis

Recurrent granulomatous dermatitis with eosinophilia

▶ Eosinophilic cellulitis

Recurrent painful bruising

▶ Gardner-Diamond syndrome

Recurring digital fibroma of childhood

▶ Infantile digital fibromatosis

Refsum disease

Synonym(s)
Heredopathia atactica polyneuritiformis

Definition
Neurocutaneous syndrome characterized biochemically by phytanic acid accumulation in plasma and tissues, resulting in peripheral polyneuropathy, cerebellar ataxia, retinitis pigmentosa, and ichthyosis

Pathogenesis
Autosomal recessive trait; mutation in the phytanoyl-CoA hydroxylase gene causes defective peroxisomal alpha-oxidation of phytanic acid; tissue accumulation of this fatty acid, which derives from exogenous sources (mainly from dietary plant chlorophyll and from animal tissues)

Clinical manifestation
Skin findings: variable ichthyosiform plaques over lower trunk and extremities
Neurologic/ocular findings: partial, intermittent, sensorimotor polyneuropathy; cataracts; nystagmus; concentric visual field constriction; sensorineural deafness; cerebellar ataxia; skeletal defects; cardiomyopathy

Differential diagnosis
Ichthyosis vulgaris; lamellar ichthyosis; X-linked ichthyosis; Sjögren-Larsson syndrome; chronic and intermittent polyneuritis; relapsing infectious polyneuritis; mitochondrial myopathies; acute intermittent porphyria; toxin exposure; hereditary motor neuropathies

Therapy
Phytanic acid-free diet*; plasmapheresis; alpha hydroxy acids

References
Wills AJ, Manning NJ, Reilly MM (2001) Refsum's disease. QJM 94(8):403–406

Regressing atypical histiocytosis

▶ Cutaneous CD30+ (Ki-1) anaplastic large-cell lymphoma

Reiter disease

▶ Reiter syndrome

Reiter syndrome

Synonym(s)
Reiter disease; Fiessinger-Leroy-Reiter syndrome; Fiessinger-Leroy syndrome; arthritis urethritica; blennorrheal idiopathic arthritis

Definition
Multisystem disorder characterized by psoriasis-like plaques, balanitis, keratoderma, conjunctivitis, urethritis, arthritis, and spondylitis, often after episode of urethritis or dysentery

Pathogenesis
Probable immunologic hypersensitivity reaction to microorganism; genetic factors far more common in men; HLA B-27 common haplotype in affected individuals

Clinical manifestation
Diarrhea and dysenteric syndrome or symptoms of urethritis prior to other findings; circinate balanitis with circular or gyrate white plaques growing centrifugally over glans penis; conjunctivitis with intense red, conjunctival injection; joint symptoms resembling rhematoid arthritis, but asymmetrical and often involving single joint; knee and tarsal joints and sacroiliac region most commonly involved; psoriasiform cutaneous lesions; palms and soles most commonly involved with keratotic papules, plaques, and pustules; keratoderma blenorrhagica, with painful, keratotic papules and plaques; distal involvement with painful and erosive lesions in the tips of the fingers and toes, with pustules; nail dystrophy; red macules and plaques, diffuse erythema, erosions, and bleeding on oral and pharyngeal mucosae; circinate lesions on tongue resembling geographic tongue; common syndrome in patients with HIV disease

Differential diagnosis
Psoriasis; pityriasis rubra pilaris; lichen planus; lupus erythematosus; dermatomyositis; Behçet's disease; arthritis associated with gonococcal disease, rheumatoid arthritis; septic arthritis; scabies; mycosis fungoides; subcorneal pustulosis of Sneddon-Wilkinson; atopic dermatitis; acute exanthematic pustulosis; other causes of erythroderma

Therapy
Topical therapy: corticosteroids, topical, super potent; coal tar 1–5 % gel applied nightly, anthralin; calcipotriene; tazarotene
Scalp therapy: corticosteroids, topical, high potency foam or lotion; anti-seborrheic shampoo used daily; phenol/saline lotion applied to wet scalp nightly under shower cap; UVB phototherapy; photochemotherapy; excimer laser therapy
Systemic therapy: methotrexate; acitretin; cyclosporine; thioguanine; mycophenolate mofetil; hydroxyurea

References
Hughes RA, Keat AC (1994) Reiter's syndrome and reactive arthritis: a current view. Seminars in Arthritis & Rheumatism 24(3):190–210

Relapsing febrile nodular nonsuppurative panniculitis

▶ Weber-Christian disease

Relapsing febrile nonsuppurative nodular panniculitis

▶ Weber-Christian disease

Relapsing fever

Synonym(s)
Tick-borne relapsing fever; louse-borne relapsing fever

Definition
Acute infectious disease transmitted by ticks or lice, caused by several species of the genus Borrelia

Pathogenesis
Louse-borne spirochetes transmitted either by bite of louse or by inoculation of louse feces; tick-borne spirochetes enter host blood stream after bite

Clinical manifestation
Acute onset of illness with fever, headache, chills, sweats, myalgias, arthralgia; dizziness, nausea, and vomiting; dry mucous membranes; petechiae on the trunk and extremities; photophobia and conjunctival injection; scleral icterus; nonproductive cough; pleuritic pain; epistaxis; blood-tinged sputum

Differential diagnosis
Lyme disease; Rocky Mountain spotted fever; leptospirosis; Colorado tick fever; trench fever; rat bite fever; dengue fever

Therapy
Tetracycline*; doxycycline; erythromycin

References
Rahlenbeck SI, Gebre-Yohannes A (1995) Louse-borne relapsing fever and its treatment. Tropical & Geographical Medicine 47(2):49–52
Shapiro ED (1997) Tick-borne diseases. Advances in Pediatric Infectious Diseases 13:187–218

Relapsing polychondritis

Synonym(s)
Polychondropathy; systemic chondromalacia; chronic atrophic polychondritis

Definition
Episodic inflammatory disease of cartilaginous structures, predominantly those of the ear, nose, and laryngotracheobronchial tree

Pathogenesis
Probably immune-mediated

Clinical manifestation
Erythema and edema overlying inflamed cartilaginous structures; vasculitis of skin and other organs; sudden onset of unilateral or bilateral auricle pain, swelling, and redness, sparing the lobules; nonerosive, seronegative inflammatory polyarthritis; acute nasal chondritis with pain and feeling of fullness over nasal bridge; episodic inflammation of the uveal tract, conjunctivae, sclerae, and cornea; respiratory tract chondritis; auricular chondritis, with sudden hearing loss, tinnitus, nausea, vomiting, nystagmus, and vertigo; cardiovascular structural changes

Differential diagnosis
Cellulitis; polyarteritis nodosa; chondrodermatitis nodularis helicis; rheumatoid arthritis; Cogan syndrome; infectious perichondritis; MAGIC syndrome; trauma; syphilis; chronic external otitis; auricular calcification from trauma; Addison disease; diabetes or hyperthyroidism

Therapy

Prednisone[*]; steroid-sparing agents: dapsone, azathioprine, methotrexate, cyclophosphamide, cyclosporine, methotrexate

References

Trentham DE, Le CH (1998) Relapsing polychondritis. Annals of Internal Medicine 129(2):114–122

REM syndrome

▶ Reticular erythematous mucinosis

Rendu-Osler syndrome

▶ Osler-Weber-Rendu syndrome

Respiratory scleroma

▶ Rhinoscleroma

Reticular erythematous mucinosis

Synonym(s)

REM syndrome; round cell erythematosus

Definition

Dermal mucinosis presenting as erythematous, infiltrated reticulated plaques

Pathogenesis

May be related to abnormal mucopolysaccharide production from populations of FXIIIa+/HAS2+ dermal dendrocytes

Clinical manifestation

Asymptomatic or slightly pruritic, erythematous, infiltrated papules, either isolated or coalescing into plaques, in the midline of the back or chest; exascerbation with sun exposure

Differential diagnosis

Generalized myxedema; pretibial myxedema; scleredema; scleromyxedema; papular mucnosis; focal mucinosis; cutaneous mucinosis of infancy; nevus mucinosis; alopecia mucinosa; lupus erythematosus

Therapy

Hydroxychloroquine[*]; pulse dye laser

References

Cohen PR, Rabinowitz AD, Ruszkowski AM, DeLeo VA (1990) Reticular erythematous mucinosis syndrome: review of the world literature and report of the syndrome in a prepubertal child. Pediatric Dermatology 7(1):1–10

Reticulate acropigmentation of Kitamura

Synonym(s)

Kitamura's reticulate acropigmentation; Kitamura's acropigmentatio reticularis

Definition

Reticulate, lentigo-like pigmenation of the dorsal aspects of the hands

Pathogenesis

Autosomal dominant inheritance; exact defect unknown

Clinical manifestation

Net-like hyperpigmentation, with atrophy, of the dorsal aspects of the hands; pigmentation at other sites as the patient ages; palmar pits may be associated

Differential diagnosis

Acromelanosis progressiva; acropigmentation of Dohi; universal acquired melanosis

Therapy
None

References

Schnur RE, Heymann WR (1997) Reticulate hyperpigmentation. Seminars in Cutaneous Medicine & Surgery 16(1):72–80

Reticulate pigmented anomaly

Synonym(s)
Dowling-Degos disease; dark dot disease; Dowling Degos Ossipowski disease

Definition
Progressive. acquired pigment disorder, characterized by flexural, pigmented reticulate macules, and comedone-like papules on the back and neck

Pathogenesis
Autosomal dominant trait; unknown gene defect

Clinical manifestation
Flexural pigmentation with onset from childhood to adult life; brownish-black color with steely-gray or navy hues; sometimes stippled in shades of brown; palpable plaques from secondary lichenification; margins may have punctate pigmented comedones; occasional speckled macules involving the dorsum of the hands, proximal nail folds, or scrotum

Differential diagnosis
Carney's syndrome; acanthosis nigricans; confluent and reticulate papillmatosis of Gougerot-Carteaud; Kitamura reticulate acropigmentation; Haber syndrome; Galli-Galli disease

Therapy
No effective therapy

References

Amichai B, Grunwald AM, Bergman R (1997) Guess what? European Journal of Dermatology 7(6): 465–466

Reye tumor

▶ Infantile digital fibromatosis

Rhabdomyoblastoma

▶ Rhabdomyosarcoma

Rhabdomyosarcoma

Synonym(s)
Malignant rhabdomyoma; myosarcoma; sarcoma botryoides; rhabdomyoblastoma

Definition
Malignant mesenchymal tumor with striated muscle differentiation

Pathogenesis
Unknown

Clinical manifestation
Mass lesion, often in infancy or early childhood, usually involving head and neck region, genitourinary tract, or deep soft tissues of the extremities

Differential diagnosis
Rhabdomyoma; lymphoma; liposarcoma; malignant fibrous histiocytoma

Therapy
Surgical excision, followed by radiation and/or chemotherapy[*]

References
Womer RB, Pressey JG (2000) Rhabdomyosarcoma and soft tissue sarcoma in childhood. Current Opinion in Oncology 12(4):337–344

Rhagades

Definition
Linear fissures of the skin, especially on the anus or at the corner of the mouth, sometimes due to syphilis

References
Parish JL (2000) Treponemal infections in the pediatric population. Clinics in Dermatology 18(6):687–700

Rheumatoid nodule

Definition
Firm, non-tender, freely-movable, subcutaneous nodule, usually in periarticular location, seen with rheumatoid arthritis

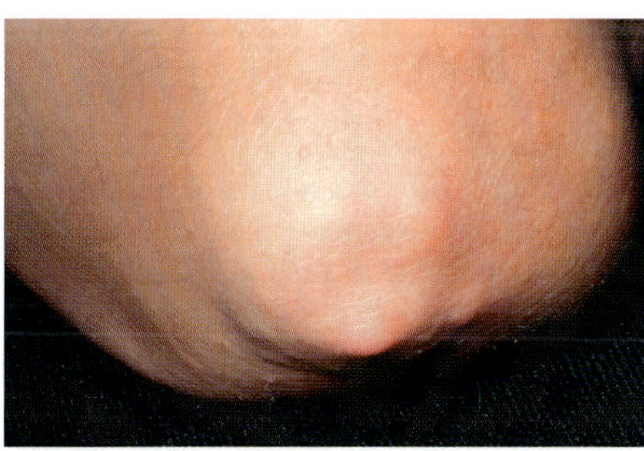

Rheumatoid nodule. Subcutaneous nodule on the elbow

References
Swezey RL (1997) The management of rheumatoid nodules. American Journal of Orthopedics 26(2):73

Rheumatoid vasculitis

▶ Leukocytoclastic vasculitis

Rhinoscleroma

Synonym(s)
Mikulicz disease; respiratory scleroma; scleroma

Definition
Chronic granulomatous disease of the nose and other structures of the upper respiratory tract, resulting from infection by the bacterium Klebsiella rhinoscleromatis

Pathogenesis
Caused by infection from bacterium Klebsiella rhinoscleromatis, contracted by direct inhalation of droplets or contaminated material

Clinical manifestation
Affects nasal cavity, nasopharynx, larynx, trachea, and bronchi
Granulomatous (hypertrophic) stage: nasal mucosa is bluish red and granular, with formation of rubbery nodules or polyps in the nose; epistaxis; deformity and destruction of the nasal cartilage (Hebra nose); thickened soft palate, with erythematous, crusted papules or nodules
Sclerotic stage: nodules replaced by fibrous tissue, leading to scarring and stenosis

Differential diagnosis
Verrucous carcinoma; leprosy; Wegener's granulomatosis; leishmaniasis; lymphoma (lethal midline granuloma); actinomycosis; syphilis; yaws; sarcoidosis; Langerhans cell histiocytosis; tuberculosis; actinomycosis; syphilis; leprosy; histoplasmosis; blastomycosis; paracoccidioidomycosis; sporotrichosis; rhinospiridiosis

Therapy
Tetracycline★; ciprofloxacin

References
Lenis A, Ruff T, Diaz JA, Ghandour EG (1988) Rhinoscleroma. Southern Medical Journal 81(12):1580–1582

Rhinosporidiosis

Synonym(s)
None

Definition
Infectious disease characterized by slow-growing, tumorlike mass, arising in the nasal mucosa or ocular conjunctivae, caused by aquatic protozoan parasite, Rhinosporidium seeberi

Pathogenesis
Caused by aquatic protozoan parasite, Rhinosporidium seeberi, after local traumatic inoculation with the organism, in people bathing or working in stagnant water

Clinical manifestation
Unilateral nasal obstruction or epistaxis; other symptoms: local pruritus, coryza with sneezing, rhinorrhea, and postnasal discharge with cough; soft, pink-to-deep-red, sessile or pedunculated polyps on the nose or eye; skin lesions begin as papillomas and gradually become verrucous

Differential diagnosis
Rhinoscleroma; condyloma acuminatum; nasal polyp; mucocele; squamous cell carcinoma

Therapy
Surgical excision★

References
Elgart ML (1996) Unusual subcutaneous infections. Dermatologic Clinics 14(1):105–111

Rhus dermatitis

▶ Contact dermatitis

Rice-field fever

▶ Leptospirosis

Richner-Hanhart syndrome

▶ Tyrosinemia II

Rickettsemia

▶ Typhus

Rickettsialpox

Synonym(s)
Gamasid rickettsiosis; vesicular rickettsiosis

Definition
Self-limited, zoonotic, febrile illness, caused by rickettsial organism, characterized by papulovesicular skin rash at the site of the mite bite

Pathogenesis
Causative agent: Rickettsia akari; vector: colorless mite, Allodermanyssus sanguineus, found on mice and other rodents

Clinical manifestation
Bite, preceding febrile illness and producing red papule with central vesicle surrmounting it; lesion dries with black

eschar; prodrome of high fever, lasting for a week, with occasional remissions in the morning; generalized exanthem; lesions on tongue, buccal mucosa, and pharynx; mild constitutional symptoms

Differential diagnosis
Varicella; scrub typhus; hand-foot-mouth disease; Boutonneuse fever; viral exanthem

Therapy
Tetracycline; doxycycline; ciprofloxacin

References
Boyd AS (1997) Rickettsialpox. Dermatologic Clinics 15(2):313–318

Riehl melanosis

▶ Riehl's melanosis

Riehl's melanosis

Synonym(s)
Riehl melanosis; pigmented cosmetic dermatitis; pigmented contact dermatitis; melanosis faciei feminae; erythroderma exfoliativa recidivans faciei; lichen ruber planus cum pigmentatione

Definition
Pigmented contact dermatitis of the face, most commonly caused by sensitizing chemicals in cosmetics

Pathogenesis
Type IV allergic reaction; basement membrane damaged by allergic reaction, causing melanin from damaged cells to fall into upper dermis to be ingested by macrophages; ultraviolet light may be a factor; inciting agents: formaldehyde, brilliant lake red R, musk ambrette, optical brighteners and analine dyes

Clinical manifestation
Sudden onset of diffuse or patchy brown pigmentation of cheeks and forehead; severe cases may be black, purple, or blue-black; reticular pigment patterning; erythematous macules or papules

Differential diagnosis
Berloque dermatitis; phytophotodermatitis; melasma; polymorphous light eruption; lupus erythematosus; lichen planus; postinflammatory hyperpigmentation

Therapy
No effective therapy

References
Hori Y, Takayama O (1988) Circumscribed dermal melanoses. Classification and histologic features. Dermatologic Clinics 6(2):315–326

Rifampin

Trade name(s)
Rifadin; Rimactane

Generic available
Yes

Drug class
Rifamycin

Mechanism of action
Inhibits bacterial RNA synthesis by inhibiting DNA-dependent RNA polymerase

Dosage form
150 mg, 300 mg capsule

Dermatologic indications and dosage
See table

Common side effects
Cutaneous: pruritus, urticaria or other eruptions
Gastrointestinal: abdominal pain, nausea, vomiting, diarrhea
Laboratory: elevated liver enzymes

R

Rifampin. Dermatologic indications and dosage

Disease	Adult dosage	Child dosage
Cutaneous tuberculosis	10 mg per kg PO daily, divided into 2 doses	10–20 mg per kg PO daily, divided into 2 doses
Leprosy, multibacillary disease	600 mg daily PO for 3 years	10–20 mg per kg daily PO for 3 years
Leprosy, paucibacillary disease	300 mg PO twice daily for 3 months	10–20 mg per kg PO daily for 3 months
Staphylococcal pyoderma, to eliminate carrier state	600 mg PO daily for 7 days	10–20 mg per kg daily PO for 7 days

Miscellaneous: reddish-orange body fluids, stained contact lenses
Neurologic: dizziness, ataxia, headache

Serious side effects
Bone marrow: thrombocytopenia, leukopenia
Gastrointestinal: hepatotoxicity
Renal: renal failure, interstitial nephritis

Drug interactions
Digoxin; chloramphenicol; warfarin; phenobarbital; phenytoin; ketoconazole; theophylline; verapamil; cyclosporine; corticosteroids; oral contraceptives; dapsone; sulfonylureas

Contraindications/precautions
Hypersensitivity to drug class or component; caution in patients with hepatic insufficiency

References
Tsankov NK, Kamarashev JA (1993) Rifampin in dermatology. International Journal of Dermatology 32(6):401–406

Right Guard Sport

▶ **Aluminium chlorohydrate**

Riley-Smith syndrome

▶ **Bannayan-Riley-Ruvalcaba syndrome**

Ringed keratolysis

▶ **Pitted keratolysis**

Ringworm

▶ **Tinea corporis**

Ringworm of the beard

▶ **Sycosis barbae**

Ringworm of the face

▶ **Tinea faciei**

Ringworm of the feet

▶ Tinea pedis

Ringworm of the groin

▶ Tinea cruris

Ringworm of the scalp

▶ Tinea capitis

Robert-Unna syndrome

▶ Cutis verticis gyrata

Robles' disease

▶ Filariasis

Rocky Mountain spotted fever

Synonym(s)
Tick fever; spotted fever; tick typhus; New World spotted fever; Sao Paulo fever

Definition
Tick-borne rickettsial disease, characterized by fever, rash, and constitutional signs and symptoms

Pathogenesis
Caused by R rickettsii, rickettsial organism transmitted from tick to human during feeding; proliferates in the endothelial lining, causing intravascular thrombi; vasculitis leads to small vessel occlusion and tissue necrosis

Clinical manifestation
Presents within 1 week of tick bite; prodrome of fever, headache, myalgias; skin and mucous membrane changes: confluent macular and papular eruption on wrists and ankles; spreads centripetally to trunk and proximal extremities and palms and soles; eruption becomes petechial after a few days; conjunctival suffusion; periorbital edema, especially in children; photophobia
Cardiovascular system: myocarditis; bradycardia; arrhythmias; occasional hypotension; congestive heart failure secondary to myocarditis
Pulmonary system: pulmonary edema in severe cases; pneumonitis
Gastrointestinal system: anorexia; abdominal pain and tenderness; jaundice in severe cases; hepatomegaly and splenomegaly; diarrhea
Musculoskeletal system: myalgia, especially in the legs, abdomen, and back; diffuse arthralgias; edema of the dorsum of hands and feet
Central nervous system: restlessness and irritability; altered mental status; meningoencephalitis; cranial neuropathies; paralysis; ataxia; meningismus

Differential diagnosis
Dengue fever; babesiosis; ehrlichiosis; mononucleosis; leptospirosis; Lyme disease; malaria; meningococcemia; bacterial sepsis; toxic shock syndrome; tularemia; other rickettsial infections; allergic vasculitis; Brill-Zinsser disease; drug hypersensitivity; atypical measles; rubeola; drug eruption

Therapy
Doxycycline[*]; chloramphenicol:
adult dose: 500 mg IV divided into 4 doses per day for 7 days;

pediatric dose: 50 mg per kg PO divided into 4 doses for 7 days and for at least 48 hours after defervescence

References

Sexton DJ, Kaye KS (2002) Rocky Mountain spotted fever. Medical Clinics of North America 86(2):351–360

Rodent ulcer

▶ Basal cell carcinoma

Romberg-Perry syndrome

▶ Morphea

Romberg's facial hemiatrophy

▶ Morphea

Rosacea

Synonym(s)
Acne rosacea

Definition
Disorder characterized by facial flushing and a spectrum of clinical signs including erythema, telangiectasia, and inflammatory papules and pustules

Pathogenesis
Genetic component; preferentially occurs in those with constitutive facial flushing; probably related to the local release of vasoac-

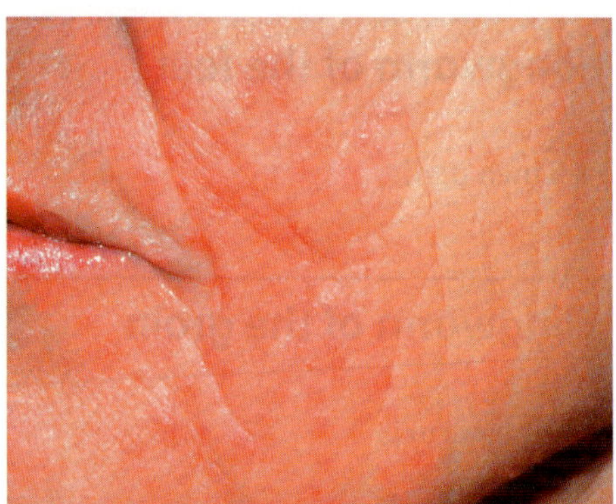

Rosacea. Red papules on the cheek

tive substances; exascerbated by local heat from hot drinks, alcohol, spicy foods and temperature changes

Clinical manifestation
Background of facial flushing; erythema and telangiectasia over the cheeks and forehead; inflammatory papules and pustules, predominantly over the nose, forehead, and cheeks; extra-facial involvement over the neck and upper chest; prominent sebaceous glands with development of thickened and disfigured nose (rhinophyma)
Ocular variant: conjunctival injection, chalazion, and episcleritis
Granulomatous variant (lupus miliaris disseminata faciei): inflammatory, erythematous or flesh-colored papules distributed symmetrically across the upper face, particularly around the eyes and nose

Differential diagnosis
Seborrheic dermatitis; lupus erythematosus; polymorphous light eruption; tinea faciei; acne vulgaris; perioral dermatitis; folliculitis; lupus vulgaris; carcinoid syndrome

Therapy
Tetracycline; minocycline; doxycycline; metronidazole; azelaic acid; tretinoin; isotretinoin; surgical therapy: permanent telangiectasia: 585-nm pulsed dye laser; rhinophyma: mechanical dermabrasion; CO_2 laser peel

References

Rebora A (2002) The management of rosacea. American Journal of Clinical Dermatology 3(7):489–496

Rosacea-like dermatitis

▶ Perioral dermatitis

Rose gardener's disease

▶ Sporotrichosis

Roseola

Synonym(s)

Roseola infantum; exanthem subitum; sixth disease

Definition

Childhood exanthematous disease caused by Human Herpesvirus-6 (HHV-6)

Pathogenesis

Main cause HHV-6B; in primary infection, replication of the virus in leukocytes and salivary glands; early invasion of the central nervous system, causes seizures and other CNS complications

Clinical manifestation

Most primary infections asymptomatic; typical presentation: 9–12-month-old child with abrupt onset of high fever (40°C), lasting for 3 days with nonspecific complaints; febrile seizures may occur; rapid defervescence of fever occurring with onset of pink morbilliform exanthem composed of either discrete, small, pale pink papules or a blanchable exanthem, lasting 2 days; enanthem (Nagayama's spots) with erythematous papules on the mucosa of the soft palate and base of the uvula

Differential diagnosis

Other viral exanthems, including mononucleosis; rubeola and rubella; scarlet fever; meningococcemia; dengue fever; medication reaction

Therapy

Antipyretic therapy such as acetaminophen

References

Blauvelt A (2001) Skin diseases associated with human herpesvirus 6, 7, and 8 infection. Journal of Investigative Dermatology. Symposium Proceedings 6(3):197–202

Roseola infantum

▶ Roseola

Rothman-Makai syndrome

Synonym(s)

Lipogranulomatosis subcutanea; adiponecrosis subcutanea; lipophagic panniculitis of childhood

Definition

Panniculitis of children, characterized by subcutaneous nodules without systemic signs or symptoms

Pathogenesis

May be a variant of Weber-Christian disease; mechanism of disease unknown

Clinical manifestation

Well-demarcated, somewhat painful, symmetrical subcutaneous nodules, most often on lower extremities and trunk; atrophy in lesions of lipophagic panniculitis variant

Differential diagnosis

Thrombophlebitis; vasculitis; sarcoidosis; alpha-1 antitrypsin deficiency panniculitis; polyarteritis nodosa; eosinophilic fasciitis; eosinophilic myalgia syndrome; erythema

R

induratum; erythema nodosum; leukemia; lipodermatosclerosis; lymphoma; pancreatic panniculitis; poststeroid panniculitis; scleroderma panniculitis; cytophagic histiocytic panniculitis; Sweet's syndrome

Therapy
No therapy indicated

References
Requena L, Sanchez Yus E (2001) Panniculitis. Part II. Mostly lobular panniculitis. Journal of the American Academy of Dermatology 45(3):325–361

Rothmund-Thomson syndrome

Synonym(s)
Poikiloderma congenitale

Definition
Hereditary disorder characterized by multisystem abnormalities and early photosensitivity, resulting in poikiloderma

Pathogenesis
Autosomal recessive trait; genetic defect on chromosome 8

Clinical manifestation
Irregular erythema of the skin progressing to poikiloderma with atrophy, telangiectasia, hyperpigmentation, and hypopigmentation; sparse hair; premature canities; dystrophic or atrophic nails; acral hyperkeratotic lesions on elbows, knees, hands, and feet; distinctive facies with frontal bossing, saddle nose, and micrognathia; short stature; sexual abnormalities; cataracts; dental abnormalities

Differential diagnosis
Bloom syndrome; lupus erythematosus; erythropoietic protoporphyria; Werner's syndrome progeria; Fanconi's anemia; acrogeria; Cockayne syndrome; xeroderma pigmentosus; Mendes da Costa syndrome

Therapy
Sun protection[*]; pulse dye laser therapy for telangiectases

References
Vennos EM, Collins M, James WD (1992) Rothmund-Thomson syndrome: review of the world literature. Journal of the American Academy of Dermatology 27(5 Pt 1):750–762

Round cell erythematosus

▶ Reticular erythematous mucinosis

Rubella

Synonym(s)
German measles; three day measles

Definition
Contagious viral infection with mild symptoms associated with eruption and lymphadenopathy

Pathogenesis
RNA virus classified as a Rubivirus in the Togaviridae family

Clinical manifestation
Spread by nasal droplet infection; incubation period of 14–19 days, with onset of rash usually on the 15th day; disease contagious from a few days before to 5–7 days after the appearance of the exanthem; most contagious when rash is erupting; may have no prodrome in children, with rash being first manifestation; in adults, fever, sore throat, and rhinitis may occur; discrete macules on the face that spread to the neck, trunk, and extremities, with coalescence into plaques; exanthem lasts 1–3 days, first leaving the face; nonspecific enanthem (Forscheimer's spots) of pinpoint red macules and petechiae visible over the soft palate and uvula just before or with the exanthem;

generalized tender lymphadenopathy involving all nodes, but most striking in the suboccipital, postauricular, and anterior and posterior cervical nodes; joint symptoms may occur in adults; congenital rubella syndrome in infants whose mothers contract the disease during the first trimester: purpura at birth, low birth weight, small head size, lethargy, irritabilitiy, deafness, seizures, developmental delay, mental retardation

Differential diagnosis
Juvenile rheumatoid arthritis; rubeola; other viral exanthems; scarlet fever; Kawasaki disease; drug eruption

Therapy
None; isolation for 7 days after onset of the eruption

References
Bullens D, Smets K, Vanhaesebrouck P (2000) Congenital rubella syndrome after maternal reinfection. Clinical Pediatrics 39(2):113–116

Rubeola

Synonym(s)
Measles; rubeola morbilli; rubeola measles

Definition
Acute, contagious, viral disease characterized by distinct red lesions in the mouth followed by a generalized eruption

Pathogenesis
Measles virus infects respiratory epithelium; transmitted via respiratory droplets; replication in lymph nodes leads to viremia; infection of endothelial cells ensues, causing enanthem (Koplik spots); infection of epithelial cells leads to skin eruption

Clinical manifestation
Incubation period from 7–14 days (average 10–11 days); communicable just before the beginning of prodromal symptoms, until approximately 4 days following the onset of the exanthem; prodrome of cough, coryza, conjunctivitis, fever, photophobia
Enanthem (Koplik spots): blue-white spots surrounded by red halo; appear on buccal mucosa opposite the premolar teeth; predate exanthem by 24–48 hours and last approximately 2–4 days.
Exanthem: begins on the fourth or fifth day after onset of symptoms; appears as slightly elevated papules beginning on face and behind the ears and spreading to trunk and extremities within 24–36 hours; initial color dark red, slowly fading to purplish hue, and then to yellow/brown lesions with fine scale, over the following 5–10 days

Differential diagnosis
Other viral exanthems, such as rubella, enterovirus, echovirus, cytomegalovirus infection, primary HIV disease; brucellosis; drug eruption; Kawasaki disease

Therapy
No specific therapy

▶ Rubella

References
Omer MI (1999) Measles: a disease that has to be eradicated. Annals of Tropical Paediatrics 19(2):125–134

Rubeola measles

▶ Rubeola

Rubeola morbilli

▶ Rubeola

Rubinstein syndrome

▶ Rubinstein-Taybi syndrome

Rubinstein Taybi broad thumb-hallux syndrome

▶ Rubinstein-Taybi syndrome

Rubinstein-Taybi syndrome

Synonym(s)
Rubinstein syndrome; broad thumb-hallux syndrome

Definition
Genetic multisystem disorder characterized by broad thumbs and great toes, characteristic facies, and mental retardation

Pathogenesis
Possible autosomal dominant inheritance in some families; gene on the short arm (p) of chromosome 16 (16p13.3); may be caused by point mutation or deletion in gene involved in regulation of CREB binding protein

Clinical manifestation
Skin changes: one or capillary hemangiomas or nevus flammeus lesions on forehead, neck nape, and/or back; cafe au lait spots; keloid formation; hypertrichosis; ingrown finger- or toenails.
Systemic changes: growth retardation; delayed bone age; mental retardation; craniofacial dysmorphism (including hypertelorism, broad nasal bridge, and "beak-shaped" nose); abnormally broad thumbs and great toes; breathing and swallowing difficulties; malformations of the heart, kidneys, urogenital system, and/or skeletal system

Differential diagnosis
Saethre-Chotzen syndrome; Trisomy 13 syndrome; Cornelia de Lange syndrome

Therapy
No specific therapy

References
De Silva B (2002) What syndrome is this? Rubenstein-Taybi syndrome. Pediatric Dermatology 19(2):177–179

Rudimentary polydactyly

▶ Supernumerary digit

Runaround abscess

▶ Paronychia

Runaround infection

▶ Paronychia

Ruvalcaba-Myhre-Smith syndrome

▶ Bannayan-Riley-Ruvalcaba syndrome

Ruvalcaba-Myhre syndrome

▶ Bannayan-Riley-Ruvalcaba syndrome

Saethre-Chotzen syndrome

▶ Acrocephalosyndactyly

Sailor's neck

▶ Actinic elastosis

Salivosudoriparous syndrome

▶ Auriculotemporal syndrome

Pathogenesis
Possible persistent fetal circulatory pattern

Clinical manifestation
Pink-to-red macule or patch on the nape of the neck, glabella, forehead, upper eyelid, or nasolabial region; present at birth in about 40% of cases

Differential diagnosis
Hemangioma; Sturge-Weber syndrome; child abuse; insect bite reaction

Therapy
No therapy indicated

References
Mallory SB (1991) Neonatal skin disorders. Pediatric Clinics of North America 38(4):745–761

Salmon patch

Synonym(s)
Stork bite; angel's kiss; nevus simplex; erythema nuchae

Definition
Vascular malformation, present in infancy, consisting of ectatic capillaries

Salmonellosis

Synonym(s)
Typhoid fever; paratyphoid fever

Definition
Infection caused by bacteria in the genus Salmonella, usually contracted by eating contaminated food

Pathogenesis
Infection caused by salmonellae, gram-negative, rod-shaped bacteria of the family Enterobacteriaceae; most common sources of bacteria: beef, poultry, eggs

Clinical manifestation
Skin signs: light red papules (rose spots) occurring in crops on trunk during second to fourth week of illness; erythema nodosum, Sweet's syndrome, pustular dermatitis and generalized erythroderma (erythema typhosum)
Gastrointestinal signs: loose stool or watery diarrhea; abdominal pain; mild hepatosplenomegaly

Differential diagnosis
Viral gastroenteritis; shigellosis; ingestion of preformed toxins ("food poisoning"); campylobacter infection; cryptosporidiosis; cyclospora infection; escherichia coli infection; listeriosis; vibrio infection

Therapy
Antibiotics only for patients with severe disease or those at high risk of invasive disease: ciprofloxacin; amoxicillin

▶ Typhoid fever

References
Stutman HR (1994) Salmonella, shigella, and campylobacter: common bacterial causes of infectious diarrhea. Pediatric Annals 23(10):538–543

San Joaquin Valley fever

▶ Coccidioidomycosis

Sandworm disease

▶ Cutaneous larva migrans

Sanfilippo syndrome

Synonym(s)
Mucopolysaccharidosis type III-A; mucopolysaccharidosis type III-B; mucopolysaccharidosis type III-C

Definition
Inherited metabolic storage disease from a deficiency of either heparan sulfate sulfamidase, N-acetyl-alpha-D-glucosaminidase, acetyl-CoA alpha-glucosamide N-acetyltransferase, or N-acetyl-alpha-D-glucosamine-6-sulfatase

Pathogenesis
Autosomal recessive trait; deficiency of either heparan sulfate sulfamidase, or N-acetyl-alpha-D-glucosaminidase, or acetyl-CoA alpha-glucosamide N-acetyltransferase, or N-acetyl-alpha-D-glucosamine-6-sulfatase, resulting in accumulation of mucopolysaccharides in the lysosomes of the cells in the connective tissue

Clinical manifestation
Onset of symptoms from age 2–6 years; organs most involved: bone, viscera, connective tissue, and brain; regression of psychomotor development and neurologic signs, including severe mental retardation, hyperactivity, autistic features, and behavioral disorders; thickened facial features; coarse hair; hirsutism; genu valgum; short neck; progressive deterioration and death, usually before age 20 years

Differential diagnosis
Hunter syndrome; Hurler syndrome; Scheie syndrome; Gaucher's disease; Niemann-Pick disease

Therapy
None

References
Yogalingam G, Hopwood JJ (2001) Molecular genetics of mucopolysaccharidosis type IIIA and

IIIB: Diagnostic, clinical, and biological implications. Human Mutation 18(4):264–281

Sao Paulo fever

▶ **Rocky Mountain spotted fever**

Sarcoidosis

Synonym(s)
Angiolupoid sarcoid; Besnier-Boeck-Schaumann disease; Boeck's sarcoid

Definition
Chronic multisystem disease, characterized by noncaseating epithelioid granulomas

Pathogenesis
May result from exposure of a genetically susceptible host to specific environmental agents, such as infectious organisms, aluminium, zirconium, talc, pine tree pollen, and clay, that the immune system is unable to effectively clear

Clinical manifestation
Skin: asymptomatic, red-brown macules and papules commonly involving the face, periorbital, nasolabial folds, extensor surfaces of extremities; round-to-oval, red-brown-to-purple, infiltrated plaques, the center of which may be atrophic; non-tender, firm, oval, flesh-colored or violaceous nodules on extremities or trunk (Darier-Roussy sarcoidosis); inflitration of scars
Pulmonary system: involvement in most patients; dyspnea; dry cough; chest tightness or pain
Lymphatic system: palpable lymph nodes
Ocular involvement: anterior uveitis, associated with fever and parotid swelling (uveoparotid fever)

Neurologic system: central nervous system involvement sometimes fatal; seventh cranial nerve palsy most frequent finding; miscellaneous findings: myocardial involvement, arthritis, proximal muscle weakness, renal failure

Differential diagnosis
Tuberculosis; lymphoma; pseudolymphoma; foreign body granuloma; drug reaction; granuloma annulare; granuloma faciale; lichen planus; lupus erythematosus; leprosy; syphilis; psoriasis; tinea corporis; necrobiosis lipoidica

Therapy
Cutaneous involvement: triamcinolone 3 mg per ml intralesional
Severe, recalcitrant disease: methotrexate; azathioprine; hydroxychloroquine
Symptomatic systemic disease: prednisone[*]

References
Vourlekis JS, Sawyer RT, Newman LS (2000) Sarcoidosis: developments in etiology, immunology, and therapeutics. Advances in Internal Medicine 45:209–257

Sarcoma botryoides

▶ **Rhabdomyosarcoma**

Savill's syndrome

▶ **Sulzberger-Garbe syndrome**

Say syndrome

▶ **Barber-Say syndrome**

Scabies

Synonym(s)
Seven-year itch

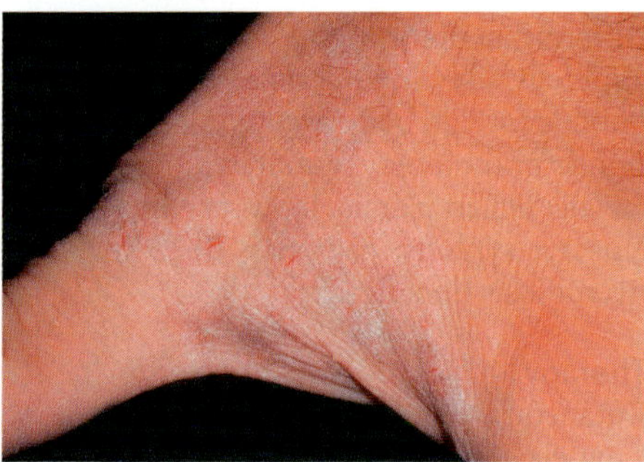

Scabies. Scaly and fissured papules and plaques in the finger web spaces

Definition
Contagious infestation of the skin by arachnid mite Sarcoptes scabiei, var hominis

Pathogenesis
Causative organism is mite, Sarcoptes scabiei; disease spreads through direct and prolonged contact between hosts; possible transmission through fomites, such as infected bedding or clothing, but less likely; delayed type IV hypersensitivity reaction to mites, eggs, or scybala (packets of feces) which causes intense pruritus

Clinical manifestation
Intense pruritus, particularly at night; slightly elevated, pink-white, linear, curved, or s-shaped line (burrow), located in webbed spaces of fingers, flexor surfaces of wrists, elbows, axillae, belt line, feet, and scrotum in men and areolae in women; burrows on the palms and soles in infants; vesicles; red papules on penile shaft
Nodular variant: pink, tan, brown, or red nodules lasting for weeks
Crusted (Norwegian) variant: occurs in immunocompromised and institutionalized patients; minimally pruritic, hyperkeratotic, crusted plaques over large areas; nail dystrophy; scalp lesions

Differential diagnosis
Atopic dermatitis; dermatitis herpetiformis; pityriasis lichenoides; lichen planus; insect bite reaction; contact dermatitis; psoriasis; ecthyma; impetigo; xerotic eczema; transient acantholytic dermatosis; linear IgA bullous dermatosis; seborrheic dermatitis; erythroderma from other causes such as Sézary syndrome and pemphigus foliaceus; Langerhans cell histiocytosis; fiberglass dermatitis; dyshidrotic eczema; pityriasis rosea; animal scabies; pediculosis; delusions of parasitosis; metabolic pruritus

Therapy
Permethrin; ivermectin; prednisone for severe symptoms

References
Wendel K, Rompalo A (2002) Scabies and pediculosis pubis: an update of treatment regimens and general review. Clinical Infectious Diseases 35(Suppl 2):S146–151

Scalded skin syndrome

▶ **Staphylococcal scalded skin syndrome**

Scalp and head syndrome

▶ **Adams-Oliver Syndrome**

Scalp cyst

▶ **Pilar cyst**

Scarlatina

▶ Scarlet fever

Scarlet fever

Synonym(s)
Scarlatina

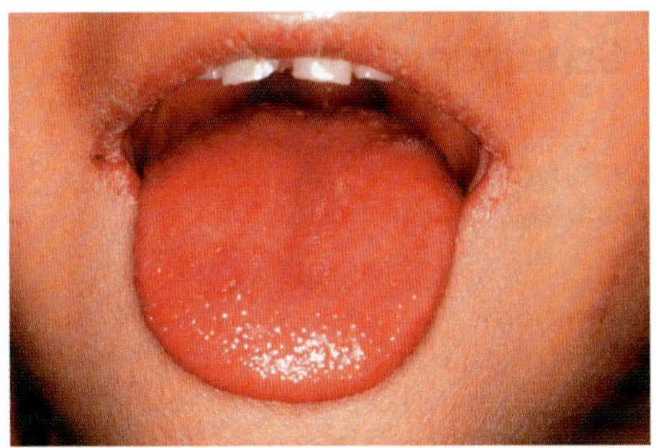

Scarlet fever. Bright red tongue with prominent papillae

Definition
Bacterial infection caused by toxin-producing group-A beta hemolytic streptococci

Pathogenesis
Eruption caused by erythemogenic toxin as consequence of local production of inflammatory mediators and alteration of the cutaneous cytokines

Clinical manifestation
Abrupt onset of fever, headache, vomiting, malaise, chills, and sore throat, with rash appearing after 1–4 days; exudative tonsillitis a common site of infection; mucous membranes usually bright red; scattered petechiae and small, red papules on soft palate; during first days of infection, white membrane coating on tongue through which edematous, red papillae protrude (white strawberry tongue); after white membrane sloughs, tongue red with prominent papillae (red strawberry tongue); exanthem consisting of fine red, punctate papules, appearing within 1–4 days following the onset of illness; first appear on upper trunk and axillae and then generalize, with accentuation in flexural areas; may appear more intense at dependent sites and sites of pressure, such as the buttocks; sandpaper feel to affected skin; transverse areas of hyperpigmentation with petechiae in the axillary, antecubital, and inguinal areas (Pastia lines); flushed face with circumoral pallor; rash fades with fine desquamation after 4–5 days

Differential diagnosis
Viral exanthem, including rubella, rubeola, fifth disease; toxic shock syndrome; Kawasaki syndrome; lupus erythematosus; drug reaction

Therapy
Penicillin VK★; benzathine penicillin G; penicillin allergy – cephalexin, erythromycin

References
Chiesa C, Pacifico L, Nanni F, Orefici G (1994) Recurrent attacks of scarlet fever. Archives of Pediatrics & Adolescent Medicine 148(6):656–660

Scarring pemphigoid

▶ Cicatricial pemphigoid

Schamberg disease

▶ Benign pigmented purpura

Schamberg's progressive pigmented purpura

▶ Benign pigmented purpura

Scheie syndrome

Synonym(s)
Mucopolysaccharidosis type I-H/S; mucopolysaccharidosis type I-S; Hurler-Scheie syndrome

Definition
Inherited metabolic storage disease arising from a deficiency of alpha-L-iduronidase

Pathogenesis
Autosomal recessive trait; deficiency of alpha-L-iduronidase, which results in accumulation of mucopolysaccharides in the lysosomes of the cells in the connective tissue

Clinical manifestation
Onset of symptoms from age 2–4 years; signs and symptoms similar to those of Hurler syndrome, but milder, with slower progression; lichenified, dry, thick skin with diminished elasticity; increased pigmentation on the dorsum of the hands; sclerodermalike changes; hypertrichosis of the extremities; pale colored hair; mild skeletal deformation and deformity of the hands; growth sometimes normal; aortic stenosis or regurgitation sometimes present; hepatosplenomegaly; intelligence usually normal

Differential diagnosis
Hurler syndrome; Hunter syndrome; Gaucher's disease; Niemann-Pick diseae; osteogenesis imperfecta

Therapy
None

References
Schiro JA, Mallory SB, Demmer L, Dowton SB, Luke MC (1996) Grouped papules in Hurler-Scheie syndrome. Journal of the American Academy of Dermatology 35(5 Pt 2):868–870

Schenck's disease

▶ Sporotrichosis

Schilder-Addison syndrome

▶ Addison-Schilder disease

Schnitzler syndrome

Synonym(s)
Schnitzler's syndrome

Definition
Disorder characterized by chronic urticaria, in association with recurrent fever, bone pain, and IgM monoclonal gammopathy

Pathogenesis
May be related to deposition of the IgM paraprotein, leading to immune complex deposition and complement activation

Clinical manifestation
Chronic urticaria; individual episode usually resolves within few hours; fevers persist for up to 24–48 hours; relapsing arthralgias; bone pain involving tibia, femur, ileum, and vertebral column; myalgias; fatigue; weight loss

Differential diagnosis
Urticarial vasculitis; lupus erythematosus; adult Still disease; Waldenström macroglobulinemia; chronic hepatitis B infection

Therapy
Acute disease flare: prednisone

References

Lipsker D, Veran Y, Grunenberger F, Cribier B, Heid E, Grosshans E (2001) The Schnitzler syndrome. Four new cases and review of the literature. Medicine 80(1):37–44

Schnitzler's syndrome

▶ Schnitzler syndrome

Schönlein-Henoch purpura

▶ Henoch-Schönlein purpura

Schwannoma

▶ Granular cell tumor

Schweninger and Buzzi, idiopathic anetoderma of

▶ Anetoderma

Scleredema

Synonym(s)

Scleredema adultorum; scleredema adultorum of Buschke; scleredema diabeticorum; scleredema diabeticorum of Buschke

Definition

Disorder characterized by nonpitting, indurated plaques and histological evidence of dermal mucin deposition

Pathogenesis

Increased procollagen synthesis

Clinical manifestation

Group 1 subtype: precedes febrile illness, particularly upper respiratory tract streptococcal infection; usually clears in 6 months to 2 years

Group 2 subtype: no prior history of febrile illness; insidious onset of skin lesions; at risk of developing paraproteinemias, including multiple myeloma

Group 3 subtype: prior history of diabetes mellitus, usually adult onset and insulin dependent, unremitting course; ill-defined, woody, nonpitting, indurated plaques; erythema, hyperpigmentation, and/or a peau d'orange appearance; usually located on face, neck, trunk, or upper extremities

Differential diagnosis

Scleroderma; lichen myxedema; generalized myxedema; sclerema neonatorum; amyloidosis; cellulitis; erysipelas

Therapy

No effective therapy

References

Tate BJ, Kelly JW, Rotstein H (1996) Scleredema of Buschke: a report of seven cases. Australasian Journal of Dermatology 37(3):139–142

Scleredema adultorum

▶ Scleredema

Scleredema adultorum of Buschke

▶ Scleredema

Scleredema diabeticorum

▶ Scleredema

Scleredema diabeticorum of Buschke

▶ Scleredema

Scleredema of Buschke

▶ Scleredema

Sclerema

▶ Sclerema neonatorum

Sclerema neonatorum

Synonym(s)
Sclerema

Definition
Disorder of the subcutaneous fat in debilitated neonates, resulting in generalized subcutaneous plaques

Pathogenesis
Prematurity, hypothermia, shock, and metabolic abnormalities increases saturated-to-unsaturated fatty acid ratio, possibly as a result of enzymatic alteration, allowing precipitation of fatty acid crystals within lipocytes; occurs with prematurity, pneumonia, septicemia, respiratory distress syndrome, congenital heart defects, gastroenteritis, and intestinal obstruction

Clinical manifestation
Firm, violaceous subcutaneous plaques appearing suddenly, first on thighs and buttocks and then spreading; may affect all parts of the body except palms, soles, and genitalia; temperature instability; restricted respiration; difficulty in feeding; decreased spontaneous movement

Differential diagnosis
Scleredema; scleroderma; subcutaneous fat necrosis of newborn; neonatal cold injury

Therapy
No specific therapy for skin disorder; institution of therapy specific for the underlying disease

References
Fretzin DF, Arias AM (1987) Sclerema neonatorum and subcutaneous fat necrosis of the newborn. Pediatric Dermatology 4(2):112–122

Scleroderma

Synonym(s)
None

Definition
Group of disorders characterized by skin thickening secondary to increased dermal collagen production

▶ **Progressive systemic sclerosus**

References
Haustein UF (2002) Systemic sclerosis-scleroderma. Dermatology Online Journal 8(1):3

Sclerodermoid fasciitis

▶ **Eosinophilia-myalgia syndrome**

Sclerodermoid myalgia

► Eosinophilia-myalgia syndrome

Scleroma

► Rhinoscleroma

Scleromyxedema

► Papular mucinosis

Scleromyxedema-like illness of hemodialysis

► Nephrogenic fibrosing dermopathy

Scleromyxedema-like illness of renal disease

► Nephrogenic fibrosing dermopathy

Sclerosing angioma

► Dermatofibroma

Sclerosing epithelial hamartoma

► Trichoepithelioma

Sclerosing hemangioma

► Dermatofibroma

Sclerosing periphlebitis of the lateral chest wall

► Mondor's disease

Scrofuloderma

► Cutaneous tuberculosis

Scrotal tongue

► Lingua plicata

Scrub typhus

Synonym(s)
Tsutsugamushi disease; tsutsugamushi fever

Definition
Acute, febrile, infectious illness caused by Rickettsia tsutsugamushi, characterized by rash and systemic signs and symptoms

Pathogenesis
Caused by Rickettsia tsutsugamushi (Rickettsia orientalis), acquired when infected chigger bites and inoculates pathogens

Clinical manifestation
High, severe headache, myalgia; ocular pain; wet cough; malaise; injected conjunctiva; eruption begins as a red, indurated

papule that eventually enlarges to 8–12 mm, vesiculates, and ruptures, developing necrosis; 5–8 days later, onset of centrifugal-spreading macular eruption on trunk, sometimes becoming papular

Differential diagnosis
Tularemia; leptospirosis; typhoid fever; other rickettsial infections; viral exanthem; dengue fever

Therapy
Doxycycline[*]; chloramphenicol – 500 mg PO 4 times daily for 7–14 days

References
Baxter JD (1996) The typhus group. Clinics in Dermatology 14(3):271–278

Scurvy

Synonym(s)
Vitamin C deficiency syndrome

Definition
Vitamin C deficiency disease manifested by gingival lesions, hemorrhage, arthralgia, loss of appetite, and listlessness

Pathogenesis
Vitamin C deficiency, after at least 3 months of severe or total lack of vitamin C, resulting in defective collagen synthesis and defective folic acid and iron utilization

Clinical manifestation
Perifollicular hyperkeratotic papules, surrounded by a hemorrhagic halo; hairs are twisted like corkscrews and may be fragmented; submucosal gingival bleeding; subperiosteal hemorrhage causes painful bones of the legs and elsewhere; arthralgia; anorexia; listlessness; conjunctival hemorrhage; poor wound healing

Differential diagnosis
Vasculitis; physical abuse; coagulation abnormalities with leukemia; platelet abnormalities; deep vein thrombosis; thrombophlebitis

Therapy
Ascorbic acid 800–1000 mg per day PO for at least 1 week, then 400 mg per day until recovery complete

References
Hirschmann JV, Raugi GJ (1999) Adult scurvy. Journal of the American Academy of Dermatology 41(6):895–906

Scutula

Definition
Dense masses of mycelium and epithelial debris forming yellowish, cup-shaped crusts, seen in the favus form of tinea capitis

References
Qianggiang Z, Limo Q, Jiajun W, Li L (2002) Report of two cases of tinea infection with scutula-like lesions caused by Microsporum gypseum. International Journal of Dermatology 41(6):372–373

Sea boot foot

▶ **Immersion foot**

Sea lice

▶ **Seabather's eruption**

Seabather's eruption

Synonym(s)
Sea lice

Definition
Pruritic, papular eruption occurring underneath the swimsuit after extended exposure to seawater

Pathogenesis
Hypersensitivity reaction to larval form of the thimble jellyfish, Linuche unguiculata; factors promoting larval venom discharge: wearing of bathing suits for prolonged periods following swimming, exposure to fresh water through showering, and mechanical stimulation

Clinical manifestation
Onset a few hours after ocean bathing; pruritic papules in a bathing suit distribution pattern; occurence in axilla and on chest in men with significant chest hair

Differential diagnosis
Cercarial dermatitis; insect bite reaction; scabies; folliculitis; jellyfish sting; urticaria

Therapy
Corticosteroids, topical, high potency; antihistamines, first generation, for sedation

References
Wong DE, Meinking TL, Rosen LB (1994) Seabather's eruption. Clinical, histologic, and immunologic features. Journal of the American Academy of Dermatology 30(3): 399–406

Sebaceoma

▶ Sebaceous epithelioma

Sebaceous adenoma

Synonym(s)
None

Definition
Benign epithelial neoplasm composed of sebaceous gland-like structures with sebaceous differentiation

Pathogenesis
Genetic predisposition exists in some cases of Muir-Torre syndrome

Clinical manifestation
Yellow, tan, or pink, speckled, smooth-surfaced, well-circumscribed papule or nodule, sometimes with central umbilication, located on face, scalp, or neck

Differential diagnosis
Basal cell carcinoma; sebaceous carcinoma; sebaceous gland hyperplasia; nevus sebaceous; xanthoma; xanthelasma; molluscum contagiosum; other adnexal neoplasms

Therapy
Surgical excision[*]

References
Iezzi G, Rubini C, Fioroni M, Piattelli A (2002) Sebaceous adenoma of the cheek. Oral Oncology 38(1):111–113

Sebaceous carcinoma

Synonym(s)
Sebaceous gland carcinoma

Definition
Aggressive, malignant, cutaneous tumor, arising from sebaceous glands in the skin

Pathogenesis
Genetic predisposition exists in some cases of Muir-Torre syndrome

Clinical manifestation
Firm, slowly enlarging, flesh-colored papule, located on upper eyelid, scalp, or neck; metastatic potential

Differential diagnosis
Keratoconjunctivitis; blepharoconjunctivitis; chalazion; squamous cell carcinoma; basal cell carcinoma; Merkel cell carcinoma; pyogenic granuloma; melanoma; metastasis; benign adnexal tumor; sarcoidosis, ocular pemphigoid

Therapy
Mohs micrographic surgery[*]

References
Snow SN, Larson PO, Lucarelli MJ, Lemke BN, Madjar DD (2002) Sebaceous carcinoma of the eyelids treated by mohs micrographic surgery: report of nine cases with review of the literature. Dermatologic Surgery 28(7):623–631

Sebaceous cyst

▶ Epidermoid cyst

Sebaceous epithelioma

Synonym(s)
Sebaceoma

Definition
Benign cutaneous tumor composed of less than 50 % of cells having sebaceous differentiation

Pathogenesis
Genetic predisposition exists in some cases of Muir-Torre syndrome

Clinical manifestation
Firm, flesh-colored or yellowish, smooth, sessile, or pedunculated papule on face, scalp, or eyelid; older lesions may form plaque and ulcerate

Differential diagnosis
Sebaceous carcinoma; squamous cell carcinoma; basal cell carcinoma; Merkel cell carcinoma; chalazion; pyogenic granuloma; melanoma; metastasis; sarcoidosis

Therapy
Surgical excision[*]

References
Brown MD (2000) Recognition and management of unusual cutaneous tumors. Dermatologic Clinics 18(3):543–552

Sebaceous gland carcinoma

▶ Sebaceous carcinoma

Sebaceous gland hyperplasia

▶ Sebaceous hyperplasia

Sebaceous hyperplasia

Synonym(s)
Sebaceous gland hyperplasia; senile sebaceous adenoma; senile sebaceous hyperplasia

Definition
Hamartomatous enlargement of facial sebaceous glands, characterized by yellow papules with central dell

Pathogenesis
Occurs commonly in organ transplant recipients, suggesting immune mechanisms in some cases

Clinical manifestation
Well-demarcated, yellow-to-flesh-colored, delled papules, most commonly on forehead and cheeks

Differential diagnosis
Sebaceous carcinoma; melanocytic nevus; sebaceous adenoma; sebaceous epithelioma; squamous cell carcinoma; basal cell carcinoma; sarcoidosis; colloid milium; fibrous papule; granuloma annulare; lipoid proteinosis; milium; molluscum contagiosum; syringoma; trichoepithelioma; xanthoma; xanthelasma

Therapy
Light electrodesiccation; liquid nitrogen cryotherapy; laser ablation; shave removal; isotretinoin for multiple lesions

References
de Berker DA, Taylor AE, Quinn AG (1996) Sebaceous hyperplasia in organ transplant recipients: shared aspects of hyperplastic and dysplastic processes? Journal of the American Academy of Dermatology 35(5 Pt 1): 696–699

Sebocystomatosis

▶ **Steatocystoma multiplex**

Seborrhea

▶ **Seborrheic dermatitis**

Seborrhea capitis

▶ **Seborrheic dermatitis**

Seborrheic blepharitis

▶ **Seborrheic dermatitis**

Seborrheic dermatitis

Synonym(s)
Seborrhea; dandruff; seborrheic eczema; seborrhea capitis; pityriasis sicca; pityriasis simplex capitis; pityriasis oleosa; pityriasis corporis; seborrheic blepharitis

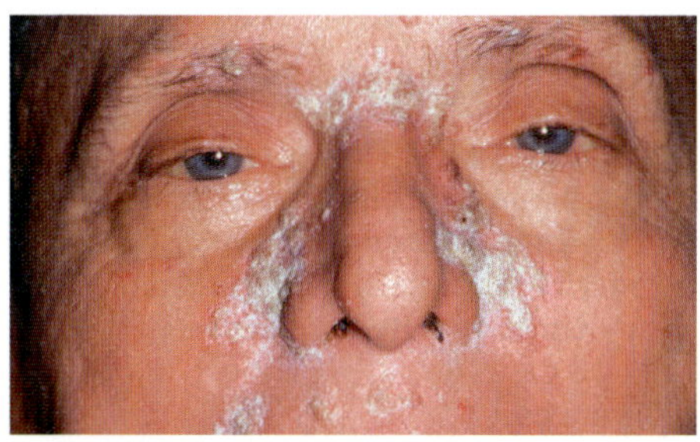

Seborrheic dermatitis. Scaly plaques on the central face

Definition
Inflammatory dermatosis in areas with high sebum flow and accumulation, such as the scalp, face, intertriginous areas, and chest

Pathogenesis
Abnormal immune response to a normal constituent of the skin flora, Pityrosporum ovale

Clinical manifestation
Scalp: appearance varies from mild, patchy scaling to widespread, thick, adherent crusts
Face: central facial erythema and scale, most prominent in skin folds
Eyelids: poorly defined, scaly, reddish-brown plaques
Presternal or interscapular area: poorly defined, red-brown, scaly papules and plaques
Intertriginous areas: fairly sharply demarcated, red, scaly plaques

Differential diagnosis
Tinea capitis; atopic dermatitis; psoriasis; intertrigo; contact dermatitis; candidiasis;

diaper dermatitis; pityriasis rosea; pityriasis lichenoides chronica; lupus erythematosus; rosacea; Darier disease; Hailey-Hailey disease; Grover's disease; pemphigus foliaceus; xerotic eczema; chronic granulomatous disease; exfoliative erythroderma; infectious eczematoid dermatitis; Letterer-Siwe disease; staphylococcal blepharitis; tinea amiantacea; vitamin B and/or zinc deficiency; glucagonoma syndrome

Therapy
Anti-seborrheic shampoo, used daily; corticosteroids, topical, low potency for face; corticosteroids, topical, mid potency for trunk; azole antifungal agents seborrheic blepharitis: scrubbing of eyelids daily with baby shampoo diluted 1 : 1 with water

References
Faergemann J (2000) Management of seborrheic dermatitis and pityriasis versicolor. American Journal of Clinical Dermatology 1(2):75–80

Seborrheic eczema

► Seborrheic dermatitis

Seborrheic keratosis

Synonym(s)
Seborrheic wart; senile wart; basal cell papilloma

Definition
Benign tumor composed of epidermal keratinocytes

Pathogenesis
Hereditary component; sunlight may be a factor in some cases

Clinical manifestation
Non-inflamed, single or multiple, sharply defined, flesh-colored, light brown, gray, blue, or black, flat papules with a velvety or finely verrucous surface; edges raised off skin surface, giving lesion a "stuck-on" appearance
Dermatosis papulosa nigra variant: small, pedunculated, heavily pigmented papule, with minimal keratotic element, on face
Stucco keratosis variant: superficial, gray-to-light-brown, flat, keratotic papules on the dorsa of the feet, ankles, hands, and forearms
Melanoacanthoma variant: deeply pigmented keratotic plaque with histologic evidence of proliferation or activation of dendritic melanocytes

Differential diagnosis
Melanocytic nevus; melanoma; acrochordon; actinic keratosis; basal cell carcinoma; squamous cell carcinoma; psoriasis; pemphigus foliaceus; wart

Therapy
Electrodesiccation and curettage; liquid nitrogen cryotherapy; shave removal; elliptical excision

References
Pariser RJ (1998) Benign neoplasms of the skin. Medical Clinics of North America 82(6):1285–1307

Seborrheic wart

► Seborrheic keratosis

Secret antiperspirant

► Aluminium chlorohydrate

Sedge pool itch

► Cercarial dermatitis

Segmental hyalinizing vasculitis

▶ Livedoid vasculitis

Seidlmayer syndrome

▶ Acute hemorrhagic edema of infancy

Seip syndrome

▶ Berardinelli-Seip syndrome

Selective serotonin reuptake inhibitor (SSRI)

Trade name(s)
Generic names in parentheses:
Celexa (citalopram); Zoloft (sertraline); Prozac (fluoxetine); Paxil (paroxetine); Luvox (fluvoxamine)

Generic available
Yes – fluoxetine; fluvoxamine

Drug class
Selective serotonin reuptake inhibitor

Mechanism of action
Inhibits serotonin reuptake at the presynaptic terminal

Dosage form
Celexa: 20 mg, 40 mg tablet
Zoloft: 25 mg, 50 mg, 100 mg tablet
Prozac: 10 mg, 20 mg tablet, 20 mg per 5 ml liquid
Paxil: 20 mg, 30 mg tablet
Luvox: 25 mg, 50 mg, 100 mg tablet

Dermatologic indications and dosage
See table

Common side effects
Cutaneous: skin eruption
Gastrointestinal: anorexia, hyperexia
Genitourinary: sexual dysfunction
Neurologic: insomnia, sedation, headache

Serious side effects
Neurologic: serotonin syndrome

Drug interactions
Buspirone; cimetidine; ergot alkaloids; ethanol; anti-psychotics, both typical and atypical; lithium; MAO inhibitors; metoprolol; phenytoin; quinidine; tricyclics; warfarin

Contraindications/precautions
Hypersensitivity to drug class or component; MAO inhibitors within 14 days; avoid rapid withdrawal

References
Gupta MA, Guptat AK (2001) The use of antidepressant drugs in dermatology. Journal of the European Academy of Dermatology & Venereology 15(6):512–518

Self-healing epithelioma

▶ Keratoacanthoma

Self-healing squamous cell carcinoma

▶ Keratoacanthoma

Selective serotonin reuptake inhibitor (SSRI). Dermatologic indications and dosage

Disease	Adult dosage	Child dosage
Burning mouth syndrome	Celexa: 20–40 mg PO once daily; Zoloft: 50–100 mg PO once daily; Prozac 10–60 mg PO once daily; Paxil 20–40 mg PO once daily; Luvox 25–100 mg PO at bedtime	Celexa: safety and effectiveness not established; Zoloft: 25 mg PO once daily (6–12 years old); Prozac 5–20 mg PO once daily; Paxil 10–30 mg PO once daily (> 8 years old); Luvox 25–50 mg PO at bedtime
Obsessive-compulsive disorders	Celexa: 20–40 mg PO once daily; Zoloft: 50–100 mg PO once daily; Prozac 10–60 mg PO once daily; Paxil 20–40 mg PO once daily; Luvox 25–100 mg PO at bedtime	Celexa: safety and effectiveness not established; Zoloft: 25 mg PO once daily (6–12 years old); Prozac 5–20 mg PO once daily; Paxil 10–30 mg PO once daily (> 8 years old); Luvox 25–50 mg PO at bedtime
Prurigo nodularis	Celexa: 20–40 mg PO once daily; Zoloft: 50–100 mg PO once daily; Prozac 10–60 mg PO once daily; Paxil 20–40 mg PO once daily; Luvox 25–100 mg PO at bedtime	Celexa: safety and effectiveness not established; Zoloft: 25 mg PO once daily (6–12 years old); Prozac 5–20 mg PO once daily; Paxil 10–30 mg PO once daily (> 8 years old); Luvox 25–50 mg PO at bedtime
Trichotillomania	Celexa: 20–40 mg PO once daily; Zoloft: 50–100 mg PO once daily; Prozac 10–60 mg PO once daily; Paxil 20–40 mg PO once daily; Luvox 25–100 mg PO at bedtime	Celexa: safety and effectiveness not established; Zoloft: 25 mg PO once daily (6–12 years old); Prozac 5–20 mg PO once daily; Paxil 10–30 mg PO once daily (> 8 years old); Luvox 25–50 mg PO at bedtime

Self-limiting acroderamatitis enteropathica

▶ Acrodermatitis enteropathica

Senile comedones

▶ Favre-Racouchot syndrome

Senile depigmented spots

▶ Idiopathic guttate hypomelanosis

Senile elastosis

▶ Actinic elastosis

Senile hemangioma of the lips

▶ Venous lake

Senile keratosis

▶ Actinic keratosis

Senile sebaceous adenoma

▶ Sebaceous hyperplasia

Senile sebaceous hyperplasia

▶ Sebaceous hyperplasia

Senile wart

▶ Seborrheic keratosis

Sertraline

▶ Selective serotonin reuptake inhibitor (SSRI)

Serum sickness

Synonym(s)
None

Definition
Self-limited immune complex disease caused by exposure to foreign proteins or haptens

Pathogenesis
With slight antigen excess, intermediate-sized immune complexes deposit in small vessels and activate complement; increased adhesion molecule expression in endothelial cells causes cytokine release and vascular injury

Clinical manifestation
Urticarial, morbilliform, or scarlatiniform eruption; palpable purpura; erythema multiforme; facial edema; pruritus and erythema at injection site; symmetrical arthritis, usually in metacarpophalangeal and knee joints; myalgias; lymphadenopathy; splenomegaly; neurologic complications, including headache, optic neuritis; cranial nerves palsies, Guillain-Barré syndrome; gastrointestinal complaints, including abdominal pain, nausea, vomiting, diarrhea; clinical recovery after 7–28 days

Differential diagnosis
Urticaria; cryoglobulinemia; hepatitis; mononucleosis; hypersensitivity vasculitis; lupus erythematosus; Henoch-Schönlein purpura; Still disease

Therapy
Antihistamines, first generation; prednisone for patients with multisystem involvement and significant symptomatology

References
Roujeau JC, Stern RS (1994) Severe adverse cutaneous reactions to drugs. New England Journal of Medicine 331(19):1272–1285

Seven-day fever

▶ Leptospirosis

Seven-year itch

▶ Scabies

Sézary's syndrome

▶ T-cell lymphoma, cutaneous

Shank fever

▶ Trench fever

Sharp syndrome

▶ Mixed connective tissue disease

Sharp's syndrome

▶ Mixed connective tissue disease

Shaving bumps

▶ Pseudofolliculitis barbae

Sheep-pox

▶ Orf

Shin spots

▶ Diabetic dermopathy

Shinbone fever

▶ Trench fever

Shingles

▶ Herpes zoster

Short anagen syndrome

▶ Loose anagen hair syndrome

Sicca syndrome

▶ Sjögren syndrome

Siemerling-Creutzfeldt syndrome

▶ Addison-Schilder disease

Sign of Leser-Trelat

Definition
Abrupt appearance and growth of multiple seborrheic keratoses, caused by an underlying malignancy

References
Schwartz RA (1996) Sign of Leser-Trelat. Journal of the American Academy of Dermatology 35(1):88–95

Silt itch

▶ Cercarial dermatitis

Sipple syndrome

▶ Mucosal neuroma syndrome

Sitosterolemia

▶ Phytosterolemia

Sixth disease

▶ Roseola

Sjögren syndrome

Synonym(s)
Sicca syndrome; Sjögren's syndrome; Gougerot-Houwer-Sjögren syndrome; keratoconjunctivitis sicca

Definition
Chronic disorder characterized by keratoconjunctivitis sicca and xerostomia

Pathogenesis
Autoimmune dysregulation, particularly polyclonal B lymphocyte hyperreactivity; genetic susceptibility; abnormality in cellular apoptosis

Clinical manifestation
Glandular symptoms: dry eye syndrome, characterized by dryness of cornea and conjunctiva; dry mouth; dry lips; red, smooth dry tongue; dental caries; recurrent oral candidiasis; recurrent salivary gland swelling; nasal dryness with recurrent infections, hoarseness, and aphonia; atrophic changes in the vulva and vagina, resulting in pruritus and vaginitis; anal and rectal mucosal dryness

Skin symptoms: xerosis; decreased sweating; dry, sparse hair; annular, red, scaly plaques, especially on face and neck; cutaneous vasculitis

Primary variant: no associated connective tissue or autoimmune disease; extraglandular involvement: lung involvement, nervous system dysfunction, renal involvement, Raynaud phenomenon, and lymphoproliferative disorders

Secondary variant: associated connective tissue or autoimmune disease; milder disease with fewer systemic manifestations

Differential diagnosis
HIV infection; drug reaction; lupus erythematosus; amyloidosis; environmental dryness

Therapy
Dry eyes: Artificial tears (e.g., methylcellulose, 1 % hyaluronic acid solution, alcohol solutions) applied 4–6 times daily

Dry mouth: frequent small drinks and mouthwashes; artificial saliva; stimulation of salivary secretion with sweets, etc.

References
Manoussakis MN, Moutsopoulos HM (2001) Sjögren's syndrome: current concepts. Advances in Internal Medicine 47:191–217

Sjögren's syndrome

▶ Sjögren syndrome

Skeeter's syndrome

▶ Amniotic band syndrome

Skin tag

▶ Acrochordon

Skin writing

▶ Dermatographism

Slapped-cheek disease

▶ Erythema infectiosum

Sleeping sickness

▶ African trypanosomiasis

Small cell carcinoma of the skin

▶ Merkel cell carcinoma

Small plaque parapsoriasis

Synonym(s)
Benign parapsoriasis; digitate dermatitis; digitate dermatosis; chronic superficial dermatitis; guttate parapsoriasis; Brocq's disease

Definition
Chronic, benign, cutaneous disease, characterized by scaly plaques resembling psoriasis

Pathogenesis
Most likely represents a reactive process of predominantly CD4+ T cells

Clinical manifestation
Well-circumscribed, slightly scaly, light salmon-colored papules or plaques scattered over the trunk and extremities
Digitate pattern: palisading, elongated fingerlike plaques following a dermatomal pattern, most prominently on the flank; active lesions for months to several years; usually resolves spontaneously

Differential diagnosis
Psoriasis; dermatophytosis; lupus erythematosus; lichen planus; pityriasis rosea; syphilis; seborrheic dermatitis; mycosis fungoides; xerosis; nummular dermatitis

Therapy
Corticosteroids, topical, high potency; UVB phototherapy; photochemotherapy

References
Lambert WC, Everett MA (1981) The nosology of parapsoriasis. Journal of the American Academy of Dermatology 5(4):373–395

Small vessel vasculitis

▶ Leukocytoclastic vasculitis

Smallpox

▶ Variola

Smoker's comedones

▶ Favre-Racouchot syndrome

Sneddon-Wilkinson disease

▶ Subcorneal pustular dermatosis

Sodoku

▶ Rat-bite fever

Soft chancre

▶ Chancroid

Soft wart

▶ Acrochordon

Solar cheilitis

▶ Actinic cheilitis

Solar comedones

▶ Favre-Racouchot syndrome

Solar elastosis

▶ Actinic elastosis

Solar keratosis

▶ Actinic keratosis

Solar urticaria

▶ Urticaria

Solid cystic hidradenoma

▶ Eccrine hidradenoma

Solitary lichen planus

▶ Lichenoid keratosis

Solitary lichen planus-like keratosis

▶ Lichenoid keratosis

Sorbsan

▶ Alginates

South African porphyria

▶ Variegate porphyria

South African tick typhus

▶ Boutonneuse Fever

South American blastomycosis

Synonym(s)
Paracoccidioidomycosis; Lutz mycosis; Brazilian blastomycosis

Definition
Systemic mycotic infection, endemic to countries in Central America and South America, caused by the fungus Paracoccidioides brasiliensis

Pathogenesis
Caused by thermally dimorphic fungus, Paracoccidioides brasiliensis; acquired by inhalation of conidia fungus that transforms into yeast cells within alveolar macrophages; fungus may disseminate, causing granulomatous disease in multiple organs; alcohol and tobacco use associated with dissemination

Clinical manifestation
Adult chronic form:
Mucous membranes: slowly progressive, painful papules or plaques ulcerate in oral, nasal, pharyngeal, and laryngeal tissue; gingival lesions cause loss of teeth; conjunctivitis and ulcerative lesions of the perianal area
Skin: occurs most commonly on the face; may have nodules, ulcerations or papillomatous lesions; most often arises from direct extension of mucous membrane lesions; hematogenous spread causes widely scattered subcutaneous abscesses; lymph nodes: extensive hypertrophic, painful lymphadenopathy with visceral and subcutaneous nodes; cervical nodes commonly affected; suppuration causes sinus tracts or skin ulcers
Respiratory: lung involvement in 70-80% of patients and often the only organ system involved; frequently resembles tuberculosis, with chronic dyspnea, cough, and sputum production
Other systemic problems: hepatosplenomegaly, adrenal insufficiency meningitis, intestinal ulcerations, and osteomyelitis
Juvenile subacute form:
Mucous membranes: rare mucosal ulcerations
Skin: acneiform eruption or subcutaneous abscesses; scrofuloderma as a result of lymph node suppuration
Lymph nodes: prominent lymphadenopathy with suppuration; mesenteric adenopathy may produce bowel obstruction
Respiratory: occasional pneumonia
Other problems: cachexia, hepatosplenomegaly, adrenal insufficiency, osteomyelitis, gastrointestinal problems

Differential diagnosis
Actinomycosis; coccidioidomycosis; leishmaniasis; sporotrichosis; syphilis; tuberculosis; histoplasmosis; North American blastomycosis; Wegener's granulomatosis; oral carcinoma; drug eruption; lymphoma; leukemia

Therapy
Trimethoprim and sulfamethoxazole*; ketoconazole; itraconazole; for severe disease: amphotericin B – 0.7–1 mg per kg IV daily for 4–8 weeks, followed by trimethoprim and sulfamethoxazole for 2–3 years

References
Rivitti EA, Aoki V (1999) Deep fungal infections in tropical countries. Clinics in Dermatology 17(2):171–190

South American pemphigus

▶ Fogo selvagem

South American trypanosomiasis

▶ American trypanosomiasis

Spanish toxic oil syndrome

▶ Toxic oil syndrome

Speckled lentiginous nevus

▶ Nevus spilus

Speckled nevus spilus

▶ Nevus spilus

Spectacle frame granuloma

▶ Acanthoma fissuratum

Sphingomyelin-cholesterol lipidoses

▶ Niemann-Pick disease

Spider angioma

Synonym(s)
Spider nevus; nevus araneus; vascular spider

Definition
Vascular lesion consisting of central arteriole with radiating, thin-walled vessels

Pathogenesis
Dilation of pre-existing vessels; sometimes occurs in patients with cirrhosis or other hepatic abnormalities; elevated blood estrogen a common characteristic

Clinical manifestation
Red macule or papule surrounded by several distinct radiating vessels, occurring most commonly on face, below eyes, and over cheekbones; central pressure causes lesion to blanch

Differential diagnosis
Telangiectatic mat; spider telangiectasia; insect bite; cherry angioma

Therapy
Destruction by electrodesiccation or laser vaporization

References
Requena L, Sangueza OP (1997) Cutaneous vascular anomalies. Part I. Hamartomas, malformations, and dilation of preexisting vessels. Journal of the American Academy of Dermatology 37(4):523–549

Spider nevus

▶ Spider angioma

Spider veins

▶ Varicose and telangiectatic leg veins

Spiegler-Fendt, pseudolymphoma of

▶ Pseudolymphoma

Spiegler-Fendt sarcoid

▶ Pseudolymphoma

Spiradenoma

Synonym(s)
Eccrine spiradenoma

Definition
Benign tumor of sweat gland origin, presenting as a solitary gray-pink papule

Pathogenesis
Unclear whether tumor arises from apocrine or eccrine epithelium

Clinical manifestation
Solitary firm, gray-pink papule, usually arising in the head and neck region or trunk; occasional pain and tenderness

Differential diagnosis
Cylindroma; basal cell carcinoma; trichoepithelioma; eccrine poroma; angiofibroma; milium

Therapy
Surgical excision★

References
Michal M (1996) Spiradenoma associated with apocrine adenoma component. Pathology, Research & Practice 192(11):1135–1139

Spirillary fever

▶ Rat-bite fever

Spironolactone

Trade name(s)
Aldactone

Generic available
Yes

Drug class
Diuretic; anti-androgen

Mechanism of action
Androgen receptor antagonist on sebaceus glands; inhibits androgen synthesis

Dosage form
25 mg, 50 mg, 100 mg tablet

Dermatologic indications and dosage
See table

Spironolactone. Dermatologic indications and dosage

Disease	Adult dosage	Child dosage
Acne vulgaris	25–100 mg PO twice daily	Not indicated
Androgenetic alopecia	25–100 mg PO twice daily	Not indicated
Hidradenitis suppurativa	25–100 mg PO twice daily	Not indicated
Hirsutism	25–100 mg PO twice daily	Not indicated

Common side effects
Dermatologic: skin eruption
Gastrointestinal: dyspepsia
Neurologic: sedation, headache
Genitourinary: sexual dysfunction, dysmenorrhea

Serious side effects
Dermatologic: anaphylaxis
Bone marrow: marrow suppression

Drug interactions
ACE inhibitors; cyclosporine; non-steroidal anti-inflammatory agents; COX-2 inhibitors; potassium salts; tacrolimus

Contraindications/precautions
Hypersensitivity to drug class or component; renal insufficiency; hyperkalemia; caution in patients with liver dysfunction

References
Thiboutot D (2001) Hormones and acne: pathophysiology, clinical evaluation, and therapies. Seminars in Cutaneous Medicine & Surgery 20(3):144–53

Splash rash

▶ Hot tub folliculitis

Sporotrichosis

Synonym(s)
Schenck's disease; Beurmann's disease; rose gardener's disease; peat moss disease

Definition
Subcutaneous or systemic fungal infection caused by soil pathogen, Sporothrix schenckii

Pathogenesis
Caused by Sporothrix schenckii, dimorphic fungus commonly found on vegetative matter, particularly in humid climates; may

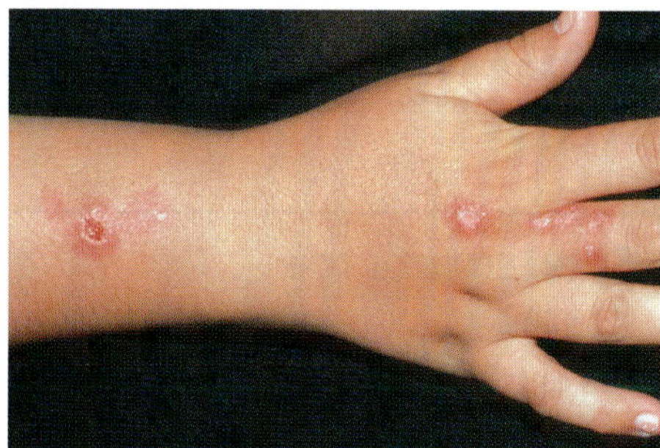

Sporotrichosis. Linear, scaly, red papules, one of which is ulcerated

gain entry through puncture wound, spreading via lymphatic vessels

Clinical manifestation
History of prick injury at site of infection, within 3 weeks of onset of signs and symptoms
Lymphocutaneous variant: subcutaneous nodule developing at site of inoculation and sometimes ulcerating after central abscess formation; satellite lesions along associated lymphatic chain with lymphadenopathy
Fixed cutaneous variant: scaly, acneform, verrucous, or ulcerative nodule remaining localized to site of inoculation
Disseminated variant: multiple organ involvement causing pyelonephritis, orchitis, mastitis, arthritis, synovitis, meningitis, osseous infection, or (rarely) pulmonary disease

Differential diagnosis
Atypical mycobacterial infection; nocardiosis; North American blastomycosis; South American blastomycosis; leishmaniasis; bacterial pyoderma; anthrax; cutaneous tuberculosis; tularemia; foreign body granuloma; herpes zoster

Therapy
Lymphocutaneous variant: itraconazole★; saturated solution of potassium iodide: 300–500 mg PO 3 times daily for 4–8 weeks
Disseminated variant: amphotericin B – 3 mg per kg per day IV until significant clinical response; itraconazole

References

Morris-Jones R (2002) Sporotrichosis. Clinical & Experimental Dermatology 27(6):427–431

Sportsman's toe

▶ Tennis toe

Spotted fever

▶ Rocky Mountain spotted fever

Spotted leg syndrome

▶ Diabetic dermopathy

Spun glass hair

▶ Uncombable hair syndrome

Squamous cell carcinoma

Synonym(s)

Epidermoid carcinoma; prickle cell carcinoma

Definition

Malignant tumor of keratinocytes, most often arising in chronically sun-exposed skin

Pathogenesis

Related closely to chronic sun exposure; other risk factors: immunosuppression, fair complexion, history of ionizing radiation or photochemotherapy, abnormal DNA repair mechanisms, infection with certain human papillomavirus virus subtypes, and local sites of chronic inflammation

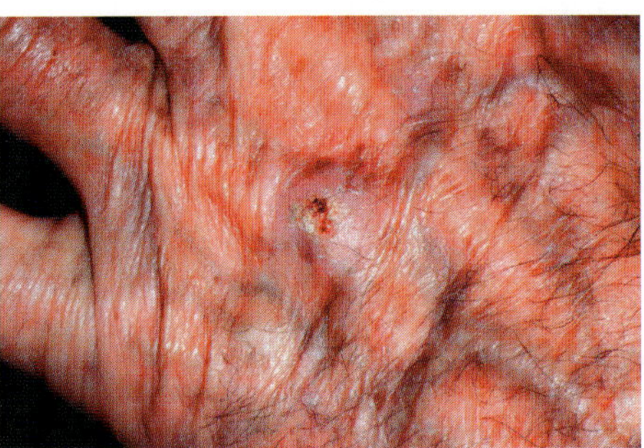

Squamous cell carcinoma. Scaly red papule with central erosion

Clinical manifestation

Elevated, firm, pink to flesh-colored, keratotic papule or plaque with or without overlying cutaneous horn or ulceration, often arising from pre-existing actinic keratosis; lip lesion: most commonly on vermillion border of lower lip; shiny, ulcerated papule or nodule

Differential diagnosis

Actinic keratosis; basal cell carcinoma; benign adnexal neoplasm; melanoma; Merkel cell carcinoma; atypical fibroxanthoma; seborrheic keratosis; wart; pyogenic granuloma; proliferating trichilemmal cyst; granular cell tumor; granulomatous diseases such as tuberculosis, leishmaniasis, coccidioidomycosis, North American blastomycosis, syphilis, and bromoderma

Therapy

Surgical excision; destruction by electrodesiccation and curettage or liquid nitrogen cryotherapy; superficial orthovoltage radiation therapy; large tumors, lesions in anatomically sensitive areas, or recurrent tumors – Mohs micrographic surgery or other form of microscopically controlled excision

References

An KP, Ratner D (2001) Surgical management of cutaneous malignancies. Clinics in Dermatology 19(3):305–320

Squamous cell carcinoma in-situ

▶ Bowen's disease

SSSS

▶ Staphylococcal scalded skin syndrome

Staphylococcal scalded skin syndrome

Synonym(s)
SSSS; scalded skin syndrome; pemphigus neonatorum

Definition
Toxin-mediated disease of young children, characterized by acute generalized skin exfoliation

Pathogenesis
Caused by toxigenic strains of Staphylococcus aureus, usually belonging to phage group 2 (types 3A, 3B, 3C, 55, or 71); two exotoxins (ETs), epidermolytic toxin A (ET-A) and epidermolytic toxin B (ET-B), responsible for the pathologic changes and blistering produced by disruption of epidermal granular cell layer

Clinical manifestation
Original focus of infection may be purulent conjunctivitis, otitis media, or nasopharyngeal infection; fever; irritability; generalized, faint, orange-red, macular erythema with cutaneous tenderness and periorificial and flexural accentuation; early positive Nikolsky sign; within 24–48 hours, rash progresses to generalized, superficial blistering eruption, with tissue paper-like surface wrinkling, followed by large, flaccid bullae in axillae, groin, and around the body orifices, sparing mucous membranes; after epidermal sloughing, moist erythematous base present; healing usually complete within 5–7 days

Differential diagnosis
Toxic shock syndrome; Kawasaki disease; scarlet fever; erythema multiforme; child abuse

Therapy
Dicloxacillin*

References
Veien NK (1998) The clinician's choice of antibiotics in the treatment of bacterial skin infection. British Journal of Dermatology 139 Suppl 53:30–36

Staphylococcal toxic shock syndrome

▶ Toxic shock syndrome

Stasis dermatitis

Synonym(s)
Venous eczema

Definition
Inflammatory disease of the lower extremities, characterized by eczematous changes in the context of chronic pedal edema

Pathogenesis
Result of venous insufficiency; disturbed function of the deep venous plexus valvular system with backflow of blood from the deep to the superficial venous system, producing venous hypertension; possibly related to leukocyte sequestration in microcirculation, with increased contact of leukocytes with the capillary endothelium and

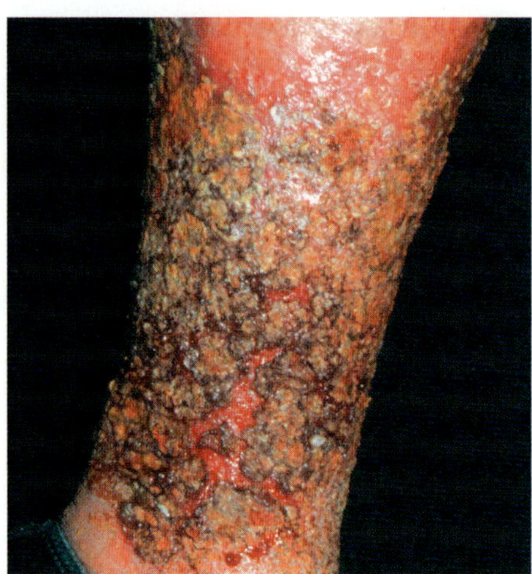

Stasis dermatitis. Scaly, crusted, and eroded plaque on the lower extremity

release of inflammatory mediators; leukocyte sludging may block dermal capillaries, leading to tissue ischemia

Clinical manifestation
Erythematous, scaling, eroded plaques of lower extremity; medial ankle most frequently and severely involved; acute flares with exudative, weeping plaques; longstanding lesions with lichenification and hyperpigmentation; skin induration sometimes progresses to significant scarring lipodermatosclerosis and violaceous plaques and nodules on the legs and dorsal feet (acroangiodermatitis)

Differential diagnosis
Contact dermatitis; cellulitis; Kaposi's sarcoma; atopic dermatitis; xerotic eczema; necrobiosis lipoidica; nummular eczema; dermatophytosis; benign pigmented purpura; pretibial myxedema

Therapy
Corticosteroids, topical, mid potency★; compression therapy with Unna boot dressings, controlled gradient compression device or compression stockings; prednisone for severe acute flares

References
Weingarten MS (2001) State-of-the-art treatment of chronic venous disease. Clinical Infectious Diseases 32(6):949–954

Steatoblepharon

▶ Dermatochalasis

Steatocystoma

▶ Steatocystoma multiplex

Steatocystoma multiplex

Synonym(s)
Steatocystoma; sebocystomatosis

Definition
Heritable disorder of pilosebaceous unit, characterized by multiple sebum-containing cysts

Pathogenesis
Autosomal dominant trait; hamartomatous formation of abortive hair follicles at site where sebaceous glands attach; associated with vellus hair cysts and trichostasis spinulosa, and sometimes existing on spectrum with these entities

Clinical manifestation
Asymptomatic, smooth, flesh-to-yellow-colored papules; occasional rupture into the dermis producing inflammation with scarring; concentrated over upper torso, proximal extremities; contents of lesion odorless, creamy or oily fluid; non-hereditary variant: solitary lesion morphologically identical to multiple lesions (steatocystoma simplex)

Differential diagnosis
Acne vulgaris; epidermoid cyst; trichilemmal cyst; eruptive vellus hair cyst; milia; syringoma; Gardner syndrome

Therapy
Tetracycline; isotretinoin; surgical excision of individual inflammatory lesions

References
Rollins T, Levin RM, Heymann WR (2000) Acral steatocystoma multiplex. Journal of the American Academy of Dermatology 43(2 Pt 2):396–369

Steatocystoma simplex

► **Steatocystoma multiplex**

Steatoma

► **Epidermoid cyst**

Steely hair syndrome

► **Menkes kinky hair syndrome**

Sterile eosinophilic pustulosis

► **Eosinophilic pustular folliculitis**

Steroid acne

► **Acne medicamentosa**

Steroid rosacea

► **Perioral dermatitis**

Stevens-Johnson syndrome

Synonym(s)
Erythema multiforme major

Definition
Systemic hypersensitivity reaction, mainly involving the skin and mucous membranes

Pathogenesis
Cell-mediated immune response, mediated by CD8 lymphocytes; may involve an HLA-DQw3-related, altered immune response; associated with medications, such as sulfonamides, penicillin, or anti-convulsants, and with infections (most commonly, herpes simplex virus infection and mycoplasma pneumonia)

Clinical manifestation
Erythematous papules, vesicles, bullae, and target-like papules, mainly on face, trunk, and mucous membranes, including oral, genital mucosa; < 35 % of body surface involved; lesions may be located on linings of respiratory and gastrointestinal tracts; conjunctivitis with photophobia; burning sensation in eyes; hepatitis; nephritis; gastrointestinal bleeding; pneumonia; myalgia; arthritis; arthralgia

Differential diagnosis
Pemphigus vulgaris, erosive lichen planus; varicella zoster infection; Behcet's disease; Reiter's syndrome; herpes simplex virus infection; bullous pemphigoid; toxic epidermal necrolysis; Henoch-Schönlein purpura; urticaria; viral exanthem; Kawasaki disease; figurate erythema; fixed drug eruption; lupus erythematosus; aphthous stomatitis

Therapy
Prednisone

References
Prendiville J (2002) Stevens-Johnson syndrome and toxic epidermal necrolysis. Advances in Dermatology 18:151–173

Stewart-Bluefarb syndrome

▶ Acroangiodermatitis

Stewart-Treves syndrome

Synonym(s)
Lymphangiosarcoma of Stewart-Treves

Definition
Malignant vascular tumor arising in an area of chronic lymphedema, particularly on upper extremity after radical mastectomy

Pathogenesis
Occurs in the context of chronic lymphedema

Clinical manifestation
Purplish patch, evolving into plaque or nodule in the area of chronic lymphedema; palpable subcutaneous mass or poorly healing eschar with recurrent bleeding and oozing; nodules may become polypoid, develop small satellite papules and become confluent; overlying epidermis sometimes ulcerates, producing recurrent episodes of bleeding and infection; high metastatic potential

Differential diagnosis
Angioendotheliomatosis; angiolymphoid hyperplasia with eosinophilia; Kaposi's sarcoma; lymphangioma; melanoma; metastasis; hemangioendothelioma; hemangiopericytoma

Therapy
Radical amputation of the limb[*]; radiation therapy

References
Chung KC, Kim HJ, Jeffers LL (2000) Lymphangiosarcoma (Stewart-Treves syndrome) in postmastectomy patients. Journal of Hand Surgery – American Volume 25(6):1163–1168

Sticker disease

▶ Erythema infectiosum

Sticker's disease

▶ Erythema infectiosum

Stomatitis areata migrans

▶ Benign migratory glossitis

Stork bite

▶ Salmon patch

Strawberry hemangioma

▶ Capillary hemangioma

Strawberry mark

▶ Capillary hemangioma

Strawberry patch

▶ Nevus flammeus

Streeter's dysplasia

▶ Amniotic band syndrome

Streeter's spots

▶ Aplasia cutis congenita

Strep toxic shock syndrome

▶ Streptococcal toxic shock-like syndrome

Strep toxic shocklike syndrome

▶ Streptococcal toxic shock-like syndrome

Streptobacillary fever

▶ Rat-bite fever

Streptococcal toxic shock-like syndrome

Synonym(s)
Strep toxic shock-like syndrome; streptococcal TSS flesh eating disease

Definition
Acute febrile illness, characterized by signs of localized infection, often in the skin; generalized erythematous eruption accompanied by shock and multiple organ dysfunction

Pathogenesis
Caused by strains of Streptococcus pyogenes; superantigen behavior of pyrogenic exotoxin-A (SPE-A); may also produce streptococcal pyrogenic exotoxin-B (SPE-B), streptococcal pyrogenic exotoxin-C (SPE-C), streptococcal superantigen and mitogenic factor, as well as non–group-A streptococci aureus; release of tumor necrosis factor-α (TNF-α) and interleukin-1b (IL-1b), which mediate signs and symptoms of disease; predisposing factors: influenza A, soft tissue wounds, varicella, pneumonia, unidentified bacteremia, surgical site infection, septic arthritis, thrombophlebitis, meningitis, pelvic infection, endophthalmitis; additional risk factors: HIV, diabetes mellitus, cancer, ethanol abuse, and other chronic diseases

Clinical manifestation
Localized pain in an extremity, rapidly progressing over 48–72 hours
Cutaneous signs: localized edema and erythema; bullous and hemorrhagic cellulitis; necrotizing fasciitis or myositis; gangrene
Other organ involvement: fever; hypotension; cardiomyopathy; nausea; vomiting; diarrhea; rhabdomyolysis; myalgias; muscle tenderness and weakness; azotemia; acute renal failure; adult respiratory distress syndrome; elevated serum glutamic oxaloacetic transaminase (SGOT) and serum bilirubin; thrombocytopenia; leukocytosis; disseminated intravascular coagulation; hypophosphatemia; hypocalcemia; and electrolyte imbalance

Differential diagnosis
Toxic shock syndrome; Stevens-Johnson syndrome; Kawasaki disease; staphylococcal scalded skin syndrome; toxic epidermal necrolysis; drug reaction; scarlet fever;

Rocky Mountain spotted fever; leptospirosis; gas gangrene; meningococcemia

Therapy
Nafcillin: 2 gm IV every 4 hours in adults; 100–200 mg per kg per day divided into 4–6 doses per day in children
Clindamycin: 600–900 mg IV every 8 hours in adults; 20–40 mg per kg per day IV divided into 3–4 doses in children
Intravenous immunoglobulin (IVIG) 1–2 gm per kg over 2–3 days

References
Levine N., Kunkel M, Thanh N; Ackerman L (2002) Emergency department dermatology. Current Problems in Dermatology 14(6):188–220

Streptococcal TSS flesh eating disease

► Streptococcal toxic shock-like syndrome

Stretch marks

► Striae

Striae

Synonym(s)
Striae distensae; striae atrophicans; striae rubra; striae alba; stretch marks

Definition
Linear dermal scars accompanied by epidermal atrophy

Pathogenesis
Results from stress rupture of dermal connective tissue framework; affects skin subjected to continuous and progressive

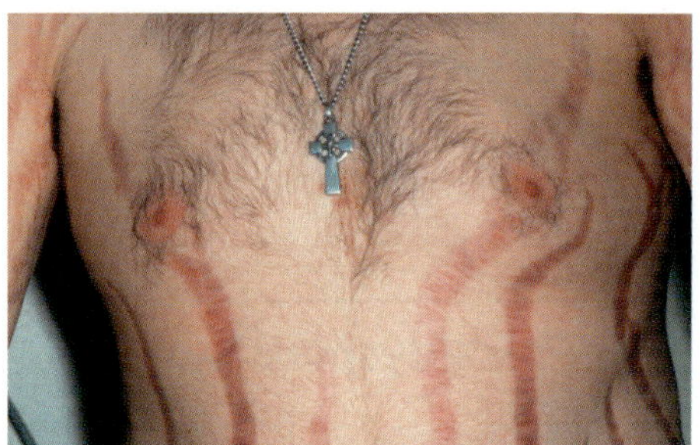

Striae. Linear, red-brown, atrophic plaques

stretching; skin distension causes excessive mast cell degranulation with subsequent damage of collagen and elastin; may develop more easily in skin with high proportion of rigid cross-linked collagen; associated with increased adrenal cortical hormone activity, such as in Cushing's disease or with exogenous glucocorticoid therapy

Clinical manifestation
Flattened, atrophic plaques with a pink hue, which enlarge in length and width and become violaceous; older striae are white, depressed, irregularly shaped bands with their long axis parallel to skin tension lines; in pregnancy, striae affect abdomen and breasts; adolescent striae occur on outer aspects of thighs and lumbo-sacral region in boys, and thighs, buttocks, and breasts in girls; flexures affected with topical corticosteroid use, especially if used under occlusion

Differential diagnosis
Linear focal elastosis; Marfan syndrome; Cushing's syndrome; external trauma

Therapy
585-nm flashlamp pumped dye laser; tretinoin; chemexfoliation with trichloroacetic acid

References
McDaniel DH, Ash K, Zukowski M (1996) Treatment of stretch marks with the 585-nm flashlamp-pumped pulsed dye laser. Dermatologic Surgery 22(4): 332–337

Striae alba

▶ Striae

Striae atrophicans

▶ Striae

Striae distensae

▶ Striae

Striae rubra

▶ Striae

Striate keratoderma

Synonym(s)
Keratoderma palmoplantaris striata; striate palmoplantar keratoderma; Brunaur-Fuhs-Siemens syndrome; palmoplantar keratoderma areata

Definition
Disorder characterized by linear or striate patterns of keratoderma radiating from the palm and extending along the fingers

Pathogenesis
Autosomal dominant trait; mutations in gene encoding for desmoglein 1 and desmoplakin

Clinical manifestation
Linear or striate keratotic plaques radiating along the digits from the palm; onset from 5–20 years of age; diffuse thickening of palms and soles and plaques or islands of increased keratin developing at pressure sites

Differential diagnosis
Wart; callus; focal nonepidermolytic palmoplantar keratoderma; focal epidermolytic palmoplantar keratoderma; focal palmoplantar and oral mucosa hyperkeratosis; tyrosinemia type II; punctate keratoderma; acrokeratoelastoidosis; focal acral hyperkeratosis

Therapy
Acitretin*

References
Helm T, Spigel GT, McMahon J, Bergfeld WF (1998) Striate palmoplantar keratoderma: a clinical and ultrastructural study. Cutis 61(1):18–20

Striate palmoplantar keratoderma

▶ Striate keratoderma

Strongyloidosis

Synonym(s)
Strongylydiasis; cutaneous strongyloidiasis; human threadworm infection; anguillulosis; Cochin China diarrhea

Definition
Parasitic infection of the organism Strongyloides stercoralis

Pathogenesis
Infection acquired when infective filariform larvae penetrate the skin during contact with contaminated soil; immunosuppression a risk factor for wide dissemination

Clinical manifestation

Mild, pruritic eruption of feet, site of inoculation of larvae; larva currens (creeping eruption), a form of cutaneous larva migrans specific to *Strongyloides* infection, and a result of autoinfection; rapidly spreading pruritic eruption in perianal region; with disseminated infection, expanding petechial and purpuric lesions, sometimes accompanied by pink macules and papules; gastrointestinal findings: abdominal tenderness; distension; hyperactive, hypoactive, or absent bowel sounds; central nervous system infection: altered mental status; meningismus; pulmonary findings: coughing; respiratory distress; wheezing

Differential diagnosis

Scabies; contact dermatitis; cat or dog hookworm infestation; pinworm infestation; bacterial pyoderma

Therapy

Intestinal stage: ivermectin★; albendazole; disseminated disease: thiabendazole 1.5 g per dose PO twice daily for 2–3 days

References

Schneider JH, Rogers AI (1997) Strongyloidiasis. The protean parasitic infection. Postgraduate Medicine 102(3):177–184

Strongylydiasis

▶ Strongyloidosis

Strübing-Marchiafava-Micheli syndrome

▶ Paroxysmal nocturnal hemoglobinuria

Struma-double lips syndrome

▶ Ascher's syndrome

Sturge-Weber syndrome

▶ Nevus flammeus

Stuttgart disease

▶ Leptospirosis

Subacute cutaneous lupus erythematosus

▶ Lupus erythematosus, subacute cutaneous

Subacute nodular migratory panniculitis

Synonym(s)

Vilanova disease; chronic erythema nodosum; erythema nodosum migrans

Definition

Disorder characterized by migrating subcutaneous nodules on the legs, occurring mostly in women

Pathogenesis

Unknown

Clinical manifestation
Solitary, discrete, erythematous subcutaneous nodule or plaque on anterolateral lower extremity, with peripheral extension later in the course and without ulceration; additional lesions may occur at other sites over time

Differential diagnosis
Erythema nodosum; erythema induratum; lupus panniculitis; traumatic fat necrosis; pancreatic panniculitis; cellulitis

Therapy
Potassium iodide: 300 mg PO 3 times daily, increased to 500–1500 mg PO 3–4 times per day as needed; dapsone

References
Ross M, White GM, Barr RJ (1992) Erythematous plaque on the leg. Vilanova's disease (subacute nodular migratory panniculitis). Archives of Dermatology 128(12):1644–1645, 1647

Subareolar adenomatosis

▶ Erosive adenomatosis of the nipple

Subcorneal pustular dermatosis

Synonym(s)
Sneddon-Wilkinson disease; subcorneal pustulosis of Sneddon and Wilkinson

Definition
Chronic relapsing eruption, characterized by flaccid pustules that coalesce into larger pustular plaques

Pathogenesis
Neutrophil chemoattractants, such as interleukin 8, leukotriene B4, and complement fragments C5a in lesional skin

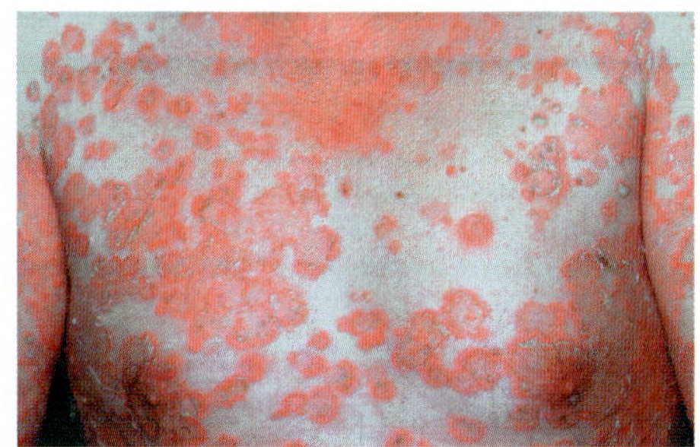

Subcorneal pustular dermatosis. Minimally eroded plaques on the chest wall, abdomen, and arms

Clinical manifestation
Variably pruritic, superficial, flaccid pustules on normal or minimally erythematous skin, typically involving axillae, groin, neck, submammary regions; pus in the lower half of the lesions; lesions isolated or grouped, and sometimes coalesce to form annular, circinate, or serpiginous plaques; heal with mild hyperpigmentation; further waves of pustulation may arise

Differential diagnosis
Impetigo; pustular psoriasis; folliculitis; pemphigus foliaceus; pemphigus vulgaris; dermatitis herpetiformis; bacterial pyoderma; acute generalized exanthematous pustulosis; dermatophytosis

Therapy
Dapsone*; corticosteroids, topical, high potency; acitretin; UVB phototherapy; photochemotherapy

References
Reed J, Wilkinson J (2000) Subcorneal pustular dermatosis. Clinics in Dermatology 18(3):301–313

Subcorneal pustulosis of Sneddon and Wilkinson

▶ Subcorneal pustular dermatosis

Subcutaneous fat necrosis

▶ Subcutaneous fat necrosis of newborn

Subcutaneous fat necrosis of newborn

Synonym(s)
Panniculitis of the newborn; subcutaneous fat necrosis

Definition
Disorder characterized by firm, erythematous nodules and plaques over the trunk, arms, buttocks, thighs, and cheeks in otherwise healthy newborn infants

Pathogenesis
Possible causative factors: underlying defect in fat composition or metabolism; neonatal stress resulting in hypothermia with secondary fat crystallization, leading to necrosis; pressure-induced necrosis occurring during delivery

Clinical manifestation
Presents in normal term neonates as an area of edema, progressing to variably circumscribed, indurated nodules and plaques; overlying skin sometimes red, purple, or flesh-colored; lesions may become fluctuant and spontaneously drain necrotic fat; antecedant birth trauma (meconium aspiration, etc.) may precede onset of lesions

Differential diagnosis
Sclerema neonatorum; cellulitis; erythema nodosum; hemangioma; lipogranulomatosis (Farber disease); neurofibroma; rhabdomyosarcoma or other sarcoma

Therapy
Self-limited process, not requiring therapy

References
Burden AD, Krafchik BR (1999) Subcutaneous fat necrosis of the newborn: a review of 11 cases. Pediatric Dermatology 16(5):384–387

Subcutaneous fibroma

▶ Knuckle pads

Subcutaneous phlebitis of the breast and chest wall

▶ Mondor's disease

Subungual exostosis

Synonym(s)
None

Definition
Acquired, benign, bony tumor of the distal phalanx, causing overlying nail plate dystrophy

Pathogenesis
Begins as a reactive fibrous growth that develops cartilage and ultimately ossifies

Clinical manifestation
Distal, subungual mass, usually on the dorsal-medial great toe; fingernail lesions rarely occur; overlying nail plate may be tented or completely destroyed

Differential diagnosis
Squamous cell carcinoma of the nail bed; glomus tumor; subungual wart; melanoma; traumatic nail dystrophy; osteochondroma; enchondroma

Therapy
Surgical excision

References
Davis DA, Cohen PR (1996) Subungual exostosis: case report and review of the literature. Pediatric Dermatology 13(3):212–218

Sudamina

▶ Miliaria

Sulzberger-Garbe syndrome

Synonym(s)
Exudative discoid and lichenoid dermatitis; lichenoid chronic dermatosis; polymorphic prurigo syndrome; polymorphous prurigo syndrome; Savill's syndrome

Definition
Chronic, pruritic dermatosis, characterized by discoid, lichenoid, exudative, and urticarial phases, occurring predominately in adult Jewish men

Pathogenesis
Suspected to have psychogenic component

Clinical manifestation
Scrotum and penis are main sites of involvement; discoid phase with round, scaly, and crusted papules; lichenoid phase with flat-topped, red-violaceosu papules and plaques; exudative phase with serous exudation from lesions; urticarial phase with wheals

Differential diagnosis
Nummular eczema; scabies; atopic dermatitis; contact dermatitis; lichen planus; lupus erythematosus; dermatitis herpetiformis; mycosis fungoides

Therapy
Prednisone*; azathioprine

References
Schmidt H, Midtgaard K (1968) The Sulzberger-Garbe syndrome. a survey and a case report. Acta Dermato-Venereologica 48(4):287–289

Sun damage

▶ Actinic elastosis

Sun spot

▶ Lentigo

Sunburn

Synonym(s)
Acute sun damage; acute sunburn reaction; erythema solare

Definition
Intense, transient inflammatory skin reaction caused by acute overexposure to ultraviolet radiation in sunlight, primarily ultraviolet B (UV-B)

Pathogenesis
Most injury from UVB spectrum of sunlight; UV-B absorbed by skin chromophores, which become excited and induce membrane lipid peroxidation and destruction; DNA in epidermal keratinocytes absorbs ultraviolet light, resulting in pyrimidine dimer formation; synthesis of cytokines (such as prostaglandins, tumor necrosis factor TNF-α), adhesion molecules, histamines, kinins, substance P, calcitonin gene-related peptide, and nitric oxide induce tissue injury

Clinical manifestation
Persons most prone are those with blue or green eye color, lighter skin, and ones who

tan poorly and freckle easily; beginning 2–6 hours after excess sun exposure, peaking at 15–36 hours, and resolving within 3–5 days; confluent erythema and warmth in exposed areas; edema, pain, and tenderness; pruritus with moderate-to-severe sun exposure; vesiculation in severe cases; scaling or peeling a few days following exposure; systemic signs and symptoms such as nausea, abdominal cramping, weakness and malaise, fever, chills, and headache with severe sunburn

Differential diagnosis
Burn from chemical or heat source; phototoxic drug eruption; toxic shock syndrome; lupus erythematosus; dermatomyositis; chronic actinic dermatitis; polymorphous light eruption; erythropoietic protoporphyria

Therapy
Ice water compresses for 20 minutes, repeated 3–4 times daily*; corticosteroids, topical, mid-potency; aloe gel, directly from plant leaf, applied 3–4 times per day

References
Rapaport MJ, Rapaport V (1998) Preventive and therapeutic approaches to short- and long-term sun damaged skin. Clinics in Dermatology 16(4):429–439

Superficial pemphigus

▶ **Pemphigus foliaceus**

Superficial porokeratosis

▶ **Porokeratosis**

Superficial thrombophlebitis

▶ **Thrombophlebitis, superficial**

Superficial white onychomycosis

▶ **Onychomycosis**

Supernumerary digit

Synonym(s)
Rudimentary polydactyly; digital duplication

Definition
Disorder manifested by a papule on the base of the ulnar side of the little finger, present from birth

Pathogenesis
Some cases manifested as autosomal dominant trait

Clinical manifestation
Smooth, flesh-colored papule at base of the fifth digit, present at birth

Differential diagnosis
Fibroma; neuroma; neurofibroma; pyogenic granuloma; wart

Therapy
Surgical removal for cosmesis only

References
Rayan GM, Frey B (2001) Ulnar polydactyly. Plastic & Reconstructive Surgery 107(6):1449–1454

Supernumerary nipple

Synonym(s)
Accessory nipple; polythelia

Definition
Congenital anomaly, characterized by additional nipples and/or related tissue in addition to the two nipples normally appearing on chest

Pathogenesis
Autosomal dominant transmission with incomplete expressivity; present in some cases of Turner syndrome, Fanconi anemia, ectodermal dysplasia, Kaufman-McKusick syndrome, and Char syndrome

Clinical manifestation
Small, pigmented or pearl-colored macule or papule or concave or umbilicated papule, often enlarging at puberty; distributed bilaterally or unilaterally, symmetrically or asymmetrically; usually located along milk line

Differential diagnosis
Nevocellular nevus; lipoma; lymphangioma; neurofibroma; wart; acrochordon

Therapy
Surgical excision for cosmesis

References
Cohen PR, Kurzrock R (1995) Miscellaneous genodermatoses: Beckwith-Wiedemann syndrome, Birt-Hogg-Dube syndrome, familial atypical multiple mole melanoma syndrome, hereditary tylosis, incontinentia pigmenti, and supernumerary nipples. Dermatologic Clinics 13(1):211–229

Suppurative fasciitis

▶ Necrotizing fasciitis

Suppurative hidradenitis

▶ Hidradenitis suppurativa

Suprarenal insufficiency

▶ Addison's disease

Sure antiperspirant

▶ Aluminium chlorohydrate

Sutton's nevus

▶ Halo nevus

Swamp fever

▶ Leptospirosis

Swamp itch

▶ Cercarial dermatitis

Sweat gland adenoma

▶ Eccrine acrospiroma

Sweating gustatory syndrome

▶ Auriculotemporal syndrome

Sweet syndrome

▶ Acute febrile neutrophilic dermatosis

Sweet's syndrome

▶ Acute febrile neutrophilic dermatosis

Swimmer's ear

▶ Otitis externa

Swimmer's itch

▶ Cercarial dermatitis

Swimming pool granuloma

▶ Mycobacterium marinum infection

Swineherd's disease

▶ Leptospirosis

Swollen veins

▶ Varicose and telangiectatic leg veins

Sycosis barbae

Synonym(s)
Tinea barbae; ringworm of the beard; barber's itch; trichophytosis barbae; tinea sycosis

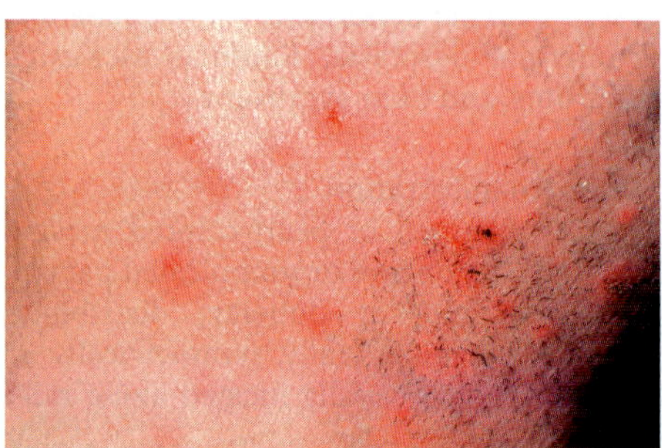

Sycosis barbae. Red papules in a beard distribution

Definition
Superficial dermatophyte infection on the bearded areas of the face and neck

Pathogenesis
Hair and hair follicles invaded by fungi, producing inflammatory response; Trichophyton species most common and include T. rubrum, T. mentagrophytes, and T. verrucosum

Clinical manifestation
Inflammatory variant (kerion): caused mostly by zoophilic dermatophytes; solitary plaque or nodule, usually localized on chin, cheeks, or neck; inflammatory reddish papule or nodule with pustules and draining sinuses, often covered by exudate and crust

Non-inflammatory variant: erythematous plaques with active border composed of papules, vesicles, and/or crusts; hairs breaking at skin surface or plugging follicle

Differential diagnosis
Acne vulgaris; actinomycosis; candidiasis; contact dermatitis; bacterial folliculitis; non-infectious folliculitis; rosacea; halogenoderma

Therapy
Terbinafine; itraconazole; griseofulvin

References
Kick G, Korting HC (1998) Tinea barbae due to Trichophyton mentagrophytes related to persistent child infection. Mycoses 41(9–10):439–441

Sycosis cruris

▶ Tinea cruris

Symmetric progressive leukopathy of extremities

▶ Idiopathic guttate hypomelanosis

Symmetrical dyschromatosis of the extremities

▶ Acropigmentation of Dohi

Syndrome of Favre-Racouchot

▶ Favre-Racouchot syndrome

Synovial cyst

▶ Digital mucous cyst

Syphilis

Synonym(s)
Lues

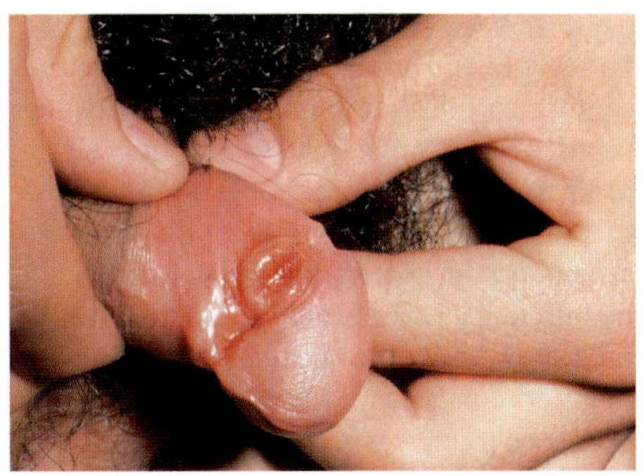

Syphilis. Indurated, red papule on the penis

Definition
Sexually transmitted or congenital infection caused by the bacterium Treponema pallidum

Pathogenesis
Caused by the spirochete, Treponema pallidum; penetrates intact mucous membranes or microscopic dermal abrasions and, within a few hours, enters lymphatics and blood to produce systemic infection; ultimate tissue injury related to obliterative endarteritis

Clinical manifestation
Primary syphilis: occurs within 3 weeks of contact with an infected individual; single ulcerated lesion with a surrounding red areola; ulcer edge and base have button-like consistency; usually heals within 4–8 weeks; painless regional lymphadenopathy
Secondary syphilis: bilaterally symmetrical, pale red to pink, discrete, round mac-

ules on trunk and proximal extremities; after several days or weeks, appearance of red, scaly papules sometimes becoming necrotic; distributed widely, with frequent involvement of the palms and soles; small papular follicular syphilids involving hair follicles sometimes result in patchy alopecia; highly infectious papules develop at mucocutaneous junctions and in moist intertriginous skin, become hypertrophic and dull pink or gray (condyloma lata); superficial mucosal erosions on the palate, pharynx, larynx, glans penis, vulva, in anal canal and rectum (mucous patches)

Late syphilis: usually solitary gummas presenting as indurated, nodular, papulosquamous or ulcerative lesions forming circles or arcs with peripheral hyperpigmentation; cardiovascular findings: diastolic murmur, secondary to aortic dilation with valvular insufficiency; symptomatic neurosyphilis, including meningovascular syphilis: cranial nerve palsies and pupillary abnormalities occurring with basilar meningitis (Argyll Robertson pupil); tabes dorsalis; ulcers of feet from loss of pain sensation

Congenital syphilis:

Early manifestations: diffuse eruption, characterized by extensive sloughing of the epithelium, particularly on palms, soles, and skin around mouth and anus; abnormal bone radiographs; hepatomegaly; splenomegaly; petechiae; anemia lymphadenopathy; jaundice; pseudoparalysis; snuffles; depressed linear scars radiating from the orifice of the mouth (rhagades or Parrot lines)

Late manifestations: interstitial keratitis; cranial nerve VIII deafness; corneal opacities; recurrent arthropathy

Congenital neurosyphilis: gummatous periostitis, saddle nose, dental abnormalities including centrally notched and widely spaced, peg-shaped, upper central incisors (Hutchinson teeth) and sixth-year molars with multiple poorly developed cusps (mulberry molars); bone findings: frontal bossing, unilateral irregular enlargement of the sternoclavicular portion of the clavicle

Differential diagnosis

Amyloidosis; chancroid; lymphogranuloma venereum; granuloma inguinale; herpes simplex virus infection; drug eruption; erythema multiforme; leprosy; tinea corporis; psoriasis; parapsoriasis; lichen planus; pityriasis rosea; lupus erythematosus; sarcoidosis; traumatic balanitis

Therapy

Penicillin G benzathine*; erythromycin; tetracycline

References

Pao D, Goh BT, Bingham JS (2002) Management issues in syphilis. Drugs 62(10):1447–1461

Syringadenoma papilliferum

▶ Syringocystadenoma papilliferum

Syringectasia

▶ Eccrine hidrocystoma

Syringocystadenoma

▶ Epidermal nevus
▶ Syringocystadenoma papilliferum

Syringocystadenoma papilliferum

Synonym(s)

Papillary syringadenoma; nevus syringadenoma papilliferum; syringadenoma papilliferum; Werther's tumor, syringocystadenoma

Definition
Benign tumor, most commonly on the scalp, characterized by one papule, several papules in a linear arrangement, or a solitary verrucous plaque

Pathogenesis
Tumor with apocrine differentiation; associated with nevus sebaceous and tubular apocrine adenoma

Clinical manifestation
Presents at birth or in early childhood with infiltrative, verrucous papule or plaque, most commonly on scalp or face; occasionally in linear pattern; alopecia over tumor when in scalp; at puberty may increase in size and become more papillomatous

Differential diagnosis
Basal cell carcinoma; kerion; wart; epidermal nevus; squamous cell carcinoma

Therapy
Surgical excision[*]

References
Mammino JJ, Vidmar DA (1991) Syringocystadenoma papilliferum. International Journal of Dermatology 30(11):763–766

Syringoma

Synonym(s)
None

Definition
Benign adnexal tumor formed by well-differentiated sweat ductal elements

Pathogenesis
May be related to eccrine elements, apocrine elements, or pluripotential stem cells

Clinical manifestation
Skin-colored or yellowish, small, dermal papules, often with a translucent or cystic appearance, most commonly on upper parts of cheeks and lower eyelids, but also on axilla, chest, abdomen, penis, and vulva

Differential diagnosis
Trichoepithelioma; basal cell carcinoma; molluscum contagiosum; milium; flat wart; xanthelasma; granuloma annulare

Therapy
Surgical removal for cosmetic reasons only: electrodesiccation and curettage; CO_2 laser vaporization; dermabrasion; TCA chemical peel

References
Frazier CC, Camacho AP, Cockerell CJ (2001) The treatment of eruptive syringomas in an African American patient with a combination of trichloroacetic acid and CO_2 laser destruction. Dermatologic Surgery 27(5):489–492

Systematized elastorrhexis

▶ Pseudoxanthoma elasticum

Systematized lichenification

▶ Lichen striatus

Systemic allergic reaction

▶ Anaphylaxis

Systemic chondromalacia

▶ Relapsing polychondritis

Systemic connective tissue disease

► Progressive systemic sclerosus

Systemic necrotizing angiitis

► Wegener's granulomatosis

Systemic sclerosis

► Progressive systemic sclerosus

Systemic vasculitis

► Wegener's granulomatosis

T-cell lymphoma, cutaneous

Synonym(s)
Mycosis fungoides

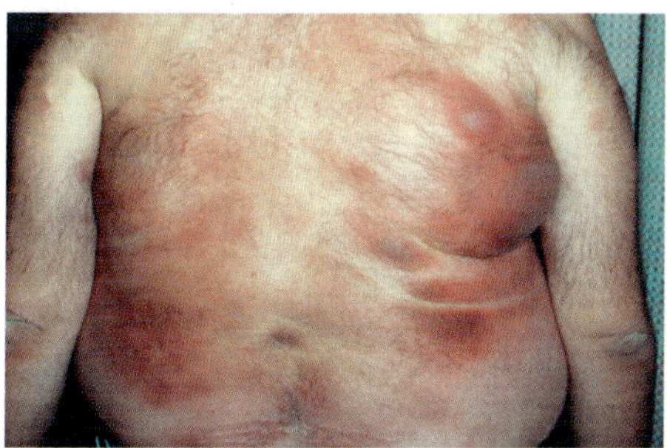

T-cell lymphoma, cutaneous. Irregular, infiltrated, violaceous plaques on the trunk

Definition
Heterogenous group of malignant T-cell lymphomas with primary manifestations in the skin

Pathogenesis
Expansion of clone of $CD4^+$ memory T cells, which home to the skin

Clinical manifestation
Patch/plaque stage: flat, erythematous patches, sometimes becoming more infiltrative and evolving into palpable, scaly plaques with irregular borders; alopecia if scalp is involved

Tumor stage: red-to-violaceous, exophytic and/or ulcerated nodules; generalized erythroderma

Pagetoid reticulosis (Woringer-Kolopp disease) variant: solitary, asymptomatic, slowly enlarging, well-defined, red, scaly plaque on the extremities

Sezary variant: large number of circulating abnormal T cells; erythroderma; lymphadenopathy

Differential diagnosis
Parapsoriasis en plaque; lymphomatoid papulosis; psoriasis; lupus erythematosus; lichen planus; atopic dermatitis; tinea corporis; other causes of exfoliative erythroderma, including drug eruption, seborrheic dermatitis

Therapy
Topical/physical modalities: corticosteroids, topical, high potency; UVB phototherapy; photochemotherapy; topical mechlorethamine (nitrogen mustard): 90 mg with 10 ml of absolute alcohol dissolved in Aquaphor QS 900 gm, applied daily. Topical carmustine (BCNU): 100 mg dissolved in 50 ml alcohol; 5 ml dissolved in 50 ml water for daily application; electron beam therapy; extracorporeal photopheresis.

Systemic modalities: prednisone; methotrexate; isotretinoin; bexarotene: 20–150 mcg PO per day; systemic chemotherapy

References
Apisarnthanarax N, Talpur R, Duvic M (2002) Treatment of cutaneous T cell lymphoma: cur-

rent status and future directions. American Journal of Clinical Dermatology 3(3):193–215

Taenia solium infestation

▶ Cysticercosis

Takatsuki syndrome

▶ POEMS syndrome

Talon noir

▶ Black heel

Tattoo, traumatic

▶ Traumatic tattoo

Tay syndrome

Synonym(s)
Trichothiodystrophy with congenital ichthyosis; Tay's syndrome; trichothio-dystrophy; IBIDS

Definition
Hereditary disorder characterized by: photosensitivity; brittle, twisted hair; ichthyosis; abnormal fingernails and toenails; multiple developmental defects

Pathogenesis
Autosomal recessive disorder; trichothiodystrophy with sulfur-containing amino acid deficiency in hair; defective repair of UV-induced DNA lesions possibly associated with photosensitivity

Clinical manifestation
Brittle, twisted hair, and ichthyosiform erythroderma; abnormal nails; loss of subcutaneous fat, resulting in prematurely aged-looking face; photosensitivity; slowed physical development; intellectual impairment; wide variety of central nervous system abnormalities, including seizures, tremors, ataxia and neurosensory deafness; underdeveloped reproductive organs; cataracts; abnormalities of bones and teeth; increased susceptibility to infection

Differential diagnosis
Progeria; Werner's syndrome; xeroderma pigmentosum; Netherton's syndrome; Sjögren-Larsson syndrome; Cockayne's syndrome; non-bullous ichthyosiform erythroderma

Therapy
Emollients for dry skin

References
Kousseff BG, Esterly NB (1988) Trichothiodystrophy, IBIDS syndrome or Tay syndrome? Birth Defects: Original Article Series 24(2):169–181, 1988

Tay's syndrome

▶ Tay syndrome

Tazarotene

Trade name(s)
Tazorac

Generic available
No

Drug class
Retinoid

Tazarotene. Dermatologic indications and dosage

Disease	Adult dosage	Child dosage
Acne vulgaris	Apply daily	Apply daily
Psoriasis	Apply daily	Apply daily
Reiter syndrome	Apply daily	Apply daily
Sun-induced skin aging	Apply daily	Apply daily

Mechanism of action
Gene transcription after membrane receptor binding and intracellular transport; modulates abnormal epidermal keratinization

Dosage form
0.05%, 0.1% gel and cream

Dermatologic indications and dosage
See table

Common side effects
Cutaneous: scaling, erythema, blistering, photosensitivity

Serious side effects
None

Drug interactions
Benzoyl peroxide; isotretinoin; photosensitizing drugs

Contraindications/precautions
Hypersensitivity to drug class or component

References
Tremblay JF, Bissonnette R (2002) Topical agents for the treatment of psoriasis, past, present and future. Journal of Cutaneous Medicine & Surgery 6(3 Suppl):8–11

Telangiectasia macularis eruptiva perstans

▶ **Mastocytosis**

Telogen defluvium

▶ Telogen effluvium

Telogen effluvium

Synonym(s)
Telogen defluvium

Definition
Reactive process resulting in nonscarring alopecia, characterized by diffuse hair shedding, caused by metabolic or hormonal stress or by medications

Pathogenesis
Large number of hairs entering telogen phase at one time; shedding occurs when new anagen hairs begin to grow; emerging hairs force some of the resting hairs out of the follicle, leading to temporary alopecia

Clinical manifestation
Acute form: relatively sudden onset of diffuse scalp hair loss, usually after a metabolic or physiologic stress 1–6 months before the start of the hair shedding; inciting stresses: febrile illness, major injury, change in diet, pregnancy and delivery, and beginning a new medication
Chronic form: hair shedding lasting longer than 6 months; onset often insidious; inciting causes: chronic illness such as malignancy, particularly lymphoproliferative malignancy; any chronic debilitating illness such as systemic lupus erythematosus;

end-stage renal disease or liver disease; hormonal changes; diet changes; heavy metal intoxication

Differential diagnosis
Alopecia areata; androgenetic alopecia; trichotillomania; tinea capitis; anagen effluvium; traumatic hair breakage

Therapy
Minoxidil 5% solution 1 ml applied twice daily

References
Sperling LC (2001) Hair and systemic disease. Dermatologic Clinics 19(4):711–726

Temporal arteritis

Synonym(s)
Giant cell arteritis; arteritis temporalis; arteritis cranialis; Horton disease; granulomatous arteritis; arteritis of the aged

Definition
Vasculitis that affects large and medium-sized arteries containing elastic tissue throughout the body, most commonly the temporal arteries

Pathogenesis
Vasculitis primarily damaging the media and destroying the internal elastic layer; panarteritis developing and intimal proliferation causing lumenal occlusion, resulting in signs and symptoms of decreased perfusion

Clinical manifestation
Constitutional symptoms, such as malaise, weight loss, fever and fatigue; temporal headache; tender scalp; jaw claudication; visual changes, including diplopia, blurred vision, amaurosis fugax, and blindness of one or both eyes; temporal arteries may be tender, inflamed, dilated, thickened or cord-like, and pulsatile; ulceration sometimes occurring over the temporal artery

Differential diagnosis
Wegener's granulomatosis; amyloidosis; polymyalgia rheumatica; polyarteritis nodosa; lupus erythematosus; rheumatoid arthritis; Takayasu arteritis

Therapy
Prednisone★

References
Salvarani C, Cantini F, Boiardi L, Hunder GG (2002) Polymyalgia rheumatica and giant-cell arteritis. New England Journal of Medicine 347(4):261–271

Tendinous xanthoma

▶ Xanthoma

Tennis heel

▶ Black heel

Tennis toe

Synonym(s)
Sportsman's toe

Definition
Acute subungual accumulation of blood from sudden blunt impact of the toe against athletic footwear

Pathogenesis
Subungual hemorrhage of the lateral nail bed caused by jamming of the toe into the front of the athletic shoe

Terbinafine. Dermatologic indications and dosage

Disease	Adult dosage	Child dosage
Black piedra	250 mg PO once daily for 1 month	250 mg PO for 1 month (> 40 kg weight); 125 mg PO for 1 month (20–40 kg weight); 62.5 mg PO daily for 1 month (< 20 kg weight)
Chromoblastomycosis	250 mg PO daily for 3-6 months	250 mg PO 3-6 months (> 40 kg weight); 125 mg PO for 3-6 months (20–40 kg weight); 62.5 mg PO daily for 3-6 months (< 20 kg weight
Majocchi granuloma	250 mg PO daily for 4–6 weeks	250 mg PO for 4–6 weeks (> 40 kg weight); 125 mg PO for 4–6 weeks (20–40 kg weight); 62.5 mg PO daily for 4–6 weeks (< 20 kg weight)
Onychomycosis	250 mg PO daily for 3 months	250 mg PO for 3 months (> 40 kg weight); 125 mg PO for 3 months (20–40 kg weight); 62.5 mg PO daily for 3 months (< 20 kg weight)
Sycosis barbae	250 mg PO daily for 4 weeks	250 mg PO for 4 weeks (> 40 kg weight); 125 mg PO for 4 weeks (20–40 kg weight); 62.5 mg PO daily for 4 weeks (< 20 kg weight
Tinea capitis	250 mg PO daily for 4–6 weeks	250 mg PO for 4–6 weeks (> 40 kg weight); 125 mg PO for 4–6 weeks (20–40 kg weight); 62.5 mg PO daily for 4-6weeks (< 20 kg weight)
Tinea corporis	250 mg PO daily for 4–6 weeks	250 mg PO for 4–6 weeks (> 40 kg weight); 125 mg PO for 4-6 weeks (20–40 kg weight); 62.5 mg PO daily for 4–6 weeks (< 20 kg weight)
Tinea cruris	Apply cream twice daily for 7 days or 250 mg PO for 2–4 weeks	Apply cream twice daily for 7 days
Tinea faciei	Apply cream twice daily for 7 days or 250 mg PO for 2–4 weeks	Apply cream twice daily for 7 days or250 mg PO for 2–4 weeks (> 40 kg weight); 125 mg PO for 2–4 weeks (20–40 kg weight); 62.5 mg PO daily for 2–4 weeks (< 20 kg weight)
Tinea nigra	Apply cream twice daily for 7 days or 250 mg PO for 2–4 weeks	Apply cream twice daily for 7 days
Tinea pedis	Apply cream twice daily for 7 days or 250 mg PO for 2–4 weeks	Apply cream twice daily for 7 days

Clinical manifestation

Pain and reddish-blue discoloration under the affected nail plate; mainly occurs in sports that require frequent, abrupt stops and quick pivoting, such as basketball, tennis, squash, and racquetball; usually affects either the great toe or second toe, whichever is longer; sometimes occurs with jogging, affecting the third, fourth, or fifth toes, secondary to repeated pounding of the foot on a firm running surface

Differential diagnosis
Melanoma; melanocytic nevus

Therapy
Puncture of the nail plate with a blunt pointed instrument, such as a heated paper clip, to express blood*

References
Elizabeth L. Tanzi, MD, Richard K. Scher (1999) Managing common nail disorders in active patients and athletes. Physician and Sportsmedicine 27(9):35–37

Terbinafine

Trade name(s)
Lamisil

Generic available
No

Drug class
Allylamine antifungal agent

Mechanism of action
Inhibition of squalene epoxidase, which blocks ergosterol synthesis

Dosage form
250 mg tablet; 1% cream

Dermatologic indications and dosage
See table

Common side effects
Cutaneous: skin eruption, pruritus (oral formulation)
Gastrointestinal: nausea and vomiting, diarrhea, dyspepsia

Laboratory: elevated liver enzymes
Neurologic: taste changes

Serious side effects
Cutaneous: Stevens-Johnson syndrome, toxic epidermal necrolysis, anaphylaxis
Gastrointestinal: hepatotoxicity
Laboratory: elevated liver enzymes, neutropenia

Drug interactions
Cimetidine; cyclosporine; rifampin; theophylline; thioridazine; tricyclic antidepressants

Contraindications/precautions
Hypersensitivity to drug class or component; caution in patients with impaired liver or renal function

References
Moosavi M, Bagheri B, Scher R (2001) Systemic antifungal therapy. Dermatologic Clinics 19(1):35–52

Terminal transverse defects of arm

▶ **Amniotic band syndrome**

Tetracycline

Trade name(s)
Sumycin; Achromycin-V; Tetracap; Panmycin

Generic available
Yes

Drug class
Tetracycline antibiotic

Tetracycline. Dermatologic indications and dosage

Disease	Adult dosage	Child dosage
Acne vulgaris	250–500 mg PO twice daily	Not indicated below age 8 years; 250–500 mg PO twice daily
Atrophoderma of Pasini-Pierini	250–500 mg PO twice daily	Not indicated below age 8 years; 250–500 mg PO twice daily
Bejel	500 mg PO 4 times daily for 15 days	Not indicated below age 8 years; 250 mg PO 4 times daily for 15 days
Bullous pemphigoid	250–500 mg PO twice daily	Not indicated below age 8 years; 250–500 mg PO twice daily
Chloracne	250–500 mg PO twice daily	Not indicated below age 8 years; 250–500 mg PO twice daily
Dermatitis herpetiformis	250–500 mg PO twice daily	Not indicated below age 8 years; 250–500 mg PO twice daily
Folliculitis	250–500 mg PO twice daily	Not indicated below age 8 years; 250–500 mg PO twice daily
Glanders	40 mg per kg daily, divided into 3 doses for 60–150 days	Not indicated below age 8 years; 40 mg per kg daily, divided into 3 doses for 60–150 days
Hidradenitis suppurativa	250–500 mg PO twice daily	Not indicated below age 8 years; 250–500 mg PO twice daily
Linear IgA bullous dermatosis	250–500 mg PO twice daily	Not indicated below age 8 years; 250–500 mg PO twice daily
Melioidosis	40 mg per kg daily, divided into 3 doses for 60–150 days	Not indicated below age 8 years; 40 mg per kg daily, divided into 3 doses for 60–150 days
Perioral dermatitis	250–500 mg PO twice daily	Not indicated below age 8 years; 250–500 mg PO twice daily
Pinta	500 mg PO 4 times daily for 15 days	Not indicated below age 8 years; 25-50 mg per kg daily PO for 15 days
Pityriasis lichenoides	250–500 mg PO twice daily	Not indicated below age 8 years; 250–500 mg PO twice daily
Protothecosis	500 mg PO twice daily for 1-6 weeks (combined with amphotericin B)	Not indicated below age 8 years; 250 mg PO twice daily for 1-6 weeks (combined with amphotericin B)
Relapsing fever	1 gm PO twice daily for 7 days after patient becomes afebrile	Not indicated below age 8 years; 500 mg PO twice daily for 7 days after patient becomes afebrile
Rhinoscleroma	500 mg PO twice daily for months to years	Not indicated below age 8 years; 500 mg PO twice daily for months to years
Rickettsialpox	500 mg PO twice daily for 5 days	Not indicated below age 8 years; 250 mg PO twice daily for 5 days
Rosacea	250–500 mg PO daily	Not indicated below age 8 years; 250–500 mg PO twice daily

T

Tetracycline. Dermatologic indications and dosage (Continued)

Disease	Adult dosage	Child dosage
Steatocystoma multiplex	250–500 mg PO twice daily	Not indicated below age 8 years; 250–500 mg PO twice daily
Syphilis	500 mg PO 4 times daily for 14 days; late latent syphilis with normal CSF examination, cardiovascular syphilis, and late benign (gumma) disease – 500 mg PO 4 times daily for 28 days	Not indicated
Tropical phagedenic ulcer	1 gm twice daily until ulcer closure	Not indicated below age 8 years; 500 mg PO twice daily until ulcer closure

Mechanism of action
Antibiotic activity: protein synthesis inhibition by binding to the 30S ribosomal subunit
Anti-inflammatory activity: unclear mechanism

Dosage form
250 mg, 500 mg capsule

Dermatologic indications and dosage
See table

Common side effects
Cutaneous: photosensitivity, stomatitis, oral candidiasis, urticaria or other vascular reaction
Gastrointestinal: nausea and vomiting, diarrhea, esophagitis
Neurologic: tinnitus, dizziness, drowsiness, headache, ataxia

Serious side effects
Gastrointestinal: pseudomembranous colitis, hepatotoxicity
Neurologic: pseudotumor cerebri
Hematologic: neutropenia, thrombocytopenia

Drug interactions
Antacids; calcium salts; oral contraceptives; digoxin; iron salts; isotretinoin; magnesium salts; warfarin

Contraindications/precautions
Hypersensitivity to drug class or component; pregnancy; patient < 8 years old; caution in patients with impaired renal or liver function

References
Sadick N (2000) Systemic antibiotic agents. Dermatologic Clinics 19(1):1–22

Thalidomide

Trade name(s)
Thalomid

Generic available
No

Drug class
Immune modulator

Mechanism of action
Immunomodulatory; anti-inflammatory; hypnotic-sedative

Dosage form
50 mg tablet

Dermatologic indications and dosage
See table

Thalidomide. Dermatologic indications and dosage

Disease	Adult dosage	Child dosage
Jessner lymphocytic infiltration of skin	100 mg PO daily for 2 months	Not indicated
Leprosy, reactional state	100–300 mg PO daily	Not indicated
Lupus erythematosus, acute	100–300 mg PO daily	Not indicated
Lupus erythematosus, discoid	100–300 mg PO daily	Not indicated
Lupus erythematosus, subacute cutaneous	100–300 mg PO daily	Not indicated
Polymorphous light eruption	50–200 mg PO daily	Not indicated
Prurigo nodularis	100–300 mg PO daily	Not indicated

Common side effects
Cutaneous: eruption, photosensitivity
Constitutional: fever, chills
Gastrointestinal: increased appetite and weight gain, diarrhea
Neurologic: somnolence, mood changes, confusion, amnesia, headache

Serious side effects
Bone marrow: neutropenia
Cardiovascular: severe hypertension, bradycardia
Cutaneous: Stevens-Johnson syndrome, toxic epidermal necrolysis
Neurologic: peripheral neuropathy, seizures
Pregnancy: severe birth defects

Drug interactions
Acetaminophen; antihistamines; antipsychotics; barbiturates; protease inhibitors; griseofulvin; rifampin; phenytoin; carbamazepine; opiates; sedative hypnotics

Other interactions
Ethanol

Contraindications/precautions
Hypersensitivity to drug class or component; pregnancy; moderate to severe pre-existing peripheral neuropathy; caution in patients with seizure disorder, cardiovascular disease, or child-bearing potential

References
Radomsky CL, Levine N (2001) Thalidomide. Dermatologic Clinics 19(1):87–103

Therapy-induced bullous photosensitivity

▶ **Pseudoporphyria**

Thioguanine

Trade name(s)
Thioguanine

Generic available
No

Drug class
Purine analog

Thioguanine. Dermatologic indications and dosage

Disease	Adult dosage	Child dosage
Pityriasis rubra pilaris	120 mg PO twice weekly to 160 mg PO 3 times weekly	Not indicated
Psoriasis	120 mg PO twice weekly to 160 mg PO 3 times weekly	Not indicated
Reiter syndrome	120 mg PO twice weekly to 160 mg PO 3 times weekly	Not indicated

Mechanism of action
Inhibition of lymphocyte synthesis

Dosage form
40 mg tablet

Dermatologic indications and dosage
See table

Common side effects
Gastrointestinal: diarrhea, nausea, vomiting
Neurologic: headache, fatigue

Serious side effects
Bone marrow: myelosuppression
Gastrointestinal: hepatotoxicity

Drug interactions
Sulfasalazine; busulfan; azathioprine

Contraindications/precautions
Hypersensitivity to drug class or component; caution with other immunosuppressants or bone marrow suppressants

References
Silvis NG, Levine N (1999) Pulse dosing of thioguanine in recalcitrant psoriasis. Archives of Dermatology 135(4):433–437

Thost-Unna disease

▶ **Unna-Thost palmoplantar keratoderma**

Three day measles

▶ **Rubella**

Thrombophlebitis, superficial

Synonym(s)
Venous clot

Definition
Inflammatory reaction with thrombus of a subcutaneous vein

Pathogenesis
Associated with intimal damage (from trauma, infection, or inflammation), stasis, or changes in blood constituents; risk factors: varicose veins, obesity, old age, cigarette smoking, and injection of caustic materials such as street drugs

Clinical manifestation
Redness and tenderness along course of vein, usually accompanied by edema; often occurs in patients with varicose veins; involvement of upper extremities at infusion sites or sites of trauma

Differential diagnosis
Deep vein thrombophlebitis; cellulitis; factitial disease; lymphangitis; pancreatic panniculitis; Weber-Christian disease; lupus

panniculitis; erythema nodosum; erythema induratum

Therapy
Elastic support dressings; for severe involvement: bedrest with elevation of the extremity and application of hot, wet compresses

References
Kalodiki E, Nicolaides AN (2002) Superficial thrombophlebitis and low-molecular-weight heparins. Angiology 53(6):659–663

Thrush

▶ Candidiasis

Thyroglossal duct cyst

▶ Cutaneous columnar cyst

Thyroid acropachy

Definition
Clubbing of fingers and toes, associated with soft tissue thickening and periosteal new bone formation of distal hands and feet in patients with hyperthyroidism

References
Niepomniszcze H, Amad RH (2001) Skin disorders and thyroid diseases. Journal of Endocrinological Investigation 24(8):628–638

Thyroid blepharochalasis syndrome

▶ Ascher's syndrome

Tick bite fever

▶ Boutonneuse fever

Tick fever

▶ Rocky Mountain spotted fever

Tick typhus

▶ Boutonneuse fever
▶ Rocky Mountain spotted fever

Tick-borne relapsing fever

▶ Relapsing fever

Tinea amiantacea

Definition
Morphologic entity characterized by thick, adherent scale on the scalp and in the hair

References
Bettencourt MS, Olsen EA (1999) Pityriasis amiantacea: a report of two cases in adults. Cutis 64(3):187–189

Tinea barbae

▶ Sycosis barbae

Tinea capitis

Synonym(s)
Ringworm of the scalp

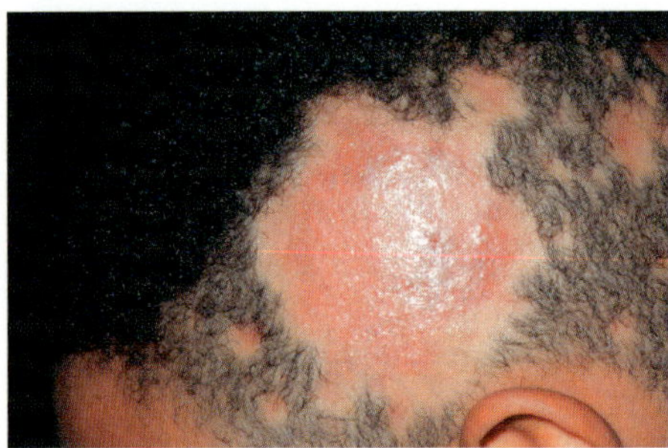

Tinea capitis. Boggy, red, alopecic plaque, studded with papules and minute pustules

Definition
Superficial fungal infection of scalp skin, eyebrows, and eyelashes, with propensity for invading hair shafts and follicles

Pathogenesis
Causative agents are fungal species of genera Trichophyton and Microsporum; after inoculation, fungal hyphae invades hair keratin as it is formed

Clinical manifestation
Red papules progressing to grayish, annular plaques consisting of perifollicular papules; pustules with crusts, exudate, matted hairs, and debris
Black dot variant: infection with fracture of the hair, leaving dark stubs visible in the follicular orifices
Kerion variant: extreme inflammation associated with boggy scalp and pustules; may progress to patchy or diffuse hair loss with scarring alopecia
Favus variant (tinea favosa): chronic infection caused most commonly by T. schoenleinii, characterized by yellow, cup-shaped crusts, termed scutula, which surround the infected hair follicles

Differential diagnosis
Psoriasis; seborrheic dermatitis; pediculosis; alopecia areata; traction alopecia; trichotillomania; folliculitis; secondary syphilis; bacterial pyoderma

Therapy
Griseofulvin; itraconazole; terbinafine; prednisone for kerion[*]

References
Al Sogair S, Hay RJ (2000) Fungal infection in children: tinea capitis. Clinics in Dermatology 18(6):679–685

Tinea corporis

Synonym(s)
Ringworm

Definition
Superficial fungal infection of glabrous skin of the trunk and extremities

Pathogenesis
Causative agent mainly fungal species of genera Microsporum (most commonly M. canis) and Trichophyton (most commonly T. rubrum); pathogens produce keratinases, allowing invasion of stratum corneum; cell wall of T rubrum contains mannan, possible inhibitor of local cell-mediated immunity; infection transmitted by fomites, such as infected pets, or by autoinoculation from reservoir elsewhere on skin

Clinical manifestation
Rapidly evolving, annular, erythematous, scaly plaques; border may have crusting, vesicle formation, and papules; intense inflammatory response with zoophilic fungi (e.g., M. canis)
Majocchi granuloma variant: granulomatous reaction secondary to fungal folliculitis, usually caused by T rubrum; plaques studded with follicular papules and/or pus-

tules; organism also occurs in the surrounding dermis

Tinea manuum variant: diffuse erythema and scale of palm, extending onto dorsum of hand

Tinea imbricata variant: caused by T concentricum; scaly plaques arranged in concentric rings

Differential diagnosis

Tinea versicolor; psoriasis; seborrheic dermatitis; lupus erythematosus; bacterial pyoderma; candidiasis; contact dermatitis; superficial pemphigus; pityriasis rosea; syphilis; nummular eczema; granuloma annulare; sarcoidosis; erythema annulare centrifugum

Therapy

Azole antifungal agents; ciclopirox; terbinafine cream; griseofulvin; itraconazole; oral terbinafine

References

Lesher JL Jr (1999) Oral therapy of common superficial fungal infections of the skin. Journal of the American Academy of Dermatology 40(6 Pt 2):S 31–34

autoinoculation from reservoir elsewhere on skin

Clinical manifestation

Almost exclusively in men; erythema with central clearing with hyperpigmentation and advancing scaly border in inguinal creases; extends distally onto medial thighs and proximally to lower abdomen and pubic area; with acute infections, moisture and exudation; scrotum spared

Differential diagnosis

Psoriasis; seborrheic dermatitis; pediculosis; bacterial pyoderma; candida intertrigo; contact dermatitis; acanthosis nigricans; erythrasma; benign familial pemphigus; Langerhans cell histiocytosis

Therapy

Azole antifungal agents; ciclopirox; terbinafine cream; griseofulvin; itraconazole; oral terbinafine

References

Weinstein A, Berman B (2002) Topical treatment of common superficial tinea infections. American Family Physician 65(10):2095–2102

Tinea cruris

Synonym(s)

Tinea inguinalis; groin dermatophytosis; ringworm of the groin; eczema marginatum; gym itch; jock itch; crotch rot

Definition

Superficial fungal infection of groin and adjacent skin

Pathogenesis

Causative agents the fungal species of genera Trichophyton (most commonly, T. Rubrum) and Epidermophyton; pathogens produce keratinases, allowing invasion of stratum corneum; infection transmitted by fomites, such as contaminated towels, or by

Tinea faciei

Synonym(s)

Ringworm of the face; facial ringworm

Definition

Superficial fungal infection of glabrous skin of face

Pathogenesis

Causative agent mainly the fungal species of genera Microsporum (most commonly, M. canis) and Trichophyton (most commonly, T. tonsurans); pathogens produce keratinases, allowing invasion of stratum corneum; infection transmitted by fomites, such as infected pets, or by autoinoculation from reservoir elsewhere on skin

Clinical manifestation

Pruritic, annular, or serpiginous erythematous scaling plaques, with active border composed of papules, vesicles, and/or crusts

Differential diagnosis

Psoriasis; seborrheic dermatitis; lupus erythematosus; bacterial pyoderma; candidiasis; contact dermatitis; superficial pemphigus; rosacea; perioral dermatitis; coccidioidomycosis; granuloma annulare; sarcoidosis

Therapy

Azole antifungal agents; ciclopirox; terbinafine cream; griseofulvin; itraconazole; oral terbinafine

References

Lesher JL Jr (1999) Oral therapy of common superficial fungal infections of the skin. Journal of the American Academy of Dermatology 40(6 Pt 2):S 31–34

Tinea favosa

▶ Tinea capitis

Tinea flava

▶ Tinea versicolor

Tinea imbricata

▶ Tinea corporis

Tinea inguinalis

▶ Tinea cruris

Tinea manuum

▶ Tinea corporis

Tinea nigra

Synonym(s)

Tinea nigra palmaris; tinea nigra plantaris; keratomycosis nigricans palmaris; dermatomycosis nigricans

Definition

Superficial fungal infection, characterized by hyperpigmented macules or patches, usually occurring on palms

Pathogenesis

Causative agent the fungal pathogen, Phaeoannellomyces werneckii; inoculation from contamination source such as soil, sewage, wood, or compost; pigmentary change due to accumulation of melanin-like substance in fungus

Clinical manifestation

Discrete, oval, round or irregular, painless, brown-to-black macule or patch, beginning as small dark spot; hyperpigmentation ranging from light brown to black and sometimes appearing mottled or velvety; varies in size, depending on the duration of infection

Differential diagnosis

Exogenous staining; melanoma; yaws; pinta; drug-induced hyperpigmentation

Therapy

Azole antifungal agents; ciclopirox; terbinafine cream

References

Shannon PL, Ramos-Caro FA, Cosgrove BF, Flowers FP (1999) Treatment of tinea nigra with terbinafine. Cutis 64(3):199–201

Tinea nigra palmaris

▶ Tinea nigra

Tinea nigra plantaris

▶ Tinea nigra

Tinea nodosa

▶ Piedra

Tinea pedis

Synonym(s)
Ringworm of the feet; athlete's feet

Definition
Superficial fungal infection of the skin of the feet

Pathogenesis
Causative agent the fungal species of genera Epidermophyton (most commonly, E. floccosum) and Trichophyton (most commonly, T. rubrum or T. mentagrophytes); pathogens produce keratinases, allowing invasion of stratum corneum; cell wall of T rubrum contains mannan, possible inhibitor of local cell-mediated immunity; temperature and serum factors, such as beta globulins and ferritin, may play role in limiting infection; hyperhidrosis a risk factor for infection

Clinical manifestation
Interdigital variant: maceration, fissuring, and scaling, most often between fourth and fifth toes; usually spares dorsal aspect of foot, but some extension onto plantar surface

Moccasin (hyperkeratotic) variant: symmetrical, asymptomatic or pruritic erythema with slight scaling; dorsal foot spared, but sometimes extends onto the sides of the foot

Vesicular variant: painful, pruritic vesicles or bullae, most often on instep or anterior plantar surfaces; clear or purulent fluid in blisters; after rupture, scaling with erythema

Ulcerative variant: rapidly spreading vesiculopustular lesions, often with secondary bacterial infection; may develop cellulitis, lymphangitis, pyrexia, and malaise

Differential diagnosis
Psoriasis; dyshidrotic eczema; atopic dermatitis; bacterial pyoderma; candidiasis; contact dermatitis; erythema multiforme; syphilis; localized bullous pemphigoid; xerosis

Therapy
Azole antifungal agents; ciclopirox; terbinafine cream; griseofulvin; itraconazole; oral terbinafine

References
Lesher JL Jr (1999) Oral therapy of common superficial fungal infections of the skin. Journal of the American Academy of Dermatology 40 (6 Pt 2):S 31–34

Tinea sycosis

▶ Sycosis barbae

Tinea unguium

▶ Onychogryphosis

Tinea versicolor

Synonym(s)
Pityriasis versicolor; chromophytosis; dermatomycosis furfuracea; tinea flava

Definition
Superficial fungal infection, characterized by hypopigmented or hyperpigmented macules, patches, and scaly papules on the chest, neck, and back

Pathogenesis
Caused by dimorphic, lipophilic organism, Malassezia furfur, normal constituent of host flora in yeast form; factors associated with conversion to mycelial morphologic form: genetic predisposition; warm, humid environments; immunosuppression; malnutrition; Cushing disease; individual variations in skin surface lipids may be factor in disease susceptibility

Clinical manifestation
Well-marginated, reticulated, finely scaly, oval-to-round, variably colored papules, coalescing into plaques; located over trunk, neck, chest, with occasional extension to abdomen and proximal extremities; more noticeable during summer months; in immunosuppressed patients, lesions in flexural regions, face, or isolated areas of extremities

Differential diagnosis
Tinea corporis; parapsoriasis; psoriasis; confluent and reticulated papillomatosis of Gougerot and Carteaud; erythrasma; pityriasis alba; seborrheic dermatitis; vitiligo

Therapy
Ketoconazole; azole antifungal agents; ciclopirox; terbinafine cream; selenium sulfide 2.5 % lotion applied every other day for 2 weeks

References
Gupta AK, Bluhm R, Summerbell R (2002) Pityriasis versicolor. Journal of the European Academy of Dermatology & Venereology 16(1):19–33

Toasted skin syndrome

▸ **Erythema ab igne**

Tomato tumor

▸ **Cylindroma**

Toriello-Carey syndrome

Synonym(s)
Corpus callosum agenesis-facial anomalies-Robin sequence syndrome

Definition
Congenital syndrome consisting of agenesis of the corpus callosum, multiple facial defects, laryngeal abnormalities, heart defect, skeletal anomalies, and developmental delay

Pathogenesis
May have X-linked inheritance

Clinical manifestation
Agenesis of the corpus callosum; telecanthus; short palpebral fissures; small nose with anteverted nares; malformed ears; redundant neck skin; laryngeal abnormalities; heart defect; short hands; hypotonia; occasional Hirschsprung disease, moderate to severe developmental delay

Differential diagnosis
None

Therapy
No effective therapy

References
Czarnecki P, Lacombe D, Weiss L (1996) Toriello-Carey syndrome: evidence for X-linked inheritance. American Journal of Medical Genetics 65(4):291–294

Torre syndrome

▶ Muir-Torre syndrome

Torulosis

▶ Cryptococcosis

Touraine-Solente-Gole syndrome

▶ Pachydermoperiostosis

Toxemic erythema of pregnancy

▶ Pruritic urticarial papules and plaques of pregnancy

Toxemic rash of pregnancy

▶ Pruritic urticarial papules and plaques of pregnancy

Toxic epidermal necrolysis

Synonym(s)
Acute disseminated epidermal necrosis; acute skin failure; Lyell syndrome

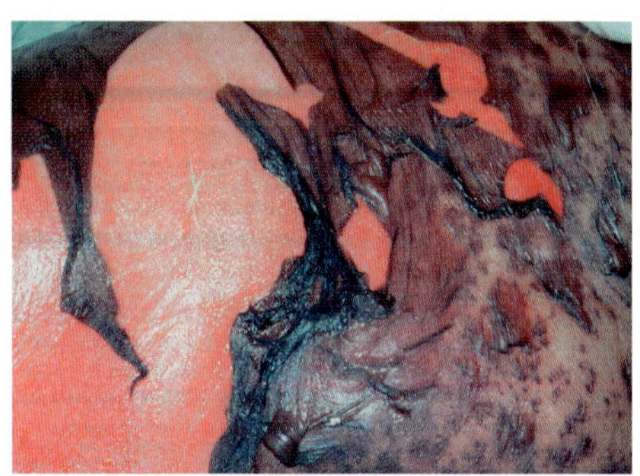

Toxic epidermal necrolysis. Full-thickness epidermal sloughing

Definition
Severe, acute, systemic disorder characterized by extensive epidermal loss

Pathogenesis
Most often drug-induced (antiepileptic drugs, sulfonamides, ampicillin, allopurinol, nonsteroidal anti-inflammatory agents); immune-related cytotoxic reaction destroys keratinocytes; TNF-α likely main mediator in epidermal destruction directly through apoptosis, indirectly by stimulating cytotoxic T cells

Clinical manifestation
Prodrome of malaise, fever, cough, sore throat, myalgia, rhinitis, and anorexia; skin lesions beginn as morbilliform eruption; epidermal sloughing in sheets, leaving moist, denuded dermis; positive Nikolsky sign; hemorrhagic crusting of the lips; conjunctivitis; pneumonia is a major complication

Differential diagnosis
Toxic shock syndrome; Stevens-Johnson syndrome; Kawasaki disease; staphylococ-

cal scalded skin syndrome; exfoliative erythroderma; bullous pemphigoid; pemphigus vulgaris; chemical or thermal burn

Therapy
Discontinuation of all suspect medications[*]; intravenous immunoglobulin (IVIG) – 2 gm per kg IV given over 3 days; plasmapheresis

References
Levine N., Kunkel M, Thanh N; Ackerman L (2002) Emergency department dermatology. Current Problems in Dermatology 14(6):188–220

Toxic erythema

▶ Erythema toxicum

Toxic erythema of newborn

▶ Erythema toxicum

Toxic oil syndrome

Synonym(s)
Spanish toxic oil syndrome

Definition
Illness resulting from consumption of adulterated rapeseed oil, characterized by intense myalgias, marked peripheral eosinophilia, pulmonary infiltrates, and scleroderma-like skin changes

Pathogenesis
Suggestion of autoimmune mechanisms; directly related to consumption of oils containing fatty acid esters of 3-(N-phenylamino)-1,2-propanediol (PAP)

Clinical manifestation
Prodrome of fever, headache, cough, dyspnea, and pruritus; after 1 month, development of extremity edema, followed by scleroderma-like changes; extreme myalgias with subsequent muscle atrophy; late alopecia, sicca syndrome, and liver abnormalities; peripheral eosinophilia; chronic changes more common in women

Differential diagnosis
Eosinophilia-myalgia syndrome; progressive systemic sclerosis; eosinophilic fasciitis; dermatomyositis; hypereosinophilic syndrome

Therapy
No effective therapy

References
Diggle GE (2001) The toxic oil syndrome: 20 years on. International Journal of Clinical Practice 55(6):371–375

Toxic shock syndrome

Synonym(s)
Staphylococcal toxic shock syndrome

Definition
Acute febrile illness, characterized by generalized erythematous eruption accompanied by hypotension and multiple organ dysfunction

Pathogenesis
Caused by strains of Staphylococcus aureus producing TSS toxin, associated with release of tumor necrosis factor- α (TNF-α) and interleukin-1 (IL-1), which mediate signs and symptoms of disease; predisposing factors: influenza, sinusiitis, intravenous drug use, HIV infection, burn or other wounds, postoperative infection

Clinical manifestation
Skin and mucous membrane changes: diffuse macular erythroderma or scarletini-

form eruption; erythema and edema of palms and soles; hyperemia of conjunctiva and mucous membranes, with strawberry tongue; delayed palm and sole desquamation

Other organ involvement: fever; hypotension; cardiomyopathy; nausea; vomiting; diarrhea; rhabdomyolysis; myalgias; muscle tenderness and weakness; azotemia; acute renal failure; adult respiratory distress syndrome; elevated serum glutamic oxaloacetic transaminase (SGOT) and serum bilirubin; thrombocytopenia; leukocytosis; disseminated intravascular coagulation; hypophosphatemia; hypocalcemia; electrolyte imbalance

Differential diagnosis

Streptococcal toxic shock-like syndrome; Kawasaki disease; staphylococcal scalded skin syndrome; toxic epidermal necrolysis; drug reaction; scarlet fever; Rocky Mountain spotted fever; leptospirosis

Therapy

Nafcillin: 1–2 gm IV every 4 hours in adults; 50–200 mg per kg per day divided into 4–6 doses per day in children

Clindamycin: 600–900 mg IV every 8 hours in adults; 20–40 mg per kg per day IV divided into 3–4 doses in children

References

Levine N., Kunkel M, Thanh N; Ackerman L (2002) Emergency department dermatology. Current Problems in Dermatology 14(6):188-220

Trabecular carcinoma

▶ Merkel cell carcinoma

Trachyonychia

▶ Twenty nail dystrophy

Traction alopecia

Synonym(s)

Traumatic alopecia marginalis; pressure alopecia; massage alopecia; ponytail band alopecia

Definition

Group of acute or chronic scalp injuries leading to patchy alopecia

Pathogenesis

Excessive traction for prolonged periods (e.g., tight braiding, wearing of ponytails) causes conversion of anagen phase to telogen phase hair growth; overprocessing, chemical treatment of hair with dyes, bleaches, or straighteners disrupts keratin structure and reduces its tensile strength, making it susceptible to breakage

Clinical manifestation

Patchy areas of hair loss; hair-pulling test results in the detachment of more than 6 strands; may have perifollicular erythema, scaling, and pustules; marginal alopecia in temporal region or occipital area; with cornrowing hair style, most affected area immediately adjacent to the braided region; reversible if causitive hair styling practice discontinued early in course

Differential diagnosis

Alopecia areata; androgenetic alopecia; trichotillomania; tinea capitis; follicular degeneration syndrome; telogen effluvium; anagen effluvium; syphilis; lupus erythematosus

Therapy

Discontinuation of practices that exert traction on hair or otherwise traumatize hair[*]

References

Sperling LC, Mezebish DS (1998) Hair diseases. Medical Clinics of North America 82(5):1155-1169

Transient acantholytic dermatosis

Synonym(s)
Grover disease; Grover's disease

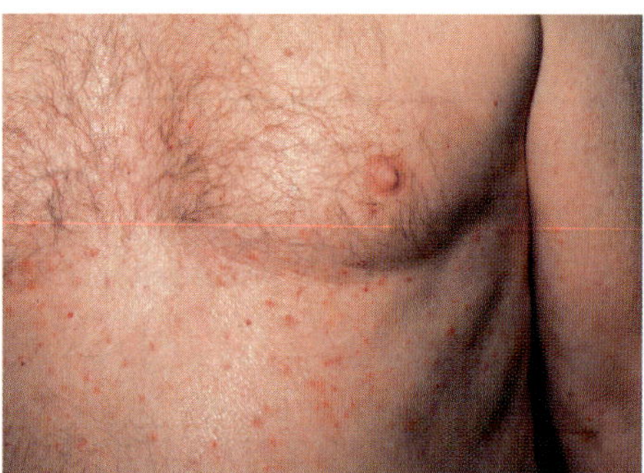

Transient acantholytic dermatosis. Multiple red, scaly, or eroded papules on the trunk

Definition
Pruritic papular disorder, characterized histologically by focal acantholysis

Pathogenesis
Association with heat and sweating

Clinical manifestation
Pruritic eruption of the skin of the anterior chest, upper back, and lower rib cage; multiple, discrete, erythematous to red-brown keratotic papules, most common in middle-aged or older men; occasionally, lesions are acneiform, vesicular, or pustular

Differential diagnosis
Folliculitis; Darier's disease; Hailey-Hailey disease; pemphigus foliaceus; insect bite reaction; scabies; dermatitis herpetiformis; tinea corporis; psoriasis; xerotic eczema; pityriasis rosea; miliaria; drug eruption

Therapy
Vitamin A 150,000 units PO daily for 30 days, repeated after a 1 month rest period; isotretinoin

References
Parsons JM (1996) Transient acantholytic dermatosis (Grover's disease): a global perspective. Journal of the American Academy of Dermatology 35(5 Pt 1):653–666

Transient bullous dermolysis of newborn

▶ Aplasia cutis congenita

Transient neonatal pustular melanosis

Synonym(s)
None

Definition
Disorder usually present at birth, characterized by vesicles, superficial pustules, and pigmented macules

Pathogenesis
Unknown

Clinical manifestation
Pustules and pigmented macules found mainly on the chin, neck, or forehead, behind the ears, or on the trunk, palms, and soles; no systemic signs or symptoms; most common in black neonates

Differential diagnosis
Mongolian spot; acropustulosis of infancy; erythema toxicum neonatorum; neonatal herpes simplex virus infection; miliaria; milia; neonatal acne; impetigo; candidiasis

Therapy
No therapy indicated

References
Van Praag MC, Van Rooij RW, Folkers E, Spritzer R, Menke HE, Oranje AP (1997) Diagnosis and

treatment of pustular disorders in the neonate. Pediatric Dermatology 14(2):131–143

Transient neonatal pustulosis

▶ Transient neonatal pustular melanosis

Transient symptomatic zinc deficiency

▶ Acrodermatitis enteropathica

Traumatic alopecia marginalis

▶ Traction alopecia

Traumatic tattoo

Synonym(s)
Accidental tattoo

Definition
Localized skin dyspigmentation secondary to deposition of colored material in the skin from a deep dirty abrasion or other penetrating injury

Pathogenesis
Deposition of material into dermis, often after high velocity penetration

Clinical manifestation
Irregular dyspigmentation at site of skin injury

Amalgam tattoo variant: punctate gray discoloration in oral mucosa secondary to penetration of dental amalgam with dental procedures; some particles may extrude without therapy

Differential diagnosis
Melanoma; melanocytic nevus; lentigo; drug-induced pigmentation; exogenous ochronosis

Therapy
Ablation by Q-switched laser; surgical excision; dermabrasion; laser resurfacing; chemical peel

References
Fusade T, Toubel G, Grognard C, Mazer JM (2000) Treatment of gunpowder traumatic tattoo by Q-switched Nd:YAG laser: an unusual adverse effect. Dermatologic Surgery 26(11):1057–1059

Trenaunay syndrome

▶ Klippel-Trenaunay-Weber syndrome

Trench fever

Synonym(s)
5–day fever; quintan fever; shinbone fever; shank fever; His-Werner disease; Wolhynia fever; urban trench fever

Definition
Blood-borne bacterial infection characterized by fever, systemic signs and symptoms, and an eruption occurring at the onset of the disease

Pathogenesis
Caused by Bartonella quintana, gram negative bacteria introduced to human host by body louse; inoculation of organism in louse feces through a skin break or a louse bite

Clinical manifestation
Fever, varying from single episode to recurrent episodes to persistently elevated body temperature for weeks; conjunctivitis; skin eruption most commonly occurring during first fever episode; groups of erythematous macules or papules on abdomen, chest, and back; splenomegaly; hepatomegaly; tachycardia

Differential diagnosis
Babesiosis; bacillary angiomatosis; cryptococcosis; Lyme disease; relapsing fever; Rocky Mountain spotted fever; HIV infection; tuberculosis

Therapy
Doxycycline; erythromycin; azithromycin

▶ **Bartonellosis**

References
Ohl ME, Spach DH (2000) Bartonella quintana and urban trench fever. Clinical Infectious Diseases 31(1):131–135

Trench foot

▶ **Immersion foot**

Trench mouth

▶ **Acute necrotizing gingivitis**

Tretinoin

Trade name(s)
Retin-A; Retin A Micro; Avita; Renova

Generic available
Yes

Drug class
Retinoid

Mechanism of action
Gene transcription after membrane receptor binding and intracellular transport; normalizes follicular keratinization

Dosage form
0.025%, 0.05%, 0.1% cream; 0.04%, 0.1% micro gel; 0.025% gel

Dermatologic indications and dosage
See table

Common side effects
Cutaneous: scaling, erythema, blistering, photosensitivity

Serious side effects
None

Drug interactions
Benzoyl peroxide; isotretinoin; photosensitizing drugs

Contraindications/precautions
Hypersensitivity to drug class or component

References
Bershad S (2001) Developments in topical retinoid therapy for acne. Seminars in Cutaneous Medicine & Surgery 20(3):154–161

Triamcinolone

▶ **Corticosteroids, topical, medium potency**

Trichilemmal cyst

▶ **Pilar cyst**

Tretinoin. Dermatologic indications and dosage

Disease	Adult dosage	Child dosage
Acanthosis nigricans	Apply once daily, preferably at bedtime; apply 20–30 minutes after washing and drying skin	Apply once daily, preferably at bedtime; apply 20–30 minutes after washing and drying skin
Acne vulgaris	Apply once daily, preferably at bedtime; apply 20–30 minutes after washing and drying skin	Apply once daily, preferably at bedtime; apply 20–30 minutes after washing and drying skin
Acrokeratoelastoidosis	Apply once daily, preferably at bedtime; apply 20–30 minutes after washing and drying skin	Not applicable
Acrokeratosis verruciformis	Apply once daily, preferably at bedtime; apply 20–30 minutes after washing and drying skin	Apply once daily, preferably at bedtime; apply 20–30 minutes after washing and drying skin
Actinic elastosis	Apply once daily, preferably at bedtime; apply 20–30 minutes after washing and drying skin	Not applicable
Actinic keratosis	Apply twice daily for up to 3 months	Apply once daily, preferably at bedtime; apply 20–30 minutes after washing and drying skin
Bowenoid papulosis	Apply twice daily for up to 3 months	Not applicable
Chloracne	Apply once daily, preferably at bedtime; apply 20–30 minutes after washing and drying skin	Apply once daily, preferably at bedtime; apply 20–30 minutes after washing and drying skin
Epidermolytic hyperkeratosis	Apply once daily, preferably at bedtime; apply 20–30 minutes after washing and drying skin	Apply once daily, preferably at bedtime; apply 20–30 minutes after washing and drying skin
Favre Racouchot disease	Apply once daily, preferably at bedtime; apply 20–30 minutes after washing and drying skin	Not applicable
Fox-Fordyce disease	Apply once daily, preferably at bedtime; apply 20–30 minutes after washing and drying skin	Apply once daily, preferably at bedtime; apply 20–30 minutes after washing and drying skin
Hairy tongue	Apply twice daily for up to 3 months	Apply once daily, preferably at bedtime; apply 20–30 minutes after washing and drying skin
Idiopathic guttate hypomelanosis	Apply once daily, preferably at bedtime; apply 20–30 minutes after washing and drying skin	Not applicable
Keratosis pilaris	Apply once daily, preferably at bedtime; apply 20–30 minutes after washing and drying skin	Apply once daily, preferably at bedtime; apply 20–30 minutes after washing and drying skin
Kyrle's disease	Apply once daily, preferably at bedtime; apply 20–30 minutes after washing and drying skin	Apply once daily, preferably at bedtime; apply 20–30 minutes after washing and drying skin

Tretinoin. Dermatologic indications and dosage (Continued)

Disease	Adult dosage	Child dosage
Lamellar ichthyosis	Apply once daily, preferably at bedtime; apply 20–30 minutes after washing and drying skin	Apply once daily, preferably at bedtime; apply 20–30 minutes after washing and drying skin
Melasma	Apply once daily, preferably at bedtime; apply 20–30 minutes after washing and drying skin	Apply once daily, preferably at bedtime; apply 20–30 minutes after washing and drying skin
Nevus comedonicus	Apply once daily, preferably at bedtime; apply 20–30 minutes after washing and drying skin	Apply once daily, preferably at bedtime; apply 20–30 minutes after washing and drying skin
Nevus verrucosus	Apply once daily, preferably at bedtime; apply 20–30 minutes after washing and drying skin	Apply once daily, preferably at bedtime; apply 20–30 minutes after washing and drying skin
Perforating folliculitis	Apply once daily, preferably at bedtime; apply 20–30 minutes after washing and drying skin	Apply once daily, preferably at bedtime; apply 20–30 minutes after washing and drying skin
Photo-aging	Apply once daily, preferably at bedtime; apply 20–30 minutes after washing and drying skin	Not applicable
Pomade acne	Apply once daily, preferably at bedtime; apply 20–30 minutes after washing and drying skin	Apply once daily, preferably at bedtime; apply 20–30 minutes after washing and drying skin
Postinflammatory hyperpigmentation	Apply once daily, preferably at bedtime; apply 20–30 minutes after washing and drying skin	Apply once daily, preferably at bedtime; apply 20–30 minutes after washing and drying skin
Reactive perforating collagenosis	Apply once daily, preferably at bedtime; apply 20–30 minutes after washing and drying skin	Apply once daily, preferably at bedtime; apply 20–30 minutes after washing and drying skin
Rosacea	Apply once daily, preferably at bedtime; apply 20–30 minutes after washing and drying skin	Apply once daily, preferably at bedtime; apply 20–30 minutes after washing and drying skin
Striae	Apply once daily, preferably at bedtime; apply 20–30 minutes after washing and drying skin	Apply once daily, preferably at bedtime; apply 20–30 minutes after washing and drying skin

Trichilemmoma

Synonym(s)
Tricholemmoma

Definition
Benign neoplasm with differentiation toward pilosebaceous follicular epithelium

Pathogenesis
Unknown

Clinical manifestation
Asymptomatic, slow growing papule and/or plaque on face, ear, or upper extremity; small, flesh-colored papules; small plaques, particularly in the nasolabial fold region; with enlargement, thick hyperkeratotic surface suggestive of wart

Differential diagnosis
Basal cell carcinoma; epidermoid cyst; wart; neurilemmoma; trichoepithelioma; trichofolliculoma; clear cell acanthoma

Therapy
Shave removal; elliptical excision

References
Tellechea O, Reis JP, Baptista AP (1992) Desmoplastic trichilemmoma. American Journal of Dermatopathology 14(2):107–114

Trichoblastoma

▶ Trichoepithelioma

Trichodiscoma

Synonym(s)
Neurofollicular hamartoma

Definition
Hamartomatous proliferation of mesodermal component of haarscheibe, slowly reacting nerve receptor around hair follicle

Pathogenesis
Unknown

Clinical manifestation
Solitary or multiple, discrete, flat-topped papules, usually located on central face

Differential diagnosis
Trichoepithelioma; trichofolliculoma; angiofibroma; syringoma; basal cell carcinoma; acrochordon

Therapy
Surgical excision*

References
Nova MP, Zung M, Halperin A (1991) Neurofollicular hamartoma. A clinicopathological study.

American Journal of Dermatopathology 13(5):459–462

Trichoepithelioma

Synonym(s)
Trichoblastoma; epithelioma adenoides cysticum; trichoepithelioma papulosum multiplex; sclerosing epithelial hamartoma; Brooke tumor

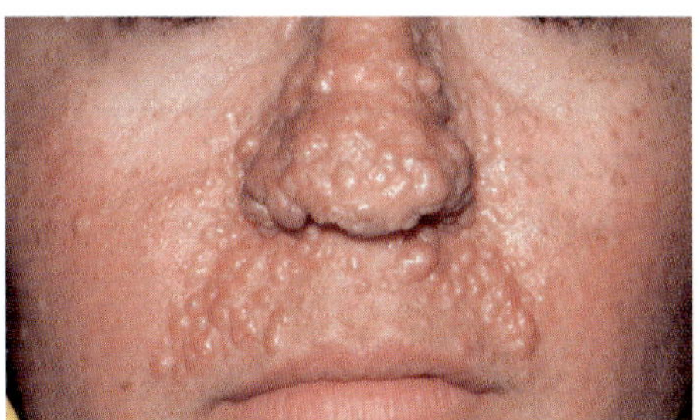

Trichoepithelioma. Multiple flesh-colored papules in the central facial area

Definition
Benign adnexal tumor with differentiation toward hair follicle epithelium

Pathogenesis
Autosomal dominant familial form related to a mutation in tumor suppressor gene, located on 9q21

Clinical manifestation
Round, skin-colored, firm papule or nodule, located mainly on nasolabial folds, nose, forehead, upper lip, and scalp; occasional lesions on neck and upper trunk; rare ulceration; multiple lesions in familial form, usually on nasolabial folds; solitary giant trichoepithelioma: large, polypoid tumor, usually in the lower trunk or in gluteal area

Differential diagnosis
Basal cell epithelioma; colloid milium; cylindroma; angiofibroma; milium; pilar

cyst; syringoma; trichilemmoma; microcystic adnexal carcinoma

Therapy
Solitary tumor: surgical excision or shave removal
Multiple tumors: CO_2 laser ablation; dermabrasion

References
Smith KJ, Skelton HG, Holland T (1992). Recent advances and controversies concerning adnexal neoplasms. Dermatologic Clinics 10(1):117–160

Trichoepithelioma papulosum multiplex

▶ Trichoepithelioma

Trichofolliculoma

Synonym(s)
Folliculoma; hair follicle nevus

Definition
Hamartoma of follicular epithelium, typically occurring on the face

Pathogenesis
May be abortive differentiation of pluripotent skin cells towards hair follicles

Clinical manifestation
Single, flesh-colored or whitish papule, typically on face, most frequently around the nose; central pore or black dot, sometimes draining sebaceous-like material; tuft of white hair sometimes emerges from central pore

Differential diagnosis
Basal cell epithelioma; colloid milium; cylindroma; angiofibroma; milium; pilar

cyst; syringoma; trichilemmoma; microcystic adnexal carcinoma; trichoepithelioma; vellus hair cyst

Therapy
Surgical excision for cosmesis only

References
Labandeira J, Peteiro C, Toribio J (1996) Hair follicle nevus: case report and review. American Journal of Dermatopathology 18(1):90-93

Tricholemmoma

▶ Trichilemmoma

Trichomalacia

Definition
Damage to anagen hair root by repeated plucking or other injury, characterized by deformed and twisted bulb, seen mainly with trichotillomania

References
Walsh KH, McDougle CJ (2001) Trichotillomania. presentation, etiology, diagnosis and therapy. American Journal of Clinical Dermatology 2(5):327–333

Trichomatricoma

▶ Pilomatricoma

Trichomatrioma

▶ Pilomatricoma

Trichomycosis axillaris and pubis

Synonym(s)
Trichomycosis nodosa; trichomycosis nodularis

Definition
Superficial bacterial colonization of the axillary hair shafts, characterized by granular concretions adhering to hair shaft

Pathogenesis
Caused by several species of the gram-positive diphtheroid Corynebacterium overgrowth on hair shafts in moist regions of the body

Clinical manifestation
Seen more often in tropical climates; sometimes associated with hyperhidrosis; concretions encircling hair shaft, giving it beaded appearance; most common on the central portion of axillary hair (trichomycosis axillaris) or inguinal region, often on scrotum (trichomycosis pubis); red, black, or yellow concretions firmly adhering to hair shaft; yellow color sometimes stains clothes yellow, black, and red

Differential diagnosis
Pediculosis; piedra; hair casts; soap or deodorant remnants

Therapy
Shaving of affected hair[*]; use of antiperspirants to prevent recurrence

References
O'Dell ML (1998) Skin and wound infections: an overview. American Family Physician 57(10):2424–2432

Trichomycosis nodosa

▶ Trichomycosis axillaris and pubis

Trichomycosis nodularis

▶ Piedra
▶ Trichomycosis axillaris and pubis

Trichophytosis barbae

▶ Sycosis barbae

Trichopoliodystrophy

▶ Menkes kinky hair syndrome

Trichorrhexis invaginata

Definition
Hair fibers having the shape of bamboo; fibers with focal nodules making them resemble a bamboo shoot; focal defects in the hair fiber, with development of a cup and ball shape; seen in Netherton's syndrome

References
Rogers M (1996) Hair shaft abnormalities: Part II. Australasian Journal of Dermatology 37(1):1–11

Trichorrhexis nodosa

Definition
Defect in the hair shaft characterized by thickening or weak points (nodes) causing the hair to break easily; precipitated by environmental insults in disorders such as argininosuccinic aciduria, Menkes' kinky hair syndrome, Netherton's syndrome, hypothyroidism, or trichothiodystrophy

References

Rogers M (1995) Hair shaft abnormalities: Part I. Australasian Journal of Dermatology 36(4):179–184

Trichosporosis

▶ Piedra

Trichostasis spinulosa

Synonym(s)
None

Definition
Dark follicular papules, caused by multiple vellus hairs imbedded in follicular orifice

Pathogenesis
Results from successive production and retention of vellus telogen club hairs from single hair matrix in single follicle

Clinical manifestation
Dark, follicular plugs or papules, sometimes with tufts or spines of fine hair protuding; most common on nose and upper trunk

Differential diagnosis
Comedonal acne; lichen spinulosus; retained dirt; keratosis pilaris

Therapy
Depilatory wax or adhesive strips; drainage with comedone extractor

References

Harford RR, Cobb MW, Miller ML (1996) Trichostasis spinulosa: a clinical simulant of acne open comedones. Pediatric Dermatology 13(6):490–492

Trichothiodystrophy

▶ Tay syndrome

Trichothiodystrophy with congenital ichthyosis

▶ Tay syndrome

Trichotillomania

Synonym(s)
Chronic hair pulling; morbid hair pulling; compulsive hair pulling

Definition
Alopecia caused by compulsive pulling and/or twisting of the hair until it breaks off

Pathogenesis
Impulse control disorder, often with underlying emotional problem; become habitual once behavior is established, regardless of initial emotional problem

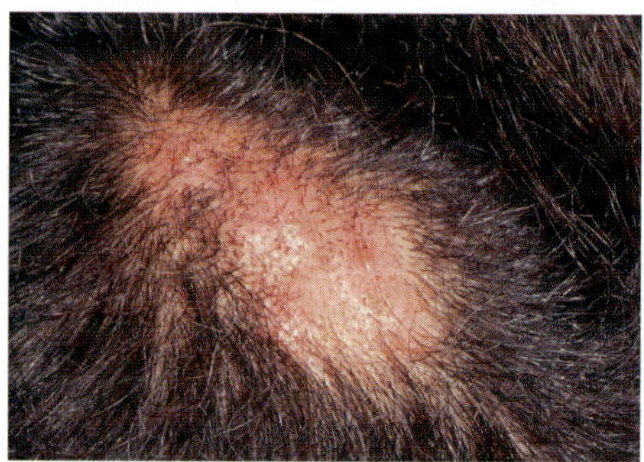

Trichotillomania. Alopecic plaque with broken hairs in the scalp

Clinical manifestation
Incomplete nonscarring alopecia, in relatively localized sites; geometric shapes of involved area, with broken hair; occurs most frequently in scalp, but sometimes involves eyebrows or eyelashes

Differential diagnosis
Alopecia areata; tinea capitis; androgenetic alopecia; syphilis; lupus erythematosus; monilethrix; traction alopecia; pili torti; temporal triangular alopecia

Therapy
Selective serotonin reuptake inhibitors in patients unable to control impulse after understanding nature of disorder

References
Hautmann G, Hercogova J, Lotti T (2002) Trichotillomania. Journal of the American Academy of Dermatology 46(6):807–821

Trichrome vitiligo

▶ Vitiligo

Triglyceride storage disease

▶ Chanarin-Dorfman syndrome

Trimethoprim-sulfamethoxazole

Trade name(s)
Bactrim; Septra

Generic available
Yes

Drug class
Antibiotic

Mechanism of action
Inhibition of enzymes involved in bacterial tetrahydrofolic acid synthesis

Dosage form
DS capsule

Dermatologic indications and dosage
See table

Common side effects
Cutaneous: urticaria or other vascular reaction, photosensitivity
Gastrointestinal: anorexia, nausea, vomiting, diarrhea
Neurologic: dizziness

Serious side effects
Bone marrow: aplastic anemia, agranulocytosis
Cutaneous: Stevens-Johnson syndrome, toxic epidermal necrolysis
Gastrointestinal: hepatitis, hepatic necrosis, pseudomembranous colitis
Renal: interstitial nephritis

Drug interactions
Oral contraceptives; dapsone; MAO inhibitors; metformin; methotrexate; phenytoin; probenecid; procainamide; sulfonylureas; warfarin

Contraindications/precautions
Hypersensitivity to drug class or component; folate deficiency; G6PD deficiency

References
Smilack JD (1999) Trimethoprim-sulfamethoxazole. Mayo Clinic Proceedings 74(7):730–734

Trimox

▶ Amoxicillin

Trimethoprim-sulfamethoxazole. Dermatologic indications and dosage

Disease	Adult dosage	Child dosage
Granuloma inguinale	DS capsule twice daily for at least 3 weeks	Not established
Melioidosis	DS capsule twice daily until ulceration heals	Not established
Mycetoma	DS capsule twice daily until ulceration heals	Not established
Mycobacterium marinum infection	DS capsule PO twice daily for 4–6 weeks after clincial resolution	Not established
Nocardiosis	DS capsule twice daily for at least 3 weeks	Not established
South American blastomycosis	DS capsule twice daily for 2–3 years	Not established

Tropical anhidrosis

▶ Miliaria

Tropical anhidrotic asthenia

▶ Acquired generalized anhidrosis

Tropical jungle foot

▶ Immersion foot

Tropical phagedenic ulcer

Synonym(s)
Vincent's ulcer; tropical sloughing phagedena; ulcus tropicum

Definition
Acute, painful, destructive skin ulceration occurring in presence of fusiform bacilli and spirochetes

Pathogenesis
Multiple contributing factors, including protein deficiency, presence of fusiform bacilli and spirochetes, and minor trauma to affected site

Clinical manifestation
Papule or vesicle at site of minor trauma, often on lower extremity; rapid evolution of necrotic, purulent, putrid ulceration often down to fascia, tendon, and bone; chronic stage with indolent, non-purulent ulceration

Differential diagnosis
Leishmaniasis; bacterial pyoderma; pyoderma gangrenosum; cutaneous diphtheria; gummatous syphilis; yaws; leprosy; chromomycosis; squamous cell carcinoma; venous stasis ulcer; atypical mycobacterial infection; venomous sting or bite

Therapy
Acute stage: Benzathine penicillin G[★]; tetracycline; metronidazole: 400 mg PO 3 times daily until healing
Chronic stage: no specific antibiotic therapy

References
Robinson DC, Adriaans B, Hay RJ, Yesudian P (1988) The clinical and epidemiologic features of tropical ulcer (tropical phagedenic ulcer).

International Journal of Dermatology 27(1):49–53

Tropical sloughing phagedena

▶ Tropical phagedenic ulcer

Tsutsugamushi disease

▶ Scrub typhus

Tsutsugamushi fever

▶ Scrub typhus

Tuberculosis, cutaneous

▶ Cutaneous tuberculosis

Tuberculosis cutis orificialis

▶ Cutaneous tuberculosis

Tuberculosis cutis verrucosa

▶ Cutaneous tuberculosis

Tuberculosis of skin

▶ Cutaneous tuberculosis

Tuberculosis verrucosa cutis

▶ Cutaneous tuberculosis

Tuberculous chancre

▶ Cutaneous tuberculosis

Tuberculous gumma

▶ Cutaneous tuberculosis

Tuberous sclerosis

Synonym(s)
Epiloia; Bourneville disease; tuberous sclerosis complex

Definition
Hereditary disorder characterized by hamartomas in multiple organs

Pathogenesis
Autosomal dominant trait; mutations of genes coding for hamartin and tuberin, involved in the regulation of cell proliferation and differentiation (hamartin) and tumor suppression (tuberin)

Clinical manifestation
Skin lesions: angiofibromas (adenoma sebaceum) often in nasolabial folds and on cheeks and chin; periungual fibromas (Koenen tumors); connective tissue nevus (Shagreen patch), presenting as flesh-colored, soft plaque in the lumbosacral area; ash leaf-shaped macules on trunk or limb; guttate leukoderma; café au lait macules; poliosis
Neurologic changes: tuberosclerotic nodules of glial proliferation in cerebral cortex,

T

basal ganglia, and ventricular walls; number of tubers appears to correlate with clinical disease severity; epilepsy; mental retardation

Other features noted: schizophrenia; autistic behavior; and attention-deficit hyperactivity disorder

Miscellaneous findings: cardiac rhabdomyomas; aortic aneurysm; renal angiomyolipoma and renal cysts; pulmonary lymphangiomatosis with cyst formation; microhamartomatous polyps in bone cysts; pituitary adrenal dysfunction; thyroid disorders; premature puberty; diffuse cutaneous reticulohistiocytosis; gigantism

Differential diagnosis

Acne; connective tissue nevus; nevus anemicus; vitiligo; warts; trichoepithelioma; syringoma; rosacea

Therapy

Pulsed dye or CO_2 laser ablation or dermabrasion for facial angiofibromas; CO_2 laser vaporization for periungual fibromas

References

Harris-Stith R, Elston DM (2002) Tuberous sclerosis. Cutis 69(2):103–109

Tuberous sclerosis complex

▶ Tuberous sclerosis

Tuberous xanthoma

▶ Xanthoma

Tufted angioma

Synonym(s)

Nakagawa's angioma; Nakagawa's angioblastoma; progressive capillary hemangioma; acquired tufted angioma; angioblastoma

Definition

Vascular skin tumor, characterized by slow angiomatous proliferation and a distinctive histologic presentation

Pathogenesis

Occasional occurrence within port wine stains

Clinical manifestation

Solitary or multifocal, sometimes painful, purplish-red to red-brown patch or plaque predominantly appearing on upper trunk, neck, or shoulders; less commonly occurring on face, scalp, or proximal extremities

Differential diagnosis

Capillary hemangioma; Kaposi's sarcoma; kaposiform hemangioendothelioma; hemangiopericytoma; pyogenic granuloma; endovascular papillary angioendothelioma; melanoma

Therapy

Surgical excision; pulse dye laser ablation

References

Okada E, Tamura A, Ishikawa O, Miyachi Y (2000) Tufted angioma (angioblastoma): case report and review of 41 cases in the Japanese literature. Clinical & Experimental Dermatology 25(8):627–630

Tularemia

Synonym(s)

Rabbit fever; deer-fly fever; wild hare disease; water-rat trapper's disease; market men's disease

Definition

Acute infectious zoonosis, characterized by skin eruption and/or ulceration, lymphadenopathy, and variable systemic signs and symptoms

Pathogenesis

Caused by aerobic gram-negative pleomorphic bacillus Francisella tularensis, after introduction of bacillus by inhalation, intradermal injection, or oral ingestion; rabbits and ticks (especially Dermatocentor and Amblyomma species) most common vectors

Clinical manifestation

Ulceroglandular variant: organism usually gaining entry via scratch or abrasion; ulcer at the site of entry begins as tender papule and eventually ulcerates; sharply demarcated border with a yellowish exudate; base of the ulcer with yellow exudate becomes black; regional lymphadenopathy
Glandular variant: similar to ulceroglandular form except for absence of skin lesion
Oculoglandular variant: organism enters via the conjunctivae after inoculation from either splashing of blood or rubbing of eyes after contact with infectious materials; unilateral, painful, purulent conjunctivitis with preauricular or cervical lymphadenopathy
Oropharyngeal variant: occurs after eating poorly cooked rabbit meat; sore throat; abdominal pain; nausea; vomiting; diarrhea; and; occasional gastrointestinal bleeding
Pneumonic variant: occurring after inhalation of organism; pneumonia also sometimes occurs after hematogenous spread in patients with ulceroglandular tularemia or typhoidal tularemia; dry cough; dyspnea; and pleuritic-type chest pain
Typhoidal (septicemic) variant: represents bacteremia; fever; chills; myalgias; malaise; weight loss, often with subsequent pneumonia

Differential diagnosis

Anthrax; orf; milker's nodule; foreign body granuloma; Q fever; Rocky Mountain spotted fever; Lyme disease; Majocchi's granuloma; sporotrichosis; coccidioidomycosis; North American blastomycosis; plague; brucellosis; diphtheria; bacterial endocarditis; legionella infection; malaria; mononucleosis; syphilis; rat bite fever; atypical mycobacterial infection

Therapy

Streptomycin: adult dose: 1–2 gm IM, given twice daily for 7–14 days or until patient is afebrile for 5–7 days; pediatric dose: 20–40 mg per kg per day IM given twice daily for 7–14 days or until patient is afebrile for 5–7 daysw; doxycycline

References

Choi E (2002) Tularemia and Q fever. Medical Clinics of North America 86(2):393–416

Tungiasis

Synonym(s)

None

Definition

Infestation by burrowing human flea

Pathogenesis

Caused by infestation with the burrowing flea, Tunga penetrans, common in Central America, South America, India, and tropical Africa; major risk factor: failure to wear shoes when walking in sand in an area with active infestation; upon contact, fleas invade unprotected skin

Clinical manifestation

Common areas of involvement: plantar foot, intertriginous regions of the toes, and periungual regions; pruritic white papule with central black dot
More advanced infestation: crusted erythematous papules, painful pruritic nodules, crateriform lesions, and secondary infection including lymphangitis and septicemia

Differential diagnosis

Insect bite reaction; scabies; cercarial dermatitis; tick bite; myiasis; fire ant sting; creeping eruption; dracunculiasis

Therapy

Surgical extirpation of the parasite using sterile needle or curette*

References
Fein H, Naseem S, Witte DP, Garcia VF, Lucky A, Staat MA (2001) Tungiasis in North America: a report of 2 cases in internationally adopted children. Journal of Pediatrics 139(5):744–746

Turban tumor

▶ Cylindroma

Turner Kieser syndrome

▶ Nail-patella syndrome

Turner phenotype syndrome

▶ Noonan's syndrome

Turner syndrome

Synonym(s)
Bonnevie-Ullrich syndrome; gonadal dysgenesis

Definition
Disorder in women caused by a chromosomal defect, producing impaired sexual development, infertility, and multiple other congenital defects

Pathogenesis
Results from lack of second *SHOX* gene on X chromosome; many features, including the short stature

Clinical manifestation
Short stature; signs of ovarian failure; hypoplastic or hyperconvex nails; many nevocellular nevi; cutis laxa; webbed neck; skeletal anomalies including cubitus valgus, scoliosis, short fourth metacarpal or metatarsal bone, shield chest, hip dislocation; eye changes including ptosis, strabismus, amblyopia and cataracts; gastrointestinal bleeding

Differential diagnosis
Noonan's syndrome; gonadal dysgenesis; autoimmune thyroiditis; XY gonadal agenesis syndrome

Therapy
No specific therapy

References
Cunniff C (2002) Turner syndrome. Adolescent Medicine State of the Art Reviews 13(2):359–366

Turner-like syndrome

▶ Noonan's syndrome

Twenty nail dystrophy

Synonym(s)
Twenty nail dystrophy of childhood; trachyonychia

Definition
Acquired nail abnormality characterized by rough linear ridges on many but not necessarily all twenty nails of the fingers and toes

Pathogenesis
Many cases with no known cause; some associated with alopecia areata, psoriasis, lichen planus, atopy, ichthyosis, or other inflammatory dermatoses

Clinical manifestation
Rough linear edges of nail plates; opalescent and frequently brittle nail plates that split at free margin; more common in chil-

dren, with tendency for improvement with increased age

Differential diagnosis
Onychomycosis; lichen planus; psoriasis; onychophagia; traumatic nail dystrophy

Therapy
No effective therapy

References
Tosti A, Bardazzi F, Piraccini BM, Fanti PA (1994) Idiopathic trachyonychia (twenty-nail dystrophy): a pathological study of 23 patients. British Journal of Dermatology 131(6):866–872

Twenty-nail dystrophy of childhood

► **Twenty nail dystrophy**

Tylosis

Synonym(s)
Keratosis palmaris et plantaris with carcinoma of the esophagus; Howell-Evans syndrome

Definition
Familial hyperkeratosis of the palms and soles associated with carcinoma of the esophagus

Pathogenesis
Autosomal dominant gene; tylosis esophageal cancer gene (TOC) localized to chromosome 17q25

Clinical manifestation
Focal palmoplantar keratoderma beginning by age 5–15 years; variable oral leukokeratosis; follicular keratosis; increased susceptibility to carcinoma of esophagus

Differential diagnosis
Tyrosinemia type II; pachyonycia congenita; focal palmoplantar and oral mucosa hyperkeratosis; acrokeratoelastoidosis; focal acral hyperkeratosis; acrokeratois of Bazex; arsenical keratosis

Therapy
Alpha hydroxy acids; emollients; urea

References
Cohen PR, Kurzrock R (1995) Miscellaneous genodermatoses: Beckwith-Wiedemann syndrome, Birt-Hogg-Dube syndrome, familial atypical multiple mole melanoma syndrome, hereditary tylosis, incontinentia pigmenti, and supernumerary nipples. Dermatologic Clinics 13(1):211–229

Type II histiocytosis

► **Langerhans cell histiocytosis**

Typhoid fever

► **Salmonellosis**

Typhus

Synonym(s)
Rickettsemia

Definition
Group of infectious diseases caused by rickettsial organisms and producing acute febrile illness

References
Cowan G (2000) Rickettsial diseases: the typhus group of fevers – a review. Postgraduate Medical Journal 76(895):269–272

Typus degenerativus amstelodamensis

▶ Cornelia de Lange syndrome

Tyrosinemia II

Synonym(s)
Richner-Hanhart syndrome; Hanhart-Richner syndrome; tyrosinosis; keratosis palmo-plantaris circumscripta

Definition
Hereditary disease characterized by tyrosinemia, palmar and plantar erosion, keratitis, and occasional mental retardation

Pathogenesis
Deficiency of hepatic tyrosine aminotransferase, leading to elevated levels of tyrosine, which crystalizes in tissues and causes inflammatory response

Clinical manifestation
Skin findings: painful erosions of the palms and soles, which become crusted and then hyperkeratotic; hyperkeratosis of the tongue.
Ocular findings: tearing and photophobia; corneal ulcerations and subsequent scarring.
Neurologic findings: mental retardation; self-mutilating behavior; fine coordination disturbances

Differential diagnosis
Other forms of focal palmo-plantar keratoderma, such as Wachter syndrome and Howel-Evans syndrome; epidermolysis bullosa; Spanlang-Tappeiner syndrome

Therapy
Low tyrosine, low phenylalanine diet, such as Mead Johnson 3200 AB[*]; acitretin

References
Rabinowitz LG, Williams LR, Anderson CE, Mazur A, Kaplan P (1995) Painful keratoderma and photophobia: hallmarks of tyrosinemia type II. Journal of Pediatrics 126(2):266–269

Tyrosinosis

▶ Tyrosinemia II

U

Ulcus tropicum

▶ Tropical phagedenic ulcer

Ulerythema

▶ Ulerythema ophryogenes

Ulerythema acneiforme

▶ Keratosis pilaris atrophicans

Ulerythema ophryogenes

Synonym(s)

Ulerythema; keratosis pilaris rubra atrophicans faciei; folliculitis ulerythema reticulata; honeycomb atrophy; atrophoderma vermiculatum; keratosis pilaris atrophicans

Definition

Disorder characterized by inflammatory keratotic facial papules with scarring, atrophy, and alopecia

Pathogenesis

May be subset of keratosis pilaris

Clinical manifestation

Erythema with follicular hyperkeratosis on cheeks and lateral aspects of eyebrows; occasional scalp involvement; generalized facial erythema with scattered open and closed comedones and milia; hyperkeratotic follicular papules with surrounding erythema evolving into coalescent follicular depressions in a honeycombed pattern; improvement with age

Differential diagnosis

Keratosis pilaris; acne vulgaris; folliculitis; rosacea; lupus erythematosus; pityriasis rubra pilaris; constitutive flushing

Therapy

585-nm pulse dye laser ablation; alpha hydroxy acids

▶ Keratosis pilaris atrophicans

References

Clark SM, Mills CM, Lanigan SW (2000) Treatment of keratosis pilaris atrophicans with the pulsed tunable dye laser. Journal of Cutaneous Laser Therapy 2(3):151–156

Ullrich-Noonan syndrome

▶ Noonan's syndrome

Uncombable hair syndrome

Synonym(s)
Spun glass hair; cheveux incoiffables; pili trianguli et canaliculi

Definition
Hereditary disorder characterized by dry, brittle, hypopigmented, spangled scalp hair

Pathogenesis
Autosomal dominant trait; hair fiber inflexible, making it difficult to lay flat against the scalp

Clinical manifestation
Most frequently develops shortly after birth but possibly any time until puberty; slow-growing scalp hair, with little or no pigment, easily pulled out; very dry; sometimes brittle; spangled appearance; eyebrow and eyelash hairs usually normal but sometimes sparse; nails sometimes short, brittle, and easy to split; teeth aberrations such as enamel defects; possibility of spontaneous recovery with advancing age

Differential diagnosis
Loose anagen hair syndrome; monilethrix; pili torti; Marie-Unna syndrome; progeria; Menke disease

Therapy
No effective therapy

References
Hicks J, Metry DW, Barrish J, Levy M (2001) Uncombable hair (cheveux incoiffables, pili trianguli et canaliculi) syndrome: brief review and role of scanning electron microscopy in diagnosis. Ultrastructural Pathology 25(2):99–103

Universal acquired melanosis

Synonym(s)
Carbon baby

Definition
Progressive generalized hyperpigmentation

Pathogenesis
Increased pigmentation secondary to increased number of melanocytes and increased melanization in the epidermis

Clinical manifestation
Onset in the first few months of life; slowly increasing pigmentation of the skin and mucous membranes

Differential diagnosis
Normal racial pigmentation; Addison's disease; bronze baby; Schilder's disease

Therapy
None

References
Ruiz-Maldonado R, Tamayo L, Fernandez-Diez J (1978) Universal acquired melanosis. The carbon baby. Archives of Dermatology 114(5):775–778

Unna-Thost palmoplantar keratoderma

Synonym(s)
Diffuse nonepidermolytic palmoplantar keratoderma; Thost-Unna disease; palmoplantar keratoderma diffusa circumscripta; congenital keratoderma of the palms and soles; hereditary palmo-plantar keratoderma; hyperkeratosis palmaris et plantaris; ichthyosis palmaris et plantaris

Definition
Hereditary keratoderma of the palms and soles, characterized by thick plaques over palms and soles

Pathogenesis
Autosomal dominant trait; linkage to type II keratin locus on 12q11–13

Clinical manifestation
Keratotic lesions confined to palms and soles; thick, horny, hard, yellowish plaques with waxy smooth surfaces; plaques sometimes pitted and verrucous, surrounded by erythematous halos; occasional corneal opacites; pili torti, sensorineural hearing loss; hypohidrosis; dental abnormalities

Differential diagnosis
Mal de Meleda; Papillon-Lefèvre syndrome; hereditary epidermolytic palmoplantar keratoderma; Vohwinkel syndrome; Richner-Hanhart syndrome; progressive keratoderma; punctate keratoderma; pityriasis rubra pilaris; xerosis

Therapy
Alpha hydroxy acids; urea; keratolytic agents such as salicylic acid 6 % gel; propylene glycol 60 %

References
Zemtsov A, Veitschegger M (1993) Keratodermas. International Journal of Dermatology 32(7):493–498

Urbach-Wiethe disease

▶ Lipoid proteinosis

Urban trench fever

▶ Bartonellosis
▶ Trench fever

Urea, topical

Trade name(s)
Aquacare; Neutraplus; Carmol; Ultramide; Ureacin

Generic available
Yes

Drug class
Emollient; keratolytic agent

Mechanism of action
Hydrophilic property allows for water retention in stratum corneum; protein solvent and denaturant; chemical hygroscopic keratolysis

Dosage form
10%, 20%, 40% cream; 25% lotion

Dermatologic indications and dosage
See table

Common side effects
Cutaneous: burning sensation, stinging, irritation

Serious side effects
None

Drug interactions
None

Contraindications/precautions
Hypersensitivity to drug class or component

Urea, topical. Dermatologic indications and dosage

Disease	Adult dosage	Child dosage
Ichthyosis	Apply twice daily	Apply twice daily
Keratoderma	Apply twice daily	Apply twice daily
Keratosis pilaris	Apply twice daily	Apply twice daily
Xerosis	Apply twice daily	Apply twice daily

References

Swanbeck G (1992) Urea in the treatment of dry skin. Acta Dermato-Venereologica (Suppl) 177:7–8

Uremic gangrene syndrome

▶ Calciphylaxis

Uremic necrosis

▶ Calciphylaxis

Uremic pruritus

Synonym(s)
None

Definition
Pruritus occurring in patients with chronic renal failure

Pathogenesis
May involve unidentified pruritogenic substances accumulating in dialysis patient as a result of molecular size; other theories: xerosis; hyperparathyroidism; hypercalcemia; hyperphosphatemia; elevated plasma histamine levels; uremic neuropathy

Clinical manifestation
Generalized or localized paroxysmal pruritus, most commonly occurring on forearm and back

Differential diagnosis
Xerosis; atopic dermatitis; scabies; drug-induced pruritus; hyperthyroidism; hyperparathyroidism; psychogenic pruritus

Therapy
UVB phototherapy*; naltrexone: 50 mg PO daily; cholestyramine: 4 gm PO twice daily; activated charcoal: 6 gm PO daily divided into 4–6 doses; antihistamines, first generation; emollients; acupuncture

References
Urbonas A, Schwartz RA, Szepietowski JC (2001) Uremic pruritus–an update. American Journal of Nephrology 21(5):343–350

Urticaria

Synonym(s)
Hives

Definition
Hypersensitivity reaction, causing transient erythema and edema

Pathogenesis
Allergic and non-allergic mechanisms operative; final common pathway histamine and other mediator release from mast cells; in allergic reactions, adjacent IgE molecules, bound to the surface of mast cells by the IgE receptors, cross-linked by allergens, lead to the release of histamine and other mediators; most commonly related to reactions to medications or infections; sometimes related to foods, food dyes and preservatives, rheumatic disorders, neoplastic diseases

Clinical manifestation
Transient, pruritic, edematous, pink or red papules or plaques (wheals) of variable size and shape, with surrounding erythema
Angioedema variant: ill-defined, subcutaneous, edematous plaques, with associated pruritus, pain, or burning sensation in lesions
Physical urticaria (dermatographism): urticarial wheal at site of light stroking or rubbing; may occur with concomitant chronic

idiopathic urticaria; pressure-induced urticaria; delayed response to pressure applied to skin

Cold urticaria: wheal at site of cold application; may occur with rapid temperature change, without extremes of cold

Solar urticaria: wheals after brief exposure to sunlight

Cholinergic urticaria: small wheals triggered by heat, exercise, or emotional stress

Exercise-induced urticaria: wheals appearing after vigorous exercise

Aquagenic urticaria: wheals appearing after exposure to water

Differential diagnosis

Urticarial vasculitis; erythema multiforme; insect bite reaction; mastocytosis; bullous pemphigoid; pruritic urticarial papules and plaques of pregnancy; Melkersson-Rosenthal syndrome

Therapy

Antihistamines, first generation; antihistamines, second generation; severely symptomatic, recalcitrant disease: prednisone; nifedipine: 10 mg PO 2–3 times daily; cyclosporine; dapsone

References

Grattan CE, Sabroe RA, Greaves MW (2002) Chronic urticaria. Journal of the American Academy of Dermatology 46(5):645–657

Urticaria neonatorum

▶ **Erythema toxicum**

Urticaria pigmentosa

▶ **Mastocytosis**

Urticarial vasculitis

Synonym(s)

Immune complex urticaria

Definition

Urticaria-like eruption with histologic findings of vasculitis

Pathogenesis

Antigen-antibody complexes deposited in the vascular lumina, resulting in complement activation and chemotaxis of neutrophils; cells release proteolytic enzymes, such as collagenase and elastase, resulting in damage to the vascular lumina

Clinical manifestation

Erythematous wheals, accompanied by a painful or burning sensation, which remain for several days; as lesions evolve, purpura may appear; lesions may resolve with postinflammatory pigmentation; associated photosensitivity, lymphadenopathy, arthralgia, angioedema, fever, abdominal pain, dyspnea, and pleural and pericardial effusions

Main identifiable causes: drug induced, such as angiotensin-converting enzyme inhibitors, penicillin, sulfonamides, fluoxetine, and thiazides; rheumatic diseases, such as lupus erythematosus and Sjögren syndrome; viral diseases, such as hepatitis B, hepatitis C, and infectious mononucleosis; hypocomplementemia occurs in patients with associated systemic diseases, such as systemic lupus erythematosus; regardless of cause, disease tends to run chronic cours

Differential diagnosis

Urticaria; allergic cutaneous vasculitis; erythema multiforme

Therapy

Antihistamines, second generation; recalcitrant disease: colchicine; hydroxychloroquine; dapsone; systemic disease: prednisone

References
Black AK (1999) Urticarial vasculitis. Clinics in
   Dermatology 17(5):565–569

Uveoencephalitis

▶ Vogt-Koyanagi-Harada syndrome

Uveomeningoencephalitic syndrome

▶ Vogt-Koyanagi-Harada syndrome

Valacyclovir

Trade name(s)
Valtrex

Generic available
No

Drug class
Anti-viral

Mechanism of action
DNA polymerase inhibition

Dosage form
500 mg, 1000 mg tablet

Dermatologic indications and dosage
See table

Common side effects
Gastrointestinal: nausea, vomiting
Neurologic: headache

Serious side effects
Bone marrow: suppression
Gastrointestinal: hepatitis
Neurologic: seizures, encephalopathy, coma

Drug interactions
Aminoglycosides; carboplatin; cidofovir; cisplatin; glyburide; metformin; mycophenolate mofetil; probenecid; nephrotoxic agents

Other interactions
None

Contraindications/precautions
Hypersensitivity to drug class or component; elderly patients or those with renal failure may need lower dose

Valacyclovir. Dermatologic indications and dosage

Disease	Adult dosage	Child dosage
Herpes simplex virus infection, first episode	1000 mg PO twice daily for 10 days	Not established
Herpes simplex virus infection, prophylaxis	500 mg-1000 mg PO daily for up to 1 year	Not established
Herpes simplex virus infection, recurrent episode	2000 mg PO twice daily for 1 day	Not established
Herpes zoster	1000 mg PO 3 times daily for 7 days	Not established
Varicella	1000 mg PO 3 times daily for 7 days	Not established

References

Baker DA (2002) Valacyclovir in the treatment of genital herpes and herpes zoster. Expert Opinion on Pharmacotherapy 3(1):51–58

Valley fever

▶ Coccidioidomycosis

Van Buren's disease

▶ Peyronie's disease

Varicella

Synonym(s)
Chickenpox; primary varicella

Definition
Exanthem caused by the varicella zoster virus

Pathogenesis
Acquired by the inhalation of airborne respiratory droplets containing virus from an infected host; viremia disseminates the virus to the skin; transmission also occurs through direct contact with virus-containing cutaneous vesicles

Clinical manifestation
Rash, malaise, and low-grade fever at the onset; small, red macules appearing on the scalp, face, trunk, and proximal limbs, with progression to pruritic papules, vesicles, and pustules; central umbilication and crust formation as lesions evolve; new crops of lesions over a few days; infectious for 1–2 days prior to the development of rash and for 4–5 days afterwards; healing without scarring, except with excoriation or secondary bacterial superinfection

Differential diagnosis
Herpes simplex virus infection; drug eruption; other viral exanthem; bullous pemphigoid; dermatitis herpetiformis; erythema multiforme; pityriasis lichenoides et varioliformis acuta; congenital syphilis

Therapy
Immunocompetent adult population: valacyclovir
Immunocompromised population: intravenous acyclovir[*]
Highly susceptible, virus-exposed immunosuppressed populations: varicella-zoster immune globulin [VZIG][*]
Healthy children: avoidance of use of salicylates; calamine lotion, oatmeal baths for pruritus; antihistamines, first generation

References
McCrary ML, Severson J, Tyring SK (1999) Varicella zoster virus. Journal of the American Academy of Dermatology 41(1):1–14

Varicose and telangiectatic leg veins

Synonym(s)
Broken capillaries; varicosities; venectasia; varicose veins; spider veins; swollen veins

Definition
Surface manifestations of an underlying venous insufficiency syndrome, characterized by dilated and tortuous vascular channels on the leg

Pathogenesis
Dilatation of normal veins under the influence of increased venous pressure, most often resulting from venous insufficiency due to valve incompetence in the deep or superficial veins; increased venous pressure from outflow obstruction, either from intravascular thrombosis or from extrinsic compression; changes during pregnancy

most often caused by hormonal changes rendering vein wall and the valves more pliable; genetic component to primary valvular failure susceptibility

Clinical manifestation
Visible distension of superficial veins, mostly along the course of greater saphenous vein on leg and over medial thigh; sometimes associated with acute varicose complications, including variceal bleeding, stasis dermatitis, thrombophlebitis, cellulitis, and ulceration

Differential diagnosis
Thrombophlebitis; cellulitis; Osler-Weber-Rendu syndrome; stasis dermatitis

Therapy
Small or superficial vein disease: support hose; intermittent leg elevation; weight loss; chemical sclerosis (sclerotherapy); transcutaneous laser therapy; intense-pulsed-light (IPL) therapy
Large and deep vein disease: ligation of saphenofemoral junction with vein stripping; phlebectomy; endovenous radiofrequency thermal ablation; endovenous laser thermal ablation

References
Weksberg F (1999) Leg vein evaluation and therapy. Journal of Cutaneous Medicine & Surgery 3 Suppl 4:S43–8

Varicose veins

▶ Varicose and telangiectatic leg veins

Varicosities

▶ Varicose and telangiectatic leg veins

Variegate dermatitis

▶ Large plaque parapsoriasis

Variegate porphyria

Synonym(s)
Porphyria variegata; South African porphyria; protocoproporphyria; mixed porphyria

Definition
Hereditary disorder of porphyrin metabolism, characterized by photosensitivity and neurologic dysfunction

Pathogenesis
Autosomal dominant trait; gene mutation encoding defective protoporphyrinogen oxidase; trigger factors: certain drugs, hormonal fluctuations, carbohydrate restriction, infections

Clinical manifestation
Skin manifestations: photosensitivity; mechanical fragility; non-inflammatory vesicles and bullae, most commonly over dorsum of hands; scarring of sun-exposed skin; hypertrichosis; hyperpigmentation
Gastrointestinal manifestations: abdominal pain; nausea and vomiting
Neurologic manifestations: confusion; disorientation; agitation; psychotic behavior; seizures; coma; peripheral neuropathy causing paresthesias, and/or paralysis; autonomic neuropathy

Differential diagnosis
Porphyria cutanea tarda; hereditary coproporphyria; erythropoietic protoporphyria; acute intermittent porphyria; lupus erythematosus; polymorphous light eruption; epidermolysis bullosa; epidermolysis bullosa acquisita; pseudoporphyria; drug-induced photosensitivity

Therapy

Acute attack management: panhematin – 3–5 mg per kg IV 1–2 times daily for 3–4 days[*]; strict avoidance of triggers, such as extreme carbohydrate-restricted dieting, certain medications, alcohol, and smoking

References

Lim HW, Cohen JL (1999) The cutaneous porphyrias. Seminars in Cutaneous Medicine & Surgery 18(4):285–292

Variola

Synonym(s)

Smallpox

Definition

Viral infection causing widespread cutaneous vesicular eruption and serious systemic illness

Pathogenesis

Caused by infection with variola virus, spread via the respiratory route; major role of cell-mediated immunity in controlling disease; virus-specific cytotoxic T cells sometimes limit viral spread

Clinical manifestation

7–17 day incubation, followed by prodrome of fever, headache, pharyngitis, backache, nausea, vomiting, and feeling of general debility; oral mucous membrane enanthem; skin eruption begins with small, red macules on face and then spreads to extremities and trunk; lesions evolve into firm papules, then vesiculate, develop into pustules, and coalesce; by day 17, pustules form crusts and heal with pitted scars; lesions tend to be in same stage of development
Variola minor variant: constitutional symptoms, with fewer and smaller skin lesions

Differential diagnosis

Varicella; other viral exanthems, including coxsackievirus, parvovirus; infectious mononucleosis, rubella and rubeola; herpes simples virus infection; disseminated herpes zoster infection; impetigo; erythema multiforme; rickettsialpox; Kawasaki disease; rat bite fever; leukemia; contact dermatitis

Therapy

Strict respiratory and contact isolation for 17 days[*]; vaccination for contacts in early incubation period

References

Patt HA, Feigin RD (2002) Diagnosis and management of suspected cases of bioterrorism: a pediatric perspective. Pediatrics 109(4):685–692

Vascular gigantism

▶ Vascular malformation

Vascular malformation

Synonym(s)

Vascular gigantism; arteriovenous malformation

Definition

Group of disorders characterized by abnormalities of arteries, veins, capillaries, or lymphatic vessels, often present at birth, producing characteristic clinical, histologic, and radiologic changes

References

Fishman SJ, Mulliken JB (1993) Hemangiomas and vascular malformations of infancy and childhood. Pediatric Clinics of North America 40(6):1177–1200

Vascular spider

▶ Spider angioma

Vegetating bromidism

▶ Granuloma gluteale infantum

Vegetating potassium bromide toxic dermatitis

▶ Granuloma gluteale infantum

Venectasia

▶ Varicose and telangiectatic leg veins

Venous clot

▶ Thrombophlebitis, superficial

Venous eczema

▶ Stasis dermatitis

Venous lake

Synonym(s)
Venous-lake angioma; Bean-Walsh angioma; venous varix; senile hemangioma of the lips

Definition
Bluish-purple papule secondary to vascular dilatation, occurring usually in elderly people with excess sun exposure

Pathogenesis
Alteration of vascular and dermal elastic fibers secondary to solar damage, causing vascular dilatation

Clinical manifestation
Well demarcated, blue-purple, soft, compressible, smooth papules, distributed on the sun-exposed surfaces of face and neck, especially on helix or antihelix of ear, posterior pinna, or vermilion border of lower lip

Differential diagnosis
Hemangioma; blue nevus; mucosal melanosis; melanoma; angiokeratoma circumscriptum; traumatic tattoo

Therapy
Cryosurgery; electrosurgery, surgical excision; flashlamp pulse dye laser ablation; intense pulse light ablation

References
Requena L, Sangueza OP (1997) Cutaneous vascular anomalies. Part I. Hamartomas, malformations, and dilation of preexisting vessels. Journal of the American Academy of Dermatology 37(4):523–549

Venous stasis dermatitis

▶ Stasis dermatitis

Venous varix

▶ Venous lake

Venous-lake angioma

▶ Venous lake

Vermiculate atrophoderma

▶ Ulerythema ophryogenes

Verruca

▶ Wart

Verruca vulgaris

▶ Wart

Verrucous carcinoma

Synonym(s)

Ackerman tumor; Ackerman's tumor; carcinoma cuniculatum; warty cancer; epithelioma cuniculatum

Definition

Low grade squamous cell carcinoma characterized by slow growth of a verrucous nodule or plaque and rare metastatic spread

Pathogenesis

May be related to human papillomavirus (HPV) infection (particularly on penis, vulva, and periungual region), chemical carcinogens, and/or chronic irritation and inflammation, such as that occurring in patients who chew tobacco or betel nuts or use snuff

Clinical manifestation

Oral florid papillomatosis variant: white, translucent plaque on erythematous base, located on buccal mucosa, alveolar ridge, upper and lower gingiva, floor of mouth, tongue, tonsil, vermilion border of lip; sometimes develops in previous areas of leukoplakia, lichen planus, chronic lupus erythematous, cheilitis, or candidiasis; lesions evolve into white, cauliflower-like papillomas with a pebbly surface, sometimes extending and coalescing over large areas of the oral mucosa; ulceration, fistulation, and invasion locally into soft tissues and bone

Anourologic type (Buschke-Loewenstein tumor): most commonly on the glans penis, mainly in uncircumcised men; may also occur in the bladder and the vaginal, cervical, perianal, and pelvic organs; large, cauliflower-like nodule

Palmoplantar variant (epithelioma cuniculatum): most commonly involves skin overlying the first metatarsal head, but also on toes, heel, medioplantar region, and amputated stumps; exophytic tumors with ulceration and sinuses draining foul-smelling discharge; pain; bleeding; difficulty walking

Differential diagnosis

Wart; keratoacanthoma; North American blastomycosis; leishmaniasis; leprosy; actinomycosis; tuberculosis; mycetoma; granular cell tumor

Therapy

Mohs micrographic surgery*; destruction by electrodesiccation and curettage or liquid nitrogen cryotherapy; local radiation therapy

References

Kanik AB, Lee J, Wax F, Bhawan J (1997) Penile verrucous carcinoma in a 37-year-old circumcised man. Journal of the American Academy of Dermatology 37(2 Pt 2):329–331

Miller SB, Brandes BA, Mahmarian RR, Durham JR (2001) Verrucous carcinoma of the foot: a review and report of two cases. Journal of Foot & Ankle Surgery 40(4):225–231

Verrucous dermatitis

► Chromoblastomycosis

Verruga peruana

► Bartonellosis

Vesicular eczema of palms and soles

► Dyshidrotic eczema

Vesicular palmoplantar eczema

► Dyshidrotic eczema

Vesicular rickettsiosis

► Rickettsialpox

Viking disease

► Dupuytren's contracture

Vilanova disease

► Subacute nodular migratory panniculitis

Vincent's ulcer

► Tropical phagedenic ulcer

Viral keratoses

► Bowenoid papulosis

Vitamin B 3 deficiency

► Pellagra

Vitamin C deficiency syndrome

► Barlow's disease
► Scurvy

Vitiligo

Synonym(s)
White spot disease

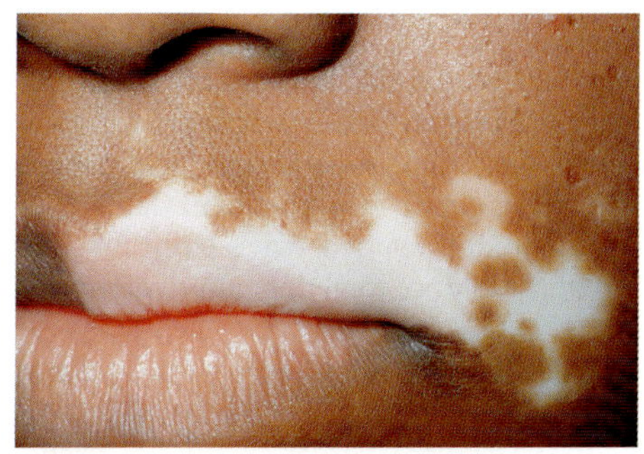

Vitiligo. Depigmented patch on the upper lip

Definition
Acquired progressive leukoderma, characterized by depigmented patches

Pathogenesis
Theories of causation: aberration of immune surveillance, melanocyte destruction by neurochemical mediator, melanocyte destruction by intermediate or metabolic product of melanin synthesis, inborn melanocyte abnormality

Clinical manifestation
Sharply circumscribed, white macules and patches, sometimes with perilesional hyperpigmentation, beginning with few lesions and expanding over time
Localized variant: restricted to one area, often in segmental distribution; onset early in life, then spreading rapidly within affected area; patches persist indefinitely
Generalized variant: bilaterally symmetrical, white macules and patches; sometimes involve mucous membranes, particularly the lip and genitalia; occur in areas of minor trauma (Koebner phenomenon), such as elbow, knee, dorsal aspect of hands; periorificial location of involvement; depigmentation of body hair, including scalp, eyebrow, and pubic and axillary hair

Differential diagnosis
Nevoid hypomelanosis; leprosy; piebaldism; tinea versicolor; post-inflammatory hypopigmentation; pityriasis alba; halo nevus; scleroderma; lichen sclerosus; tuberous sclerosis

Therapy
Photochemotherapy; corticosteroids, topical, superpotent; skin transplants for local areas of depigmentation; widespread involvement: 20 % monobenzylether of hydroquinone applied twice daily for 3–12 months to induce total depigmentation

References
Shaffrali F, Gawkrodger D (2000) Management of vitiligo. Clinical & Experimental Dermatology 25(8):575–579

Vogt-Koyanagi-Harada syndrome

Synonym(s)
Harada syndrome; uveoencephalitis; uveomeningoencephalitic syndrome

Definition
Syndrome involving various organs containing melanocytes, producing uveitis in association with cutaneous, neurologic, and auditory abnormalities

Pathogenesis
May be a post-viral syndrome, perhaps secondary to Epstein-Barr virus; possibly an autoimmune disorder; susceptibility related to presence of HLA-DR4 antigen and DRB*0405 allele

Clinical manifestation
Prodromal stage: non-specific symptoms, including headache, vertigo, nausea, nuchal rigidity, vomiting, and low-grade fever
Meningoencephalitis phase: generalized muscle weakness; hemiparesis; hemiplegia; dysarthria; aphasia, and other mental status changes
Ophthalmic-auditory phase: decreased acuity; eye pain and irritation; dysacusis, usually bilateral; tinnitus
Convalescent phase: cutaneous signs developing after uveitis begins to subside; poliosis; vitiligo; halo nevi; alopecia

Differential diagnosis
Alezzandrini's syndrome; piebaldism; vitiligo; alopecia areata

Therapy
Hypopigmentation: photochemotherapy; corticosteroids, topical, superpotent; eye inflammatory changes: prednisone

References
Read RW (2002) Vogt-Koyanagi-Harada disease. Ophthalmology Clinics of North America 15(3):333–341

Vohwinkel syndrome

Synonym(s)
Vohwinkel's syndrome; keratoderma hereditaria mutilans; palmoplantar keratoderma mutilans

Definition
Disorder characterized by hyperkeratosis of the palms and soles with a honeycomb appearance, constrictions of the skin around the digits, and hyperkeratotic plaques over the dorsal aspects of the extremities

Pathogenesis
Autosomal dominant trait; phenotype due to abnormal gap junctions caused by the mutation D66H in the gene GJB2 encoding connexin 26; possibly also insertional mutation of the loricrin gene

Clinical manifestation
Honeycomb-like hyperkeratosis of the palms and soles; constriction of skin around digits, causing autoamputation (pseudo-ainhum); starfish-shaped hyperkeratotic plaques on the dorsum of the hands and feet, elbows, and knees; occasional deafness

Differential diagnosis
Erythropoetic protoporphyria; discoid lupus erythematosus; mal de Meleda; pachyonychia congenita; palmoplantar keratoderma of Sybert; Olmsted syndrome; palmoplantar keratoderma of Gamborg Nielsen; hereditary bullous acrokeratotic poikiloderma of Weary-Kindler; Clouston syndrome; psoriasis

Therapy
Surgical release of constriction bands to preserve digits[*]; acitretin

References
Solis RR, Diven DG, Trizna Z (2001) Vohwinkel's syndrome in three generations. Journal of the American Academy of Dermatology 44(2 Suppl):376–378

Vohwinkel's syndrome

▶ Vohwinkel syndrome

Von Frey's syndrome

▶ Auriculotemporal syndrome

Von Recklinghausen disease

▶ Neurofibromatosis

Von Recklinghausen's disease

▶ Neurofibromatosis

Vulvodynia

Definition
Vulvar discomfort, characterized by itching, burning, stinging, or stabbing in the area around the opening of the vagina

References
Masheb RM, Nash JM, Brondolo E, Kerns RD (2000) Vulvodynia: an introduction and critical review of a chronic pain condition. Pain 86(1-2):3–10

Waardenburg syndrome

Synonym(s)
Klein-Waardenburg syndrome; Waardenburg's syndrome

Definition
Hereditary disease characterized by deafness in association with pigmentary abnormalities and other defects of neural crest-derived tissues

Pathogenesis
Autosomal dominant inheritance; unclear cause, but may be related, in part, to developmental defect of neural crest

Clinical manifestation
Type I variant: dystopia canthorum; nasal and other facial abnormalities; strabismus
Type II variant: normally placed canthi; sensorineural hearing loss; heterochromic irides; white forelock; hypopigmented skin patches
Type III variant: changes of type I variant and the following – musculoskeletal abnormalities; mental retardation; microcephaly
Type IV variant: association of changes of Waardenburg's syndrome with Hirshsprung disease

Differential diagnosis
Oculocutaneous albinism; piebaldism; vitiligo; Woolf syndrome; Fisch syndrome; Rozlycki syndrome

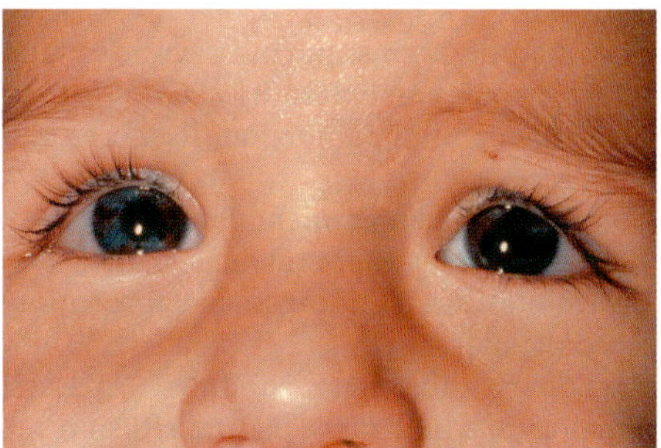

Waardenburg syndrome. Heterochromic irides

Therapy
No effective therapy

References
Newton VE (2002) Clinical features of the Waardenburg syndromes. Advances in Oto-Rhino-Laryngology 61:201–208

Waardenburg's syndrome

▶ Waardenburg syndrome

Waldenström macroglobulinemia

Synonym(s)
Waldenström's macroglobulinemia; Waldenström's hypergammaglobulinemia; Waldenström hypergammaglobulinemia

Definition
B lymphoma that causes overproduction of monoclonal macroglobulin

Pathogenesis
IgM-induced hyperviscosity of blood and neoplastic lymphoplasmacytic cell infiltratration of tissue, leading to many of the symptoms and signs of the disease

Clinical manifestation
Insidious constitutional signs and symptoms skin
Skin manifestations: purpura; vesicles; and bullae; papules on extremities; chronic urticaria; Raynaud phenomenon; livedo reticularis; acrocyanosis
Neurologic findings: mental status change; visual changes; peripheral neuropathy
Gastrointestinal findings: malabsorption; bleeding; diarrhea
Pulmonary findings: nodules, masses, parenchymal infiltrates; pleural effusion

Differential diagnosis
Myeloma; other hyperviscosity syndromes; polyarteritis nodosa; Churg-Strauss syndrome; antiphospholipid antibody syndrome; serum sickness; septic vasculitis; systemic lupus erythematosus; sarcoidosis

Therapy
Symptomatic hyperviscosity: plasmapheresis*; lymphoma: chemotherapy; splenectomy

References
Alexanian R, Weber D (2001) Recent advances in treatment of multiple myeloma and Waldenström's macroglobulinemia. Biomedicine & Pharmacotherapy 55(9-10):550–552

Waldenström's hypergammaglobulinemia

▶ Waldenström macroglobulinemia

Waldenström's macroglobulinemia

▶ Waldenström macroglobulinemia

Warfarin skin necrosis

▶ Coumarin necrosis

Wart

Synonym(s)
Verruca

Definition
Virally induced, benign proliferation of skin and mucosa

Pathogenesis
Caused by human papilloma virus (HPV); various wart subtypes have tendency to be site-specific; viral replication in differentiated epithelial cells in upper epidermis

Clinical manifestation
Common variant (verruca vulgaris): hard papules with a rough, irregular, scaly surface, most commonly seen on hands
Filiform variant: elongated, slender papules with filiform fronds, usually seen on face, around the lips, eyelids, or nares
Palmoplantar warts (myrmecia): small, shiny papules, progressing to deep endophytic, sharply defined, round papules or plaques with keratotic surface, surrounded by a smooth collar of thickened horn; plantar lesions usually found on weight-bearing areas, such as metatarsal head and heel; hand lesions often are subungual or periungual
Flat wart (plane wart, verruca plana) variant: flat or slightly elevated, flesh-colored,

smooth or slightly hyperkeratotic papules; sometimes become grouped or confluent; may appear in linear distribution as a result of scratching or trauma (Koebner phenomenon)

Butcher's wart variant: seen in people who handle raw meat; similar morphology to common warts, most commonly on the hands

Mosaic variant: plaque of closely grouped warts, usually seen on palms and soles

Anogenital (condyloma accuminata) variant: pink-to-brown, exophytic, cauliflower-like papules or nodules of genitalia, perineum, crural folds, and/or anus; discrete, flesh-colored or hyperpigmented papules on the shaft of the penis; lesions may extend into the vagina, urethra, cervix, perirectal epithelium, anus, and rectum

Differential diagnosis

Acquired digital fibrokeratoma; actinic keratosis; squamous cell carcinoma; arsenical keratosis; seborrheic keratosis; acrochordon; lichen planus; molluscum contagiosum; prurigo nodularis; callus; lichen nitidus; acne vulgaris

Therapy

Salicylic acid 5–40 % solution applied daily for weeks to months; cantharidin applied once every 3–6 weeks; squaric acid applied 1–2 times weekly after sensitization; trichloroacetic acid 80 % applied once every 4–6 weeks; podofilox; imiquimod; bleomycin: 0.5–1 unit per ml intralesional injection; liquid nitrogen cryotherapy; destruction by electrodesiccation and curettage; CO_2 laser vaporization; hypnotherapy; hyperthermia

References

Allen AL, Siegfried EC (2000) What's new in human papillomavirus infection. Current Opinion in Pediatrics 12(4):365–369

Warty cancer

▶ Verrucous carcinoma

Warty dyskeratoma

Synonym(s)
Focal acantholytic dyskeratosis

Definition
Solitary, benign, epithelial neoplasm, characterized by papule with depressed and crusted center containing a keratotic plug

Pathogenesis
Localized abnormal keratinization, with unknown stimulus

Clinical manifestation
Flesh-colored to brown papule with central keratotic plug, occurring in association with the pilosebaceous unit, especially on scalp, face, neck, and axilla; most often occurs in older men

Differential diagnosis
Wart; keratoacanthoma; squamous cell carcinoma; actinic keratosis; Darier disease; Hailey-Hailey disease; epidermal nevus; Grover's disease

Therapy
Surgical excision[*]

References
Kaddu S, Dong H, Mayer G, Kerl H, Cerroni L (2002) Warty dyskeratoma – "follicular dyskeratoma": analysis of clinicopathologic features of a distinctive follicular adnexal neoplasm. Journal of the American Academy of Dermatology 47(3):423–428c

Wasp sting

▶ Hymenoptera sting

Water wart

▶ Molluscum contagiosum

Water-rat trapper's disease

▶ Tularemia

Watson syndrome

Synonym(s)
Watson's syndrome; neurofibromatosis-Noonan syndrome; neurofibromatosis with Noonan phenotype; pulmonic stenosis; café au lait spots syndrome

Definition
Hereditary condition characterized by clinical elements of both Noonan's syndrome and neurofibromatosis

Pathogenesis
Autosomal dominant trait; may be associated with NF-1 gene mutation

Clinical manifestation
Café-au-lait macules; axillary freckling; Lisch nodules; pulmonary stenosis; low intelligence; short stature

Differential diagnosis
Neurofibromatosis; Noonan's syndrome; Turner's syndrome

Therapy
No effective therapy

References
Conway JB, Posner M (1994) Anaesthesia for caesarean section in a patient with Watson's syndrome. Canadian Journal of Anaesthesia 41(11):1113–1116

Watson's syndrome

▶ Watson syndrome

Weber-Christian disease

Synonym(s)
Idiopathic lobular panniculitis; relapsing febrile nodular nonsuppurative panniculitis; nodular nonsuppurative panniculitis; Pfeifer-Weber-Christian syndrome

Definition
Spectrum of disorders characterized by nodular panniculitis and additional symptoms and signs involving multiple organ systems of the body

Pathogenesis
Unknown

Clinical manifestation
Erythematous, edematous, and tender symmetrical, subcutaneous nodules, usually on the lower extremities, resolving over a few weeks, leaving atrophic depressed scar; occasional breakdown of nodules with discharge of oily liquid; hepatomegaly; splenomegaly; systemic symptoms: malaise, fever, nausea, vomiting, abdominal pain, weight loss, bone pain, myalgia, and arthralgia

Differential diagnosis
Thrombophlebitis; vasculitis; sarcoidosis; alpha-1-antitrypsin deficiency panniculitis; polyarteritis nodosa; eosinophilic fasciitis; eosinophilic myalgia syndrome; erythema induratum; erythema nodosum; leukemia; lipodermatosclerosis; lymphoma; pancreatic panniculitis; poststeroid panniculitis; scleroderma panniculitis; cytophagic histiocytic panniculitis; Sweet's syndrome

Therapy
Prednisone; hydroxychloroquine; azathioprine; thalidomide; cyclophosphamide; mycophenolate mofetil

References
Enk AH, Knop J (1998) Treatment of relapsing idiopathic nodular panniculitis (Pfeifer-Weber-Christian disease) with mycophenolate mofetil.

Journal of the American Academy of Dermatology 39(3):508–509

Wegener granulomatosis

▶ Wegener's granulomatosis

Wegener's disease

▶ Wegener's granulomatosis

Wegener's granulomatosis

Synonym(s)
Wegener granulomatosis; Wegener's disease; systemic vasculitis; systemic necrotizing angiitis; necrotizing granulomatous inflammation of the respiratory tract; necrotizing glomerulonephritis

Definition
Multisystem disease characterized by necrotizing granulomatous inflammation of the upper and lower respiratory tract, kidneys, and skin, and by necrotizing vasculitis affecting small- and medium-sized vessels

Pathogenesis
Probably an autoimmune inflammatory process, antineutrophil cytoplasmic antibodies (c-ANCA) directed at neutrophil proteinase 3 (PR-3) may be involved; endothelial cell damage and activation of neutrophils produce inflammatory mediators, leading to recruitment of monocytes and T cells and endothelial damage

Clinical manifestation
Non-specific constitutional symptoms and signs

Skin findings: variable and usually nonspecific; palpable purpura; papules; subcutaneous nodules; ulcerations resembling pyoderma gangrenosum; petechiae; vesicles; pustules; hemorrhagic bullae; livedo reticularis; lower extremities most commonly affected
Ocular findings: conjunctivitis; scleritis; proptosis
Ear, nose, and throat findings: sinusitis and disease in the nasal mucosa, with purulent or sanguinous nasal discharge; otitis media; deformation or destruction of the pinnae or nose
Oral findings: mucosal ulcerations; gingival hyperplasia with petechiae
Renal findings: oliguria; hematuria; glomerulonephritis; chronic renal insufficiency
Cardiac and neurologic involvement

Differential diagnosis
Churg-Strauss disease; acute febrile neutrophilic dermatosis; polyarteritis nodosa; cryoglobulinemic vasculitis; lethal midline granuloma; lymphomatoid granulomatosis; Henoch-Schönlein purpura; pyoderma gangrenosum

Therapy
Cyclophosphamide★; prednisone

References
Regan MJ, Hellmann DB, Stone JH (2001) Treatment of Wegener's granulomatosis. Rheumatic Diseases Clinics of North America 27(4):863–886

Weil disease

▶ Leptospirosis

Well's syndrome

▶ Eosinophilic cellulitis

Wells syndrome

▶ Eosinophilic cellulitis

Wells' syndrome

▶ Eosinophilic cellulitis

Wen

▶ Epidermoid cyst
▶ Pilar cyst

Werther's tumor

▶ Syringocystadenoma papilliferum

Whirlpool folliculitis

▶ Hot tub folliculitis

White folded gingivostomatitis

▶ White sponge nevus

White piedra

▶ Piedra

White sponge nevus

Synonym(s)
Oral epithelial nevus; white folded gingivostomatitis; hereditary leukokeratosis; Cannon's disease; nevus of Cannon

Definition
Developmental mucosal disorder, characterized by sponge-like, white plaque on buccal mucosa and other mucosal sites

Pathogenesis
Autosomal recessive trait; mutation in the mucosal keratin K4

Clinical manifestation
Bilateral, white, keratotic plaques, most commonly on buccal mucosal surface and sometimes on labial, lingual, and other mucosal sites; thick, white, often corrugated plaque, sometimes covering much of buccal mucosa; occasional less thick lesions with semitransparent appearance

Differential diagnosis
Hereditary benign intraepithelial dyskeratosis; Witkop's disease; pachyonychia congenita; dyskeratosis congenita; leukoedema; smokeless tobacco keratosis; chronic cheek bite keratosis; leukoplakia

Therapy
Surgical excision for cosmesis only

References
Marcushamer M, King DL, McGuff S (1995) White sponge nevus: case report. Pediatric Dentistry 17(7):458–459

White sponge nevus of Cannon

▶ White sponge nevus

White spot disease

▶ Vitiligo

Whitmore disease

▶ Glanders and melioidosis

Wild hare disease

▶ Tularemia

Wilson disease

Synonym(s)
Hepatolenticular degeneration; Wilson's disease

Definition
Inherited disorder of copper metabolism, characterized by cirrhosis and central nervous system degenerative changes

Pathogenesis
Autosomal recessive trait; gene linked to the long arm of chromosome 13; defective protein (p-type adenosine triphosphatase) responsible for copper transport; organ dysfunction from inadequate biliary copper excretion and subsequent copper deposition, most notably in liver and central nervous system

Clinical manifestation
Skin changes: hyperpigmentation; bluish discoloration over proximal fingernails
Gastrointestinal changes: hepatic insufficiency and cirrhosis, with subsequent ascites, spider angiomas, palmar erythema, digital clubbing, and jaundice
Ocular findings: copper granules in the stromal layer of the eye (Kayser-Fleischer rings); golden brown, brownish green, bronze color in the limbic area of the eye
Central nervous system changes: drooling; dysphagia; dystonia; incoordination; difficulty with fine motor tasks; masklike facies; gait disturbance
Skeletal abnormalities: highly variable, including osteoporosis, osteomalacia, rickets, spontaneous fractures, and polyarthritis

Differential diagnosis
Autoimmune hepatitis; viral hepatitis; glycogen storage disease; multiple sclerosis; Huntington disease; Parkinson disease; leukodystrophy; hemochromatosis

Therapy
Penicillamine: 250 mg PO 4 times daily[*]; dietary copper restriction

References
Subramanian I, Vanek ZF, Bronstein JM (2002) Diagnosis and treatment of Wilson's disease. Current Neurology & Neuroscience Reports 2(4):317–323

Wilson's disease

▶ Wilson disease

Winer's dilated pore

▶ Dilated pore

Winer's pore

▶ Dilated pore

Winter erythrokeratolysis

▶ **Keratolytic winter erythema**

Winter itch

▶ **Asteatosis**
▶ **Asteatotic eczema**

Wiskott-Aldrich syndrome

Synonym(s)
Aldrich syndrome

Definition
Hereditary disorder, characterized by immunodeficiency, thrombocytopenia, eczema, and recurrent pyogenic infections

Pathogenesis
X-linked trait; mutations in WASP gene, important transcription factor of lymphocyte and platelet function; eczema related to the abnormal T-cell function and humoral immune responses

Clinical manifestation
Eczema with onset in first month of life, indistinguishable from atopic dermatitis; thrombocytopenia and platelet dysfunction at birth, with bloody diarrhea, hematuria, epistaxis, and cutaneous petechiae; recurrent bacterial infections beginning in infancy, with susceptibility to wide variety of bacterial infections, including septicemia, pneumonia, meningitis, pansinusitis, conjunctivitis, furunculosis, otitis externa, and otitis media

Differential diagnosis
Atopic dermatitis; Leiner disease; DiGeorge syndrome; seborrheic dermatitis; Langerhans cell histiocytosis

Therapy
Eczema: corticosteroids, topical, mid potency; platelet transfusions as needed; antibiotics for recurrent pyogenic infections; bone marrow transplantation for severe involvement

References
Ochs HD (2001) The Wiskott-Aldrich syndrome. Clinical Reviews in Allergy & Immunology 20(1):61–86

Wolhynia fever

▶ **Trench fever**

Woolsorter's disease

▶ **Anthrax, cutaneous**

Wooly hair nevus

Synonym(s)
None

Definition
Sporadic anomaly of hair growth, characterized by coarse, lusterless, and wiry patch of hair

Pathogenesis
Unknown

Clinical manifestation
Localized area of coarse, wiry hair, usually limited to scalp; begins in early childhood and stable throughout life; sometimes seen with incontinentia pigmenti

Differential diagnosis
Menke's kinky hair syndrome; uncombable hair syndrome

Therapy
No effective therapy

References
Al Harmozi SA; Somaia FM, Ejeckam GC (1992) Woolly hair nevus syndrome. Journal of the American Academy of Dermatology 27(2Pt1):259–260

Woringer-Kolopp disease

▶ T-cell lymphoma, cutaneous

Wyburn-Mason syndrome

Synonym(s)
Bonnet-Dechaume-Blanc syndrome

Definition
Disease characterized by arteriovenous malformations in the central nervous system and the retina and ipsilateral cutaneous vascular abnormalities

Pathogenesis
Alterations in capillary and arteriolar networks by unknown mechanisms

Clinical manifestation
Subtle port wine stain in the region of the affected eye; intracranial vascular malformations; retinal arterial-venous malformations

Differential diagnosis
Sturge-Weber syndrome; capillary hemangioma

Therapy
Flash-pumped dye laser ablation of port wine stain

References
Patel U, Gupta SC (1990) Wyburn-Mason syndrome. A case report and review of the literature. Neuroradiology 31(6):544–546

X

X-linked chronic granulomatous disease

▶ Chronic granulomatous disease

X-linked dominant type

▶ Conradi disease

X-linked ichthyosis

Synonym(s)
Ichthyosis nigricans

Definition
Hereditary disorder of keratinization, characterized by severe scaling, especially on the extremities

Pathogenesis
X-linked trait; caused by a steroid sulfatase deficiency resulting from abnormalities in its coding gene (*STS*); retention hyperkeratosis from delayed dissolution of desmosomes in the stratum corneum

Clinical manifestation
Onset at birth or in neonatal period; adherent brown scaling in widespread distribution produces dirty-appearing skin; scaling of scalp, preauricular skin, and posterior neck; flexures sometimes involved, but palms and soles usually spared; scaling becomes more evident and assumes a dirty-yellow or brown color with dark, polygonal, firmly adherent scale; tends to fade on head but more prominent on trunk and extremities, particularly on the extensor surfaces of the legs; asymptomatic corneal opacities; occasional cryptorchidism

Differential diagnosis
Ichthyosis vulgaris; lamellar ichthyosis; xerosis; atopic dermatitis; hygiene problem with resultant dirty skin

Therapy
Alpha hydroxy acids; emollients

References
Hernandez-Martin A, Gonzalez-Sarmiento R, De Unamuno P (1999) X-linked ichthyosis: an update. British Journal of Dermatology 141(4):617–627

Xanthelasma

▶ Xanthoma

Xanthogranuloma

▶ Juvenile xanthogranuloma

Xanthoma

Synonym(s)
Xanthomatosis

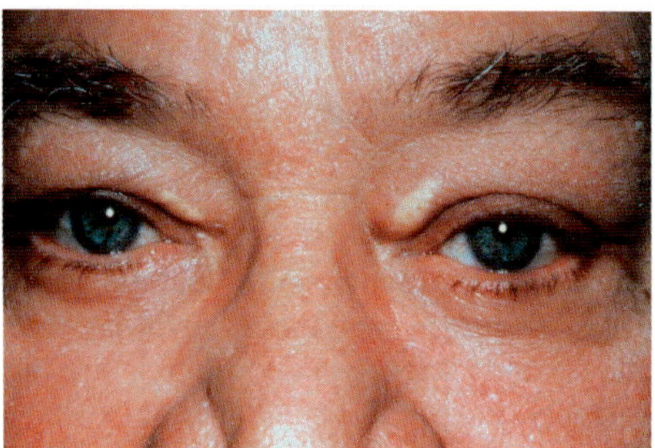

Xanthoma. Yellow-white papules on the upper eyelids

Definition
Group of disorders characterized by skin lesions with lipid-laden macrophages

Pathogenesis
Alterations in lipoproteins from genetic mutations yield defective apolipoproteins (primary hyperlipoproteinemia) or from systemic disorder, such as diabetes mellitus (secondary hyperlipoproteinemia); distribution pattern and morphology of lesions depend on specific genetic type or underlying disease

Clinical manifestation
Xanthelasma palpebrarum variant: asymptomatic, symmetrical, soft, velvety, yellow, flat-topped, polygonal papules on and around eyelids, most commonly in upper eyelid near the inner canthus; may have no associated lipid abnormality or may be associated with hyperlipidemia, where any type of primary hyperlipoproteinemia can be present; occasional association with secondary hyperlipoproteinemias, such as cholestasis

Tuberous xanthoma variant: asymptomatic, firm, red-yellow papules or nodules usually developing in pressure areas, such as knees, elbows, or buttocks; may coalesce to form multilobated tumors; associated with hypercholesterolemia and increased levels of LDL, with familial dysbetalipoproteinemia and familial hypercholesterolemia or with secondary hyperlipidemias (e.g., nephrotic syndrome, hypothyroidism)

Tendinous xanthoma variant: slowly enlarging subcutaneous nodules around tendons or ligaments, often over extensor tendons of the hands, the feet, and the Achilles tendons; sometimes occurs after trauma; associated with severe hypercholesterolemia and elevated LDL levels, particularly in the type IIa form, or secondary hyperlipidemias such as cholestasis

Eruptive xanthoma variant: sudden onset of crops of small, pruritic, red-yellow papules on an erythematous base, most commonly over buttocks, shoulders, and extensor surfaces of extremities; may spontaneously resolve over weeks; associated with hypertriglyceridemia, particularly with types I, IV, and V (high concentrations of VLDL and chylomicrons) or with secondary hyperlipidemias, particularly in diabetes

Plane xanthoma variant: flat, yellowish papules, occurring in any site, and sometimes covering large areas of face, neck, thorax, and flexures; when palmar creases involved, type III dysbetalipoproteinemia likely diagnosis; may occur with secondary hyperlipidemias, especially in cholestasis, with monoclonal gammopathy and hyperlipidemia, particularly hypertriglyceridemia

Xanthoma disseminatum variant: occurs in normolipemic patients; begins in adults as red-yellow papules and nodules with a predilection for flexures; sometimes also occurs on mucosa of the upper part of the aerodigestive tract; usually resolves spontaneously

Verruciform xanthoma variant: normolipemic patients with predominantly oral cavity, solitary, papillomatous yellow nodule or plaque

Differential diagnosis
Juvenile xanthogranuloma; amyloidosis; lipoid proteinosis; erythema elevatum diutinum; sarcoidosis; granuloma annu-

lare; necrobiosis lipoidica; necrobiotic xanthogranuloma; calcinosis cutis; Langerhans cell histiocytosis; rheumatoid nodules; gouty tophi; mastocytosis; lymphoma

Therapy
Xanthelasma: topical trichloroacetic acid; electrodesiccation; laser therapy; excision; verruciform xanthoma; local excision; control of underlying lipid defect or other illness causing lesions to arise

References
Vermeer BJ, Gevers Leuven J (1991) New aspects of xanthomatosis and hyperlipoproteinemia. Current Problems in Dermatology 20:63–72

Xanthoma disseminatum

▶ Xanthoma

Xanthoma multiplex

▶ Juvenile xanthogranuloma

Xanthoma naviforme

▶ Juvenile xanthogranuloma

Xanthoma striatum palmare

▶ Xanthoma

Xanthoma, tendinous

▶ Xanthoma

Xanthoma, tuberous

▶ Xanthoma

Xanthomatosis

▶ Xanthoma

Xerac-AC

▶ Aluminium chloride

Xeroderma

▶ Ichthyosis vulgaris

Xeroderma of Hebra

▶ Xeroderma pigmentosum

Xeroderma pigmentosum

Synonym(s)
Kaposi's dermatosis; xeroderma of Hebra; angioma pigmentosum et atrophicum; atrophoderma pigmentosum; melanosis lenticularis progressiva

Definition
Disease characterized by extreme photosensitivity, pigmentary changes, premature skin aging, and development of malignant tumors

Pathogenesis

Defect in nucleotide excision repair, leading to deficient repair of DNA damaged by ultraviolet radiation; seven XP repair genes with seven complementation groups; local immunosuppression may be a factor in increased skin malignancies

Clinical manifestation

Stage 1: after the age of 6 months, onset of diffuse erythema, scaling, and freckle-like areas of increased pigmentation
Stage 2: poikiloderma causes an appearance similar to chronic radiation dermatitis
Stage 3: numerous malignancies, including squamous cell carcinoma, basal cell carcinoma, malignant melanoma, and fibrosarcoma
Ocular findings: photophobia; conjunctivitis; eyelid solar lentigines; ectropion; symblepharon with ulceration; vascular pterygia; fibrovascular pannus of the cornea; epitheliomas of the lids
Neurologic findings: electroencephalographic abnormalities; microcephaly; spasticity; hyporeflexia or areflexia; ataxia; chorea; motor neuron signs or segmental demyelination; sensorineural deafness; supranuclear ophthalmoplegia; mental retardation
De Sanctis Cacchione syndrome: changes of xeroderma pigmentosum; neurologic abnormalities; hypogonadism; dwarfism

Differential diagnosis

Basal cell nevus syndrome; porphyria; Bloom syndrome; Cockayne syndrome; progeria; Rothmund-Thomson syndrome; lupus erythematosus; polymorphous light eruption; LEOPARD syndrome; hydroa vacciniforme

Therapy

Absolute protection from sun exposure from the time of birth; surgical excision of skin malignancies*; isotretinoin; genetic counseling for families at risk*

References

Moriwaki S, Kraemer KH (2001) Xeroderma pigmentosum – bridging a gap between clinic and laboratory. Photodermatology, Photoimmunology & Photomedicine 17(2):47–54

Xerosis

▶ Asteatosis

Xerotic eczema

▶ Asteatotic eczema

Yaws

Synonym(s)
Pian; frambesia tropica; bouba; parangi; paru

Definition
Infectious, nonvenereal, treponemal disease, characterized by involvement of skin and bones

Pathogenesis
Caused by Treponema pallidum, subspecies pertenue, serologically and morphologically indistinguishable from organism causing syphilis

Clinical manifestation
Primary stage: incubation period of 9–90 days; primary lesion (mother yaw) at site of inoculation after a scratch, bite, or abrasion, most commonly on legs, feet, or buttocks; nontender, occasionally pruritic, red papule or nodule that ulcerates; satellite lesions may coalesce to form plaque; lymphadenopathy; fever; joint pain; mother yaw resolves spontaneously in 2–9 months, leaving atrophic scar with central hypopigmentation
Secondary stage: beginning 6–16 weeks after primary stage, skin lesions (daughter yaws) resembling mother yaw but smaller; periorificial location; lesions expand, ulcerate, and exude a fibrinous fluid that dries into a crust; red, scaly papules and plaques that resemble syphilis over any part of the body; moist lesions in axillae, groin, mucous membranes; papillomas on plantar surfaces; macules or hyperkeratotic papules on palms and soles; skeletal involvement: painful osteoperiostitis; fusiform soft tissue swelling of the metatarsals and metacarpals; may develop relapses after healing up to 5 years following infection
Late stage: occurs after 5–15 years of latency; progressively enlarging, painless, subcutaneous nodules that ulcerate, with well-defined edges and indurated base with granulation tissue and yellowish slough; keratoderma of palms and soles; juxtaarticular ulcerated gummatous nodules; skeletal lesions consisting of hypertrophic periostitis, gummatous periostitis, osteitis, and osteomyelitis

Differential diagnosis
Atopic dermatitis; tuberculosis; leishmaniasis; leprosy; psoriasis; sarcoidosis; scabies; tungiasis; warts; syphilis; keratodermas from other causes; insect bite reaction; nutritional deficiency

Therapy
Penicillin G benzathine*; erythromycin; doxycycline

References
Walker SL, Hay RJ (2000) Yaws-a review of the last 50 years. International Journal of Dermatology 39(4):258–260

Yellow jacket sting

▶ Hymenoptera sting

Z

Zinc deficiency syndrome

▶ Acrodermatitis enteropathica

Zinc depletion syndrome

▶ Acrodermatitis enteropathica

Zinsser-Cole-Engman syndrome

▶ Dyskeratosis congenita

Zinsser-Engman-Cole syndrome

▶ Dyskeratosis congenita

Ziprkowski-Margolis syndrome

Synonym(s)
Albinism-deafness syndrome

Definition
Hereditary syndrome consisting of congenital deafness and partial albinism

Pathogenesis
X-linked trait; possibly related to Waardenburg syndrome; specific pattern of hearing impairment in carrier females

Clinical manifestation
Patchy hypopigmentation and hyperpigmentation; congenital neurosensory deafness; no ocular changes

Differential diagnosis
Piebaldism; oculocutaneous albinism; chemical leukoderma; onchocerciasis; pinta; yaws; Waardenburg syndrome; Alezzandrini syndrome; leprosy; Vogt-Koyanagi-Harada syndrome

Therapy
No effective therapy

References
Shiloh Y, Litvak G, Ziv Y, Lehner T, Sandkuyl L, Hildesheimer, M, Buchris, V, et al. Genetic mapping of X-linked albinism-deafness syndrome (ADFN) to Xq26.3–q27.1. American Journal of Human Genetics 47: 20–27

Zonal dermatosis

▶ Lichen striatus

Zoon balanitis

Synonym(s)
Zoon's balanitis; plasma cell balanitis of Zoon; Zoon's disease; Zoon's plasma cell balanitis; balanitis circumscripta plasmacellularis; plasma cell balanitis; plasma cell mucositis

Definition
Benign inflammatory dermatosis of the penis in uncircumcised men, with histologic findings of plasma cells in the dermal infiltrate

Pathogenesis
Theories of causation: friction; trauma; heat; poor hygiene; chronic infection with Mycobacterium smegmatis; reactive response to an unknown exogenous or infectious agent; immediate hypersensitivity response mediated by immunoglobulin E class antibodies; hypospadias

Clinical manifestation
Solitary, shiny, red-orange-to-violaceous plaque of the glans or prepuce of an uncircumcised male

Differential diagnosis
Erythroplasia of Queyrat; candidiasis; lichen sclerosus; lichen planus; syphilis; psoriasis; fixed medication reaction

Therapy
Circumcision*

References
Mallon E, Hawkins D, Dinneen M, Francics N, Fearfield L, Newson R, Bunker C (2000) Circumcision and genital dermatoses. Archives of Dermatology 136(3):350–354

Zoon's balanitis

▶ Zoon balanitis

Zoon's disease

▶ Zoon balanitis

Zoon's plasma cell balanitis

▶ Zoon balanitis

Zoster

▶ Herpes zoster

Zygomycosis

▶ Mucormycosis

Appendix

Tab. 1. Generics and common trade names mentioned in the book

Generic	Trade Name
▶ Adapalene	Differin
▶ Acyclovir	Zovirax
▶ Antihistamines, first generation	Benadryl
	Chlor-Trimeton
	Comtrex
	Dermarest
	Dimetane
	Periactin
	Phenergan
	Polaramine
	Pyribenzamine
	Sinequan
	Sominex
▶ Antihistamines, second generation	Allegra
	Claritin
	Clarinex
	Zyrtec
▶ Anthralin	Anthro-derm
	Drithocreme
	Dritho-Scalp
	Micanol
▶ Auranofin	Ridaura
▶ Aurothioglucose	Solganol
▶ Azathioprine	Imuran
▶ Azelaic acid	Azelex
▶ Azithromycin	Zithromax
▶ Azole antifungal agents	Exelderm
	Lamisil AT
	Lotrimin
	Micatin
	Mycelex
	Nizoral
	Oxistat
	Spectazole

Tab. 1. Generics and common trade names mentioned in the book (continued)

Generic	Trade Name
▶ Bacitracin	Baciguent
	Betadine antibiotic ointment
	Gold Bond Triple Action
	Mycitracin
	Neosporin
	Polysporin
	Spectrocin Plus
▶ Benzoyl peroxide	Benoxyl
	Benza-Gel
	Benzac AC
	BenzaClin
	Benzamycin
	Brevoxyl
	Desquam-E
	Duac
	PanOxyl
	Persa-Gel
	Triaz
▶ Calcipotriene	Dovonex
▶ Cantharidin	Canthacur
▶ Capsaicin	Zostrix
	Zostrix HP
▶ Cephalexin	Biocef
	Keflex
	Keftab
▶ Ciclopirox	Loprox
	Penlac
▶ Ciprofloxacin	Cipro
▶ Clarithromycin	Biaxin
▶ Clindamycin, systemic	Cleocin
▶ Corticosteroids, topical, high potency	Cyclocort
	Diprosone
	Halog
	Lidex
	Topicort
▶ Corticosteroids, topical, low potency	Aclovate
	Cortaid
	DesOwen

Tab. 1. Generics and common trade names mentioned in the book (continued)

Generic	Trade Name
▶ Corticosteroids, topical, medium potency	Cloderm
	Cordran
	Cutivate
	Dermatop
	Diprosone
	Elocon
	Locoid
	Synalar
	Uticort
	Valisone
	Venalog
	Westcort
▶ Corticosteroids, topical, super potency	Cordan Tape
	Diprolone
	Florone
	Temovate
	Ultravate
▶ Cyclophosphamide	Cytoxan
	Neosar
▶ Cyclosporine	Neoral
	Sandimmune
	SangCya
▶ Depilatories, chemical	Nair
	Neet
	Nudit
	Magic Shaving Powder
	Royal Crown Shaving Powder
▶ Dicloxacillin	Dynapen
▶ Doxycycline	Doryx
	Monodox
	Vibra-Tabs
	Vibramycin
▶ Eflornithine	Vaniqa
▶ Erythromycin, systemic	E-mycin
	EES
	Eryc
	Ilosone
	PCE

Tab. 1. Generics and common trade names mentioned in the book (continued)

Generic	Trade Name
▶ Erythromycin, topical	Emgel
	Erycette
	EryDerm
	Erymax
	Erythra-Derm
	Staticin
	T-Stat
	Theramycin
▶ Famciclovir	Famvir
▶ Finasteride	Propecia
▶ Fluconazole	Diflucan
▶ Fluorouracil, topical	Adrucil
	Carac
	Efudex
	Fluoroplex
▶ Griseofulvin	Fulvicin P/G
	Grifulvin V
	Gris-PEG
▶ Hydroquinone	Eldopaque
	Eldoquin
	Esoterica
	Esoterica
	Lustra
	Melanex
	Nuquin
	Porcelana Fade Cream
	Solaquin Forte
	Tri-Luma
▶ Hydroxychloroquine	Plaquenil
▶ Hydroxyurea	Hydrea
▶ Imiquimod	Aldara
▶ Interferon-α	Intron A
	Roferon A
▶ Isotretinoin	Accutane
	Amnesteem
▶ Itraconazole	Sporanox
▶ Ivermectin	Stromectol
▶ Ketoconazole	Nizoral
▶ Methotrexate	Rheumatrex

Tab. 1. Generics and common trade names mentioned in the book (continued)

Generic	Trade Name
▶ Methoxsalen	Oxsoralen lotion
	Oxsoralen Ultra
▶ Metronidazole, topical	MetroCream
	MetroGel
	MetroLotion
	Noritate
▶ Minocycline	Dynacin
	Minocin
	Vectrin
▶ Minoxidil, topical	Rogaine
▶ Mupirocin	Bactroban
▶ Mycophenolate mofetil	CellCept
▶ Naftifine	Naftin
▶ Penicillin G benzathine	Bicillin LA
▶ Penicillin VK	Pen-Vee K
	Veetids
▶ Permethrin	Elimite
	Nix
▶ Podofilox	Condylox
▶ Prednisone	Deltasone
	Sterapred
▶ Rifampin	Rifadin
	Rimactane
▶ Spironolactone	Aldactone
▶ Selective serotonin reuptake inhibitor (SSRI)	Celexa
	Luvox
	Paxil
	Prozac
	Zoloft
▶ Tazarotene	Tazorac
▶ Tetracycline	Achromycin-V
	Lamisil
	Panmycin
	Sumycin
	Tetracap
▶ Thalidomide	Thalomid
▶ Thioguanine	Thioguanine

Tab. 1. Generics and common trade names mentioned in the book (continued)

Generic	Trade Name
▶ Tretinoin	Avita
	Renova
	Retin A Micro
	Retin-A
▶ Trimethoprim-sulfamethoxazole	Bactrim
	Septra
▶ Urea, topical	Aquacare
	Carmol
	Neutraplus
	Ultramide
	Ureacin
▶ Valacyclovir	Valtrex

Tab. 2. Trade names mentioned in the book and their generics

Trade Name	Generic
Accutane	▶ Isotretinoin
Achromycin-V	▶ Tetracycline
Adrucil	▶ Fluorouracil, topical
Alclometasone 0.05%	▶ Corticosteroids, topical, low potency
Aldactone	▶ Spironolactone
Aldara	▶ Imiquimod
Allegra	▶ Antihistamines, second generation
Amcinonide	▶ Corticosteroids, topical, high potency
Amnesteem	▶ Isotretinoin
Anthro-derm	▶ Anthralin
Aquacare	▶ Urea, topical
Augmented betamethasone diproprionate	▶ Corticosteroids, topical, super potency
Avita	▶ Tretinoin
Azelex	▶ Azelaic acid
Baciguent	▶ Bacitracin
Bactrim	▶ Trimethoprim-sulfamethoxazole
Bactroban	▶ Mupirocin
Benadryl	▶ Antihistamines, first generation
Benoxyl	▶ Benzoyl peroxide
Benzac AC	▶ Benzoyl peroxide
BenzaClin	▶ Benzoyl peroxide
Benza-Gel	▶ Benzoyl peroxide
Benzamycin	▶ Benzoyl peroxide

Tab. 2. Trade names mentioned in the book and their generics (continued)

Trade Name	Generic
Betadine antibiotic ointment	▶ Bacitracin
Betamethasone benzoate	▶ Corticosteroids, topical, medium potency
Betamethasone dipropionate	▶ Corticosteroids, topical, high potency
Betamethasone valerate	▶ Corticosteroids, topical, medium potency
Biaxin	▶ Clarithromycin
Bicillin LA	▶ Penicillin G benzathine
Biocef	▶ Cephalexin
Brevoxyl	▶ Benzoyl peroxide
Canthacur	▶ Cantharidin
Carac	▶ Fluorouracil, topical
Carmol	▶ Urea, topical
Celexa	▶ Selective serotonin reuptake inhibitor (SSRI)
CellCept	▶ Mycophenolate mofetil
Chlor-Trimeton	▶ Antihistamines, first generation
Cipro	▶ Ciprofloxacin
Clarinex	▶ Antihistamines, second generation
Claritin	▶ Antihistamines, second generation
Cleocin	▶ Clindamycin, systemic
Clobetasol	▶ Corticosteroids, topical, super potency
Clocortolone	▶ Corticosteroids, topical, medium potency
Comtrex	▶ Antihistamines, first generation
Condylox	▶ Podofilox
Cytoxan	▶ Cyclophosphamide
Deltasone	▶ Prednisone
Dermarest	▶ Antihistamines, first generation
Desonide 0.05%	▶ Corticosteroids, topical, low potency
Desoximetasone	▶ Corticosteroids, topical, high potency
Desquam-E	▶ Benzoyl peroxide
Differin	▶ Adapalene
Diflorasone diacetate	▶ Corticosteroids, topical, super potency
Diflucan	▶ Fluconazole
Dimetane	▶ Antihistamines, first generation
Doryx	▶ Doxycycline
Dovonex	▶ Calcipotriene
Doxepin	▶ Antihistamines, first generation
Drithocreme	▶ Anthralin
Dritho-Scalp	▶ Anthralin
Duac	▶ Benzoyl peroxide
Dynacin	▶ Minocycline
Dynapen	▶ Dicloxacillin

Tab. 2. Trade names mentioned in the book and their generics (continued)

Trade Name	Generic
EES	▶ Erythromycin, systemic
Efudex	▶ Fluorouracil, topical
Eldopaque	▶ Hydroquinone
Eldoquin	▶ Hydroquinone
Elimite	▶ Permethrin
Emgel	▶ Erythromycin, topical
E-mycin	▶ Erythromycin, systemic
Eryc	▶ Erythromycin, systemic
Erycette	▶ Erythromycin, topical
EryDerm	▶ Erythromycin, topical
Erymax	▶ Erythromycin, topical
Erythra-Derm	▶ Erythromycin, topical
Esoterica	▶ Hydroquinone
Exelderm	▶ Azole antifungal agents
Famvir	▶ Famciclovir
Fluocinolone	▶ Corticosteroids, topical, medium potency
Fluocinonide	▶ Corticosteroids, topical, high potency
Fluoroplex	▶ Fluorouracil, topical
Flurandrenolide	▶ Corticosteroids, topical, medium potency
Flurandrenolide tape	▶ Corticosteroids, topical, super potency
Fluticasone	▶ Corticosteroids, topical, medium potency
Fulvicin P/G	▶ Griseofulvin
Gold Bond Triple Action	▶ Bacitracin
Grifulvin V	▶ Griseofulvin
Gris-PEG	▶ Griseofulvin
Halcinonide	▶ Corticosteroids, topical, high potency
Halobetasol	▶ Corticosteroids, topical, super potency
Hydrea	▶ Hydroxyurea
Hydrocortisone 1%	▶ Corticosteroids, topical, low potency
Hydrocortisone butyrate	▶ Corticosteroids, topical, medium potency
Hydrocortisone valerate	▶ Corticosteroids, topical, medium potency
Ilosone	▶ Erythromycin, systemic
Imuran	▶ Azathioprine
Intron A	▶ Interferon-α
Keflex	▶ Cephalexin
Keftab	▶ Cephalexin
Lamisil	▶ Terbinafine
Lamisil AT	▶ Azole antifungal agents
Loprox	▶ Ciclopirox
Lotrimin	▶ Azole antifungal agents

Tab. 2. Trade names mentioned in the book and their generics (continued)

Trade Name	Generic
Lustra	▶ Hydroquinone
Luvox	▶ Selective serotonin reuptake inhibitor (SSRI)
Magic Shaving Powder	▶ Depilatories, chemical
Melanex	▶ Hydroquinone
MetroCream	▶ Metronidazole, topical
MetroGel	▶ Metronidazole, topical
MetroLotion	▶ Metronidazole, topical
Micanol	▶ Anthralin
Micatin	▶ Azole antifungal agents
Minocin	▶ Minocycline
Mometasone	▶ Corticosteroids, topical, medium potency
Monodox	▶ Doxycycline
Mycelex	▶ Azole antifungal agents
Mycitracin	▶ Bacitracin
Naftin	▶ Naftifine
Nair	▶ Depilatories, chemical
Neet	▶ Depilatories, chemical
Neoral	▶ Cyclosporine
Neosar	▶ Cyclophosphamide
Neutraplus	▶ Urea, topical
Nix	▶ Permethrin
Nizoral	▶ Ketoconazole
Noritate	▶ Metronidazole, topical
Nudit	▶ Depilatories, chemical
Nuquin	▶ Hydroquinone
Oxistat	▶ Azole antifungal agents
Oxsoralen lotion	▶ Methoxsalen
Oxsoralen Ultra	▶ Methoxsalen
Panmycin	▶ Tetracycline
PanOxyl	▶ Benzoyl peroxide
Paxil	▶ Selective serotonin reuptake inhibitor (SSRI)
PCE	▶ Erythromycin, systemic
Penlac	▶ Ciclopirox
Pen-Vee K	▶ Penicillin VK
Periactin	▶ Antihistamines, first generation
Persa-Gel	▶ Benzoyl peroxide
Phenergan	▶ Antihistamines, first generation
Plaquenil	▶ Hydroxychloroquine
Polaramine	▶ Antihistamines, first generation
Polysporin	▶ Bacitracin

Tab. 2. Trade names mentioned in the book and their generics (continued)

Trade Name	Generic
Porcelana Fade Cream	► Hydroquinone
Prednicarbate	► Corticosteroids, topical, medium potency
Propecia	► Finasteride
Prozac	► Selective serotonin reuptake inhibitor (SSRI)
Pyribenzamine	► Antihistamines, first generation
Renova	► Tretinoin
Retin A Micro	► Tretinoin
Retin-A	► Tretinoin
Rheumatrex	► Methotrexate
Ridaura	► Auranofin
Rifadin	► Rifampin
Rimactane	► Rifampin
Roferon A	► Interferon-α
Rogaine	► Minoxidil, topical
Royal Crown Shaving Powder	► Depilatories, chemical
Sandimmune	► Cyclosporine
SangCya	► Cyclosporine
Septra	► Trimethoprim-sulfamethoxazole
Solaquin Forte	► Hydroquinone
Solganol	► Aurothioglucose
Sominex	► Antihistamines, first generation
Spectazole	► Azole antifungal agents
Spectrocin Plus	► Bacitracin
Sporanox	► Itraconazole
Staticin	► Erythromycin, topical
Sterapred	► Prednisone
Stromectol	► Ivermectin
Sumycin	► Tetracycline
Tazorac	► Tazarotene
Tetracap	► Tetracycline
Thalomid	► Thalidomide
Theramycin	► Erythromycin, topical
Thioguanine	► Thioguanine
Triamcinolone	► Corticosteroids, topical, medium potency
Triaz	► Benzoyl peroxide
Tri-Luma	► Hydroquinone
T-Stat	► Erythromycin, topical
Ultramide	► Urea, topical
Ureacin	► Urea, topical
Valtrex	► Valacyclovir

Tab. 2. Trade names mentioned in the book and their generics (continued)

Trade Name	Generic
Vaniqa	▶ Eflornithine
Vectrin	▶ Minocycline
Veetids	▶ Penicillin VK
Vibramycin	▶ Doxycycline
Vibra-Tabs	▶ Doxycycline
Zithromax	▶ Azithromycin
Zoloft	▶ Selective serotonin reuptake inhibitor (SSRI)
Zostrix	▶ Capsaicin
Zostrix HP	▶ Capsaicin
Zovirax	▶ Acyclovir
Zyrtec	▶ Antihistamines, second generation

Printing: Mercedes-Druck, Berlin
Binding: Stein+Lehmann, Berlin

Homerton Health Library, Peterborough
Education Centre, PDH
Thorpe Road, Peterborough PE3 6DA
Telephone: 01733 874766

WITHDRAWN

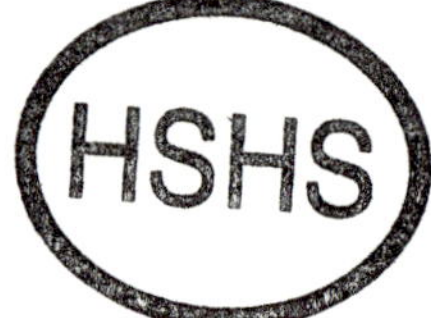